WL620
05/11

Physical Management for Neurological Conditions

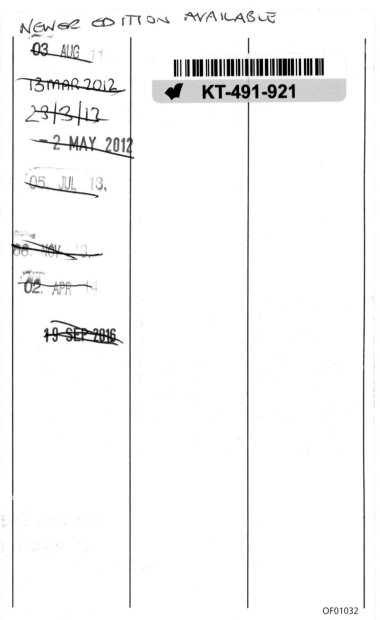
Books should be returned to the SDH Library on or before
the date stamped above unless a renewal has been arranged

Salisbury District Hospital Library

Telephone: Salisbury (01722) 336262 extn. 4432 / 33
Out of hours answer machine in operation

Commissioning Editor: *Rita Demetriou-Swanwick*
Development Editor: *Catherine Jackson*
Project Manager: *Beula Christopher*
Designer: *Stewart Larking*
Illustration Manager: *Merlyn Harvey*
Illustrator: *Richard Prime*

Physical Management for Neurological Conditions

Third Edition

Edited by

Maria Stokes, PhD, MCSP

Professor of Neuromusculoskeletal Rehabilitation, Faculty of Health Sciences,
University of Southampton
Southampton, UK

Emma Stack, GradDipPhys, MSc, PhD

Parkinson's Disease Society Senior Research Fellow, Faculty of Medicine,
University of Southampton
Southampton, UK

ELSEVIER
CHURCHILL
LIVINGSTONE

ELSEVIER
CHURCHILL
LIVINGSTONE

First edition 1998
Second edition 2004
Third Edition 2011

ISBN 978 0 7234 3560 0

British Library Cataloguing in Publication Data
A catalogue record for this book is available from the British Library

Library of Congress Cataloging in Publication Data
A catalog record for this book is available from the Library of Congress

ELSEVIER your source for books, journals and multimedia in the health sciences
www.elsevierhealth.com

Working together to grow libraries in developing countries
www.elsevier.com | www.bookaid.org | www.sabre.org
ELSEVIER   BOOK AID International   Sabre Foundation

The Publisher's policy is to use **paper manufactured from sustainable forests**

Printed in China

Dedication

Dedicated to my sons, Nicholas, Robin and William

Emma Stack

Contents

Contents

Preface

This book is intended to provide undergraduate students in health professions, primarily physiotherapy, with a basic understanding of neurological conditions and their physical management. Qualified therapists may also find it a useful resource, particularly for conditions they only see rarely in routine clinical practice.

Since publication of the previous edition in 2004, research has enabled neurological rehabilitation to advance considerably in certain areas, such as involvement in physical activity and exercise programmes. All chapters are based on research, as far as possible, and refer extensively to the scientific and clinical literature, to ensure clinical practice is evidence-based, although some areas still lack evidence.

This book is complimented by the *Pocketbook of Neurological Physiotherapy* (Lennon & Stokes, 2009), as detailed in Chapter 1, which also explains the layout of this book. Common themes throughout this book, the principles of which are discussed in specific chapters, include:

- a non-prescriptive, multidisciplinary, problem-solving approach to patient management
- involvement of the patient and carer in goal-setting and decision-making (client-centred practice)
- an eclectic approach in the selection of treatments and consideration of their theoretical basis
- scientific evidence of treatment effectiveness
- use of outcome measures to evaluate the effects of treatment in everyday practice
- use of case studies to illustrate clinical practice (chapters on specific conditions).

Terms are defined in a Glossary in Appendix 1. An important area of care is to provide patients and carers with information and support, which includes directing them to appropriate specialist organisations (see Appendix 2).

CURRENT ISSUES AFFECTING CLINICAL AND RESEARCH PRACTICE

Important initiatives that the clinician needs to remain updated with, relating to the management and conduct of practice, include the following:

Clinical and research governance

Clinical governance was introduced in the UK by the Department of Health (DoH) in the late 1990s and is defined by the Chief Medical Officer as: 'A system through which NHS organizations are accountable for continuously improving the quality of their services and safeguarding high standards of care, by creating an environment in which clinical excellence will flourish' (DoH website for clinical governance). To achieve such excellence, systems need to be in place which: are patient-centred; monitor quality; assess risk and deal with problems early; have clear lines of accountability; are transparent; and provide information to professionals and the public. The clinical governance initiative recognizes the importance of education and research being valued.

The *Research Governance Framework for Health and Social Care* was released by the DoH in 2002 and 'is intended to sustain a research culture that promotes excellence, with visible research leadership and expert management to help researchers, clinicians and managers apply standards correctly' (DoH website for research governance). The framework sets out targets for achieving compliance with national standards, developing and implementing research management systems covering general management arrangements, ethical and legal issues, scientific quality, information systems, finance systems, and health and safety issues. In addition to closer monitoring of research activities, the framework involves other requirements, such as involving consumers, informing the public and ownership of intellectual property. As well as reassuring the public by minimizing fraud and misconduct, these robust, transparent management systems should also provide a healthy environment for all grades of researchers to be suitably supported and recognized, thus enhancing the quality and productivity of clinical research.

National standards and guidelines for clinical practice

Practice standards and guidelines have been produced by the DoH through NICE (National Institute for Clinical Excellence; NICE, 2010) and national service frameworks for different clinical conditions, e.g. cancer, coronary heart disease (DoH website for national service frameworks). Guidelines for the physical management of specific conditions are also produced by other organizations, such as the Stroke Association, the Intercollegiate Working Party on Stroke and the Association of Chartered Physiotherapists Interested in Neurology (ACPIN), endorsed by the Chartered Society of Physiotherapy (CSP); and are referred to in relevant chapters throughout this book.

International Classification of Functioning, Disability and Health

The revised international classification of functioning (ICF), which is discussed in Chapter 11, focuses on how people live with their health conditions and how these conditions can be improved to achieve a productive, fulfilling life (World Health Organization (WHO), 2001).

This book aims to address issues involved in creating optimal conditions for individuals to express their natural abilities and live as full a life as possible, within the limitations of their disabilities, specifically relating to physical management.

We hope that having read this book, practitioners will understand the basic principles of rehabilitation and the strengths and weaknesses of the current evidence base. In light of this understanding, they will be able to evaluate what they see in the clinic, as well as the new ideas they are continuously exposed to by patients, colleagues, journals and the media throughout their careers.

Maria Stokes, Emma Stack
Southampton, 2010

REFERENCES

Department of Health, Clinical Governance, 2010. Available online at: www.doh.gov.uk/clinicalgovernance.

Department of Health, National Service Frameworks, 2010. Available online at: www.doh.gov.uk/nsf.

Department of Health, Research Governance Framework for Health and Social Care, 2010. Available online at: www.doh.gov.uk/research.

Lennon, S., Stokes, M. (Eds.), Pocketbook of Neurological Physiotherapy. Elsevier Ltd, London.

NICE, 2010. NHS Evidence – neurological conditions

http://www.library.nhs.uk/neurological/.

World Health Organization, 2001. International Classification of Functioning, Disability and Health: ICF. WHO, Geneva. http:/www.who.int/classification/icf.

Acknowledgements

Our thanks go to the authors for kindly sharing their knowledge and expertise, despite busy workloads as senior clinicians and academics. It was obvious how much effort had been put into producing chapters and it was a pleasure to edit their work. We also thank colleagues who peer-reviewed chapters, and the team at Elsevier for their help and support, particularly Catherine Jackson and Beula Christopher.

From Maria Stokes – I am very grateful to Emma for seeing the editing of this book through to the end, despite facing major challenges that will become evident below; a big 'Thank You' for not leaving me holding the baby! I thank my family and friends for encouraging, entertaining and supporting me throughout this project. The example set by my young nephews and nieces to live in the present moment is invaluable. Special thanks go to Philip Bryden for helping me stay focused on the task and relieving the stress at crucial times, with enjoyable distractions and a keen sense of humour. Your drive and determination to succeed are inspirational, and your expertise certainly accounts for my healthy golf handicap! I value your patience, love and support.

From Emma Stack – I would like to offer Maria some very special thanks. When you invited me to join you on this project, *no one (really, no one)* would have imagined that I was going to become the mother of triplets halfway through. Thank you for the invitation and for showing me how to edit a book; I have learned so much (and working with you has been far more enjoyable than anyone said it would be)! Heartfelt thanks for your constant and sensitive support throughout the scary moments with the boys; you shouldered far more of the load than we had planned. For keeping meetings and deadlines to a minimum, phone calls short and e-mails long, thank you. I spent some of my planning, writing and editing time perched beside cots on the Neonatal Unit at the Princess Anne Hospital, Southampton and on the High Dependency Unit at Southampton General Hospital. To the staff on those Units I offer my thanks for your total support and for demonstrating excellence in practice every single day (quite a motivator when you are editing a book like this one). My family is rather larger and more distracting than it was when I began editing this book; thank you all, especially Dorit, for being so wonderful and such a source of strength.

Maria Stokes & Emma Stack
Southampton
April 2010

Abbreviations

5HT	5-hydroxytryptamine
ABG	arterial blood gas
ABI	acquired brain injury
ACA	anterior cerebral artery
ACC	anterior cingulate cortex
ACE	angtiotensin-converting enzyme
Ach	acetylcholine
ACPIN	Association of Chartered Physiotherapists Interested in Neurology
ACPIVR	Association of Physiotherapists with an Interest in Vestibular Rehabilitation
ACPOPC	Association of Chartered Physiotherapists in Oncology and Palliative Care
ACTH	adrenocorticotrophic hormone
ADEDMD	autosomal dominant Emery Dreifuss muscular dystrophy
ADEM	acute disseminated encephalomyelitides
ADHD	attention deficit–hyperactivity disorder
ADHD-MD	attention deficit-hyperactive disorder and motor dysfunction
ADL	activities of daily living
AFO	ankle–foot orthosis
AGSD	Association for Glycogen Storage Disorders
AIDP	acute inflammatory demyelinating polyradiculopathy
AIDS	acquired immune deficiency syndrome
AIMS	Alberta infant motor scale
ALS	amyotrophic lateral sclerosis
ALSFRS	amyotrophic lateral sclerosis functional rating scale
AMPA	α-amino-3-hydroxy-5-methyl-4-isoxazole propionate
AMRC	Association of Medical Research Charities
AMT	adverse mechanical tension
ANT	adverse neural tension
ARGO	advanced reciprocal gait orthosis
ART	applied relaxation training
ASBAH	Association for Spina Bifida and Hydrocephalus
ASCS	Advice Service Capability Scotland
ASIA	American Spinal Injury Association
ASPIRE	Association of Spinal Injury Research, Rehabilitation and Reintegration
ATNR	asymmetric tonic neck response
ATP	adenosine triphosphate
ATPase	adenosine triphosphatase
AVM	arteriovenous malformation
BAEP	brainstem auditory evoked potential
BAN	British approved name
BDNF	brain-derived nerve growth factor
BIPAP	bivalent/bilevel intermittent positive airway pressure
BMD	Becker muscular dystrophy
BOT	Bruininks Oseretsky test
BP	blood pressure
BPL	brachial plexus lesion
BPPV	benign paroxysmal positional vertigo
BSID	Bayley scales of infant development
BSRM	British Society of Rehabilitation Medicine
BTS	British Thoracic Society
Ca	calcium
cAMP	cyclic adenosine monophosphate
CAOT	Canadian Association of Occupational Therapists
CBIT	Children's Brain Injury Trust
CDC	Child Development Centre
CHART	Craig handicap assessment and reporting technique
CIC	clean intermittent catheterization
CIDP	chronic inflammatory demyelinating polyradiculopathy/polyneuropathy
CIMT	constraint-induced movement therapy
CISC	clean intermittent self-catheterization
CK	creatine kinase
CLA	Chailey levels of ability
CMAP	compound muscle action potential
CMD	congenital muscular dystrophy
CMT	Charcot–Marie–Tooth
CNPS	central neuropathic pain syndrome
CNS	central nervous system
CO_2	carbon dioxide
COMT	catechol-O-methyltransferase

COPD	chronic obstructive pulmonary disease	FO	foot orthosis
COX2	cyclo-oxygenase 2	FSH	fascioscapulohumeral muscular dystrophy
CPG	central pattern generator	FVC	forced vital capacity
CPK	creatine phosphokinase	GABA	gamma-aminobutyric acid
CPM	continuous passive movement	GAP43	growth-associated protein
CPP	cerebral perfusion pressure	GAS	goal attainment scaling
CPTII	carnitine palmitoyl transferase type II deficiency	GBS	Guillain–Barré syndrome
		GCS	Glasgow coma scale
CRPS	complex regional pain syndrome	GEF	guanine nucleotide exchange factor
CSF	cerebrospinal fluid	GFR	glomerular filtration rate
CSP	Chartered Society of Physiotherapy	GHJ	glenohumeral joint
CST	cranial sacral therapy	glu	glutamate
CT	computed tomography	GMCS	gross motor classification scale
CTSIB	clinical test of sensory interaction and balance	GMFM	gross motor function measure
		GP	general practitioner
CVA	cerebrovascular accident	GPe	globus pallidus external nucleus
DA	dopamine	GPi	globus pallidus internal nucleus
DAG	diacylglycerol	GSDV	glycogen storage disease type V
DAI	diffuse axonal injury	H reflex	Hoffman reflex
DAMP	disorders of attention, motor and perception	HASO	hip and spinal orthoses
DCD	developmental coordination disorder	HCO_3	bicarbonate
DEBRA	Dystrophic Epidermolysis Bullosa Research Association	HD	Huntington's disease
		HDSA	Huntington's Disease Society of America
DL	dorsolateral		
DLF	Disabled Living Foundation	HFCWO/C	high frequency chest wall oscillator/ compressor
DM	dermatomyositis		
DM1	dystrophic myotonica	HGO	hip guidance orthosis
DMD	Duchenne muscular dystrophy	Hist	histamine
DMSA	dimercaptosuccinic acid	HIV	human immunodeficiency virus
DNA	deoxyribonucleic acid	HKAFO	hip–knee–ankle–foot orthosis
DoH	Department of Health	HLA	human leukocyte antigen
DRG	dorsal root ganglion	HMSN	hereditary motor and sensory neuropathy
DSD	detrusor sphincter dyssynergia	HO	heterotopic ossification
DTPA	diethylenetriamine penta-acid	HOT	hyperbaric oxygen therapy
DVT	deep venous thrombosis	HR-QoL	health-related quality of life
ECG	electrocardiogram	IASP	International Association for the Study of Pain
ECHO	echocardiogram		
EDMD	Emery Dreifuss muscular dystrophy	IBM	inclusion body myositis
EEG	electroencephalography	ICD-10	International Classification of Diseases
EMG	electromyography	ICF	International Classification of Functioning, Disability and Health
enc	encephalin		
ENG	electronystagmography	ICIDH	International Classification of Impairments, Disabilities, and Handicaps
EP	evoked potential		
EPP	expert patient programme	ICP	integrated care pathway
EPIOC	electric-powered indoor/outdoor chair	ICP	intracranial pressure
ES	electrical stimulation	IgG	immunoglobulin G
ESD	early supported discharge	IN	irradiation neuritis
ESR	erythrocyte sedimentation rate	IP_3	inositol triphosphate
$ETCO_2$	end-tidal carbon dioxide	IPA	impact on participation and autonomy
FAM	functional assessment measure	IPPB	intermittent positive-pressure breathing
FCMD	Fukuyama congenital muscular dystrophy	IPPV	intermittent positive-pressure ventilation
FES	functional electrical stimulation	IPV	intrapulmonary percussive ventilator
FET	forced expiratory technique	KAFO	knee–ankle–foot orthosis
FIM	functional independence measure	KP	knowledge of performance
FLAIR	fluid-attenuated inversion recovery	KR	knowledge of results
FMRP	fragile X-linked mental retardation protein	LACI	lacunar infarcts

LCAD	long-chain acyl-CoA dehydrogenase deficiency
LEA	local education authority
LGMD	limb girdle muscular dystrophy
LHS	London handicap scale
LMN	lower motor neurone
LOC	loss of consciousness
LSA	learning support assistant
LSO	lumbar-sacral orthosis
LTC	long-term condition
MAI	movement assessment of infants
MAP	mean arterial blood pressure
MAS	modified ashworth scale
MAS	motor assessment scale
MBD	minimal brain dysfunction
MCA	manual cough assist
MCA	middle cerebral artery
MCP	metacarpo-phalangeal
MCS	minimally conscious state
MDT	multidisciplinary team
MELAS	mitochondrial encephalomyopathy, lactic acidosis and stroke
MHC	major histocompatibility
MIE	mechanical insufflation/exsufflation
MND	motor neurone disease
MNDA	Motor Neurone Disease Association
MPTP	N-methyl-4-phenyl-1,2,3,6-tetrahydropyridine
MPVI	motor free visual perception test
MRC	Medical Research Council
MRI	magnetic resonance imaging
mRNA	messenger RNA
MRP	motor relearning programme
MS	multiple sclerosis
MSA	multiple system atrophy
MTI	magnetisation transfer imaging
Na	sodium
NA	noradrenaline (norepinephrine)
NCAS	national congenial abnormality system
NCS	nerve conduction studies
NDT	neurodevelopmental therapy
NGF	nerve growth factor
NGST	neuronal group selection theory
NICE	National Institute for Clinical Excellence
NICU	neonatal intensive care unit
NIH	National Institutes of Health
NIPPV	non-invasive positive-pressure ventilation
NMDA	N-methyl-D-aspartate/acid
NTD	neural tube defect
O_2	oxygen
OBPP	obstetric brachial plexus palsy
ODD	oppositional defiance disorder
OLS	one-leg stance
OSF	Oswestry standing frame
PACI	partial anterior circulation infarcts
PCA	posterior cerebral artery
PCF	peak cough flow
PCI	physiological cost index
PD	Parkinson's disease
PDMS	Peabody development motor scales
PDS	Parkinson's Disease Society
PEDI	pediatric evaluation of disability index
PEG	percutaneous endoscopic gastrostomy
PET	positron emission tomography
PHAB	physically handicapped and able bodied
PIP	proximal interphapangeal
PKA	protein kinase A
PKB	prone knee bending
PKC	protein kinase C
PM	polymyositis
PNF	proprioceptive neuromuscular facilitation
PNS	peripheral nervous system
PO	parietal operculum
PaO_2	arterial oxygen
$PaCO_2$	arterial carbon dioxide
PO_2	partial pressure of oxygen
POCI	posterior circulation infarcts
POMR	problem-oriented medical records
PP1	protein phosphatase 1
PPN	pedunculopontine nucleus
PPR	posterior parietal region
PPS	post-polio syndrome
PROM	passive range of movement
PSCC	posterior semicircular canal
PSP	progressive supranuclear palsy
PTA	post-traumatic amnesia
QoL	quality of life
RADAR	Royal Association for Disability and Rehabilitation
RCA	regional care adviser
RCT	randomised control trial
RDA	Riding for the Disabled Association
RIG	radiological insertion of a gastrostomy
rINN	recommended international non-proprietary name
RNA	ribonucleic acid
RNOH	Royal National Orthopaedic Hospital
ROM	range of movement
RSD	reflex sympathetic dystrophy
RSS	rigid spine syndrome
SaO_2	oxygen saturation
SAH	subarachnoid haemorrhage
SCC	semicircular canal
SCI	spinal cord injury
SDR	selective dorsal rhizotomy
SEN	special educational needs
SHT	5-hydroxytryptamine (serotonin)
SIGN	Scottish Intercollegiate Guidelines Network
SF-36	Short Form-36
SIP	sickness impact profile
SIU	spinal injuries unit
SLE	systemic lupus erythematosus

SLR	straight-leg raising	TMS	transcranial magnetic stimulation
SLT	speech and language therapist	TNS	transcutaneous nerve stimulation
SMA	spinal muscular atrophies	TORCH	toxoplasmosis, rubella, cytomegalovirus and herpes simplex virus
SMA	supplementary motor area		
SMART	specific, measurable, achievable/ambitious, relevant and timed (in relation to goals)	TTX	tetrodoxin
		TVPS	test of visual perceptual skills
SMR	standardised mortality ratio	TVR	tonic vibration reflex
SN	substantia nigra	UDS	urodynamic studies
SNAP	sensory nerve action potential	UHDRS	unified Huntington's disease rating scale
SNIP	sniff nasal pressure	UKABIF	UK Acquired Brain Injury Foundation
SNpc	substantia nigra pars compacta	ULNT	upper-limb neurodynamic test
SNpr	substantia nigra pars reticulata	ULTT	upper-limb tension test
SNR	substantia nigra reticulata	UMN	upper motor neurone
SOD	superoxide dismutase	VA	ventriculoatrial
SPKB	slump-prone knee-bending	VC	vital capacity
SPOD	sexual and performance difficulties of the disabled	VEP	visual evoked potential
		VL	ventrolateral
SRR	Society for Research in Rehabilitation	VLCAD	very-long-chain acyl-CoA dehydrogenase deficiency
SSEP	somatosensory evoked potential		
SSRI	selective serotonin reuptake inhibitor	VM	ventromedial
STN	subthalamic nucleus	VMI	visual motor integration
TA	tendo-achilles	VOR	vestibulo-ocular reflex
TACI	total anterior circulation infarcts	VP	ventriculoperitoneal
TBI	traumatic brain injury	VS	vegetative state
TENS	transcutaneous electrical nerve stimulation	VSR	vestibulospinal reflex
TEV	talipes equinovarus	WHO	World Health Organization
TIA	transient ischaemic attack	WISCI	walking index for spinal cord injury
TLSO	thoracolumbosacral orthoses		

Contributors

Ann Ashburn, PhD, MCSP
Professor of Rehabilitation
Faculty of Health Sciences
University of Southampton
Southampton, UK

Amanda Austin, MSc, PgCertLTHE, MCSP
Lecturer in Physiotherapy
School of Health Professions
University of Plymouth
Plymouth, UK

David Bates, MA, MB, FRCP
Consultant Neurologist and Senior Lecturer
Department of Neurology
Royal Victoria Infirmary
Newcastle upon Tyne, UK

J. Graham Beaumont, BA, MPhil, PhD,
CPsychol, FBPsS
Head of Clinical Psychology
Royal Hospital for Neuro-disability
London, UK
Honorary Professor
University of Surrey
Roehampton, UK

Anne Bruton, PhD, MA(Cantab), MCSP
Reader in Respiratory Rehabilitation
Faculty of Health Sciences
University of Southampton
Southampton, UK

Monica Busse, PhD, MSc(Med), BSc(Med),
Hons BSc (Physio)
Senior Lecturer
Department of Physiotherapy
Cardiff University
Cardiff, UK

Maggie Campbell, PhD, MCSP, SRP
LTNC Strategy and Specifications Manager
NHS Sheffield
Sheffield, UK

Elizabeth Cassidy, MSc, MCSP
Lecturer in Physiotherapy
Centre for Research in Rehabilitation
School of Health Sciences and Social Care
Brunel University West London
Middlesex, UK

Lorraine De Souza, BSc, MSc, GradDipPhys, PhD, FCSP
Professor of Rehabilitation and Head of School of Health
Sciences and Social Care,
Brunel University West London
Middlesex, UK

Bernhard Haas, BA(Hons), MSc, ILTM, MCSP
Associate Professor and Deputy Head of School of Health
Professions
University of Plymouth
Plymouth, UK

Joanna Jackson, EdD, BSc(Hons), MSc CertEd(FE),
MCSP DipTP
Head of School of Health and Human Sciences
University of Essex
Essex, UK

Diana Jones, PhD, BA, GradDipPhys, MCSP
Reader
School of Health, Community and Education Studies
University of Northumbria
Newcastle upon Tyne, UK

Fiona Jones, MSc, PGCertEd DipPhys, ILTM, MCSP
Reader in Rehabilitation
Faculty of Health and Social Care Sciences
St George's University of London and Kingston University
London, UK

Contributors

Cherry Kilbride, PhD, MSc, MCSP
Lecturer in Physiotherapy
Centre for Research in Rehabilitation
School of Health Sciences and Social Care
Brunel University West London
Middlesex, UK

Dorit Kunkel, PhD, MCSP
Senior Research Fellow
Faculty of Health Sciences
University of Southampton
Southampton, UK

Sheila Lennon, PhD, BSc, MSc, MCSP
Senior Lecturer in Physiotherapy
School of Health Sciences and Health and Rehabilitation
Sciences Research Institute
University of Ulster
Northern Ireland, UK

Rory McConn Walsh, MA, MD, FRCS(ORL)
Consultant Otolaryngologist
Beaumont Hospital
Dublin, Ireland

Dara Meldrum, BSc, MSc, MISCP
Lecturer in Physiotherapy
Royal College of Surgeons in Ireland
Dublin, Ireland

Frederick Middleton, FRCP
Retired Medical Director of a Spinal Injuries Unit
Middlesex, UK

Samantha Orridge, BSc(Hons), MCSP
Clinical Lead Physiotherapist – Neurosciences
King's College Hospital
London, UK

Sue Paddison, GradDipPhys, MCSP, SRP
Superintendent/Clinical Specialist, Physiotherapist
Spinal Cord Injury – Spinal Injuries Unit
Royal National Orthopaedic Hospital NHS Trust
Middlesex, UK

Jeremy Playfer, MD, FRCP
Consultant Physician in Geriatric Medicine
Royal Liverpool University Hospital
Liverpool, UK

Oliver Quarrell, BSc, MD, FRCP
Consultant in Clinical Genetics
Sheffield Children's Hospital
Sheffield, UK

Ros Quinlivan, BSc(Hons), MBBS, DCH, FRCPCH, FRCP
Consultant in Neuromuscular Disease,
The National Hospital for Neurology and Neurosurgery
London, UK

Lori Quinn, PT, EdD
Honorary Research Fellow
Department of Physiotherapy
Cardiff University
Cardiff, UK

Gita Ramdharry, PhD, MCSP
Senior Lecturer
St George's School of Rehabilitation Sciences
Faculty of Health and Social Care Science
St George's University of London and Kingston University
London, UK

Emma Stack, PhD, GradDipPhys, MSc
Parkinson's Disease Society Senior Research Fellow
Faculty of Medicine
University of Southampton
Southampton, UK

Emma Stebbings, MCSP
Senior Physiotherapist in Neurology
King's College Hospital
London, UK

Maria Stokes, PhD, MCSP
Professor of Neuromusculoskeletal Rehabilitation
Faculty of Health Sciences
University of Southampton
Southampton, UK

Nicola Thompson, MSc, MCSP
Clinical Specialist in Gait Analysis
Oxford Gait Laboratory
Nuffield Orthopaedic Centre NHS Trust
Oxford, UK

Geert Verheyden, PT, PhD
Roberts Fellow – Neurosciences
Faculty of Health Sciences
University of Southampton
Southampton, UK

Paul Watson, PhD, MCSP
Professor of Pain Management and Rehabilitation
Department of Health Sciences
University of Leicester
Leicester, UK

Chapter | 1 |

Rehabilitation in practice: how this book can help you to help your patients

Emma Stack, Maria Stokes

INTRODUCTION

As McLellan wrote in 1997, rehabilitation is more akin to the active process of education than it is to the traditionally more passive concept of treatment. He defined rehabilitation as:

> *A process of active change by which a person who has become disabled acquires the knowledge and skills needed for optimal physical, psychological and social function.*

Rehabilitation professionals *also* need to acquire considerable knowledge and skills if they are to be useful supporters of patients making those active changes.

Rehabilitation: The key skills

The Brain Injury Association of Queensland (2009) highlights the 'unique role and skills that neurological physiotherapists offer'. They argue that, while 'vitally concerned with movement', like all physiotherapists, the neurological specialists' interventions may be 'predominantly in teaching and training' their clients. Developing skills, of course, requires extensive *(hands on)* practice, though many authors *discuss* the rehabilitation therapists' requisite skills throughout this textbook, especially:

- assessment skills:
  - understanding the science of measurement
  - observational skills (including recognizing the response to intervention)
  - movement analysis
  - recording
- problem-solving skills:
  - risk assessment
  - goal-setting
- communication skills
- handling techniques
- educational skills.

Rehabilitation: The knowledge base

Coupled with good practical opportunities to learn and hone one's skills under the guidance of clinical experts, this book will provide beginners in rehabilitation with many options for the management of patients. Students of rehabilitation (at any level) would do well to reflect on their own experiences as learners, as they evolve into knowledgeable and skilled professionals capable of contributing to their patients' rehabilitation (see Figure 1.1).

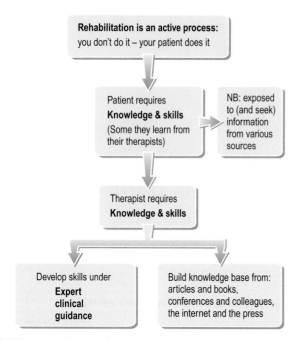

Figure 1.1 Rehabilitation in Practice: the Skills and Knowledge

This book will provide students of rehabilitation with an explanation of the theories, tools and techniques that underpin rehabilitation in practice. Recently, Lennon and Bassile (2009) identified eight guiding principles for neurological physiotherapy. Sheila Lennon discusses all eight principles in Chapter 11 of this textbook and the reader will find that many of the other chapters also address these topics. In particular, four of these principles run throughout this textbook, illustrating their significance in current rehabilitation management:

- Teamwork
- Patient-centred care
- Skill acquisition
- Self-management.

Therapists moving into rehabilitation today are entering a field in which the knowledge base is expanding as the quality of studies improves. In 2002, Moseley et al. surveyed a physiotherapy evidence database (PEDro) and found 'a significant body' of high-level evidence (randomized controlled trials and systematic reviews) for all areas of physiotherapy. They further concluded that there remains scope for improving not just the conduct, but also the reporting of trials. These are the same conclusions that they reached in an earlier (Moseley et al., 2000) analysis that was focused specifically on neurological physiotherapy.

HOW TO MAKE THE MOST OF THIS BOOK

The book has three complementary sections, which, when read together with this chapter, offer a comprehensive insight into the challenges of rehabilitation (Figure 1.2). For example, practitioners seeking information about the return of functional mobility after stroke will find relevant details in the chapters on Stroke (Ch. 2 in Section 1), abnormal movement (Ch. 14 in Section 2) and activity and falls (Chs 18 & 20 in Section 3).

Wherever possible, chapters are cross-referenced: readers seeking information about exercise or self-management, for example, will find additional information in the condition-specific chapters (of Section 1) that supplement the in-depth information of Section 3.

Example case studies (in Section 1) illustrate how, in practice, therapists tailor assessment, goal-setting and management to an individual patient's circumstances, history and presentation.

All chapters are heavily referenced, with pointers toward further resources and reading. This book is complimented by the *Pocketbook of Neurological Physiotherapy* (Lennon & Stokes, 2009), which covers several other topics in detail, including:

- evidence-based practice
- patient- and carer-centred care
- the wider context of neurorehabilitation
- motor control
- neuroplasticity
- motor impairments and impact on activity
- neurological assessment
- outcome measurement
- continuity of care
- communication considerations
- orthotic management
- neurological investigations
- drug treatments.

NEUROLOGICAL CONDITIONS

Section 1 of this textbook contains chapters devoted to conditions that form the basis of neurological rehabilitation in practice. It is important to understand how variable the presentation and progression of neurological disorders can be. As De Souza and Bates emphasize in Chapter 5, for example, multiple sclerosis (MS) can mean anything from a mild and temporary focal deficit to a severe permanent disability of rapid onset. Whether a condition is common in the typical caseload (e.g. acquired brain damage, MS, Parkinson's disease, spinal cord injury, stroke) or relatively rare (e.g. Huntingdon's disease, motor

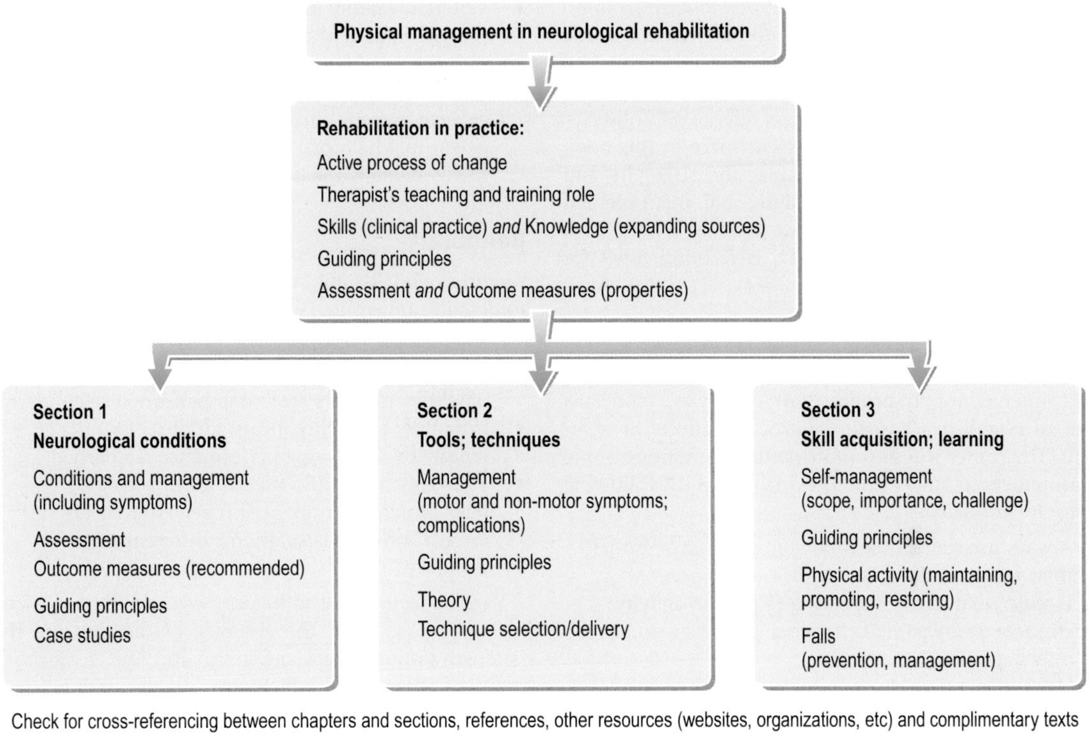

Figure 1.2 Topics in Rehabilitation (and the structure of this book)

neurone disease, muscle disorders, polyneuropathies), the authors have gathered as much up-to-date literature as possible in each case on:

- the condition (cause, epidemiology, pathology, signs, symptoms and prognosis)
- assessment and outcome measures
- management (medical, physical, multidisciplinary and patient-centred).

This type of information is essential to understand:

- how the tools of rehabilitation need be applied differently from condition to condition (or where there is less need to be condition-specific)
- how physical therapy fits into a patient's wider (multidisciplinary- and self-) management.

The state-of-the-art changes constantly (and certainly between consecutive editions of a textbook): a vast quantity of research (of variable quality) into the diagnosis and management of neurological conditions is being completed and published continuously in journals and online, worldwide. Whilst time constraints often make it difficult for clinicians to stay current (and to judge the quality of reporting), some patients avidly follow developments, particularly using the internet. Clinicians must be prepared to offer an opinion when confronted by a patient who wants to discuss an article. One resource that clinicians may wish to explore is the 'NHS Evidence –

Neurological Conditions' website (NICE, 2010). Though targeted at health professionals, the site is accessible to everyone. It includes lists of professional and patient organizations and annual evidence updates.

REHABILITATION TOOLS AND TECHNIQUES

Patient assessment

Patient assessment precedes goal setting and guides intervention. The reader will find a more detailed description of the process underpinning clinical decision making in Ryerson (2009). In summary, assessment has two parts:

- Subjective: gathering information from patient, carers, colleagues and records
- Objective: e.g. observing activity and movement; examining the performance of specific tasks; testing status of body systems, such as musculoskeletal (muscle strength), cardiovascular (e.g. blood pressure) or respiratory (e.g. lung capacity).

A complete assessment should reveal the problems that contribute to the patient's levels of activity and participation (the targets of intervention). Although the basic principles are the same across conditions, chapters in

Section 1 outline specific considerations to keep in mind during the assessment of patients with different diagnoses. Walking is an activity central to human function and, as such, gait analysis is frequently necessary during patient assessment. Though several chapters refer to gait observation and analysis, there is insufficient space in this book to discuss the process, in particular the strengths and limitations of observational analysis and instrumented (laboratory-based) analysis. A text such as Whittle's *An Introduction to Gait Analysis* (2007) is recommended for interested readers.

Outcome measurement

Once intervention is proposed or underway, clinicians need to establish a baseline and/or the effects of treatment. The reader will find more guidance about outcome measurement in Stokes (2009), which offers the following advice in summary:

- Always use standardized outcome measures, rather than invent them
- Decide what needs measuring (e.g. is an activity effective; is the patient changing?) and how to use the information
- Use sufficient measures to meet every need (e.g. indicate change, predict an outcome, provide a problem list), but *do not try to measure everything.*

The chapters in Section 1 of this textbook list appropriate measures for patients with different diagnoses and different treatment plans. Among the essential properties of a good outcome measure, the reader will most frequently see or hear 'validity' and 'reliability' being discussed. Gigerenzer (2002) defines reliability as 'the extent to which a test produces the same results under different conditions (such as repeated measurements)' and validity as 'the extent to which a test measures what it was intended to measure'. Gigerenzer points out that high reliability does not guarantee high validity and *vice versa.* These concepts are outlined below but it is important to remember that other qualities, such as responsiveness, sensitivity and clinical utility (time, space and equipment requirements, costs, etc.) are also important determinants of whether or not a measure is appropriate.

Validity

If a measure is valid, it measures what it claims to measure! The student will encounter references to different types of validity when reading about outcome measures (see Streiner & Norman [2008] for a fuller explanation, with examples):

- Face validity implies that a measure is inherently sensible and understandable, and 'looks like it is going to work', as opposed to 'has been shown to work'
- Content validity implies that it measures all aspects of the condition that are relevant to the patient

- Criterion validity implies that results agree with the 'gold standard' measures in the field and/or how well one variable can be predicted from another variable
- Construct validity implies that a measure gives the expected results when comparing groups; i.e. the extent to which practical tests developed from a theory actually measure what the theory says they do.

Reliability

As with 'valid', 'reliable' can mean many things when used to describe a measure (see Portney & Watkins [2000] for a thorough explanation):

- Inter-rater reliability means that different observers or raters score one performance similarly
- Intra-rater reliability means an observer/rater repeatedly scores one performance similarly
- Test-retest reliability means an observer/rater scores performances repeated after an interval of time (usually on different days) similarly.

Various factors will influence how reliable a particular measure is, such as: the accuracy of the measure itself (strength testing system, questionnaire); the environment; status of the person, which can vary depending on the time of day or how much activity they have undertaken prior to being assessed; the skill and experience of the operator/observer (Portney & Watkins, 2000).

Recommended outcome measures

Rehabilitation professionals should use published, standardized, valid and reliable measures whenever possible. When deciding which outcome measures to use, it is more efficient to consult expert reviews or consensus statements rather than personally evaluate the properties of individual measures. Several chapters include lists of recommended outcome measures. In Chapter 2, for example, Verheyden and Ashburn outline both Van Peppen et al.'s (2007) recommended set of valid, reliable and easy-to-administer clinical measures for people with stroke, and Tyson and Connell's (2009) specific recommendations for measuring balance post-stroke. In Chapter 6, Jones and Playfer direct the reader to the consensus on measures for overall health status and specific core areas of physiotherapy for people with Parkinson's disease (PD; Keus et al., 2004). Regardless of the patient's condition, balance assessment will always necessitate a battery of measures to cover the scope of potential deficits. In Chapter 18, Haas and Austin outline measures of physical activity and fitness (Tables 18.1 and 18.2).

Intervention

The second section of this book focuses on treatment approaches, with an emphasis on the management of motor symptoms. However, even when a patient's impaired mobility may seem to dominate their problems, focusing assessment and intervention solely on movement would be to neglect other crucial aspects of the patient's life and their rehabilitation potential. The reader will find information about symptoms that are either non-motor or include non-motor aspects throughout this book, including:

- autonomic disturbance (including bladder and bowel dysfunction)
- drooling and swallowing difficulty
- mental health problems
- sensory disturbance (including pain)
- sexual dysfunction
- sleep disorders
- speech and communication disorders.

Neurological rehabilitation is, afterall, about optimizing an individual's physical, mental *and* social wellbeing. Chapter 11 will help the reader to understand the theory and process of rehabilitation, and Chapters 13 to 17 will help them make informed choices about the techniques appropriate when a patient presents any of the following:

- Abnormal tone and movement
- Neuropsychological consequences
- Pain
- Respiratory complications
- Vestibular disorders.

It is important to remember that beyond deciding which interventions are appropriate in any particular case, the rehabilitation professional must also consider timing, environment and delivery of treatment (see Chapter 12). In other words, therapists must seek to optimize when, where and how they contribute to a patient's rehabilitation, for example:

- Should the patient meet the therapist at diagnosis or later in the disease course; and if the latter, what should trigger the consultation?
- What are the advantages and disadvantages of seeing the patient in their home versus the clinic?
- Is the patient better served by individual or group therapy and how will intervention end, if at all?

THE PATIENT AT THE CENTRE

McLellan's definition of rehabilitation as an active process still holds true today. If anything, the emphasis on self-management is gathering momentum and Lennon and Bassile (2009) consider it a 'guiding principle' of neurological rehabilitation. However, as Fiona Jones points out in Chapter 19, facilitating the move from reliance on the 'expert' to recognition of the importance of 'self' is rarely easy for clinician or patient. The third section of this book, Skill Acquisition and Learning, concerns areas of neurological rehabilitation where the patient and their carers must be active and in control:

- Exercise and physical activity
- Falls prevention
- Self-management.

With this emphasis on self-management, unlike in previous editions of *Physical Management in Neurological Rehabilitation*, this edition focuses on the adult patient. Some disorders of childhood onset will persist into adulthood, such as muscle disorders (see Ch. 10), but for a discussion of their management in childhood and of developmental neurology, we direct the reader to Shepherd's *Physiotherapy in Paediatrics* (1995). Also not included in this edition is the topic of peripheral nerve injuries, for which the reader is referred to Birch (2003) and Burke et al. (2006).

CONCLUSION

Rehabilitation is an active process whereby a patient makes changes (i.e. acquires skills), appropriately supported by a team of specifically skilled and knowledgeable professionals. Rehabilitation professionals develop their range of technical, inter-personal and educational skills through ongoing practical experience. They continuously expand their knowledge by consulting a variety of peer-reviewed sources (such as journal articles and textbooks). The evidence base is evolving; it is increasingly good, but there remains room for improvement.

Armed with a solid understanding of neurological conditions, treatments and research methods, professionals can evaluate any new information to which they and/or their patients are exposed. Most neurological therapists can expect patients with brain or spinal cord injuries, MS, PD or stroke to dominate their caseload, but they will also encounter patients with rarer conditions. Whatever the diagnosis, patients with neurological impairments present motor- and non-motor symptoms that progress (deteriorate or improve) in a variety of ways, so rigid adherence to assessment and intervention schedules is inappropriate (hence there are no 'recipes' in this book). Only by understanding a condition, how it impacts on the individual and its total management will a therapist be able to select and deliver an appropriate intervention, and monitor progress using appropriate measurement tools. Review articles and consensus statements (on generic and condition-specific treatments and measures) are useful resources in this aim for busy clinicians.

Regardless of how professionals justify their involvement in a patient's rehabilitation, the patient must always be central and expert clinicians must be honest with themselves about how challenging it can be to practice that way. The patient (and the people close to them) lives with their condition 24 hours a day; their attitude, willingness and ability to change when guided will undoubtedly influence the outcome of their care.

REFERENCES

Birch, R., 2003. Management of Brachial Plexus Injuries. In: Greenwood, R.J., Barnes, M.P., McMillan, T.M., Ward, C.D. (Eds.), Handbook of Neurological Rehabilitation, second ed. Psychology Press, Hove and New York, pp. 663–695.

Brain Injury Association of Queensland, 2009. Neurological Physiotherapy Fact Sheet. http://braininjury.org.au/portal/post-acute-phase/neurological-physiotherapy—fact-sheet.html.

Burke, S.L., Higgins, J.P., Mc Clinton, M.A., Saunders, R.J., Valdata, L. (Eds.), 2006. Hand and Upper Extremity Rehabilitation: A Practical Guide, third ed. Elsevier, Churchill Livingstone, Edinburgh.

Gigerenzer, G., 2002. Reckoning with Risk. The Penguin Press, London.

Keus, S.H.J., Hendriks, H.J.M., Bloem, B.R., et al., 2004. KNGF Guidelines for physical therapy in Parkinson's disease. Dutch Journal of Physiotherapy 114 (Suppl. 3), 1–86.

Lennon, S., Bassile, C., 2009. Guiding principles for neurological physiotherapy. In: Lennon, S., Stokes, M. (Eds.), Pocketbook of Neurological Physiotherapy. Churchill Livingstone, Edinburgh, pp. 97–112.

Lennon, S., Stokes, M. (Eds.), 2009. Pocketbook of Neurological Physiotherapy. Churchill Livingstone, Edinburgh.

McLellan, D.L., 1997. Rehabilitation Studies Handbook (Wilson, B., McLellan, D.L., Eds.). Cambridge University Press, Cambridge.

Moseley, A.M., Herbert, R.D., Sherrington, C., Maher, C.G., 2002. Evidence for physiotherapy practice: A survey of the Physiotherapy Evidence Database (PEDro). Aus. J. Physiother. 48, 43–49.

Moseley, A., Sherrington, C., Herbert, R., Maher, C., 2000. The Extent and quality of evidence in neurological physiotherapy: an analysis of the physiotherapy evidence database (PEDro). Brain Impairment 1, 130–140.

NICE, 2010. NHS Evidence – neurological conditions. http://www.library.nhs.uk/neurological/.

Portney, L.G., Watkins, M.P., 2000. Statistical measures of reliability. In: Portney, L.G., Watkins, M.P. (Eds.), Foundations of Clinical Research: Applications to Practice, second ed. Prentice-Hall Health, London, pp. 557–565.

Ryerson, S., 2009. Neurological assessment: the basis of clinical decision making. In: Lennon, S., Stokes, M. (Eds.), Pocketbook of Neurological Physiotherapy. Churchill Livingstone, Edinburgh.

McLellan, D.L., 1997. Rehabilitation Studies Handbook (Wilson, B., McLellan, D.L., Eds.). Cambridge University Press, Cambridge, pp. 113–126 (Chapter 9).

Shepherd, R.B., 1995. Physiotherapy in Paediatrics, third ed. Butterworth Heinnemann, Oxford.

Stokes, E.K., Outcome measurement. In: Lennon, S., Stokes, M. (Eds.), Pocketbook of Neurological Physiotherapy. Churchill Livingstone, Edinburgh, 2009. pp 192–201 (Chapter 11).

Streiner, D., Norman, G., 2008. Health Measurement Scales: A Practical Guide to their Development and Use, fourth ed. Oxford University Press, Oxford.

Tyson, S.F., Connell, L.A., 2009. How to measure balance in clinical practice. A systematic review of the psychometrics and clinical utility of measures of balance activity for neurological conditions. Clin Rehabil 23 (9), 824–840. Epub 2009 Aug 5.

Van Peppen, R.P.S., Hendriks, H.J.M., Van Meeteren, N.L.U., et al., 2007. The development of a clinical practice stroke guideline for physiotherapists in The Netherlands: a systematic review of available evidence. Disabil. Rehabil. 10, 767–783.

Whittle, M.W., 2007. An Introduction to Gait Analysis, fourth ed. Butterworth-Heinemann, Oxford.

Section | 1 |

Neurological and neuromuscular conditions

Chapter | 2 |

Stroke

Geert Verheyden, Ann Ashburn

CONTENTS

INTRODUCTION – TIME IS BRAIN

According to The Stroke Association (2010), every 5 minutes, someone in the UK has a stroke. This means that in Great Britain alone, approximately 150,000 people have a stroke every year. Stroke is the third biggest cause of death and the biggest cause of adult disability.

A stroke is a medical emergency and anyone suspected of having a stroke should be taken to Accident & Emergency immediately. The UK Stroke Association aims to raise stroke awareness and has organized the FAST campaign (Figure 2.1). FAST is an acronym standing for Face, Arm, Speech, Time to call 999. When you suspect someone is having a stroke, test facial weakness (can the person smile?), arm weakness (can the person raise both arms?) and speech problems (can the person speak clearly and understand what you say?). If the answer to any of these questions is no, the person might have a stroke so it is time to call 999 – because stroke is a medical emergency.

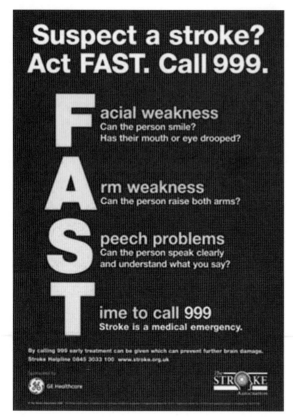

Figure 2.1 The FAST campaign leaflet (origin: The Stroke Association, with permission)

Making a prognosis directly after stroke is difficult and depends on a variety of factors, which will be presented later in this chapter. Overall, approximately 20% of patients having their first stroke are dead within a month, and of those alive at 6 months approximately one-third are dependent on others for activities of daily living (Warlow, 1998).

It is important to consider that various limitations (such as motor and sensory impairments, cognitive deficits, emotional disturbances, etc.) can cause restricted activities of daily living and participation after stroke. Rehabilitation of people after stroke should address all impairments resulting in functional restrictions; however, this chapter will focus on the physical management of people after stroke.

KEY POINTS

Time is brain: stroke is a medical emergency!
If you suspect someone is having a stroke, call 999.

DEFINITIONS

A stroke or cerebrovascular accident (CVA) is typically defined as an accident with 'rapidly developing clinical signs of focal or global disturbance of cerebral function, with symptoms lasting 24 hours or longer or leading to death, with no apparent cause other than of vascular origin' (WHO, 1988).

A transient ischaemic attack (TIA) is sometimes called a mini-stroke and patients present similar symptoms which last only minutes or hours and are gone within 24 hours.

Since the majority of strokes happen in one of the two brain hemispheres, the typical clinical sign of a person after stroke is a sensory-motor hemiparesis or hemiplegia, contralateral to the side of lesion in the brain. Hemiparesis is typically defined as weakness on one side of the body, whereas hemiplegia is total paralysis of the arm, leg and trunk on one side of the body. Of course, this focus on only motor impairment is too limited, as will become clear throughout this chapter.

KEY POINTS

A stroke is a brain attack of vascular origin, typically characterized by a sensory-motor impairment of the contralesional side of the body.

CLASSIFICATION AND AETIOLOGY OF STROKE

Strokes are classified into two main categories: ischaemic or haemorrhagic (Amarenco et al., 2009). An ischaemic stroke is caused by an interruption of the blood supply. A haemorrhagic stroke is caused by a ruptured blood vessel. The majority of strokes are ischaemic accidents (approximately 80%).

In an ischaemic stroke, blood supply to a certain area of the brain is decreased, which causes dysfunction of the brain area supplied by the affected blood vessel.

The main causes of ischaemic stroke are:

- thrombosis: obstruction of a blood vessel by a blood clot formed locally
- embolism: obstruction of a blood vessel caused by blood clot (embolus) coming from somewhere else in the body
- systemic hypoperfusion (e.g. when a person is in shock) or
- cerebral venous sinus thrombosis (caused by blood clot of the sinuses that drain blood from the brain).

A haemorrhagic stroke can be an intracerebral or intracranial accident. An intracerebral haemorrhage is a stroke where blood is leaking directly into the brain tissue, building up a haematoma. An intracranial haemorrhage is the build-up of blood anywhere within the skull, typically somewhere between the skull and the meninges surrounding the brain and spinal cord. Haemorrhagic strokes are most common in small blood vessels and potential causes are hypertension, trauma, bleeding disorders, drug use and vascular malformations.

Strokes are thus typically classified as ischaemic or haemorrhagic. Ischaemic strokes are commonly further classified according to the Oxford Community Stroke Project (OCSP) classification, also known as the Oxford or Bamford classification (Bamford et al., 1991). This classification distinguishes between a:

- total anterior circulation infarct (TACI)
- partial anterior circulation infarct (PACI)
- lacunar infarct (LACI) and
- posterior circulation infarct (POCI).

KEY POINTS

- ◆ Most strokes follow a blocked blood vessel (ischaemic).
- ◆ The minority of strokes follow a bleed in the brain (haemorrhagic).
- ◆ Ischaemic strokes are frequently classified according to the part and extent of the brain circulation that is affected (Oxford or Bamford classification).

ANATOMY AND PATHOPHYSIOLOGY

The arteries that supply blood to the brain are arranged in a circle called the Circle of Willis (Figure 2.2), after Thomas Willis (1621–1673), an English physician. All the principal arteries of the Circle of Willis give origin to secondary vessels which supply blood to the different areas of the brain (Figure 2.3).

If a stroke occurs in one of the brain arteries, the area normally supplied by the blood will be affected. The OCSP classification proposes the following symptoms for the different types of ischaemic accident:

- TACI: all of the following:
  - Higher dysfunction (e.g. speech or visuospatial impairments)
  - Visual impairments (homonymous hemianopia) and
  - Severe sensory-motor deficit in face, arm, trunk and leg.
- PACI: any one of these:
  - Two out of three as TACI
  - Higher dysfunction alone or
  - Limited sensory-motor impairments in face, arm, trunk and leg.

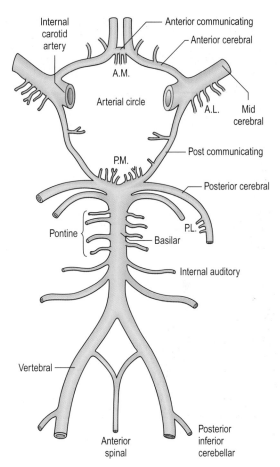

Figure 2.2 Diagram of the arterial circulation at the base of the brain. A.L. Antero-lateral. A.M. Antero-medial. P.L. Postero-lateral. P.M. Posteromedial ganglionic branches. (Origin: Henry Gray. Anatomy of the human body 1918 Fig. 519, from Bartleby.com with permission)

- LACI: any one of these:
  - Pure motor impairments in face, arm, trunk and leg
  - Pure sensory impairments in face, arm, trunk and leg
  - Sensory-motor impairments in face, arm, trunk and leg or
  - Ataxic hemiparesis.
- POCI: any of these:
  - Cranial nerve palsy and sensory-motor impairments
  - Bilateral sensory or motor impairment
  - Conjugate eye movement deficit
  - Isolated cerebellar dysfunction or
  - Isolated homonymous hemianopia.

When an ischaemic stroke occurs and part of the brain suffers from lack of blood, the ischaemic cascade starts.

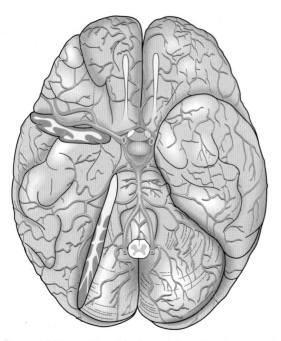

Figure 2.3 The arteries of the base of the brain. The temporal pole of the cerebrum and a portion of the cerebellar hemisphere have been removed on the right side (Origin: Henry Gray. Anatomy of the human body 1918, Fig. 516, from Bartleby.com with permission)

Without blood the brain tissue is no longer supplied with oxygen and after a few hours in this situation, irreversible injury could possibly lead to tissue death. Because of the organization of the Circle of Willis, collateral circulation is possible, so there is a continuum of possible severity. Part of the brain tissue may die immediately while other parts are potentially only injured and could recover. The area of the brain where tissue might recover is called the penumbra. Ischaemia triggers pathophysiological processes which result in cellular injury and death, such as the release of glutamate or the production of oxygen free radicals. Neuroscience research is constantly studying ways to inhibit these pathophysiological processes by means of developing neuroprotective agents (Ginsberg, 2008).

A haemorrhagic stroke causes tissue injury by compression of tissue from an expanding haematoma or blood pool. This can result in tissue injury and, consequently, the increased pressure might lead to a decreased blood supply into the surrounding tissue (and eventually infarction).

KEY POINTS

Symptoms after stroke link to the Oxford or Bamford classification.

DIAGNOSIS

The diagnosis of stroke is based on a clinical assessment and imaging techniques such as computed tomography (CT) or magnetic resonance imaging (MRI) scans. For diagnosing an ischaemic stroke in the acute setting, an MRI scan is preferred, as sensitivity and specificity are higher in comparison with CT imaging (Chalela et al., 2007). For diagnosing ischaemic strokes, CT and MRI scan have comparable sensitivity and specificity.

When a stroke has been diagnosed, determining the underlying aetiology is important with regard to secondary stroke prevention. Common techniques include:

- ultrasound of the carotid arteries to determine carotid stenosis
- electrocardiogram (ECG) to detect arrhythmias of the heart which may send clots in the heart to the blood vessels of the brain
- Holter monitor to identify intermittent arrhythmias
- angiogram of the blood vessels of the brain to detect possible aneurysms or arteriovenous malformations and
- blood test to examine the presence of hypercholesterolemia (high cholesterol).

EARLY MEDICAL TREATMENT

In the case of an ischaemic stroke, the more rapidly the blood flow is restored to the brain, the fewer brain cells die (Saver, 2006). Hyperacute stroke treatment is aimed at breaking down the blood clot by means of medication (thrombolysis) or mechanically removing the blood clot (thrombectomy). Other acute treatments focus on minimizing enlargement of the clot or preventing new clots from forming by means of medication such as aspirin, clopidogrel or dipyridamole. Furthermore, blood sugar levels should be controlled and the patient should be supplied with adequate oxygen and intravenous fluids.

Thrombolysis is performed with the drug tissue plasminogen activator (tPA); however, its use in acute stroke is controversial. It is a recommended treatment within 3 hours of onset of symptoms as long as there are no contraindications, such as high blood pressure or recent surgery. tPA improves the chance of a good neurological outcome (The National Institute of Neurological Disorders and Stroke rt-PA Stroke Study Group, 1995). In a recent study, thrombolysis has been found beneficial even when administered 3 to 4.5 hours after stroke onset (The European Cooperative Acute Stroke Study, 2008). However, another recent study showed mortality to be higher among patients receiving tPA versus those who did not (Dubinsky & Lai, 2006).

Another intervention for acute ischaemic stroke is the mechanical removal of the blood clot. This is done by inserting a catheter into the femoral artery, which is then directed into the cerebral circulation next to the thrombus. The clot is then entrapped by the device and withdrawn from the body. Studies have shown beneficial effects of thrombectomy in restoring the blood flow in patients where thrombolysis was contraindicated or not effective (Flint et al., 2007).

In case of a haemorrhagic stroke, being able to stop the bleeding as early as possible is of paramount importance and patients sometimes do require neurosurgical intervention to achieve this. Drug interventions used in ischaemic stroke (such as anticoagulants and antithrombotics) can make bleeding worse and therefore cannot be used in haemorrhagic stroke.

KEY POINTS

◆ For ischaemic strokes the key is to restore blood flow. This can be done with medication or mechanically.
◆ For haemorrhagic strokes the key is to stop the bleeding. This may require surgery.

PROGNOSIS AND RECOVERY

Van Peppen and colleagues (2007) have performed a systematic review of prognostic factors of functional recovery after stroke. They investigated walking ability, activities of daily living, and hand and arm use after stroke.

Walking ability (defined as a Functional Ambulation Category (Holden et al., 1984) score ≥4) at 6 months after stroke was best predicted by initial walking ability in the first 2 weeks after stroke, degree of motor paresis of the paretic leg, homonymous hemianopia, sitting balance, urinary incontinence, older age and initial ADL functioning in the first 2 weeks after stroke (Kwakkel et al., 1996).

The Barthel Index score (Mahoney & Barthel, 1965) in the first 2 weeks after stroke appeared to be the best prognostic factor for recovery of independence in activities of daily living at 6 months after stroke. Other contributing predictors were urinary incontinence in the first 2 weeks after stroke, level of consciousness in the first 48 hours after stroke, older age, status following recurrent stroke, degree of motor paresis, sitting balance in the first 2 weeks after stroke, orientation in time and place, and level of perceived social support (Kwakkel et al.,1996; Meijer et al., 2003).

The best clinical predictor of recovery of dexterity of the paretic arm 6 months after stroke appeared to be severity of arm paresis at 4 weeks after stroke, measured by Fugl-Meyer Arm Assessment (Kwakkel et al., 2003).

Other studies also identified severity of the upper extremity paresis, voluntary grip function of the hemiplegic arm, voluntary extension movements of the hemiplegic wrist and fingers within the first 4 weeks after stroke, and muscle strength of the paretic leg (Heller et al., 1987; Kwakkel et al., 2003; Sunderland et al.,1989).

KEY POINTS

Initial motor and functional ability is the most important predictor of long-term motor and functional performance after stroke.

Hendricks et al. (2002) conducted a systematic review of the literature of motor recovery after stroke. They concluded that approximately 65% of the hospitalized stroke survivors with initial motor deficits of the lower extremity showed some degree of motor recovery. For patients with paralysis, complete motor recovery occurred in less than 15% of cases, both for the upper and lower extremities. The recovery period in patients with severe stroke appeared twice as long as in patients with mild stroke.

There are several studies indicating that most of the overall improvement in motor function occurs within the first month after stroke, although some degree of motor recovery can continue in patients for up to 6 months after stroke. Verheyden et al. (2008) compared the recovery pattern of trunk, arm, leg and functional abilities in people after ischaemic stroke. They assessed participants at 1 week, 1 month, and 3 and 6 months after stroke. There appeared to be no difference in the recovery pattern of trunk, arm, leg and functional ability and, for all measurements, most (significant) improvement was noted between 1 week and 1 month after stroke. There was still a significant improvement between 1 month and 3 months after stroke, but between 3 and 6 months participants showed no more significant improvement. Further exploration of this latter period saw some participants stagnate in trunk, arm, leg and functional recovery and others deteriorate. Deterioration in people after stroke has been demonstrated in other (long-term) studies (van de Port et al., 2006). But despite evidence of stagnation, deterioration or a plateau phase, there is substantial secondary evidence concerning late recovery, i.e. several months after stroke, although most of these studies were in (outpatient) rehabilitation centres and thus included selected patient populations. Nevertheless, Demain et al. (2006) suggested that the notion 'plateau' is conceptually more complex than previously considered and that 'plateau' not only relates to the patients' physical potential, but is also influenced by how recovery is measured, the intensity and type of therapy, patients' actions and motivations, therapist values and service limitations.

KEY POINTS

Most significant motor and functional recovery is observed in the first month after stroke. Recovery after this initial period does happen, sometimes long after stroke.

OUTCOME MEASURES

Milestones of stroke rehabilitation should be documented by means of standardized outcome measures (Stokes, 2009). There is an increasing number of tools available. Van Peppen et al. (2007) have performed a systematic review of outcome measures for people with stroke. They propose a core set of outcome tools based on consistency with the International Classification of Functioning, Disability and Health (WHO, 2001); high-level psychometric properties (i.e. inter- and intrarater reliability, validity and responsiveness); good clinical utility (easy and quick to administer); minimal overlap of the measures and consistency with current physiotherapy practice. The core outcome measures proposed for people with stroke based on their review were:

1. The Motricity Index (Collin & Wade, 1990; Demeurisse et al., 1980) evaluates voluntary motor activity or maximal isometric muscle strength of the hemiparetic arm and leg. The test is performed from a seated position and evaluates pinch grip, elbow flexion and shoulder abduction for the upper extremity and ankle dorsiflexion, knee extension and hip flexion for the lower extremity. All six tasks are assessed on an ordinal scale ranging from 0 to 33. The total scale for the arm and leg section is 100, with a summed total score of 200; a higher score indicating a better performance.

2. The Trunk Control Test (Collin & Wade, 1990) evaluates trunk control by asking the patient to perform four tasks: from supine, rolling to the weak side, from supine, rolling to the strong side, sitting up from lying down and balance in a sitting position on the side of the bed. Each task is scored on a 3-point ordinal scale ranging from 0 to 25 points. The total score ranges from 0 to 100 points; a higher score indicating a better performance.

3. The Berg Balance Scale (Berg et al., 1995) evaluates static and dynamic balance in a functional way. The scale consists of 14 items scored on a 5-point ordinal scale (0–4 points). The items include sitting to standing, standing unsupported, sitting unsupported, standing to sitting, transfers, standing with eyes closed, standing with feet together, forward reach, picking an object from the floor, turning to look behind, turning 360°, placing the alternate foot on

a stool, standing with one foot in front and standing on one leg. The total score ranges from 0 to 56 points; a higher score indicating a better performance.

4. The Functional Ambulation Category (Holden et al., 1984 and 1986) evaluates the degree of dependency during walking. There are six categories and the patient is assigned to one of them:
   (0) Unable to walk
   (1) Dependent Walker Level 2 – support from one person needed with carrying weight and balance
   (2) Dependent Walker Level 1 – support from one person needed with balance or coordination
   (3) Dependent Walker Supervision – requires only verbal supervision or stand-by help without physical contact
   (4) Independent Walker on Level Ground – requires help on stairs, slopes or uneven surfaces and
   (5) Independent Walker – can walk anywhere.

5. The comfortable Ten Metre Walk (Wade, 1992) gives an indication of the comfortable walking speed. The patient is asked to walk comfortably over a distance of 10 m and the time to walk this distance is recorded. Normally the mean of three trials is noted. Patients can be assessed using walking aids or wearing orthotics.

6. The Frenchay Arm Test (DeSouza et al., 1980; Heller et al., 1987) evaluates the use of the hemiparetic arm and hand. The patient sits at a table for this test and is asked to use the affected hand for the following tasks: (1) stabilizing a ruler while drawing a line with the pencil held in the other hand; (2) grasping a cylinder placed in front of the patient, lifting it up about 30 cm and replace it without dropping; (3) picking up a glass of water, drinking some water and replacing the glass without spilling any water; (4) removing and replacing a sprung clothes peg from a dowel; and (5) combing his/her hair or imitating this action. The patient scores 1 for each task completed successfully, thus the total score ranges from 0 to 5.

7. The Barthel Index (Collin et al., 1988; Mahoney & Barthel, 1965) evaluates the degree of dependency during activities of daily living including grooming, toilet use, feeding, transfers, mobility, dressing, stairs, bathing, and bladder and bowel function. The activities are scored on a 2-, 3- or 4-point ordinal scale and the total Barthel Index score ranges from a minimum of 0 to a maximum of 20 points. Frequently, the 0- to 100-point version is used in the literature where essentially every score is multiplied by five.

Van Peppen et al. (2007) also propose a set of 18 optional outcome measures, to be used to evaluate a specific function or activity in people with stroke. These optional outcome measures are:

The Modified Rankin Scale
Neutral-0-Method
Numeric Pain Rating Scale
Nottingham Sensory Assessment
Modified Ashworth Scale
Testing the cranial nerves
Brunnstrom-Fugl-Meyer assessment
Hand volumeter
Trunk Impairment Scale
Action Research Arm Test
Nine Hole Peg Test
Timed Balance Test
Rivermead Mobility Index
Falls Efficacy Scale for Stroke
Timed Up&Go Test
Six Minutes Walk
Nottingham Extended ADL-index and
Frenchay Activities Index.

Clinical utility of an outcome measure is probably a key aspect and often authors have neglected this area in the past. A recent study by Tyson and Connell (2009) looked at how to measure balance in clinical practice. They performed a systematic review of measures of balance activity for neurological conditions. They scored not only psychometric properties, but also clinical utility by assigning scores to the time taken to administer, analyse and interpret the test, the costs of the tool, whether the measure needs specialist equipment and training, and whether the measurement tool is portable. They evaluated 30 measures and after excluding 11 based on limited psychometric analysis or inappropriate statistical tests used, they recommended the following balance tools for people with stroke:

Forward Reach (Duncan et al., 1990)
Arm raise tests in sitting and standing (Tyson & DeSouza, 2004b)
Step/tap test (Hill et al., 1996)
Weight shift test and step-up test (Tyson & DeSouza, 2004b)
Brunel Balance Assessment (Tyson & DeSouza, 2004a)
Berg Balance Scale (Berg et al., 1995) and
Trunk Impairment Scale (Verheyden et al., 2004).

KEY POINTS

- Standardized outcome measures should be used in stroke rehabilitation.
- Proposed core outcome measures assess voluntary motor activity, trunk control, balance, walking and walking speed, arm and hand function, and level of independence.

PRINCIPLES OF PHYSICAL MANAGEMENT

The aim of physical management following a stroke is to maximize the return of movement and independence in everyday life and to minimize unwanted secondary complications, in particular those that create risk of injury. Throughout the rehabilitation process, the purpose is to facilitate and encourage an individual to actively participate, to maximize their physical potential and to return to a life in the community.

A physiotherapist plays a major role in the physical management of people after a stroke. She/he will adopt several roles and requires an understanding of scientific measurement, assessment and handling techniques, and evidence-based therapy. As an assessor the therapist will utilize observational skills and scientific knowledge of recording and analysing movement and functional ability. For treatment the therapist has to be able to interpret assessments, problem solve and utilize educational skills and manual handling techniques to retrain movement. The therapist needs to be able to develop the expertise of recognizing positive and negative responses to therapeutic strategies, so that unwanted outcomes can be avoided and positive results encouraged. The personality and needs of the person with a stroke must be acknowledged, which requires a broad understanding of the psychosocial factors that influence people and their goals in life.

Time course

The National Clinical Guidelines for Stroke (Intercollegiate Working Party for Stroke, 2008) and the National Strategy for Stroke (Department of Health, 2007) include recommendations that people who have had a stroke are ideally managed in a stroke unit by a specialist multidisciplinary team. Even so, there are different types of clinical services, pathways and, indeed, stroke units throughout the country with varying criteria for admission and discharge. Organized services with specialist multidisciplinary teams have been identified as key to a positive outcome. A physiotherapist should expect to work with other health-care staff dedicated to the care of people with stroke and to contribute to the process of problem solving and decision making involved in the overall management. Although stroke rehabilitation commences in the acute stage on admission to hospital, active participation in the relearning of mobility and independence broadly takes place during the sub-acute and long-term stages post stroke. These three stages are rarely distinctive, they frequently overlap and do not always follow the same time frame or order for everyone, but there are common patterns. In addition, the process of transferring from hospital or rehabilitation setting and discharge from services requires structured management and should be carefully planned to be effective.

Acute stage

Patients in the acute stage can be at different levels of consciousness; they may be sedated and intubated (Kilbride & Cassidy, 2009a) or they may be able to communicate with or without difficulty. It is essential to find out if the person is medically stable before commencing physiotherapy treatment; talk to key members of the hospital team and read the medical notes. Find out the age of the patient, the type of stroke, blood pressure, ability to communicate, if an injury occurred at the time of their stroke and information about their medical history, for example have they experienced a previous stroke or do they have dementia? An outline of their social environment may also provide a guide on cultural issues and language differences. It is important to be informed of those potential risk factors that may influence what a physiotherapist does and the treatment planned. It is essential to report to nursing staff and therapists before commencing treatment. Assume all patients understand you even though they may not appear to. At a later stage, many patients describe conversations overheard between members of staff who were either talking about them or ignoring them in the early period. Remember a stroke is an event that happens suddenly; the previous day your patient could have been a director of a company, a highly skilled worker, or an independent active mother or grandmother. The change in situation can be frightening and a shock. If members of the family are present when you visit, they are also likely to be shocked and confused. Introduce yourself and say what you will be doing.

The emphasis during the early days is on ensuring normal respiratory function, skin care and management of mobility; initially this may comprise positioning or passive movements to ensure the maintenance of the length of soft tissue and range of movement, particularly when muscles work over more than one joint (Kilbride & Cassidy, 2009a). All people with stroke impairments after 24 hours should receive a full multidisciplinary assessment using an agreed procedure within five working days and this should be documented in the notes (Intercollegiate Working Party for Stroke, 2008).

When the medical condition stabilizes, mobilization should start and the person with stroke should be helped to sit up as soon as possible. In the process of helping a patient to sit up or to transfer, the physiotherapist needs to assess how much help is required (two people should be available to assist initially), how much can the individual do on their own and if they can follow commands. Remember if two people are assisting a person with a stroke, one therapist must take the lead, explain the task and set the commands. A confused person in the acute

stage of a stroke will be more confused during a treatment session if several commands are given (plus feedback) by different people at the same time.

Passive and active mobilizing can be assessed in the early stages in more than one position when the condition permits, for example lying, side lying and sitting. Through observation and handling during the process of moving the patient into the different positions, the physiotherapist will be able to judge the amount of impairment an individual has, their ability to control movement in particular head and trunk posture and their ability to initiate movement and to follow commands. Control of head and trunk position in the upright posture in the first few days is a positive indicator of future functional independence (Intercollegiate Working Party for Stroke, 2008).

> ### KEY POINTS
>
> Medically stable patients in the acute stage after stroke should be encouraged to mobilize (transfer from bed, sit in chair) as soon as possible.

Sub-acute stage

The sub-acute stage can start at any time between a few hours to days post stroke. People at this stage are medically stable having been assessed in a number of ways, which may include the use of brain scans, Glasgow coma scale, neurological signs, blood pressure, heart rate, respiratory rate, blood gases, swallowing and glucose levels (Kilbride & Cassidy, 2009a). Intervention at this the stage is characterized by programmes of rehabilitation including physiotherapy. The emphasis is on determining progress through assessment and active participation in treatments. The first assessment is the baseline against which recovery or deterioration and the effectiveness of treatment can be measured.

The core impairments include loss or reduction of movement and postural control, altered sensation, abnormalities of tone, fatigue, comprehension, ability to communicate, spatial awareness, visual neglect, visual field impairment, pain, swelling, functional independence and safety. Assessments should identify abilities and potential as well as impairment and damage. Findings from global assessments of comprehension or communication may indicate where more in-depth assessments from specialist professionals are required which in turn underlines the importance of team work and multi-professional staff. The person with stroke and their carers are members of the team. Active participation in physical programmes during and between sessions should be encouraged with practice sessions in hospital or in the community. People with stroke may range from having no activity in their limbs and trunk to advanced movement skills and could experience considerable variability in the degrees of impairment across the body.

Early supported discharge schemes are designed to reduce the amount of time people with stroke spend in hospital and provide the right environment for them to return home and a similar level of intensity of care as in a stroke unit. This approach is not suitable for everyone, but there is evidence to demonstrate cost and clinical effectiveness when organized by specialist stroke rehabilitation services (Early Supported Discharge Trialists, 2004; Langhorne et al., 2005). The meta-analysis by Langhorne and colleagues found that the greatest benefit was demonstrated in those trials evaluating multidisciplinary early supported discharge teams and in stroke patients with mild to moderate disability. The findings showed a reduction in long-term dependency and admission to institutional care as well as shortening hospital stays.

Stroke occurs at all ages but is predominantly a condition of the older population, although approximately one-quarter are aged less than 65 years (Intercollegiate Working Party for Stroke, 2008). Younger people with stroke will have different psychological and social needs to the average older person with stroke. Rehabilitation plans should be carefully negotiated with the individual. Many young people with stroke want to return to work and to indulge in leisure activities. Some barriers to these needs may be associated with fear and ignorance about stroke among the general public (Department of Health, 2007; Kersten et al., 2002).

> ### KEY POINTS
>
> Physiotherapy in the sub-acute stage should be part of multidisciplinary therapy aiming at restoring functional abilities through active patient participation, while receiving face-to-face treatment as well as through self-practice.

Long-term stage

Although most recovery takes place in the first few months post stroke, improvements, adaptation and behavioural changes can continue for many years. The impact of a stroke lasts a lifetime and most people want to return to their previous roles and to be involved in their community (Ellis-Hill et al., 2009; Parker et al., 1997). There is evidence that coordinated community stroke teams prevent people from deteriorating once they are home and that targeted interventions can be effective (Walker et al., 2004). Recommendations in the National Stroke Strategy reinforce the importance of having a review system of health and social care needs and the integration of long-term rehabilitation in society through health and social support services (Department of Health, 2007).

A long-term role of rehabilitation services is to help individuals to identify the tasks that are important to them and to help them adjust and change their role and identity over time. At 12 months post stroke, individuals will begin to discover which of their valued activities they wish to resume (Robison et al., 2009). There is a need for a balance between maintaining hope for continued improvement and accepting limitations that may lead to a change in identity. A strong multidisciplinary team is required.

> ### KEY POINTS
>
> Long-term care should deal with health and social care needs of patient integration back into the community.

Discharge from hospital or therapy

For a person with stroke there are at least two critical points in the rehabilitation process where they experience a change in service delivery. The first happens when they leave hospital to return to live in the community, either at home or in a care home. The second point of transfer or discharge happens at the end of the physiotherapy programme. These stages in the life of a person with stroke are stressful and are often reported to be times of confusion by the individual and their carers. In the process of moving from being an inpatient to being an outpatient many people with stroke report feeling afraid, unsupported, forgotten and alone. Ellis-Hill et al. (2009) reported that, although patients found going home was important in their recovery, they were not prepared for continuing their recovery and life at home and highlighted poor communication, limited liaisons and a narrow focus of rehabilitation as barriers to success. They said that patients and families had their own ideas and expectations about recovery and discharge, and they said that these ideas change over time as patients and families face new situations. For successful rehabilitation, they recommended exploring each patient and family model, and suggest that improved communication and support would limit anxiety and fears and facilitate activity.

With specific respect to physiotherapy, patients are rarely prepared for the change from inpatient to outpatient. There are differences in the frequency of sessions and aims of treatment and people often feel abandoned (Wiles et al., 2004). They may not have been warned that a delay or waiting period can occur after they have left hospital and before treatment starts as an outpatient. In hospital, they may be seen daily or every other day by the physiotherapist who in the early stages, will work to maximize recovery. In the community, treatment sessions may be booked only once or twice a week and the aim of therapy may change to an emphasis on working for function. Preparation for these changes in service is important and communication should take place between the person with stroke and their carers, and between staff in the different settings.

Communication is also essential at the second point of discharge; the end of the treatment programme. The stopping of treatment must be planned, structured and communicated over time. The literature suggests that explicit discussions between physiotherapists and patients about the anticipated extent of recovery tends to be avoided during physiotherapy, making discharge from therapy difficult, and this is the point when differing expectations might be expected to be confronted (Wiles et al., 2004). Patients believe physiotherapy is effective but disappointment with the extent of recovery reached at point of discharge is likely to be linked to expectations of recovery. The result of over-optimistic expectations about recovery is a feeling of distress and abandonment when physiotherapy ends (Wiles et al., 2002). There is evidence that patients and their carers want a clear and honest appraisal of their condition and information about likely recovery. Physiotherapists need to be aware that even if they work to actively avoid raising expectations for recovery, patients will maintain high expectations of outcome of treatment. The challenge to physiotherapists is to find ways of encouraging realistic expectations of treatment without destroying the process of active rehabilitation and skill acquisition. The discharge experience could be improved by health-care professionals understanding and exploring patients' individual models of recovery. This would allow professionals to (a) access patients concerns, (b) develop programmes addressing these, (c) correct misinterpretations, (d) keep people fully informed, and (e) share and validate the experience to reduce their sense of isolation (Ellis-Hill et al., 2009). At this point, the individual should be provided with clear instructions on how to contact services for reassessment and ensure continuing support for health maintenance is provided if required. They should be informed about the events that might require further contact (Intercollegiate Working Party for Stroke, 2008). Physiotherapists should ensure that individuals know the details of their self-practice programme and that they are reminded that this means their treatment is on-going; they should also be told if there is automatic access to on-going review and where appropriate further physiotherapy.

KEY POINTS

- ◆ Discharge from hospital or therapy is often a stressful time for patients and carers.
- ◆ Communication and support should be optimized for a smoother transition.

Physical management

Setting

An acute or rehabilitation stroke unit is a dedicated area with specialist staff for managing people with stroke. The length of stay on an acute unit can vary from a few hours to several days; following medical stabilization, patients are usually referred to a rehabilitation unit for 1 or 2 weeks or several months. Patients may be referred to outpatient rehabilitation services or the domiciliary service when transferred from inpatient care. Some patients may be discharged early from a stroke unit to be cared for in the community through early supported discharge services but patients should only be discharged early if there is specialist stroke rehabilitation in the community.

Somewhere between 5% and 15% of people with stroke are discharged into residential care or nursing homes. These people with stroke rarely receive any rehabilitation (Intercollegiate Working Party for Stroke, 2008).

Core principles

The role of the physiotherapist is to enable people with stroke to achieve their optimal physical potential and functional independence. The process comprises the use of techniques to facilitate the relearning of movements, use of strategies to enhance adaptation, the prevention of secondary complications, and the maintenance of ability and function (Lennon & Bassile, 2009). The relearning or restorative process is predominantly educational and reliant on active participation by the person with stroke. The treatment demands effort from the patient and the quality of the rehabilitation process is reliant on the quality of the working partnership between the physiotherapist and the person with stroke. The skill of the physiotherapist is in understanding the movement problem and responding appropriately to the responses of the patient to the therapeutic intervention, i.e. handling, positioning, facilitating activity and practice. The physiotherapist must learn to judge the abilities and disabilities of the person with stroke and monitor fluctuations in motor control and tone as a consequence of recovery, independence and treatment. In the early stages, she/he must watch for changes in medical stability and at all stages she/he needs to be aware of risks to safety while being able to identify how much the patient can do independent of help.

Problem-solving approach

The problem-solving approach to treatment creates an evolving structure for planning an individual's management (Figure 2.4). Information gathered from the assessments is used to set short- and long-term treatment goals. Patients and carers should be given an explanation of the movement problems and then together with the physiotherapist agree on joint treatment goals, which are documented for communication with the wider team. Assessment of the effects of intervention during and after treatment sessions allows for the adjustment of treatment, and then further assessment and modification of goal setting. A pattern of regular re-assessments during treatment should ensure the monitoring of change or lack of change in the physical status of a patient over time. In addition to the cycle of re-assessments, the use of reflection on practice and the patient's response to treatment will ensure the on-going development of the treatment package.

1. Assessment

The initial database should comprise personal details such as age, contact details, medical history, function and motor control, sensation, and psychological, social and family status. Descriptions of what happened at the time of stroke and since that period should be recorded. The purpose of the initial assessment is to both identify the level of impairment and individual experiences and their ability in terms of sensation, posture, movement, function, attention, comprehension and previous skills. Standardized measures of these characteristics are used for the comparative evaluation of recovery over time.

The initial assessment may be performed over more than one session if the person with stroke is tired and unable to complete all the measures. Equally the physiotherapist may need to observe the impact of the impairments experienced by the individual over several sessions before prioritizing a problem and setting a goal for treatment. For example the therapist may need to decide if the problem with the sequence of motor control during walking results from a loss of initiation of a component muscle group or as a result of abnormal tone. After the initial formal assessment, patient information about subsequent treatment sessions needs to be documented through a system such as Problem Orientated Medical Records (POMR). Under this system, the notes are referred to as SOAP:

S – subjective: what the patient thinks
O – objective: results of evaluation, what can be observed and tested
A – assessment: analysis and interpretation of limitations and abilities and
P – plan for therapy.

Throughout the assessment process, it is essential for the physiotherapist to observe patient postures and patterns of movement, establish what individuals can do for themselves and record what happens when they are handled and assisted. If an unwanted response emerges as a result of handling or exercise then the proposed treatment needs to be reconsidered and modified.

Following the initial assessment, immediate and long-term goals for physiotherapy should be set and formally reassessed at specific time points. An example of a short-term goal would be to achieve safe transfers within 2 weeks, while a long-term goal would be to be independent in walking inside the house in 4 months. Goal setting should follow rules. Patients and carers should be involved in the process and agree with the targets set. Goals should be specific, measurable, achievable, realistic and timed.

2. Clinical reasoning and treatment planning

Clinical decisions are built on the basis of information gathered. Clinical hypotheses for explaining movement deficits or functional difficulties are stated and used to prioritize goals and planning of treatment. For example, weakness in the trunk or the hip muscles may explain the inability to balance and perform washing and dressing in sitting (Kilbride & Cassidy, 2009b).

It is important to note that an informal process of assessment continues throughout the treatment programme. The nature of physiotherapy for people with stroke means that there is a constant monitoring of responses. The treatment plan is dependent on the responsiveness of the individual to intervention and handling. Not only is the physiotherapist aiming to facilitate a change in movement, but also she/he is teaching the individual to learn how to move and, in so doing, she/he wants them to be able to recognize a poor movement and a good movement. People need to know when they have achieved the movement and task correctly. Also the physiotherapist needs to be certain her/his patient has remembered to practice the task set. Remembering the task and the importance of practice are positive signs for active participation and potential for improvement.

3. Therapy

Physiotherapists practice in different ways. They can work on their own with a patient or they can work with one or more colleagues if a patient needs a lot of support and guidance. They will also work with carers, and teach and encourage self-practice.

General therapy principles

To maximize movement retraining, the person who is learning needs to have a clear understanding of what she/he is expected to do and what she/he is aiming to achieve. Clear instructions are essential, but it is even more important to check that the patient understands what is required. Knowledge of performance is also paramount in the learning process and comes from internal sensory feedback, but if after stroke the sensory system has been damaged, the patient will rely more heavily on verbal guidance and instruction from the physiotherapist (Schmidt, 1991). Positive reinforcement by the physiotherapist of corrected movements will assist in achieving the targeted goal. Repeated and task-specific practice has been shown to be the most effective feature of movement re-training. Recommendations in the Stroke Guidelines (Intercollegiate Working Party for Stroke, 2008) are that patients should undergo as much therapy as they are able to tolerate in the early stages and a minimum of 45 minutes. Practice of their new skills should be encouraged by the whole team with performance in different settings and task-specific training should be used to improve mobility such as standing up and sitting down, and gait speed and gait endurance (French et al., 2004). A review of 151 clinical trials by Van Peppen and colleagues (2004) found small to large effect sizes for task-orientated exercise training, particularly when applied intensively and early after stroke onset. In contrast, when therapy for impairments was observed, improvements were shown but they did not generalize to function.

Early physiotherapy

Evidence-based physiotherapy in the early stages post stroke emphasizes the importance of maintaining optimal posture, range of movement and the return of balance control. When the person with stroke has limited movement and no independent sitting balance, treatment should emphasize optimal positioning in lying and sitting in order to minimize the risk of respiratory complications, shoulder pain, contractures and pressure sores (Tyson & Nightingale, 2004). Splinting (Intercollegiate Working Party for Stroke, 2008), passive movements and stretching help to maintain range of movement and can be taught to carers, patients and staff. Loss of, or limited balance control is common after stroke (due to reduced limb and trunk movements, sensation and spatial perceptual disturbance) but intensive progressive balance training in sitting and standing is important (Marigold et al., 2005; Verheyden et al., 2009) and should begin in the early stages when patients are medically stable. The return of balance control in sitting is a strong positive indicator for future function (Verheyden et al., 2007). Always check the symmetry of posture in sitting and standing and the position of the head. Abnormal head postures can be linked to visuospatial neglect, loss of attention and lack of confidence and fatigue. Greater challenges to balance can be introduced by changing the posture and increasing the complexity of movement. Normal movements (pattern of coordination and sequencing of components) provide a valuable guideline for identifying abnormalities among people with stroke.

Physiotherapy for locomotor and upper limb recovery

When movement and activity in the limbs is more evident, therapy should follow repetitive, task-specific training particularly for 'standing up and sitting down' and for gait (French et al., 2007). The emphasis should be on repetitive practice with specialist guidance. Patients who have some ability to walk independently in the first few months may benefit from partial body-weight supported treadmill training, but this is not appropriate for everyone. Patients should be assessed and taught how to use walking aids and ankle-foot orthosis for footdrop and they should be individually fitted (Intercollegiate Working Party for Stroke, 2008). Opportunities to practice mobilizing inside and outside should be made widely available. Strength training should also be included both to improve selected muscles and gait speed and endurance (Ada et al., 2006; Morris et al., 2004). There is no evidence to support the fears that resisted exercises worsen increase in tone (Intercollegiate Working Party for Stroke, 2008). Functional Electrical Stimulation (FES) should not be recommended on a routine basis and should only be prescribed by specialist teams familiar with its use and evaluation (Intercollegiate Working Party for Stroke, 2008; Robbins et al., 2006). In patients where there is some arm movement, repetition of practice should be encouraged. Constraint-induced therapy is inappropriate for most people. For this therapy, individuals need some finger extension, be able to walk, be at least 2 weeks post stroke and be committed to the rigours of the regime. Finally, all patients should be given some training in self-management skills and problem solving (Kendall et al., 2007).

Fitness and aerobic training should be considered for people with stroke who have some independence of mobility (see Ch. 18). Many of the previously considered activities can also be progressed as recovery takes place through increased complexity of tasks, whole-body movements and increased repetitions. All progressions need to be considered within the context of the person's ability to move, to learn and their functional independence and safety.

KEY POINTS

Repetitive, task-oriented training appears to be most effective throughout the stroke rehabilitation literature.

4. Re-assessment and review

On the one hand, while on treatment, patients should be re-assessed and reviewed routinely. If necessary, for instance when patients are not progressing and might not achieve the proposed short- or long-term goal suggested, goal setting should be re-adjusted based on the re-assessment of the patient. On the other hand, following discharge from therapy, people after stroke should be reassessed within 6 months to 1 year and have access via primary care for further follow-up.

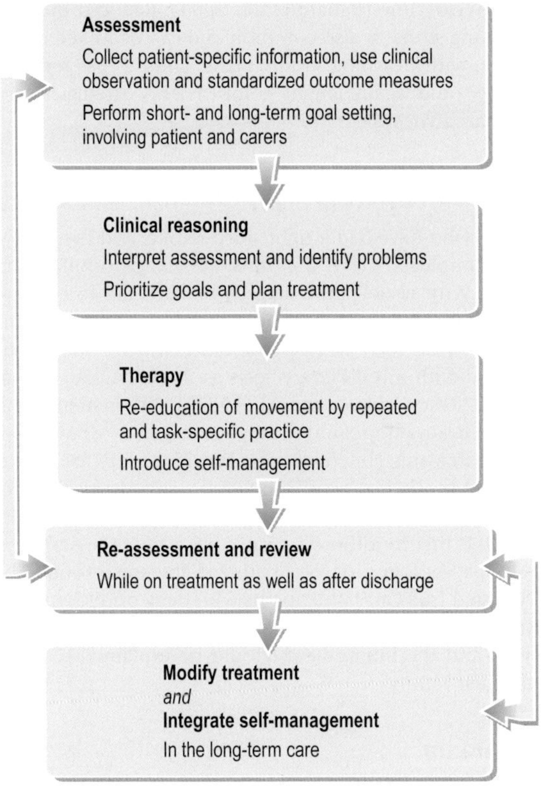

Assessment

Collect patient-specific information, use clinical observation and standardized outcome measures

Perform short- and long-term goal setting, involving patient and carers

Clinical reasoning

Interpret assessment and identify problems

Prioritize goals and plan treatment

Therapy

Re-education of movement by repeated and task-specific practice

Introduce self-management

Re-assessment and review

While on treatment as well as after discharge

Modify treatment
and
Integrate self-management
In the long-term care

Figure 2.4 Proposed structure for problem-solving approach of physical management of people after stroke

5. Modify treatment and integrate self-management

As part of the treatment programme and considering the long-term care of people after stroke, physiotherapists should ensure that they modify treatment and have provided their patients with a list of self-practice activities, which may or may not involve carer input (see Ch. 19). If carers are to be recruited to the task they should be taught what to do as they may play a crucial part in assisting with self-practice sessions. The activities should be monitored by the physiotherapist over time and regular re-assessment and review should take place in order to optimize long-term service delivery.

GENERAL MANAGEMENT ISSUES

Respiratory care

The aim of physiotherapy for respiratory care in the overall management of stroke is to maintain a clear airway, stimulate a cough reflex and assist with removal of secretions (see Ch. 15). Respiratory problems are most likely to occur in the acute and sub-acute stages. Patients may arrive with a chest infection or may be infected during their hospital stay. People with stroke may be more predisposed to these difficulties due to the considerable reduction in their mobility, the greater likelihood of supine positioning, stroke severity and difficulties with swallowing which may lead to aspiration. Positioning of patients may help with optimal oxygen saturation (Tyson & Nightingale, 2004).

Visual impairments

Visual impairments following stroke are wide ranging and encompass low vision (age-related deteriorating vision), eye movement and visual-field abnormalities and visual-perceptual difficulties (Rowe et al., 2009). Reports have indicated that a high proportion of these visual problems have frequently been unrecognized (Pollock, 2000) despite the disabling impact. Visual impairments can influence the way people with stroke perform everyday functional activities and place them at risk of falls. Individuals should be assessed by a specialist for visual impairments.

Neuropathic pain

Pain can be generated following damage to neural tissues (neuropathic pain). Estimates vary from 5 to 20%, but those who are sufferer find it extremely unpleasant. This type of pain may be associated with sensory loss and tone abnormalities. If the pain cannot be controlled pharmaceutically it may be necessary to refer individuals for specialist pain management (Intercollegiate Working Party for Stroke, 2008).

Fatigue

Fatigue after stroke is common (Staub & Bogousslavsky, 2001) and may limit a patient's tolerance of rehabilitation sessions (Morley et al., 2005). The cause of fatigue is unknown but a link with physical de-conditioning is a possible explanation, although this has not been proven. Further research into the aetiology and management is needed but with current knowledge physiotherapists need to ensure people with stroke have adequate rests during rehabilitation. Care is also needed to ensure individuals are taking sufficient nutrition.

Communication problems and swallowing disorders

These are predominantly assessed and managed by speech and language therapists. Physiotherapists working with people with stroke who experience communication difficulties must consult their colleagues for advice on developing management strategies. These deficits are distressing and can have a major impact on the re-education of movement and physical independence. When teaching or relearning any new skill it is important to establish a partnership between the teacher (physiotherapist) and the student (patient). Knowledge of the level of accuracy of understanding and response is important. A clear and consistent approach to communication is usually helpful. Remember to greet people and to involve them in the rehabilitation process. People need to be given extra time to respond and any questions or commands should be simple. Communication aids may be required. Studies have shown that people who have communication difficulties are more likely to be isolated and are not consulted about their care (Gordon et al., 2009). Communication problems commonly associated with stroke are:

- dysphasia, which affects the understanding of speech or use of the correct words
- aphasia or the inability to understand written or spoken language or to express oneself
- dysarthria, which is a problem of articulation and can result in the slurring of speech.

Approximately half of people following stroke will have swallowing difficulties or dysphagia (Smithard et al., 1997). The main swallowing difficulties of approximately one-third will have been resolved in the first 7 days. A specialist swallowing assessment should be carried out within the first 72 hours. Physiotherapists may be asked to provide help and guidance with upright posture during feeding or facilitate facial movements. Physiotherapists should be aware of the impact of restricted nutrition and hydration on energy levels and physical activity. Sometimes patients are fed through a nasogastric tube (NGT) or via a percutaneous endoscopic gastrostomy tube (PEG).

Cognitive problems

Many patients in the early stages following stroke are likely to have some cognitive loss. Poor levels of alertness are common in the first few days and more so with right hemisphere lesions (Intercollegiate Working Party for Stroke, 2008). Patients not progressing as expected should be referred for detailed cognitive assessment. Hyndman and colleagues (2008) demonstrated that attention deficits persist a long time after the initial onset of stroke. Difficulties with reduced attention span will affect physiotherapy intervention because the ability to attend is a prerequisite for learning. It may be necessary for the physiotherapist to keep treatment sessions short with rests and to minimize background distraction (Intercollegiate Working Party for Stroke, 2008). A physiotherapist should work with the psychologist to develop strategies for teaching compensation (see Ch. 17). Impaired expressive language performance and the presence of attention deficits have been reported to be associated with a higher risk of cognitive decline (Ballard et al., 2003). Reduced memory following stroke is also common and can be linked to difficulty with learning. Individuals should be formally assessed and again taught compensatory strategies in a familiar environment.

Spatial and perceptual problems

People who have had a right-sided stroke, and therefore a left hemiplegia, have the most severe perceptual problems. With visuospatial neglect, patients fail to respond to stimuli presented on the hemiplegic side and any patient with such a suspected impairment should be assessed with a test battery such as the Behavioural Inattention Test (Wilson et al., 1987). Any patient with impaired attention should be encouraged to draw attention to that side (Intercollegiate Working Party for Stroke, 2008). Agnosia is the difficulty in recognizing for instance objects, people or sounds with your senses (Kandel et al., 2000). If this condition is suspected, a formal assessment by a psychologist or occupational therapist should be requested (see Ch. 17). Patients who deny or disown their affected limbs should be encouraged to observe their limbs and the impairment should be explained to them and their family.

Dyspraxia

Dyspraxia is the difficulty in executing purposeful movements on demand despite adequate limb movements and sensation. The difficulty may be most apparent with functional tasks such as making a drink or getting dressed (Intercollegiate Working Party for Stroke, 2008; Smania et al., 2006). Formal assessment and teaching strategies for compensation (e.g. dividing up a larger task in clearly defined smaller tasks) is recommended.

Psychosocial issues

Mood disturbance is commonly manifested as depression or anxiety; the severity is frequently associated with severity of cognitive and motor impairments and the amount of restricted activities. In addition, existing psychological problems may also impact on the rehabilitation process. People who are depressed may suffer from fatigue and lack of attention, both of which have a negative effect on learning (see Ch. 17).

Emotional lability is common after a stroke (House et al., 1991). Individuals experience outbursts of crying or laughing inappropriately. Expert guidance should be sought, but at all times the physiotherapist should approach the problem with tact and care.

The return to valued activities and participation in community life is significantly disrupted post stroke and research increasingly indicates that social factors such as perceived stigma might contribute to people's reluctance to leave the house and mix with the community. Stroke has been found to significantly affect people's wellbeing and quality of life (Secrest & Thomas, 1999). Physical disabilities account for some of the problems as mobility remains a major concern for people (Ellis-Hill et al., 2009), but fear and attitudes of the general public may add to the barriers to integration.

Bladder and bowel dysfunction

Bladder and bowel dysfunction is common in the acute stage of stroke, but if both persist beyond 2 weeks the cause of the impairment needs further investigation. Both of these problems will influence or limit physiotherapy sessions and cause embarrassment for the individual. Persistent deficits may reflect stroke severity or difficulties with communication.

Carer support

The word carers can be used for formal paid carers and informal unpaid carers. At all times the patient's view on the involvement of their family and other carers should be sought (Intercollegiate Working Party for Stroke, 2008). With the patient's agreement, carers can provide additional information, and additional help with treatment practice and everyday tasks.

KEY POINTS

- Adequate respiratory care is key for people early after stroke.
- Visual impairments are commonly unnoticed in people after stroke and require specialist care.
- Pain relief should be sought for people experiencing post-stroke pain.
- People after stroke experiencing fatigue should be monitored carefully.
- Adequate communication is key for active involvement of patients in their rehabilitation process.
- Cognitive problems require an adjusted approach when providing stroke physiotherapy.
- Spatial and perceptual problems should be explained to relatives and integrated into the treatment by the multidisciplinary team.
- Dyspraxia requires a different approach in the treatment of the person with stroke.
- Psychosocial issues might have a negative impact on a patient's treatment and should therefore be addressed by the appropriate health-care professional.
- The presence of urinary incontinence in the sub-acute stage is a common predictor of poorer motor and functional ability after stroke.
- Carers should be integrated into stroke rehabilitation.

Secondary complications

Soft-tissue damage

Soft-tissue problems may involve skin breakdown and reduced range of movement, which can lead to joint contractures. Severely reduced levels of mobility following a stroke and restricted postures in bed and the chair can lead to pressure sores and soft-tissue shortening. The physiotherapist can help to prevent these secondary complications by regularly assisting people with stroke to vary their postures and positions in lying, side lying and when sitting out in a chair. Also the physiotherapist should work to ensure full range of movement at all joints of the affected limbs, but in particular shoulder, ankle, knee and extending those muscles crossing two joints (Kilbride & Cassidy, 2009b; also see Ch. 14).

Shoulder pain

The weak, affected arm of people with stroke is at risk of damage during the acute and sub-acute stages. While 5% of the stroke community is reported as having persistent pain, many more may have pain at different stages; this is often associated with an initial subluxation at the shoulder and later spasticity in the upper limb (Intercollegiate Working Party for Stroke, 2008). Physiotherapists should always carefully assess an affected arm and monitor for pain. Overhead arm slings should be avoided, and staff and carers should be trained in carefully handling the arm and in correct positioning of the limb. In addition, the lack of movement and muscle activity, and the downward hanging of the arm in the upright posture can lead to swelling of the hand.

Falls

Falls amongst the stroke population are common and have been reported to affect as many as 50 to 70% of those with stroke living in the community (Hyndman et al., 2002). The percentage varies according to the stage of recovery with more in the 6-month period after discharge from hospital. Factors such as inability to walk, visuospatial deficits, apraxia, use of sedatives and greater body sway (Andersson et al., 2006) have been associated with falls in the acute stage. At the point of leaving hospital, those who have upper limb impairment and have experienced near-falls in hospital are at greater risk of falls in the community (Ashburn et al., 2008). In the sub-acute and long-term stages, the association is not with specific stroke impairments but with reduced mobility and balance problems, particularly while performing complex tasks such as dressing (Lamb, 2003). See Chapter 20 for more information about falls and their prevention.

Multidisciplinary team

In the last few years, specialist stroke services have been seen as a priority throughout the UK and they have been shown to be more cost and clinically effective if they are well organized with specialist staff. Health-care providers with expert knowledge of managing people with stroke are recommended for the multidisciplinary teams. Teams may work in acute or rehabilitation stroke units or settings or in the primary care trust. The range of disciplines represented in a team reflects the range of impairments that can emerge following a stroke. People with a suspected stroke should be seen by a specialized physician for diagnosis and be managed by staff with expertise in stroke and rehabilitation (Intercollegiate Working Party for Stroke, 2008). A team typically includes: consultant physician(s), nurses, physiotherapists, occupational therapists, speech and language therapists, psychologists, dieticians and social workers. Stroke teams should meet at least once a week to agree on the management of patient problems and documentation of the plan and assessments to be completed. There should be education and specialist training programmes with access to services such as provision of assistive devices. The person with stroke and their carers are also part of the team and should be involved and consulted in the process of identifying and solving problems and setting treatment goals.

CASE STUDY

MT is a 55-year-old teacher who lives in a terraced house (which has one flight of stairs) with one of her two sons. She got divorced 10 years ago. She has a history of hypertension, she smokes and is overweight. Her hobbies are gardening and twice a week she plays bridge at her local club.

Presenting history

She woke up and was unable to get out of bed or to talk properly. Fortunately, her son was at home and realized his mother was making strange noises and was not making sense when she tried to talk to him. He called an ambulance and she was taken to the local district hospital.

On admission to the A&E department, she was paralyzed on the right side of her body with low tone and reduced reflexes and could not speak. She also showed facial weakness in the right lower side of her face. Her sensation on the right side was also decreased and MT developed anxiety while lying in the A&E department. An MRI scan was made and confirmed an ischaemic stroke, classified as a PACI. She was immediately given antihypertensive medication.

Acute stage – key physiotherapy problems:

• MT is bedridden, unable to sit upright without help of two persons and has reduced active movement
• Low tone on the right side of the body
• Decreased sensation on the right side of the body.

Acute stage – physiotherapy treatment plan:

• Positioning strategies together with nursing staff to prevent secondary complications and increase sensation through different positions
• Passive mobilizations with progression to active-assisted mobilizations where possible
• Whenever patient is medically stable (adequate blood pressure control), transfer of patient into sitting by means of two therapists.

After 1 week

MT has improved since being on the acute ward; she has regained some activity in the trunk and in the proximal joints of the arm and leg (leg>arm). She can come and sit on the side of the bed with help of one therapist but can only stand up with help of two therapists. Her sensation is still decreased as is the motor control in the right lower half of her face. She has a Broca's dysphasia which means that she understands language but has difficulties producing language and this frustrates her.

Key physiotherapy problems after 1 week:

• Reduced movement on the right side
• Reduced sensation on the right side
• Reduced tone on the right side (distal>proximal).

Physiotherapy treatment plan after 1 week:

• Increase the time of bringing her in the seated and upright position, maybe even by using a tilting table
• Increase the active-assisted movements and integrate them into functional movements or even movements related to her hobbies (e.g. playing cards) in order to integrate normal sensation stimuli
• Improve sitting balance by putting increasing demands on MT while in sitting (e.g. narrowing the base of support, using uneven surfaces to sit on, moving more and more to the limits of the base of support).

MT will also receive frequent occupational therapy and speech and language therapy in order to start integrating personal and functional activities (e.g. washing, grooming) and to improve communication and facial asymmetry, respectively.

After 1 month

MT is now on the rehabilitation ward. She is able to get up on the side of the bed by herself but needs active support of one therapist to transfer onto the wheelchair. She can stand up with help of one person, but is unable to walk without the help of two people. She developed increased tone in her right arm and has very little active and selective movements in this arm. Her sensation increased in her right leg but is still decreased in her right arm. She can communicate by using simple sentences with a few words.

Physiotherapy treatment plan after 1 month:

- Make the transfer from bed to wheelchair independently and increase stability of the sit-to-stand performance
- Make sure she can independently drive and steer the wheelchair
- Increase the time she spends in standing (by using maybe a standing frame) and focus on early gait rehabilitation by performing gait-related exercises in supine, sitting and standing.

After 3 months

MT is discharged from the rehabilitation ward and wants to go back home. Her son has agreed to take care of her. She still has to use a wheelchair but can walk with a walking stick in the house and on even surfaces. They have positioned a bed downstairs for her to sleep in but this is far from ideal because of space constraints. MT receives community physiotherapy.

Physiotherapy treatment plan after 3 months:

- Improve walking ability in and around the house so MT can enjoy walking in her garden

- Strong focus on learning to use the stairs again – initially with instruction of her son to facilitate her walking up- and downstairs
- Integrating exercises for self-management with a focus on stretches for the arm and leg and basic transfers (e.g. in and out of bed, sit-to-stand).

After 6 months

MT is at home and is able to get up- and downstairs with help from her son. She can also walk outside her house. However, MT has fallen three times in the past 3 months; twice while walking outside the house and once while getting out of bed at night. She continues to receive community physiotherapy.

Physiotherapy treatment plan after 6 months:

- With MT experiencing multiple falls, an extensive general, motor, sensory and cognitive assessment should take place in order to determine the cause(s) of her falls. It appeared that she was performing dual tasks while she fell the two times in the garden and that she forgot to switch on the light when she fell during the night and tripped over her shoes.
- Treatment was focused on integrating different aspects contributing to her falls but it appeared that impaired balance because of motor and sensory deficits together with the decreased attention that goes to her motor performance while doing dual tasks were the most important factors and thus the focus during treatment.
- Treatment also incorporated teaching MT, together with her son, how to get back up from the floor in case she were to experience another fall.
- As community physiotherapy will stop after this month, another set of self-management exercises is derived with a focus on improving MT's balance and a continued increase in mobility in- and outdoors.

REFERENCES

Ada, L., Dorsch, S., Canning, C., 2006. Strengthening interventions increase strength and improve activity after stroke: a systematic review. Aust. J. Physiother. 5, 241–248.

Amarenco, P., Bogousslavsky, J., Caplan, L.R., Donnan, G.A., Hennerici, M.G., 2009. Classification of stroke subtypes. Cerebrovas. Dis. 27, 493–501.

Andersson, A.G., Kamwendo, K., Seiger, A., Appelros, P., 2006. How to identify potential fallers in a stroke unit: validity indexes of four test methods. J. Rehabil. Med. 38, 186–191.

Ashburn, A., Hyndman, D., Pickering, R., et al., 2008. Predicting people with stroke at risk of falls. Age Ageing 37, 270–276.

Ballard, C., Rowan, E., Stephens, S., et al., 2003. Prospective follow-up study between 3 and 15 months after stroke: improvements and decline in cognitive function among dementia-free stroke survivors 75 years of age. Stroke 34, 2440–2444.

Bamford, J., Sandercock, P., Dennis, M., et al., 1991. Classification and natural history of clinically identifiable subtypes of cerebral infarction. Lancet 337, 1521–1526.

Berg, K., Wood-Dauphinee, S., Williams, J.I., 1995. The Balance Scale: reliability assessment with elderly residents and patients with an acute stroke. Scand. J. Rehabil. Med. 27, 27–36.

Chalela, J., Kidwell, C., Nentwich, L., et al., 2007. Magnetic resonance imaging and computed tomography in emergency assessment of patients with suspected acute stroke: a prospective comparison. Lancet 369, 293–298.

Collin, C., Wade, D.T., Davies, S., Horne, V., 1988. The Barthel ADL Index: A reliability study. Int. J. Disabil. Stud. 10, 61–63.

Collin, C., Wade, D., 1990. Assessing motor impairment after stroke: A pilot reliability study. J. Neurol. Neurosurg. Psychiatry 53, 576–579.

Demain, S., Wiles, R., Roberts, L., McPherson, K., 2006. Recovery plateau following stroke: Fact or fiction. Disabil. Rehabil. 28, 815–821.

Demeurisse, G., Demol, O., Robaye, E., 1980. Motor evaluation in vascular hemiplegia. Eur. J. Neurol. 19, 382–389.

Department of Health, 2007. A new ambition for Stroke – a consultation on a national strategy. Department of Health, London.

DeSouza, L.H., Langton-Hewer, R., Miller, S., 1980. Assessment of recovery of arm control in hemiplegic stroke patients. Arm function test. Int. J. Rehabil. Med. 2, 3–9.

Dubinsky, R., Lai, S.M., 2006. Mortality of stroke patients treated with thrombolysis: analysis of nationwide inpatient sample. Neurology 66, 1742–1744.

Duncan, P., Weiner, D., Chandler, J., 1990. Functional reach: a new clinical measure of balance. J. Gerontol. 45, M192–M197.

Early Supported Discharge Trialists, 2004. Services for reducing duration of hospital care for acute stroke. In: Cochrane Library, Issue 1. J Wiley & Son Ltd, Chichester.

Ellis-Hill, C., Robison, J., Wiles, R., et al., 2009. Going home to get on with life: Patients and carers experiences of being discharged from hospital following stroke. Disabil. Rehabil. 31, 61–72.

Flint, A.C., Duckwiler, G.R., Budzik, R.F., et al., 2007. Mechanical thrombectomy of intracranial internal carotid occlusion: pooled results of the MERCI and multi MERCI part I trials. Stroke 38, 1274–1280.

French, B., Thomas, L., Leathley, M., et al., 2007. Repetitive task training for improving functional ability after stroke: a systematic review. Cochrane Database Sys. Rev. 4, CD006073.

Ginsberg, M.D., 2008. Neuroprotection for ischemic stroke: past, present and future. Neuropharmacology 55, 363–389.

Gordon, C., Ellis-Hill, C., Ashburn, A., 2009. The use of conversational analysis: exploring the processes underlying nurse-patient interaction in communication disability following a stroke. J. Adv. Nurs. 65, 544–553.

Heller, A., Wade, D.T., Wood, V.A., et al., 1987. Arm function after stroke: Measurement and recovery over the first three months. J. Neurol. Neurosurg. Psychiatry 50, 714–719.

Hendricks, H.T., van Limbeek, J., Geurts, A.C., Zwarts, M.J., 2002. Motor recovery after stroke: A systematic review of the literature. Arch. Phys. Med. Rehabil. 83, 1629–1637.

Hill, K.D., Bernhardt, J., McGann, A.M., et al., 1996. A new test of dynamic standing balance for stroke patients: reliability, validity and comparison with healthy elderly. Physiother. Can. 48, 257–262.

Holden, M.K., Gill, K.M., Magliozzi, M.R., et al., 1984. Clinical gait assessment in the neurologically impaired. Reliability and meaningfulness. Phys. Ther. 64, 35–40.

Holden, M.K., Gill, K.M., Magliozzi, M.R., 1986. Gait assessment for neurologically impaired patients. Standards for outcome assessment. Phys. Ther. 66, 1530–1539.

House, A., Dennis, M., Morgridge, L., et al., 1991. Mood disorders in the year after first stroke. Br. J. Psychiatry 158, 83–92.

Hyndman, D., Ashburn, A., Stack, E., 2002. Fall events among people with stroke living in the community: circumstances of falls and characteristics of fallers. Arch. Phys. Med. Rehabil. 83, 165–170.

Hyndman, D., Pickering, R., Ashburn, A., 2008. The influence of attention deficits on functional recovery post stroke during the first 12 months after discharge from hospital. J. Neurol. Neurosurg. Psychiatry 79, 656–663.

Intercollegiate Working Party for Stroke, 2008. National Clinical Guidelines for Stroke, third ed. Royal College of Physicians, London.

Kandel, E.R., Schwartz, J.H., Jessel, T.M., 2000. Essentials of Neural Science and Behaviour. Appleton & Lange, New York.

Kendall, E., Catalano, T., Kuipers, P., et al., 2007. Recovery following stroke: the role self-management education. Soc. Sci. Med. 64, 735–746.

Kersten, P., Low, J., Ashburn, A., et al., 2002. The unmet needs of young people who have had a stroke: results of a national survey. Disabil. Rehabil. 24, 860–866.

Kilbride, C., Cassidy, E., 2009a. The acute patient before and during stabilisation: stroke, TBI and GBS. In: Lennon, S., Stokes, M. (Eds.), Pocketbook of Neurological Physiotherapy. Churchill Livingstone Elsevier, Edinburgh (Chapter 10.2).

Kilbride, C., Cassidy, E., 2009b. The stable acute patient with potential for recovery: stroke, TBI and GBS. In: Lennon, S., Stokes, M. (Eds.), Pocketbook of Neurological Physiotherapy. Churchill Livingstone Elsevier, Edinburgh (Chapter 10.1).

Kwakkel, G., Wagenaar, R.C., Kollen, B.J., Lankhorst, G.J., 1996. Predicting disability in stroke – a critical review of the literature. Age Ageing 25, 479–489.

Kwakkel, G., Kollen, B.J., Van der Grond, J., Prevo, A.J., 2003. Probability of regaining dexterity in the flaccid upper limb: Impact of severity of paresis and time since onset in acute stroke. Stroke 34, 2181–2186.

Lamb, S.E., Ferrucci, L., Volapto, S., et al., 2003. For women's health & ageing study. Risk factors for falling in home-dwelling older women with stroke. Stroke 34, 494–500.

Langhorne, P., Taylor, G., Murray, G., et al., 2005. Early supported discharge services for stroke patients: a meta-analysis of individual patients' data. Lancet 365, 455–456.

Lennon, S., Bassile, C., 2009. Guiding principles for neurological physiotherapy. In: Lennon, S., Stokes, M. (Eds.), Pocketbook of Neurological Physiotherapy. Churchill Livingstone Elsevier, Edinburgh (Chapter 8).

Mahoney, F., Barthel, D., 1965. Functional evaluation: the Barthel index. Md. State Med. J. 14, 61–65.

Marigold, D.S., Eng, J., Dawson, A., et al., 2005. Exercise leads to faster postural reflexes, improved balance and mobility and fewer falls in older persons with chronic stroke. J. Am. Geriatr. Soc. 53, 416–423.

Meijer, R., Ihnenfeldt, D.S., de Groot, I.J., et al., 2003. Prognostic factors for ambulation and activities of daily living in the subacute phase after stroke. A systematic review of the literature. Clin. Rehabil. 17, 119–129.

Morley, W., Jackson, K., Mead, G., 2005. Fatigue after stroke: neglected but important. Age Ageing 34, 313.

Morris, S., Dodd, K., Morris, M., 2004. Outcomes of progressive resistance strength training following stroke: A systematic review. Clin. Rehabil. 18, 27–39.

Parker, C.J., Gladman, J.R., Drummond, A.E., 1997. The role of leisure in stroke rehabilitation. Disabil. Rehabil. 19, 1–5.

Pollock, L., 2000. Managing patients with visual symptoms of cerebrovascular disease. Eye News 7, 23–26.

Robbins, S., Houghton, P., Woodbury, M., Brown, J., 2006. The therapeutic effect of functional and transcutaneous electric stimulation on improving gait speed in stroke patients: a meta-analysis. Arch. Phys. Med. Rehabil. 87, 853–859.

Robison, J., Wiles, R., Ellis-Hill, C., et al., 2009. Resuming previously valued activities post-stroke: who or what helps? Disabil. Rehabil. 31, 1555–1566.

Rowe, F., Brand, D., Jackson, C., et al., 2009. Visual impairment following stroke: do stroke patients require vision assessment? Age Ageing 38, 188–193.

Saver, J.L., 2006. Time is brain – quantified. Stroke 37, 263–266.

Schmidt, R.A., 1991. Motor learning principles for physical therapy. In: Lister, M.J. (Ed.), Contemporary management of motor control problems. Proceedings of the II Step Conference. USA Foundation for Physical Therapy, pp. 49–63.

Secrest, J., Thomas, S., 1999. Continuity and discontinuity: the quality of life following stroke. Rehabil. Nurs. 24, 240–246.

Smania, N., Aglioti, S.M., Girardi, F., Tinazzi, M., Fiaschi, A., Cosentino, A., et al., 2006. Rehabilitation of limb apraxia improves daily life activities in patients with stroke. Neurology 67, 2050–2052.

Smithard, D.G., O'Neill, P., England, R., et al., 1997. The natural history of dysphagia following stroke. Dysphagia 12, 188–193.

Staub, F., Bogousslavsky, J., 2001. Fatigue after stroke: a major but neglected issue. Cerebrovasc. Dis. 12, 75–81.

Stokes, E.K., 2009. Outcome measurement. In: Lennon, S., Stokes, M. (Eds.), Pocketbook of Neurological Physiotherapy. Churchill Livingstone, pp. 192–201.

Sunderland, A., Tinson, D., Bradley, L., Hewer, R.L., 1989. Arm function after stroke. An evaluation of grip strength as a measure of recovery and a prognostic indicator. J. Neurol. Neurosurg. Psychiatry 52, 1267–1272.

The European cooperative acute stroke study (ECASS), 2008. Thrombolysis with alteplase 3 to 4.5 hours after acute ischemic stroke. N. Engl. J. Med. 359, 1317–1329.

The National Institute of Neurological Sisorders and Stroke rt-PA Stroke Study Group, 1995. Tissue plasminogen activator for acute ischemic stroke. The national institute of neurological disorders and stroke rt-PA stroke study group. N. Engl. J. Med. 333, 1581–1587.

The Stroke Association, http://www.stroke.org.uk/information/did_you_know.html (accessed 27.01.10).

Tyson, S.F., Connell, L.A., 2009. How to measure balance in clinical practice. A systematic review of the psychometrics and clinical utility of measures of balance activity for neurological conditions. Clin. Rehabil. Aug 5, Epub ahead of print.

Tyson, S.F., DeSouza, L.H., 2004a. Development of the Brunel Balance Assessment: a new measure of balance disability post stroke. Clin. Rehabil. 18, 801–810.

Tyson, S.F., DeSouza, L.H., 2004b. Reliability and validity of functional balance tests post stroke. Clin. Rehabil. 18, 916–923.

Tyson, S.F., Nightingale, P., 2004. The effects of positioning on oxygen saturation in acute stroke: a systematic review. Clin. Rehabil. 18, 863–871.

Van de Port, I., Kwakkel, G., van Wijk, I., Lindeman, E., 2006. Susceptibility to deterioration of mobility long-term after stroke: a prospective cohort study. Stroke 37, 167–171.

Van Peppen, R.P.S., Kwakkel, G., Wood-Dauphinee, S., et al., 2004. The impact of physical therapy on functional outcomes after stroke: what's the evidence? Clin. Rehabil. 18, 833–862.

Van Peppen, R.P.S., Hendriks, H.J.M., Van Meeteren, N.L.U., et al., 2007. The development of a clinical practice stroke guideline for physiotherapists in The Netherlands: A systematic review of available evidence. Disabil. Rehabil. 10, 767–783.

Verheyden, G., Nieuwboer, A., Mertin, J., et al., 2004. The Trunk Impairment Scale: a new tool to measure motor impairment of the trunk after stroke. Clin. Rehabil. 18, 326–334.

Verheyden, G., Nieuwboer, A., De Wit, L., et al., 2007. Trunk performance after stroke: an eye catching predictor of functional outcome after stroke. J. Neurol. Neurosurg. Psychiatry 78, 694–698.

Verheyden, G., Nieuwboer, A., De Wit, L., et al., 2008. Time course of trunk, arm, leg, and functional recovery after ischemic stroke. Neurorehabil. Neural Repair 22, 173–179.

Verheyden, G., Vereeck, L., Truijen, S., et al., 2009. Additional exercises improve trunk performance after stroke: a pilot randomized controlled trial. Neurorehabil. Neural Repair 23, 281–286.

Wade, D.T., 1992. Measurement in neurological rehabilitation. Oxford University Press, Oxford.

Walker, M., Leonardi-Bee, J., Bath, P., et al., 2004. An individual patient meta-analysis of randomised controlled trials of community occupational therapy for stroke patients. Stroke 35, 2226–2232.

Warlow, C.P., 1998. Epidemiology of stroke. Lancet 352 (Suppl. 3), 1–4.

WHO, 2001. ICF-introduction, the International Classification of Functioning, Disability and Health.

Geneva. http://www.who.int/classification/icf/intros/ICF-ENG-Intro.pdf.

WHO MONICA project principal investigators, 1988. The world health organization MONICA project (monitoring trends and determinants in cardiovascular diseases: a major international collaboration). J. Clin. Epidemiol. 41, 105–114.

Wiles, R., Ashburn, A., Payne, S., Murphy, C., 2002. Patients' expectations of recovery following stroke: a

qualitative study. Disabil. Rehabil. 24, 841–850.

Wiles, R., Ashburn, A., Payne, S., Murphy, C., 2004. Discharge from physiotherapy following stroke: the management of disappointment. Soc. Sci. Med. 59, 1263–1273.

Wilson, B., Cockburn, J., Halligan, P., 1987. The Behavioural Inattention Test. Thames Valley Test Company, Titchfield.

Chapter | 3 |

Acquired brain injury: trauma and pathology

Maggie Campbell

CONTENTS

INTRODUCTION

Acquired brain injury (ABI) is an overarching term applied to describe insults to the brain that are not congenital or perinatal in nature. Usually the term ABI is used to describe the outcome of a distinct traumatic injury or a single-event pathology, such as a subarachnoid haemorrhage or a cerebral abscess, but is not applied to the results of progressive disorders or degenerative disease. The most frequent cause of ABI in young adults and adolescents is trauma and this chapter, therefore, takes traumatic brain injury (TBI) as the primary focus for discussion.

Other common pathologies producing a similar scope of neural deficits to TBI, and that are amenable to a comparable approach in terms of physiotherapy management, are also included.

Discussion of physical management is confined to rehabilitation, recovery and adjustment. The management of ABI in the context of terminal illness is not addressed. Physiotherapists most commonly encounter individuals who have survived injuries at the more severe end of the spectrum: those who are admitted for extended periods of hospital care and those who continue to have significant impairments of motor performance following hospital discharge. However, the effects of brain injury extend far beyond overt physical disability (Table 3.1) and may impact on both family members and wider social networks. An adequate understanding of this extended effect is essential if physiotherapists are to work effectively with other health- and social-care professionals to assist a person's re-establishment within the community.

TRAUMATIC BRAIN INJURY

Different types of TBI and their general management are discussed here. The physiotherapist's role in the rehabilitation of patients with ABI is discussed after the section on pathological conditions, as physical management is similar for patients regardless of the cause.

Mechanisms of injury

TBI occurs when there is a direct high-energy blow to the head or when the brain comes into contact with the inside of the skull as a result of a sudden acceleration or deceleration of the body as a whole. The brain is predisposed to certain types of injury by virtue of its structure and design, and because of irregularities on the inside of the skull. The type of brain injury sustained is a product of the circumstances generating the external force that reacts with the

Table 3.1 Definitions of traumatic brain injury

ORGANIZATION	DEFINITION
Medical Disability Society, UK	Brain injury caused by trauma to the head (including the effects upon the brain of other possible complications of injury notably hypoxaemia and hypotension, and intracerebral haematoma)
National Head Injury Foundation, USA	Traumatic head injury is an insult to the brain, not of degenerative or congenital nature but caused by an external force, that may produce a diminished or altered state of consciousness, which results in impairment of cognitive abilities or physical functioning. It can also result in the disturbance of behaviour or emotional functioning. These impairments may be either temporary of permanent and cause partial or total functional disability or psychosocial maladjustment.

brain tissue, the amount of energy involved and how that energy is dissipated throughout the brain substance.

The brain has most of its mass in two large cerebral hemispheres, above the narrower brainstem and spinal cord (Nolte, 2001a). The brain and spinal cord are suspended within three layers of membranes known as the meninges and are further protected by a layer of cerebrospinal fluid between the inner two layers, the arachnoid and pia mater. The outer layer, the dura mater, is the most substantial layer and provides most of the mechanical strength of the meninges (Nolte, 2001b). The dura mater is attached to the inner surface of the skull. During normal activities the brain is constrained to move with the head but as it is not directly anchored within the skull this does not apply during sudden, swift movements or high-energy impacts. The brain substance is composed of cells and axonal connections forming areas of different densities that move and respond to force in different ways. Thus, the brain is free to move independent of the skull and in the presence of high energy it does so in an irregular manner, causing stretching and shearing of brain tissue. Further damage is inflicted on the soft brain structure as it moves across the irregularities on the internal surface of the skull (Jennet & Teasdale, 1981).

Types of injury and associated damage

Primary damage

External forces are expressed via three main mechanisms of primary brain injury:

1. Direct impact on the skull
2. Penetration through the skull into the brain substance
3. Collision between the brain substance and the internal skull structure.

TBI can occur without disruption of the skull and this is described as a *closed injury*. Alternatively, the skull may crack in a simple linear fracture, be depressed into the brain tissue or be pierced by a sharp or high-velocity missile. Such *penetrating injuries* may be complicated by fragments of bone, skin and hair being pushed into the brain tissue, increasing the damage and raising the risk of infection. In the case of high-velocity injuries, such as gunshot wounds, damage also occurs wide of the tract created by the course of the missile, as energy is dissipated within the brain substance.

Closed injuries can result in local impact, polar impact, shearing, laceration, axonal or blood vessel damage. Local impact damage occurs immediately below the site of impact and can affect the scalp and meninges, as well as the brain substance in different measure, depending on the velocity of the impact and the flexibility of the skull. The brain may collide with the skull at the opposite pole to the site of primary impact and oscillate between the two, producing additional shearing damage. Where shearing forces affect the long axonal tracts, such as in hyperextension or rotational injuries, axons may be stretched or severed within their myelin sheaths (Adams et al., 1977). This is known as *diffuse axonal injury* (DAI). When DAI is widespread it is associated with severe injury but has also been shown to occur in mild injuries (Povlishock et al., 1983; Yokota et al., 1991).

Lacerations most commonly occur adjacent to the internal areas of the skull that are irregular, producing damage to the frontal and temporal lobes of the brain (Currie, 1993). Perfusions studies in mild injuries have identified frequent frontal, temporal and midbrain lesions (Abdel-Dayem et al., 1998; Abu-Judeh et al., 1999). Hyperextension injuries can cause damage to the carotid or vertebral arteries interrupting blood flow as a result of dissection or occlusion (Auer et al., 1994; Sprogoe-Jakobsen & Falk, 1990). Cerebral vessels can also be torn or ruptured and result in a local collection of blood. When this occurs in the immediate aftermath of an injury it is known as an *acute haematoma*. A slower accumulation of blood, known as a *chronic haematoma*, is most frequently found in the very young or in older adults.

Secondary damage

Secondary damage results from biochemical and mechanical factors. As soon as the injury occurs, the tissue damage and cell death that result spark a pathological process leading to chemical damage to adjacent but previously uninjured brain tissue and the development of oedema. The presence of oedema or a significant haematoma will result in displacement and distortion of other brain tissue. There is little internal capacity within the skull to accommodate the swelling or distorted brain and further damage occurs as the brain is pressed against the skull or pushed into adjacent intracranial compartments. As well as compression of brain substance, this can also result in occlusion of major arteries.

Secondary damage may be aggravated by infection or complications associated with systemic dysfunction, which may result from the effects of the brain injury or be caused by coexisting injuries. Around 40% of severely injured patients will have other significant injuries (Gentleman et al., 1986).

Epidemiology of traumatic brain injury

Studies reporting the incidence of TBI in Western countries produce a range of values of around 200–300 new cases presenting for medical evaluation per 100 000 population each year; for example, in the USA (Sorenson et al., 1991), the UK (Jennett & MacMillan, 1981; Tennant, 2005) and Australia (Hillier et al., 1997). The peak risk of injury is between the ages of 16 and 25, declining until late middle age before beginning to rise again around age 65 (Sorenson et al., 1991). Males are almost three times more likely to be injured and to have more severe injuries, resulting in an injured survivor ratio of around 2:1 male to female (Kraus et al., 1996). In 1998 the number of people living in the UK with significant disability after TBI was estimated to be between 50 000 and 75 000 (Centre for Health Service Studies, 1998). The figure given by the Department of Health in 2005 for those living with long-term effects of TBI in England was significantly higher at 420 000 (Department of Health, 2005).

Risk factors and preventive measures

Sporting accidents and falls are the primary causal factors for those under 20 years, with transport accidents accounting for less than 15% of injuries in one study focusing on an adolescent sample (Body et al., 1996). In adult populations transport accidents are commonly responsible for around 50–60% of injuries, with falls and assaults being the other major causal factors. In older adults there is a very high level of falls and a more even level of occurrence across genders (Miller et al., 1990).

Injury prevention can be considered on three levels (Kraus et al., 1996):

1. Reduction of the frequency of any hazard, for example, games rule changes that reduce sporting collisions or improved vehicle design leading to the prevention of crashes, or the degree of exposure to that hazard, such as wearing protective clothing, physical restraints or the use of airbags
2. Limitation of the immediate effects of an injury (see 'Principles of acute management of TBI', below)
3. Limitation of the longer-term impact by preventing the development of additional problems; for example, by providing physical, psychological and vocational rehabilitation.

Positive effects have been reported for motorcyclists wearing helmets (Gabella et al., 1995; Kraus et al., 1994) and following the introduction of compulsory bicycle helmets in the USA (Thompson et al., 1989) and Australia (McDermott, 1995). Increasing awareness of the potential for enduring problems following minor brain injury and the cumulative effects of repeated minor trauma has led to the development of guidelines for the management of concussion injuries in sport (Fick, 1995; Leblanc, 1995; Leclerc et al., 2009; McCrory et al., 2005). However, there remains a great deal to do in terms of educating healthcare providers, and youth and sports organizations to ensure that guidelines are followed and the correct advice given (Genuardi & King, 1995).

The Pashby Sports Safety Concussion website (Leclerc et al., 2009) gives definitions, explanations and advice, so that the effects of concussion can be recognized by those involved in sport at any level and to encourage return to participation to be appropriately paced. There is also now an internatioanlly agreed method of post concussion evaluation, the Sport Concussion Assessment Tool or SCAT (McCrory et al., 2005).

In terms of individual risk factors, substance misuse and, particularly, exposure to alcohol are widely recognized as prominent contributory factors in accidental (Jennett, 1996) and violent injury (Drubach et al., 1993). However, although there is some evidence that withdrawal from chronic alcohol use may exacerbate toxic cell damage following trauma, the net effects of the presence of alcohol at the time of injury at an individual level have not yet been defined (Kelly, 1995). There is emerging counter-intuitive evidence of no specific negative impact of alcohol on cognitive performance (Lange et al., 2008) or functional status (Vickery et al., 2008). There is some evidence of a relationship between previous alcohol abuse or dependency and disorders of mood and emotional disturbance following TBI (Jorge et al., 2005) and that having a first injury associated with drinking alcohol is predictive of recurrent TBI (Winqvist et al., 2008).

Measures and diagnoses of severity

The severity of TBI ranges from mild concussion with transient symptoms to very severe injury resulting in death. The two domains most frequently taken as indicators of injury severity are coma (depth and duration) and posttraumatic amnesia (PTA).

Coma

Coma is defined as 'not obeying commands, not uttering words and not opening eyes' (Teasdale & Jennett, 1974). The Glasgow Coma Scale (GCS; Teasdale & Jennett, 1974, 1976) is the most widely used measure of depth and duration of coma. The GCS has three subscales, giving a summated score of 3–15:

- Eye opening (rated 1–4)
- Best motor response (rated 1–6)
- Verbal response (rated 1–5).

Although a general impression of a person's conscious level can be gleaned from a summated score, retaining the scores at subscale level gives a more accurate clinical picture. For example, knowledge of the lowest motor response rating and the pattern of improvement over time can provide physiotherapists with a valuable insight into the initial severity of damage to brain tissue associated with physical performance. Regarding summated GCS scores the convention is to categorize injuries into mild, moderate or severe (Table 3.2) using the lowest score in the first 24 hours.

Duration of coma is also used as an indicator of severity, where coma is generally numerically defined as a GCS score of 8 or less (Bond, 1990). This convention introduces a further grading of very severe (Table 3.3), reflecting the increasing knowledge that may be gained from longitudinal review.

Postcoma states (vegetative and minimally conscious states) are discussed below (see 'Loss of consciousness').

Table 3.2 Traumatic brain injury severity: lowest summated Glasgow Coma Score in the first 24 hours post injury

GRADE	SUMMATED GCS SCORE
Mild	13–15
Moderate	9–12
Severe	3–8

GCS, Glasgow Coma Scale. (After Bond, 1986.)

Table 3.3 Traumatic brain injury severity: duration of coma

GRADE	DURATION OF COMA (GCS ≤ 8)
Mild	< 15 minutes
Moderate	> 15 minutes, < 6 hours
Severe	> 6 hours, < 48 hours
Very severe	> 48 hours

GCS, Glasgow Coma Scale. (After Bond, 1986.)

Posttraumatic amnesia

The definition and assessment of PTA remain controversial. The original concept was developed by Russell and taken to be the period from injury until the return of day-to-day memory on a continuous basis (Russell, 1932). Most analyses now identify disturbances in three domains: orientation, memory and behaviour. For example, 'the patient is confused, amnesic for ongoing events and likely to evidence behavioural disturbance' (Levin et al., 1979, p. 675). However, Russell's categorization of levels of severity is still used today (Table 3.4).

Tate and colleagues (Tate et al., 2000) discussed the relative merits of currently available scales for prospective assessment of duration of PTA, addressing issues of orientation and memory, and highlighting in particular the difficulties in assessing the memory component. Andriessan and colleagues suggest that the memory component is best assessed by a memory test that incorporates the free recall of words after a long delay (Andriessen et al., 2009). Retrospective assessment of PTA duration has been shown to be as reliable as prospective assessment in a severe population (McMillan et al., 1996), although

Table 3.4 Traumatic brain injury severity: duration of posttraumatic amnesia

GRADE	PTA
Mild	< 1 hour
Moderate	> 1 hour, < 24 hours
Severe	> 1 day, < 7 days
Very severe	> 7 days

PTA, posttraumatic amnesia. From Russell W.R., Cerebral Involvement in Head Injury: a study based on the examination of two hundred cases (1932), published by Oxford University Press. Reprinted with permission.

Gronwall and Wrightson (1980) found that one-quarter of mildly injured patients changed their estimation at a second interview after 3 months.

In practice, severity, particularly after the acute period, is currently assessed with reference to all three factors discussed above and with additional consideration given to early computed tomographic (CT) scans and later magnetic resonance imaging (MRI) scans when available.

Service provision

Improvements in surgical techniques and medical management, particularly since the 1970s, have resulted in substantially improved survival rates, and there is clarity and consensus on many medical management issues. Precise guidelines for the early management of those who sustain a TBI are now available, for example, the Scottish national clinical guideline (Scottish Intercollegiate Guideline Network, 2009) and the English National Institute for Health and Clinical Excellence (NICE) guideline (National Institute for Health and Clinical Excellence, 2007). However, services beyond the acute phase have been very slow to develop in the UK (see Campbell, 2000a, 2000f, for discussion) and while there are areas of good practice, there has been a growing recognition of the geographical inequalities and overall inadequacies of current provision (House of Commons, 2001) and some policy action to standardize and improve service delivery (Department of Health, 2005).

Worldwide, a number of models of service provision have been proposed, based on clinical experience and available evidence (Burke, 1987; Eames & Wood 1989; McMillan & Greenwood 1993; Oddy et al., 1989). Across these proposals there are a number of recurring themes, including the need for: organizational integration; inter-disciplinary team work; professionals with advanced knowledge and skills; and a systematic programme of service evaluation and innovative research (Campbell, 2000f). Furthermore, there is acknowledgement of the need for multiple service components across health and social care, including options for supported living, and for services to be flexible in response, so that individuals may access them at a time of need and on more than one occasion, if appropriate (Department of Health, 2005).

Principles of acute management of traumatic brain injury

The aims of initial emergency and early medical management are to limit the development of secondary brain damage, and to provide the best conditions for recovery from any reversible damage that has already occurred. This is achieved by establishing and maintaining a clear airway with adequate oxygenation and replacement fluids to ensure a good peripheral circulation with adequate blood volume. It is essential to achieve this before an accurate neurological assessment can be made.

During the initial evaluation, movement of the cervical spine is minimized until any fractures have been excluded. Where appropriate, prophylactic antibiotic therapy is commenced immediately (Bullock & Teasdale, 1990a, 1990b). Except for the management of immediate seizures, the routine early use of anticonvulsant therapy is not now recommended (Hernandez & Naritoku, 1997).

Patients who exhibit breathing difficulties are assisted by intubation and ventilation (Bullock & Teasdale, 1990a). In addition, elective ventilation is often the treatment of choice in the presence of facial, chest or abdominal injuries, and for those with a summated GCS score of less than 9. Ventilation is usually achieved via endotracheal tube and tracheostomy is only performed where facial or spinal fractures determine this course of action or in the few cases when respiratory support is required over a more extended period. Even when ventilation is not indicated, oxygen therapy is recommended to help meet the injured brain's increased energy requirements (Frost, 1985).

Those with significant injuries are at risk of breakdown of the normal process of cerebral autoregulation that ensures blood flow to the brain is consistently maintained, independent of the normal fluctuations in systemic blood pressure (Aitkenhead, 1986). When this protective mechanism is lost, cerebral perfusion pressure (CPP) becomes directly related to the systemic mean arterial blood pressure (MAP) and the intracranial pressure (ICP). Breathing patterns and fluid volumes can be manipulated in a ventilated and sedated patient. With the prescription of appropriate drug therapy, optimum blood gas levels, systemic blood pressure and, as far as possible, cerebral blood flow can be achieved, minimizing the development of additional brain damage.

The physical position and management of the patient are also important in the control of raised ICP and, in particular, the prevention of additional cerebral congestion due to obstruction of venous drainage. A slightly raised head position (avoiding neck flexion and compression of the jugular veins) is recommended (Feldman et al., 1992), although the maintenance of neutral alignment may be sufficient if raising the head threatens cerebral perfusion by lowering the systemic blood pressure (Rosner & Colley, 1986).

Activities that raise intrathoracic pressure also raise ICP and need to be minimized. This has particular relevance for respiratory care where the objective of preventing the organization of secretions must be achieved, with minimal use of interventions likely to raise ICP, such as manual hyperinflation. When a problematic chest requires vigorous attention, pretreatment sedation may be indicated, allowing bronchial suction with minimal provocation of cough. There is some evidence that slow percussive techniques may help reduce ICP (Garrad & Bullock, 1986). The principles of intervention for respiratory health are considered in detail by Ada and colleagues

(1990), Roberts (2002) and in brief below (see 'The role of the physiotherapist in the acute phase').

Neurosurgical intervention after traumatic brain injury

In closed TBIs, surgery is undertaken as a matter of urgency to evacuate any significant haematoma and so decompress the injured brain (Jennet & Lindsay, 1994a). Where there is a depressed fracture or a penetrating wound, surgery will also be undertaken to remove any debris, clean the wound and restore the normal contour of the skull as far as possible. In some centres, minor procedures to insert an ICP-monitoring device will be performed, according to local protocols (Pickard & Czosnyka, 2000), though their use and effectiveness remains controversial (Cremer, 2008; Shafi et al., 2008; Smith, 2008).

Physical management

Beyond intervention to save life and promote the ideal conditions for cerebral repair and recovery, the next most important issue is the prevention of secondary physical changes and the provision of optimum conditions to promote physical recovery. Patients may benefit from being cared for on a special pressure-relieving mattress (Moseley, 2002) and from intensive management of nutritional input (Taylor & Fettes, 1998). Sedated patients are paralysed and vulnerable to muscular and other soft-tissue changes associated with immobility and inactivity. They are also exposed to consistent environmental stimuli, which if left unmanaged will result in significant muscle length changes. For example, the combined effects of gravity and the weight of bedding over extended periods in lying can lead to the development of foot plantarflexion.

It is vital that physiotherapists are involved in developing a physical management plan to guide the management of physical factors over the full 24-hour period and that this occurs at the earliest possible point following hospital admission. Common physical deficits and their management are described later in this chapter.

Pathological conditions

Cerebral aneurysms

A cerebral aneurysm is an abnormal dilation or ballooning of a cerebral artery, which is usually due to a congenital or acquired weakness in the wall of the vessel (Jennet & Lindsay, 1994b). It is not usually possible to identify a single cause for the development of an aneurysm, although hypertension and arteriosclerosis are seen as risk factors. A rare form, mycotic aneurysm, results from a blood-borne infection.

Presentation

Often the first indication of the presence of an aneurysm is when it ruptures and bleeds into or around the brain. Bleeding is most commonly into the subarachnoid space (subarachnoid haemorrhage), but rupture may also result in bleeding directly into brain tissue. The incidence of subarachnoid haemorrhage in the UK is given as 10 per 100 000 population per annum (Mitchell et al., 2004), with aneurysm rupture accounting for around 75% of cases (Lindsay & Bone, 2004). Higher incidences are reported in Sweden (19 per 100 000) (Stegmayr et al., 2004) and Japan (22 per 100 000) (Ikawa et al., 2004), with a higher incidence for women reported in both studies (24% and 26% respectively). The mortality rate is reported as being between 22% (Ikawa et al., 2004) and 50% (Mitchell et al., 2004). Aneurysm rupture is most common between the ages of 40 and 60, a more mature population than the peak occurrence of TBI, but a younger age group than the mean age of 70 for stroke caused by cerebral infarct (Dombovy et al., 1998a).

Unruptured aneurysms may produce neurological symptoms due to their size or location and be diagnosed following medical investigation, including MRI brain scan. For example, a lesion on an internal carotid artery at the level of the optic chiasm can produce peripheral blurred vision (de Chigbu, 2003). Some are discovered incidentally when investigations are performed for other reasons. The diagnosis of a cerebral aneurysm is usually confirmed by angiogram, a procedure that involves injecting a radiopaque substance into the blood vessels and taking X-rays of the head (Tavernas, 1996).

Complications

Before the advent of effective surgery, almost one-third of those with a ruptured aneurysm would bleed again within 1 month. The risk of a rebleed if surgery is not undertaken remains high for 6 months. Whether or not surgery is undertaken after subarachnoid haemorrhage, there is a risk of vasospasm causing ischaemia or infarction, with resultant additional neurological damage. This most frequently occurs between four and 12 days after the initial bleed.

Extracranial complications include cardiac arrhythmias, myocardial infarction, pulmonary oedema and stress ulcers. Hydrocephalus may occur in the early postbleed period but is also reported as a late complication in 10% of cases (Lindsay & Bone, 2004).

Medical management of aneurysms and subarachnoid haemorrhage

Subarachnoid haemorrhage is graded into five levels of severity (Table 3.5). Until the mid-1980s surgery for all grades was routinely delayed for 1–2 weeks after a bleed for fear of provoking vasospasm. However, reappraisal of

Table 3.5 Grades of subarachnoid haemorrhage

GRADE	GCS	ADDITIONAL DESCRIPTORS
I	15	No motor deficit
II	13–14	No motor deficit
III	13–14	With motor deficit
IV	7–12	With or without motor deficit
V	3–6	With or without motor deficit

GCS, Glasgow Coma Scale. (After Teasdale et al., 1988.)

the risk of a rebleed within this period and improved surgical and non-surgical techniques has encouraged more aggressive management. In most centres, intervention will be undertaken for grades I and II within 3 days (Lindsay & Bone, 2004) and in some centres early intervention is becoming routine for the majority of cases (Dombovy et al., 1998a).

Intervention for subarachnoid haemorrhage or intact aneurysms traditionally involved surgical clipping, that is, open brain surgery and the placing of a small metallic clip across the base of the aneurysm preventing blood flow into the weakened area, or embolization (Jennet & Lindsay, 1994b). Embolization is a more recent vascular technique whereby a metal coil or balloons are introduced into the artery to block off the aneurysm via the arterial system at the groin, under radiological guidance (Pile-Spellman, 1996). The choice of intervention is determined by the size and position of the aneurysm.

Physical management postintervention will vary, depending on the extent of damage caused by the prior SAH and the nature of the intervention. Endovascular treatment is usually followed by 24-hour bed rest and then mobilization. Following open surgery, management may be similar to that after surgery for TBI (see 'Rehabilitation after brain injury', below).

Arteriovenous malformations

An arteriovenous malformation (AVM) is an abnormal tangle of blood vessels lacking in capillary vessels and is thought to be a congenital abnormality. Within the central nervous system they can occur within the brain, associated with the dural layer of the meninges or within the spinal cord. As dural AVMs carry a low risk of haemorrhage and spinal AVMs produce symptoms more closely related to incomplete spinal lesions, we will only consider cerebral AVMs here.

A total of 40–60% of cerebral AVMs are discovered following haemorrhage, which produces symptoms such as seizures, neurological deficits or headache. Symptomatic

AVMs present most frequently in the 20–40 age group and the mortality rate is lower than SAH at 10–20%. The risk of rebleed is also much less than following an aneurysmal haemorrhage and is highest for small lesions (Lindsay & Bone, 2004). Haematomas associated with AVMs are often visible on CT or MRI scans. Otherwise diagnosis will be confirmed via angiography.

Medical management of ateriovenous malformations

If and when an AVM is thought to be amenable to direct intervention, there are a number of possible options. These include surgical resection, stereotactic radiosurgery and embolization (Jennet & Lindsay, 1994b). Any one of these interventions may be regarded as the treatment of choice or, in some cases, a combination of these interventions may be used in a stepwise progression. Stereotactic radiosurgery is a method of precisely delivering radiation to a brain lesion while sparing the surrounding brain tissue (Pollock, 2002).

Infectious processes

Primary brain damage can result from meningitis, encephalitis or brain abscess.

Brain abscess

This condition is now relatively rare, with an incidence rate of 2–3 per 1000 000 population per annum (Lindsay & Bone, 2004). The infection can have its source in such things as dental caries, sinusitis, mastoiditis, subacute endocarditis or pulmonary disease.

The abscess can accumulate in the extradural space or in the brain substance or in the subdural space, when it may be called empyema. With antibiotics and surgical drainage there is now a 90% survival rate, although around half of those who survive will experience subsequent seizures.

Meningitis

Meningitis has a range of bacterial and viral sources, and a variety of presentations, associated complications and outcomes (Johnson, 1998; Kroll & Moxon, 1987). Drug therapy is commenced immediately in any suspected case, even before the infective organism is identified, and continued up to 2 weeks after pyrexia has settled.

Encephalitis

The most common form of sporadic viral encephalitis results from the herpes simplex virus which selectively affects the inferior frontotemporal lobes of the brain. This can result in extremely amnesic survivors, although treatment with acyclovir has increased survival rates to 80% and lessened resultant deficits (Lindsay & Bone, 2004).

Cerebral tumours

Primary brain tumours have an incidence level of 6 per 100 000 population with slightly less than 10% of these occurring in children (Lindsay & Bone, 2004). There are many different kinds of tumours with names reflecting the cells of origin and situation of growth. It is beyond the scope of this book to detail the treatment and prognostic factors for each kind, but it is important to note that even large tumours can be benign, resulting in a stable neurological deficit. It is clearly important to understand the nature of the tumour involved and to have the best prediction of outcome in order to structure rehabilitative intervention appropriately (see Thomas, 1990 and Al-Mefty, 1991 for further reading). The importance of developing appropriate rehabilitation and support for people with central nervous system tumours is increasingly recognized (National Institute for Health and Clinical Excellence, 2006).

DEFICITS ASSOCIATED WITH ACQUIRED BRAIN INJURY

There is a wide range of commonly occurring deficits after TBI that present in a variety of mixes and severities. These affect psychosocial domains, core cognitive and sensorimotor skills and specific integrative cognitive functions that, in the presence of adequate psychosocial function, allow the core skills to be used in the organization, planning and implementation of functional activities. Recent work has begun to document a similar range of impairments between this population and those who survive a significant subarachnoid bleed (Dombovy et al., 1998a, 1998b; Hellawell et al., 1999).

Impairments resulting from other sources of ABI may not necessarily encompass such a wide range of effects at an individual level, but the same range of impairments will certainly be reflected across each population.

For the sake of clarity in this discussion, we will focus primarily on recovery following severe TBI and add further structure by considering rehabilitation as occurring in three consecutive phases as described by Mazaux and Richer (1998) (Table 3.6).

Not all impairments are observable immediately following injury and the context within which assessment takes place will influence what residual impairments may be expected or detected at all stages of recovery. Time since onset is not on its own a guiding factor, even within the severe TBI subpopulation, and other potential influences to consider are injury mechanism, additional injuries, treatment received and the progress already made.

Table 3.6 Objectives of three phases of rehabilitation after brain injury

	PHASE 1: ACUTE	PHASE 2: SUBACUTE	PHASE 3: POSTACUTE
Objectives	Prevent orthopaedic and visceral complications Provide appropriate sensory stimulation	Accelerate recovery of impairments Compensate for disabilities	Maximize independence Maximize community reintegration Maximize psychosocial adjustment and self-acceptance
Common domains of focus	Global physical and sensory systems	Mobility Cognition Behaviour Personality Affect	Physical Domestic Social
Anticipated approach	Supportive of medical management preparatory for subsequent interventions	Holistic Addressing physical independence Addressing psychological independence Addressing self-awareness	Personalized

(Compiled from information in Mazaux & Richer, 1998.)

REHABILITATION AFTER BRAIN INJURY

Given the complex array of deficits that can occur, it should be apparent that physiotherapists do not have the knowledge or skills independently to address rehabilitation issues in this client group. Indeed, publications emanating from specialist provision advocate an interdisciplinary (Body et al., 1996; Children's Trust at Tadworth, 1997; New Zealand National Health Committee, 1998; Powell et al., 1994) or transdisciplinary (Jackson et al., 1995) team approach. The role of the physiotherapist within an interdisciplinary team is described in detail by Campbell (Campbell, 2000g), setting the assessment approach described by Body and colleagues (1996) in a wider context, and adding further material to guide goal-setting and intervention planning.

Client- and family-centred approach

The particular interdisciplinary approach described by Campbell (Campbell, 2000g) includes a collaborative team assessment process that attempts to place the individual and close associates at the centre of that process. This is seen as crucial to effective service delivery and as an organizational mechanism to ensure a consistent standard of information gathering.

The design of the assessment process, which includes a multiprofessional assessment case discussion, facilitates the development of agreed team goals that are feasible to deliver and relevant to the injured person as an individual. For each individual, as well as standard assessments to identify impairments and strengths, the preinjury cultural base, lifestyle and aspirations are acknowledged and incorporated into goal development. Psychosocial functioning, including the level of self-awareness and stage of adjustment to their new circumstance, is given prominent consideration and included in the discussion of assessment findings *by the whole team*.

Each team member, including the physiotherapist, contributes to the prioritization of the intervention goals based on the global assessment findings. These recommendations are then fully discussed with the client and carer, and a plan of action is then agreed. This is an inclusive method of assessment, using multiple informants, both professional and personal, to the injured person. It uses professional expertise to synthesize and interpret assessment findings, but there is also a formal process for referral back to, and discussion with, the client and family at the initial assessment stage and throughout the period of contact. In this way it is hoped to establish an effective collaborative relationship with all of those who have an interest in each case. Client-centred practice is discussed in Chapter 11.

Professional collaboration

The importance of professional collaboration in the development and delivery of services for this client group cannot be sufficiently stressed. It is important to address the range of deficits that occur, to avoid duplication of effort and ensure all aspects are addressed. Innovative ways of working have evolved, for example, to deal with those difficulties that clients encounter that are not seen as the traditional area of practice for any specific profession.

Many specialist centres use a *key worker system*, where one team member will take on some additional, mainly organizational, tasks to ensure that the wider needs of clients are met. Services for different phases of recovery are often provided on different hospital and community sites and the nature of the clients' and carers' needs demand the inclusion of specialist social work support for extended periods of time.

The complexities of health- and social-care services are challenging even for the professionals involved in their delivery, and cross-agency working, extending into other areas such as education, housing or vocational training, is required if effective service delivery is to be achieved. Various organizational mechanisms are used to help facilitate effective and, where possible, seamless service delivery including *integrated care pathways*, *multiprofessional planning groups* and collaborative funding arrangements. Within the NHS in England, formal commissioning of cohesive care pathways and linked models of service delivery is in progress.

Physiotherapists have a unique body of knowledge to contribute to the team process, but we have also much to learn from service users and from other professional groups. Learning for all is accelerated when knowledge is effectively shared and so we have a responsibility to be proactive in this regard to improve the delivery of care.

Impact on families and other social networks

At the beginning of this chapter reference was made to the wider impact of ABI on close relationships and wider social networks. These effects have been studied in reasonable depth since early work in the 1970s and 1980s first began to document carer distress and burden (Brooks, 1984; Brooks et al., 1987; Romano, 1974; Rosenbaum & Najenson, 1976). There is now little doubt of the intense early trauma, and for many the continuing stresses, that family and friends can endure.

Campbell (Campbell, 2000h) discussed the impact of this trauma in practical terms, using case examples and with reference to a model of response described by Douglas (1990); see Table 3.7. Not all families make it through this five-stage process (Ponsford, 1995) and not all family members are able to progress at the same speed (Campbell, 2000h). It is important to consider, along

Table 3.7 Family response to traumatic brain injury: a five stage model		
Inpatient care	Shock	Confusion Anguish Frustration Helplessness
	Expectancy	Exaggerated optimism about recovery Denial Hope
Community-base care	Reality	Depression Anger Guilt Withdrawal from socialization Disruption of family relationships and existing roles
	Mourning	Awareness of permanence of the situation Acceptance of changes in the injured family member Grieving for what might have been
	Adjustment	Readjusting expectations Redefining relationships and roles Restructuring the family environment
(After Douglas, 1990.)		

with other team members, where carers are in this process before making demands on them to actively contribute to the rehabilitation programme.

Treatment goals that presume active assistance from a family member who does not have either the physical or emotional resources to respond appropriately are unlikely to be achieved. It is also important to interpret carer behaviours in the light of the trauma they are experiencing and with reference to how they may be coping with the difficulties presented. Families have individual characteristics and coping styles before the advent of the brain injury; each family member has an established role within that family, and each family is at its own particular stage of progress with reference to normal life changes and developments (Turnbull & Turnbull, 1991). All of these factors will influence how, and how well, each will cope with the early trauma and the ongoing demands.

Physiotherapists do not have the role of assessing family systems or of providing intervention or support programmes to facilitate successful carer engagement. However, it is essential that they have a strong awareness of the issues involved so that they may function effectively within the wider team structure and understand the impact of the demands they make on carers as well as patients.

Issues emerging in the acute phase

Loss of consciousness

As described earlier, sudden neural dysfunction or significant damage is likely to result in loss of consciousness. This may be short lived or may extend over weeks or months, and in some cases even years. There is often confusion about terminology of coma and postcoma:

- Coma is the state where there is no verbal response, no obeying commands and the patient does not open the eyes either spontaneously or to any stimulus (Jennet & Teasdale, 1977). Coma rarely lasts longer than 1 month; the patient either dies or emerges into the vegetative state.
- The vegetative state (VS; Jennett & Plum, 1972) is defined as 'a clinical condition of complete unawareness of the self and the environment, accompanied by sleep–wake cycles with either complete or partial preservation of hypothalamic and brainstem automatic functions' (Multi-Society Task Force, 1994, p. 1500).
- The minimally conscious state (MCS) is a condition that has been described more recently. This is 'a condition of severely altered consciousness in which minimal but definite behavioural evidence of self or environmental awareness is demonstrated' (Giacino et al., 2002, pp. 350–351). One or more of four diagnostic criteria confirm MCS and include:

(1) following simple commands; (2) yes/no responses; (3) intelligible verbalization; and (4) purposeful behaviour. Such meaningful interaction with the environment is not consistent but is reproducible or sustained enough to distinguish it from reflexive behaviour.

These three conditions are part of the continuum from coma through to emergence of awareness. The patient may remain in the VS or MCS as a transient phase or the condition may be permanent.

It is now recognized that patients may be misdiagnosed as being in VS when, in fact, they have significant levels of awareness. For example, Childs et al. (1993) reported that 37% of patients admitted more than 1 month post injury with a diagnosis of coma or persistent VS had some level of awareness. In a group of longer-term patients in a nursing home, Tresch et al. (1991) found that 18% of long-term nursing home residents diagnosed as being in the persistent VS were aware of themselves or their environment.

Andrews et al. (1996) reviewed the records of 40 consecutive patients admitted to their specialist profound brain injury unit after 6 months following their brain injury and found that 43% had been misdiagnosed (41% of these for more than a year, including three for more than 5 years). The levels of cognitive functioning present in this misdiagnosed group at the time of discharge were such that 60% were oriented in time, place and person; 75% were able to recall a name after 15 minute delay; 69% were able to carry out simple mental arithmetic; 75% were able to generate words to communicate their needs; and 86% were able to make choices about their daily social activities.

The implications of misdiagnosis involve legal as well as clinical aspects, given the practice of applying to the courts to withdraw nutrition and hydration from patients diagnosed as being in VS. Precise estimates of the incidence and prevalence of VS and MCS are not available and the relative rarity of the conditions means that most clinicians will have little or no experience in assessing such patients. It is recommended that the clinician contemplating a diagnosis of VS in any individual case should seek the views of two other doctors, one a neurologist, before confirming such a diagnosis (British Medical Association, 1996).

Increased muscle tone

Prior to sedation, during the period of emergence from coma or when sedation is withdrawn, abnormalities of motor behaviour may begin to be observed. In its most dramatic form this is seen as excessively raised muscle tone, producing rigid trunk and limbs. The quality and intensity of this raised muscle tone is strikingly different from that seen after stroke (see Ch. 2). In the lower limbs it is often highly organized across opposing muscle groups preventing hip and knee flexion and ankle dorsiflexion. In the upper limbs, there can be similar levels of extension or the same intensity of activity may be seen predominantly in the flexor muscle groups, resulting in a fixed flexed position with the limbs almost adhering to the chest wall. Another primary difference from stroke is that the increase in muscular tone can develop within a very short time of the injury, particularly in severe cases, unlike after stroke where there is often a period of low tone in the early stages.

When muscle tone is high there is usually a global effect involving the back and neck extensors as well as the limb muscles. One side of the body may be more affected than the other, but this may only become apparent when the overall level of tone begins to drop. At this stage, or in cases where the initial injury has not produced the dramatic high-tone picture described above, limb weakness will be observed, evidenced by lack of automatic movement. The use of elective ventilation has limited to some extent the frequency of occurrence of the severe tonal states described.

Experience of the speed of development of secondary soft-tissue changes has also led to the promotion of the use of preventive casting (Edwards & Charlton, 1996), applied before weaning off the ventilator. It is important to note, however, that although there may be very dramatic increases in tone in the acute phase and that without management this will result in hugely disabling secondary physical changes, the overall pattern of recovery often leads eventually to *low* levels of resting tone, sometimes complicated by contracture, giving the appearance of a continuing high-tone state. It is therefore important to limit early interventions to those with short-term or reversible effects and, in particular, to avoid radical orthopaedic surgical intervention.

Behavioural observation

In addition to motor performance, behavioural observation during this period may point to other transitory or potentially longer-lived deficits in cognition and communication and efforts are currently under way to develop a scale to formalize this type of observation and ultimately increase our understanding of patterns of recovery (Sheil et al., 2000).

The role of the physiotherapist in the acute phase

Mazaux and Richer (1998) identified the objectives of the acute phase of rehabilitation as the prevention of visceral and orthopaedic complications. This is clearly a multidisciplinary task, but for physiotherapists it translates primarily into the promotion of respiratory and cardiovascular health and musculoskeletal integrity. Campbell

(2000b) described a working model to guide intervention in the acute phase, as applied to a case example of severe TBI without additional injury. This discussion included reference to established clinical practice and supporting evidence. It is clear that, while much of established intervention techniques have not been tested at the level of clinical trials, many have been logically deduced from other knowledge areas such as pathophysiology and the basic sciences.

Treatment goals

Common treatment goals and approaches for Campbell's (2000b) sample case were identified as:

- continuous assessment (Campbell, 2000e)
- respiratory care of the ventilated patient and the promotion of optimum blood oxygenation (Ada et al., 1990; Roberts, 2002)
- positioning and assisted movement (Gill-Body & Giorgetti, 1995), including proactive or reactive casting (Edwards & Charlton, 1996), to preserve the integrity of soft tissues, skin and range of motion (see Ch. 14)
- graded sensory stimulation (Wood, 1991)
- provision of information and education for family and friends
- the use of frequent, short-duration treatments with the gradual reintroduction of antigravity positioning and the experience of movement.

Physiotherapy assessment for respiratory and musculoskeletal health in the very acute period includes consideration of the level of intervention required and may result initially in an advisory-only role, for example, when there is no respiratory compromise in an electively ventilated patient (Roberts, 2002). However, the patient must be kept under direct review via routine auscultation, as well as by monitoring nursing and medical observations, so that advice is regularly updated and active intervention is commenced immediately if it is considered necessary. Careful monitoring of vital signs in this way will also provide the parameters within which interventions must take place. In any case, treatments should be well planned, of minimal duration and interspersed with adequate rest periods (Roberts, 2002).

Early observations focused on respiratory health also provide the opportunity to monitor physical status. It remains imperative within the limitations imposed by medical instability to identify any threats to soft-tissue extensibility and prevent venous stasis.

Movement through full range may be possible in a sedated and medically stable patient, but access to all joints may not be possible. Some positions and movements may need to be avoided because of threats to medical status, for example, avoidance of neck flexion, a dependent head position or increased thoracic pressure to limit increases in ICP. Subtle alterations to classic nursing positions, for example, the use of foam wedges to modify supine (see Ch. 14), will help prevent the organization of excess extensor activity. In those with moderately increased tone, the introduction of a degree of trunk flexion in side-lying has similar effects but this position is difficult to sustain in higher-tone states, when the judicious use of positioning supports to allow a semiprone position is effective in moderating tone and can have a positive impact on breathing patterns. In the severely injured, it is essential to consider proactive management of increased tone, which may potentially develop when sedation is decreased during the process of weaning from the ventilator.

The application of lower-limb casts with the feet in an appropriate plantargrade position is considerably easier before sedation is decreased than after, when tone is difficult to control, and the patient may be in a state of agitation or confusion. The ability to adopt plantargrade is an important factor in achieving stable sitting and standing positions, essential milestones in the reintroduction of the experience of normal movement and an essential prerequisite of task-orientated rehabilitation programmes which have been shown to lead to earlier and better functional abilities (Hellweg & Johannes, 2008).

The hospital environment is noisy and often lit throughout the 24-hour period. A patient in intensive care or in a high-dependency unit also undergoes a plethora of interventions involving handling and movement. It may be necessary to *limit* rather than increase sensory stimulation to ensure periods of rest, for example, the use of eye-patching to promote normal diurnal rhythms (Ada et al., 1990). It is important that this concept of regulated sensory stimulation is imparted to friends and family members so that they may appropriately contribute to the promotion of recovery.

Feedback from families beyond the acute stage is that they appreciate accurate and timely information about the effects of the pathology, the rationale for interventions, what progress may be reasonably anticipated and what the next stage in the process is likely to be. Not many individuals want to read detailed information about long-term outcomes at this time, but they do want to understand what local services are available to them and to feel that everything possible is being done.

While formal treatment sessions may need to be short and paced throughout the day, the physiotherapist should provide direct advice and guidance to the whole team with regard to physical management objectives and strategies for the full 24-hour period. Environmental controls need to be negotiated and agreed with other team members, for example, splints or casts with the occupational therapist, the use of T-rolls and the arrangement of positioning pillows with the nursing staff. Agreed plans should be clearly documented and easily accessible to all staff.

KEY POINTS

For the physiotherapist in acute care:
- Initial treatment focuses on promoting respiratory health and preventing secondary adaptive changes in the musculoskeletal system.
- The physiotherapist may provide direct treatment, specific advice to other team members or a combination of both to ensure effective 24-hour management.
- Treatments are of short duration with frequent review but allowing rest periods throughout the day.
- In severe cases, proactive lower-limb casts should be considered to limit the negative effects of severe tonal states.
- It is important to keep families informed of treatment objectives.

Impact of early physical management on longitudinal outcome

There are no formal prospective studies comparing the effects of early active physical management against no intervention or comparing the relative merits of different types of physical management on long-term outcome. However, as pointed out by McMillan and Greenwood (1993), there is a stark contrast between outcomes now and those reported by Rusk and colleagues on a series of 127 patients in the 1960s (Rusk et al., 1966; Rusk et al., 1969), with 40 pressure sores, 200 joint contractures, 30 frozen shoulders and multiple urinary and respiratory complications. However, while it may be accepted that the convention for early active management of the effects of brain damage on the musculoskeletal system has improved the overall standard of physical outcomes, the need for a significant number of postacute remedial interventions, such as surgery (Marwitz et al., 2001), argues against any complacency in this area.

Similarly, we have to ensure that the potential for long-term negative effects of limited intervention, for those who carry an initially poor prognosis but go on to confound medical science, is fully taken into account and that optimum skeletal alignment and muscular balance are achieved wherever possible as the best basis for ongoing progress (Campbell, 2000e). With clinical experience extending over 30 years, the author can testify to the improved physical outcomes brought about by advances in medical care and changes in rehabilitation practice. Two significant factors can be singled out in the latter: the advent of proactive management of muscle length imbalance and postural alignment by way of casting to facilitate early antigravity activity, and the development of organized subacute rehabilitation programmes.

Issues emerging in the subacute phase

In this phase, the patient becomes medically stable and the period of disorientation and confusion begins to settle. It then becomes possible for all members of the team to undertake more extensive and accurate assessment across domains, and so begin to log specific impairments, and either observe or project their functional effects.

Time since injury

There are no hard and fast temporal indicators of when the subacute period begins or ends in any of the pathologies we have considered so far. It is also important to realise that what constitutes the subacute phase in each individual case, even within a pathology-specific population, can vary enormously and may, therefore, require a differential response from service provision.

Case histories

The different needs of two individuals at the same time after injury are illustrated by two comparative case histories, outlined in Table 3.8.

Julian and Angela were both 5 weeks post injury but there were clear differences in the responses that were required from the service, the type of information that could be gathered from them and the scope of assessment that was appropriate to undertake. There were also several differentiating factors concerning the impact of their residual impairments on function, and the potential for physiotherapy and other professional involvement. The comparison of the two cases illustrates some of the difficulties in focusing on time since injury as an indicator of likely progression. Julian's case also clearly illustrates the interdependent nature of cognitive and physical impairments in the early recovery period. Intervention to control for, or improve, his awareness and orientation

Table 3.8 Case histories of traumatic brain injury, Julian and Angela

	JULIAN	ANGELA
Age	18	26
Time since onset	5 weeks	5 weeks
Summary	Road traffic accident GCS 3 at the scene Required neurosurgery to evacuate a large subdural haematoma Ventilated for 7 days Evidence of disturbed motor performance all four limbs Normal sleep and wake cycle now re-established Only occasional vocalization, no recognizable words	Fell from ladder at home LOC unknown, presented as confused to husband in another room of the house GCS on arrival at hospital 14 (E=4, M=6,V=4) No skull fracture on X-ray, discharged Troublesome headache for 2–3 days, rested in bed Visited GP 5, 12 and 19 days post Referred to follow-up clinic
Place of residence	Sub-acute rehabilitation facility	Home
Self-report of current concerns	None verbal Grimaces Fluctuating levels of muscle tone, ? partly in response to discomfort	Unable to return to work Poor concentration Feels unsteady Intolerant of busy or noisy environments
Commentary	Julian is unable to express his own objectives or, indeed give verbal direction to guide the scope of assessment. The professional team will have the full responsibility to decide the scope and detail of his assessment and to set management objectives on his behalf.	Initially, Angela was not regarded as having a significant injury and so did not expect to be away from work for so long. Work return is her key objective and she can easily express this within the assessment process. She is also aware, even within the context of home-based activities that she has not fully recovered from the effects of her fall and can give clear direction towards at least some of the domains requiring analysis.

GCS, Glasgow Coma Scale (summated score: GCS = E+M+V (E= Eyes, M= Motor, V= Verbal)); LOC, Loss of consciousness.

would be of equal importance to work focused on preventing the development of additional complications (physical and behavioural) and ensuring optimal conditions to drive any potential recovery.

Physical impairments

Depending on the degree of cooperation that is feasible to elicit, it may be possible to detect the limitations of cranial nerve function and to begin to document underlying motor performance difficulties, and, to some degree, the disruption of sensory perception. The sense of smell is frequently lost following TBI, especially if there has been a fracture of the anterior fossa.

The visual system may be affected at the level of the optic nerve, or processing or interpretation of visual stimuli (Narayan et al., 1990). Eye movements and the control of binocular vision may be affected via damage to the oculomotor, trochlear or abducens nerves or to the cerebral areas involved in the processing of two images into one. Individuals may report double vision (diploplia) or a squint may be observed but not reported (strabismus). Oculomotor nerve damage may also affect pupillary reaction and result in difficulties with accommodation to light. The chances of some form of visual disturbance in diffuse injuries is high, since around one-third of the brain is involved in the processing of vision (Stein, 1995). This is an important observation for physiotherapists, given the role of vision in the guidance of movement and the maintenance of balance (see Ch. 13).

Facial bone fractures can result in damage to the trigeminal nerve, producing facial numbness or hypersensitivity. Facial nerve damage (facial palsy) may develop from temporal bone trauma (Narayan et al., 1990). Direct or indirect impacts in the temporal area can also cause vestibulocochlear nerve damage resulting in neural deafness. Direct damage to the bony chain or bleeding into the middle ear may produce conduction deafness. Trauma in and around the temporal bone region may also directly damage the vestibular apparatus or create a perilymph fistula, disrupting balance function and inducing dizziness (see Ch. 13). Occasionally damage to lower cranial nerves may occur, associated with basal skull fractures or neck trauma.

Symptoms more commonly associated with whiplash injuries may also be observed and, although rare, traumatic dissection of the carotid artery associated with neck trauma may also occur, producing a range of additional neurological symptoms relative to the level of ischaemia that results.

A variety of distinct or combined motor disorders may become apparent as sedation is withdrawn or as attempts are made to undertake functional activities. Presentations vary depending on the site and distribution of damage but may include:

- hypertonicity
- ataxia
- dyskinesia (involuntary movement)
- failure to initiate movement or sustain posture due to weakness
- dyspraxia (difficulty actioning purposeful movement despite having intact sensation and motor activity)
- sensory inattention.

Commonly after TBI, aspects of these disorders will be seen in complex mixtures, thus clearly differentiating this population from those with stroke or other more localized cerebral pathologies.

Heterotopic ossification (HO; extra periarticular bone growth) may be seen after severe TBI, more commonly in children and young adults (Hurvitz et al., 1992) and often associated with extended periods of coma (Anderson, 1989). Length of coma has recently been confirmed as a risk factor for recurrence following surgical excision but not (against received wisdom) early excision (Chalidis et al., 2007); also see Chapter 14.

Cognitive and behavioural impairments

Structured observation across team members and the beginnings of formal assessment by occupational therapists, speech and language therapists and neuropsychologists will enable the development of a clearer picture of cognitive and communicative abilities. To some degree, the cognitive level, and, therefore, the ability to engage with formal assessment, will dictate the extent or limitations of assessment during the subacute phase. It is important for physiotherapists to appreciate this and, in particular, to note that even if cognitive limitations have not been identified via formal assessment they may still be present.

The frequent occurrence of lesions in the temporal and frontal lobes means that disorders of memory, attention and reasoning are common in this population along with many other cognitive and behavioural difficulties (Mazaux & Richer, 1998). All therapists working with patients at this stage need to develop excellent skills of behavioural observation and make allowances within their practice to accommodate for likely cognitive limitations.

The role of the physiotherapist in the subacute phase

The objectives for rehabilitation in the subacute phase as defined by Mazuax and Richer (1998) are to accelerate recovery of impairments and compensate for disabilities.

Case example

The physiotherapist's role can be illustrated by considering the case example of Jamie, an adolescent male with a TBI that resulted in a 2-hour loss of consciousness. In addition to the TBI, he also sustained a left femoral fracture (surgically fixed) and an undisplaced pelvic fracture. His aftercare was provided on an orthopaedic ward. Initial assessment revealed that he had:

- no apparent difficulties in maintaining his own respiration
- minor limitation of left knee flexion and moderate limitation of left hip range associated with postoperative oedema and pain
- no other obvious restrictions of joint range or soft-tissue extensibility
- decreased muscle tone without loss of the ability to initiate movement in the limbs
- poor limb-girdle stability
- initial difficulty achieving and sustaining unsupported sitting
- distress in supported standing
- repeated eye-closure in antigravity positions.

Treatment goals

The goals for initial intervention were to:

- provide orientation and reassurance
- monitor respiratory function
- preserve the integrity of soft tissues, skin and range of motion
- assess further the factors provoking distress in standing
- promote active participation in meaningful tasks (to facilitate functional use of limbs and explore balance control)
- provide information and education to Jamie and his family and friends
- provide education for professional colleagues (particularly with regard to factors provoking distress in standing)
- ensure onward referral to a TBI-aware service.

Each contact session with Jamie included a reminder of the therapists' names until he began to use their names routinely. Similarly, a simple explanation of the objective of each part of each session was given immediately before proceeding. This applied particularly to those activities that had previously caused distress, such as movement into sitting and up into standing.

Jamie was encouraged to describe what he was experiencing at the time or soon afterwards, when that was not possible. From this process it became apparent that the eye-closure was an attempt to escape from a feeling of environmental movement (the world spinning around him). It also became clear that he experienced alignment in the primary upright position as being tipped forward so, even at times in standing when he was not dizzy, he felt on the verge of falling flat on his face.

Jamie had appeared uncooperative with nursing staff trying to encourage him to assist them with his personal care activities. This situation was improved when strategies to allow recovery from dizziness following positional change were introduced and physical support was provided to maintain upright sitting, allowing him free use of his arms. Jamie also required verbal reassurance of his safety, as he was initially fearful of attempting functional tasks without supervision.

This assessment and communication role again illustrates the extent to which the physiotherapist's role extends beyond direct therapy sessions. For Jamie it was important to ensure that seating arrangements and, in time, methods of assisted walking contributed positively to the physical management objectives of reinforcing correct alignment, providing the optimum environment to facilitate antigravity activity in the trunk and encouraging positional change to drive sensory recalibration (see Ch. 13). Collaborative working during formal sessions was also beneficial, for example, working with an occupational therapist at an early stage within the context of washing and dressing. This facilitated Jamie's engagement while he was still confused and increased the range of possible therapeutic activities that could be attempted with an extra pair of hands.

By the time of his transfer to the neurorehabilitation ward, almost 5 weeks post injury Jamie had greatly improved hip mobility and was able to identify upright alignment in sitting during therapy sessions, but he still preferred to rest in a backward-leaning position. He was beginning to attempt to use his arms functionally, away from his body, in unsupported sitting. Reports of dizziness were much decreased but anxiety during standing and walking was still a live issue. Jamie's preference was to have physical contact during walking but he had begun to master walking with two sticks, within the confines of the therapy space and, to a lesser extent, on the ward.

KEY POINTS

For the physiotherapist in subacute care:

- Assessment of early residual sensorimotor deficits.
- Treatment focuses on providing an appropriate environment to assist functional recovery and on assisted practice of meaningful tasks, relevant to ability.
- A full range of treatment modalities may be used, including manual techniques, positioning and guided movement.
- Collaborative sessions with other disciplines are often appropriate.
- Effective communication with patient and family remains essential.

Issues emerging in the postacute phase

Significant motor performance deficits will already be documented and interventions to manage or reduce their functional effects will be established within the sub-acute period. Cognitive deficits and limitations affecting social behaviour may not begin to be fully quantified until much later in the recovery process, until the need to engage in social and community-based activities is encountered. This is true following any degree of injury and preinjury normality cannot be assumed until routine functional activities have been achieved and family and work roles are successfully re-established. It is also important to apply similar caution to considerations of normality in physical function, particularly concerning those who are in physically demanding employment, who like to engage in physical leisure pursuits or, as in the case of Angela, our second case history, those who bypass formal subacute provision.

Even at the minor or moderate end of the spectrum, complaints of fatigue and cognitive limitations are not uncommon (King et al., 1997). Information processing and capacity problems may mean that, although individuals can successfully perform single tasks, they may experience problems where attention has to be given to more than one task simultaneously or when their lifestyle demands performance of a number of tasks in series without respite. Although it is not the only reason for balance difficulties after moderate or minor injuries, a parallel difficulty in dual-tasking may be observed during demanding physical tasks, such as carrying a squirming toddler while walking downstairs, or when physical and cognitive demands occur together, for example, maintaining balance or holding on to an object when required to respond to an unexpected verbal enquiry or a sudden change in the environment.

A subpopulation of individuals return to normal activity levels within a relatively short period of sustaining a brain injury and it is only after a period of return to full-scale activities that problems become apparent to themselves or to those around them. They may cope at work but growing levels of fatigue may interfere with their role and relationships at home. Alternately, they may cope with the demands made at home but encounter problems in the workplace. Work difficulties may only become apparent when they attempt to undertake new or more demanding duties and failure may not immediately be related to the brain injury. The development of late medical problems can include posttraumatic epilepsy, a 2.5–5% risk (Jennett, 1990), and hormonal imbalances as a result of hypothalamic or pituitary stalk damage. Some aspect of the latter may also be latent, emerging only when there is variance from normal age-related changes (Horn & Garland, 1990).

The role of the physiotherapist in the postacute phase

Mazaux and Richer's (1998) objectives for this phase are to maximize independence, community reintegration, psychosocial adjustment and self-acceptance. While on the face of it these objectives may seem to relate more to the skills of other professions such as occupational therapy and psychology, the physiotherapist has much to contribute to the achievement of these objectives within the context of the interdisciplinary team.

The neurophysiotherapeutic role may be most easily recognized for those who continue to experience significant physical restrictions. Commonly these will be a mixture of limitations of primary motor skills and the impact of secondary musculoskeletal changes. Interventions are, therefore, targeted at reversing secondary changes and promoting improvement in specific motor skills. A third facet of treatment relates to translating the physical recovery already achieved into functionally oriented movement, with emphasis on improving performance for real-life functional goals.

The challenge for physiotherapists is that each individual presents with an almost unique mix of biomechanical and sensorimotor limiting factors and successful intervention is dependent on developing a clear hypothesis of the underlying and primary influencing factors in each case, so that intervention is focused. Therapists need to be able to apply a range of intervention strategies encompassing manual techniques (see Ch. 12), practice of isolated and task-specific movements (see Ch. 11) and the therapeutic use of functional activities requiring coordination of skilled movement, appropriately targeted to be demanding but achievable.

Intervention follows a cyclic pattern of movement analysis, work on subcomponents and skills and application to functional tasks. Work may be undertaken on a continuous basis over many months tackling several functional goals or may happen intermittently, prompted by the demands of new physical tasks or changes in personal circumstances, for example, a move to new accommodation or meeting the demands of getting about on a large educational campus. Even when there are regular intervention sessions, the limitation of direct contact time between therapist and client needs to be recognized and managed. It is important to empower individuals to contribute to their own physical progress (see Ch. 11) and to promote the development of a regular exercise habit, including the application of newly achieved or otherwise vulnerable motor skills. The strategies used will depend on clients' cognitive ability and the structure of their support network (Campbell, 2000c) but will always necessitate education sessions for clients and carers, clear and appropriate documentation (paper, electronic, audio, video) and regular review.

Demands for home practice need to be feasible (Campbell, 2000d) and supported by cognitive strategies for planning and actioning, if appropriate. Simple records of actual frequency of practice to be completed by the client provide a degree of motivation and aid programme evaluation.

For some the ultimate target may be functional mobility within the home, when intervention will focus on gait re-education. For others it may be to climb and work up a ladder, requiring work on speed of action, coordination and high-level balance skills, which have been shown to be affected even after apparently minor injuries (Campbell, 2008b). There is increasing recognition of the impact of sensory dysfunction in limiting physical recovery after brain injury (Campbell & Parry, 2005) and physiotherapy practice needs to develop to be more inclusive of the analysis of sensory dysfunction (Campbell, 2008a, 2008b), including visual and vestibular factors (see Ch. 13).

In addition to developing our skills of recognition of more subtle disorders of motor performance that act as barriers to return to preinjury work or leisure pursuits, application of wider physiotherapeutic knowledge and skills should translate into work for the promotion of cardiovascular health. Successful community reintegration is a multifactorial process and there is clearly a physical dimension not only in terms of overcoming physical barriers but also in developing the client's skills, confidence and ability to undertake regular physical leisure activities. The role of exercise and strength-training in neurological disorders is discussed in Chapter 18.

KEY POINTS

For the physiotherapist in postacute care:
- Physiotherapists may contribute to programmes for individuals with a range of residual sensorimotor deficits.
- Treatment for those with significant physical restrictions may still focus on reversing secondary adaptive changes and improving specific motor skills.
- Treatment includes helping to translate physical recovery into success with real-life functional goals.
- Programme success is dependent on skilled sensorimotor assessment and the application of knowledge gleaned from a collaborative assessment process, which includes all disciplines, clients and carers.
- Some individuals will require a lifelong physical management programme, some access to planned review and others an appropriate response at times of crisis.

Provision for those not admitted for inpatient care

Physiotherapists have, to date, gained most experience in working with those with significant physical difficulties and in the early months after injury. Current services and referral patterns in the UK focus provision on those whose injuries are severe enough to require initial hospitalization. However, in health-care systems where service provision for those with moderate and minor injuries is better established, for example in New Zealand, work is beginning to develop on appropriate physiotherapy response (Quinn & Sullivan, 2000), with some evidence of need documented in the developing literature (Campbell, 2008a, 2008b, 2008c). In the second case described in Table 3.8, Angela had a physical component within her list of residual symptoms but it was unlikely that she would be seen by a physiotherapist, or given any physiotherapy-generated advice, within current UK provision. Although her residual impairments were significantly less than Julian's, they were sufficient to prevent her return to normal activity levels and are illustrative of the need in all cases to consider residual impairments as limiting factors to achieving immediate functional goals including, at the appropriate time, return to meaningful occupation.

Long-term management of established deficits over time

There is little published literature either documenting the need for long-term management of physical deficits or proposing effective management strategies (Watson, 1997). The author's experience of contributing to postacute services within the National Health Service and in the independent sector in the UK has identified a subpopulation of survivors where ongoing proactive management is required in order to prevent specific physical deterioration and/or declining levels of physical activity. This is one of the many areas of brain injury that warrants research and evaluation.

Within this subpopulation, a spectrum of needs exists. At the most severe end of the spectrum are those with complex disabilities, who remain very physically restricted (essentially confined to bed and chair) and who may be only minimally aware, or in some cases relatively well preserved from a cognitive point of view. In terms of the overall incidence of brain injury, the numbers of those who remain very severely affected are small and there is therefore limited expertise in their holistic management. Many will benefit from a period of assessment and management planning from a specialist centre, such as the Royal Hospital for Neuro-disability in London, where:

- the level of awareness can be ascertained (Gill-Thwaites, 1997)
- medical complications can be managed
- nutritional requirements and feeding can be assessed appropriately and managed
- potential to use environmental controls or communication systems can be assessed

- appropriate seating can be prescribed (Pope, 2002)
- methods of managing pressure areas and soft-tissue vulnerability can be identified.

Some people will continue to require specialist residential care for the remainder of their lives and their level of dependency will demand continuous proactive management to prevent the development of pressure sores and soft-tissue contracture.

An alternative, or secondary, approach is to establish specialist care, and rehabilitation if appropriate, in a suitable home environment. Such packages require a consistent source of funding and can be complex to manage but, under the direction of a skilled case manager, and with the aid of an appropriately trained care team, a high quality of life can be achieved (Parker, 2006). In addition, personalized social contact and opportunities to pace care and activity appropriate to the individual, in a way that is not possible in any residential facility, provide an ideal environment to pursue any incremental progress that may be possible.

Ongoing physical management needs are not confined to the most severely disabled. In the presence of cognitive restrictions or behavioural difficulties, relatively minor physical deficits, such as a biomechanical imbalance from a residual weakness, can become incrementally more troublesome. This may show itself in the development of painful conditions or in diminishing levels of functional activity, contributing to increased behavioural problems or reduced social participation. Where there is an adequate support network, these factors can be proactively managed by including exercise or other forms of physical leisure within the weekly programme. Where this is not possible, or in cases when the client is unable to see

the value in preventive measures, service provision that can respond quickly and appropriately at the time of crisis is required.

Challenges to the delivery of effective physical management after acquired brain injury

There are many challenges to effective physical management following brain injury but there are four key factors that are to some degree interdependent:

1. The high incidence of coexisting cognitive limitations and behavioural factors
2. Fragmented services, across agencies and within service components
3. Limitations of service provision
4. Lack of detailed evidence to support the development of service provision.

The high incidence of coexisting deficits makes each case complex in its presentation. There are specific strategies that physiotherapists can adopt to help control for these confounding factors (Campbell, 2000c), but these are insufficient in the absence of action to link professional support for clients and carers at each rehabilitation phase and across all aspects of service delivery. Service provision and evaluation, particularly in the area of postacute care, need to develop further so that the service is both accessible and effective. There is great potential for physiotherapists to make a significant contribution to the development of services for this rewarding client group.

REFERENCES

Abdel-Dayem, H.M., Abu-Judeh, H., Kumar, M., Atay, S., Naddaf, S., El-Zeftawy, H., 1998. SPECT brain perfusion abnormalities in mild or moderate traumatic brain injury. Clin. Nucl. Med. 23, 309–317.

Abu-Judeh, H.H., Parker, R., Singh, M., El-Zeftawy, H., Atay, S., Kumar, M., et al., 1999. SPET brain perfusion imaging in mild traumatic brain injury without loss of consciousness and normal computed tomography. Nucl. Med. Commun. 20, 505–510.

Ada, L., Canning, C., Paratz, J., 1990. Care of the Unconscious Head-Injured Patient. In: Ada, L., Canning, C. (Eds.), Key Issues in Neurological Physiotherapy. Butterworth-Heinemann, London, pp. 249–287.

Adams, J., Mitchell, D., Graham, D., et al., 1977. Diffuse brain damage of the immediate impact type. Brain 100, 489–502.

Aitkenhead, A., 1986. Cerebral Protection. Br. J. Hosp. Med. 35, 290–298.

Al-Mefty, O. (Ed.), 1991. Meningiomas. Raven Press, New York.

Anderson, B.J., 1989. Heterotopic Ossification: a review. Rehabil. Nurs. 14, 89–91.

Andrews, K., Murphy, L., Munday, R., et al., 1996. Misdiagnosis of the vegetative state: retrospective study in a rehabilitation unit. Br. Med. J. 131, 13–16.

Andriessen, T.M., de Jong, B., Jacobs, B., van der Werf, S.P., Vos, P.E., 2009. Sensitivity and specificity of the

3-item memory test in the assessment of post traumatic amnesias. Brain Inj. 23, 345–352.

Auer, R.N., Krcek, J., Butt, J.C., 1994. Delayed symptoms and death after minor head trauma with occult vertebral artery injury. J. Neurol. Neurosurg. Psychiatry 57, 500–502.

Body, C., Leatham, J., 1996. Incidence and aetiology of head injury in a New Zealand adolescent sample. Brain Inj. 10, 567–573.

Body, R., Herbert, C., Campbell, M., Parker, M., Usher, A., 1996. An integrated approach to team assessment in head injury. Brain Inj. 10, 311–318.

Bond, M.R., 1986. Neurobehavioural sequelae of closed head injury. In: Grant, I., Adams, K.M. (Eds.), Neuropsychological Assessment of Neuropsychiatric Disorders. Oxford University Press, New York, pp. 347–373.

Bond, R., 1990. Standardised Methods for Assessing and Predicting Outcome. In: Rosenthal, M., Griffith, E., Bond, M., Miller, J. (Eds.), Rehabilitation of the Adult and Child with Traumatic Brain Injury. F A Davis, Philadelphia, pp. 59–74.

British Medical Association, 1996. Treatment decisions for patients in persistent vegetative state. British Medical Association, London. June.

Brooks, D., 1984. Closed Head Injury: Psychological, Social and Family Issues. Oxford University Press, Oxford.

Brooks, D., Campsie, L., Symington, C., Beattie, A., McKinlay, W., 1987. The effects of severe head injury on patient and relative within seven years of injury. J. Head Trauma Rehabil. 2, 1–13.

Bullock, R., Teasdale, G., 1990a. Head injuries -1. Br. Med. J. 300, 1515–1518.

Bullock, R., Teasdale, G., 1990b. Head injuries -2. Br. Med. J. 300, 1576–1579.

Burke, D., 1987. Planning a system of care for head injuries. Brain Inj. 1, 189–198.

Campbell, M., 2000a. About this book. In: Campbell, M. (Ed.), Rehabilitation for traumatic brain injury: physical therapy practice in context. Churchill Livingston, Edinburgh, pp. 1–13.

Campbell, M., 2000b. Applying neurophysiotherapeutic principles. In: Campbell, M. (Ed.), Rehabilitation for Traumatic Brain Injury: physical therapy practice in context. Churchill Livingston, Edinburgh, pp. 169–205.

Campbell, M., 2000c. Cognitive, behavioural and individual influences in programme design. In: Campbell, M. (Ed.), Rehabilitation for Traumatic Brain Injury: physiotherapy practice in context. Churchill Livingston, Edinburgh, pp. 207–230.

Campbell, M., 2000d. Defining goals for intervention. In: Campbell, M. (Ed.), Rehabilitation for Traumatic Brain Injury: physical therapy practice in context. Churchill Livingstone, Edinburgh, pp. 151–165.

Campbell, M., 2000e. Initial considerations in the process of assessment. In: Campbell, M. (Ed.), Rehabilitation for traumatic brain injury: physical therapy practice in context. Churchill Livingstone, Edinburgh, pp. 75–100.

Campbell, M., 2000f. Policy, planning and proactive management. In: Campbell, M. (Ed.), Rehabilitation for traumatic brain injury: physical therapy practice in context. Churchill Livingstone, Edinburgh, pp. 233–251.

Campbell, M., 2000g. Rehabilitation for Traumatic Brain Injury: physical therapy practice in context. Churchill Livingstone, Edinburgh.

Campbell, M., 2000h. Understanding the impact of the traumatic event and the influence of life context. In: Campbell, M. (Ed.), Rehabilitation for Traumatic Brain Injury: physical therapy practice in context. Churchill Livingstone, Edinburgh, pp. 45–72.

Campbell, M., 2008a. Key issues for the assessment of balance disorder after traumatic brain injury (TBI): Findings from a multifactorial study. Brain Inj. 22, 135–136.

Campbell, M., 2008b. New insights into the nature of balance disorder after traumatic brain injury (TBI): Findings from a multifactorial study. Brain Inj. 22, 134–135.

Campbell, M., 2008c. Towards a better understanding of MTBI and post-concussion syndrome: Insights from a study focused on balance disorder. Brain Inj. 22, 136.

Campbell, M., Parry, A., 2005. Balance disorder and traumatic brain injury: Preliminary findings of a multifactorial observational study. Brain Inj. 19, 1095–1104.

Centre for Health Service Studies, 1998. National Traumatic Brain Injury Study. Warwick University.

Chalidis, B., Stengel, D., Giannoudis, P., 2007. Early Excision and Late Excision of Heterotopic Ossification after Traumatic Brain Injury Are Equivalent: A Systematic Review of the Literature. J. Neurotrauma. 24, 1675–1686.

Children's Trust at Tadworth, R. T, 1997. Format and procedure for writing an interdisciplinary rehabilitation report. British Journal of Therapy and Rehabilitation 4, 70–74.

Childs, N.L., Mercer, W.N., Childs, H.W., 1993. Accuracy of diagnosis of persistent vegetative state. Neurology 43, 1465–1467.

Cremer, O.L., 2008. Does ICP monitoring make a difference in neurocritical care? Eur. J. Anaesthesiol. 42, 87–93.

Currie, G., 1993. The Management of Head Injuries. Oxford University Press, Oxford.

de Chigbu, G., 2003. Visual field defect: a case of cerebral aneurysm. Optometry Today 24–26.

Department of Health, 2005. The National Service Framework for Long-Term Conditions. Department of Health, London.

Dombovy, M.L., Drew-Cates, J., Serdans, R., 1998a. Recovery and rehabilitation following subarachnoid haemorrhag. Part I: outcome after inpatient rehabilitation. Brain Inj. 12, 443–454.

Dombovy, M.L., Drew-Cates, J., Serdans, R., 1998b. Recovery and rehabilitation following subarachnoid haemorrhage: part II long-term follow-up. Brain Injury 12, 887–894.

Douglas, J.M., 1990. Traumatic brain injury and the family. Paper presented at the Making Headway: NZSTA Biennial Conference, Christchurch, NZ.

Drubach, D.A., Kelly, M.P., Winslow, M.M., Flynn, J.P., 1993. Substance abuse as a factor in the causality, severity and recurrence of traumatic brain injury. Md. Med. J. 42, 989–993.

Eames, P., Wood, R., 1989. The structure and content of a head injury rehabilitation service. In: Wood, R.L., Eames, P. (Eds.), Models of Brain Injury Rehabilitation. Chapman & Hall, London, pp. 31–58.

Edwards, S., Charlton, P., 1996. Splinting and the use of orthoses in the management of patients with neurological disorders. In: Edwards, S. (Ed.), Neurological Physiotherapy: A Problem Solving Approach. Churchill Livingstone, New York, pp. 161–188.

Feldman, Z., Kanter, M.J., Robertson, C. S., Contant, C.F., Hayes, C., Sheinberg, M.A., et al., 1992. Effects of head elevation on intra-cranial pressure, cerebral perfusion pressure and cerebral blood flow in head injury patients. J. Neurosurg. 76, 207–211.

Fick, D.S., 1995. Management of concussion in collision sports. Guidelines for the sidelines. Postgrad. Med. 97, 53–56 59–60.

Frost, E.A.M., 1985. Management of head injury. Canadian Anaesthetic Society Journal 32, 532.

Gabella, B., Reiner, K.L., Hoffman, R.E., Cook, M., Stallones, L., 1995. Relationship of helmet use and head injuries among motorcycle crash victims in El Paso County, Colorado, 1989-1990. Accid. Anal. Prev. 27, 363–369.

Garrad, J., Bullock, M., 1986. The effect of respiratory therapy on intracranial pressure in ventilated neurosurgical patients. Aust. J. Physiother. 32, 107–111.

Gentleman, D., Teasdale, G., Murray, L., 1986. Cause of severe head injury and risk of complications. Br. Med. J. 292, 449.

Genuardi, F.J., King, W.D., 1995. Inappropriate discharge instructions for youth athletes hospitalised for concussion. Paediatrics 95, 216–218.

Giacino, J., Ashwal, S., Childs, N., Cranford, R., Jennet, B., Katz, D.I., et al., 2002. The minimally conscious state: definition and diagnostic criteria. Neurology 58, 349–353.

Gill-Body, K.M., Giorgetti, M.M., 1995. Acute care and prognostic outcome. In: Montgomery, J. (Ed.), Physical Therapy for Traumatic Brain Injury. Churchill Livingstone, New York, pp. 1–31.

Gill-Thwaites, H., 1997. The Sensory Modality Assessment Rehabilitation Technique – a tool for assessment and treatment of patients with severe brain injury in a vegetative state. Brain Inj. 11, 723–734.

Gronwall, D., Wrightson, P., 1980. Duration of post-traumatic amnesia after mild head injury. J. Clin. Neuropsychol. 2, 51–60.

Hellawell, D., Taylor, R., Pentland, B., 1999. Persisting symptoms and carers' views of outcome after subarachnoid haemorrhage. Clin. Rehabil. 13, 333–340.

Hellweg, S., Johannes, S., 2008. Physiotherapy after traumatic brain injury: a systematic review of the literature. Brain Inj. 22, 365–373.

Hernandez, T.D., Naritoku, D.K., 1997. Seizures, epilepsy, and functional recovery after traumatic brain injury: a reappraisal. Neurology 48, 803–806.

Hillier, S., Hiller, J., Metzer, J., 1997. Epidemiology of traumatic brain injury in South Australia. Brain Inj. 11, 649–659.

Horn, L.J., Garland, D.E., 1990. Medical and Orthopedic Complications Associated with Traumatic Brain Injury. In: Rosenthal, M., Griffith, E.R., Bond, M.R., Miller, J.D. (Eds.), Rehabilitation of the Adult and Child with Traumatic Brain Injury. F A Davis, Philadelphia, pp. 107–126.

House of Commons, 2001. Select Committe on Health 3rd Report: Head Injury Rehabilitation. Parliamentary Publications, London.

Hurvitz, E.A., Mandac, B.R., Davidoff, G., Johnson, J.H., Nelson, V.S., 1992. Risk factors for heterotopic ossification in children and adolescents with severe traumatic brain injury. Arch. Phys. Med. Rehabil. 73, 459–462.

Ikawa, F., Ohbayashi, N., Imada, Y., Matsushige, T., Kajihara, Y., Inagawa, T., et al., 2004. Analysis of subarachnoid haemorrhage according to the Japanese Standard Stroke Registry Study – incidence, outcome, and comparison with the International Subarachnoid Aneurysm Trial. Neurol. Med. Chir. (Tokyo) 44, 275–276.

Jackson, H.F., Davies, M., 1995. A transdisciplinary approach to brain injury rehabilitation. British Journal of Therapy and Rehabilitation 2, 65–70.

Jennett, B., 1990. Post-traumatic Epilepsy. In: Rosenthal, M., Griffith, E.R., Bond, M.R., Miller, J.D. (Eds.), Rehabilitation of the Adult and Child with Traumatic Brain Injury. F A Davis, Philadelphia, pp. 89–93.

Jennett, B., 1996. Epidemiology of head injury. J. Neurol. Neurosurg. Psychiatry 60, 362–369.

Jennet, B., Lindsay, K.W., 1994a. Complications after head injury. In: Jennet, B., Lindsay, K.W. (Eds.), An Introduction to Neurosurgery. Butterworth-Heinemann, Oxford, pp. 211–235.

Jennet, B., Lindsay, K.W., 1994b. Surgery for vascular lesions. In: Jennet, B., Lindsay, K.W. (Eds.), An Introduction to Neurosurgery. Butterworth-Heinemann, Oxford, pp. 142–171.

Jennett, B., MacMillan, R., 1981. Epidemiology of head injury. Br. Med. J. 282, 101–104.

Jennet, B., Plum, F., 1972. Persistent vegetative state after brain damage: a syndrome in search of a name. Lancet 1, 734–737.

Jennet, B., Teasdale, G., 1977. Aspects of coma after severe head injury. Lancet I, 878–881.

Jennet, B., Teasdale, G., 1981. Structural pathology. In: Jennett, B., Teasdale, G. (Eds.), Management of Head Injuries, vol. 20. F A Davis, Philadelphia, pp. 19–43.

Johnson, R.T., 1998. Meningitis, encephalitis and poliomyelitis. In: Johnson, R.T. (Ed.), Viral Infections of the Nervous System. Lippincott-Raven, Philadelphia, pp. 87–132.

Jorge, R.E., Starkstein, S.E., Arndt, S., Moser, D., Crespo-Facorro, B., Robinson, R., 2005. Alcohol Misuse and Mood Disorders Following Traumatic Brain Injury. Arch. Gen. Psychiatry 62, 742–749.

Kelly, D.F., 1995. Alcohol and head injury: an issue revisited. J. Neurotrauma. 12, 883–890.

King, N.S., Crawford, S., Wenden, F.J., Moss, N.E.G., Wade, D.T., 1997. Interventions and service need following mild and moderate head injury: The Oxford Head Injury Service. Clin. Rehabil. 11, 13–27.

Kraus, J., Sorenson, S., 1994. Epidemiology. In: Silver, J., Yudofsky, S., Hales, R. (Eds.), Neuropsychiatry of Traumatic Brain Injury. American Psychiatric Press, Washington, pp. 3–41.

Kraus, J.F., McArthur, D.L., 1996. Epidemiological Aspects of Brain Injury. Neurol. Clin. 14, 435–450.

Kroll, J.S., Moxon, E.R., 1987. Acute bacterial meningitis. In: Kennedy, P.G.E., Johnson, R.T. (Eds.), Infections of the nervous system. Butterworth, London, pp. 3–22.

Lange, R.T., Iverson, G.L., Franzen, M.D., 2008. Effects of day-of-injury alcohol intoxication on neuropsychological outcome in the acute recovery period following traumatic brain injury. Arch. Clin. Neuropsychol. 23, 809–822.

Leblanc, K.E., 1995. Concussion in sports: guidelines for return to competition. Am. Fam. Physician. 50, 801–808.

Leclerc, S., Shrier, I., Johnston, K., 2009. Pashby Sports Safety Concussion Site. [Web page]. Available: http://www.Thinkfirst.Ca/Downloads/Concussion/Drtompashbysportssafetyconcussionsite.Pdf (accessed 23.03.2009).

Levin, H., O'Donnell, V., Grossman, R., 1979. The Galveston Orientation and Amnesia Test: a practical scale to assess cognition after head injury. J. Nerv. Ment. Dis. 167, 675–684.

Lindsay, K.W., Bone, I., 2004. Neurology and neurosurgery illustrated. Churchill Livingston, New York.

Marwitz, J.H., Cifu, D.X., Englander, J., High, W.M., 2001. A Multi-Centre Analysis of Rehospitalizations Five Years After Brain Injury. J. Head Trauma Rehabil. 16, 307–317.

Mazaux, J.M., Richer, R., 1998. Rehabilitation after traumatic brain injury in adults. Disabil. Rehabil. 20, 435–447.

McCrory, P., Johnston, K., Meeuwisse, W., et al., 2005. Summary and agreement statement of the 2nd International Conference on Concussion in Sport, Prague 2004. Clinical Journal of Sports Medicine 15, 48–55.

McDermott, F.T., 1995. Bicyclist head injury prevention by helmets and mandatory wearing legislation in Victoria, Australia. Ann. R. Coll. Surg. Engl. 77, 38–44.

McMillan, T., Greenwood, R., 1993. Models of rehabilitation programmes for the brain-injured adult. II: model services and suggestions for change in the UK. Clin. Rehabil. 7, 346–355.

McMillan, T., Jongen, E., Greenwood, R., 1996. Assessment of post-traumatic amnesia after severe closed head injury: retrospective or prospective? J. Neurol. Neurosurg. Psychiatry 60, 422–427.

Miller, J., Jones, P., 1990. Minor Head Injury. In: Rosenthal, M., Griffith, E., Bond, M., Miller, J. (Eds.), Rehabilitation of the Adult and Child with Traumatic Brain Injury. F A Davis, Philadelphia, pp. 236–247.

Mitchell, P., Hope, T., Gregson, B.A., Mendelow, A.D., 2004. Regional differences in outcome from subarachnoid haemorrhage: comparative audit. Br. Med. J. 328, 1234–1235.

Moseley, A., 2002. Physical Management and Rehabilitation of Patients with Traumatic Head Injury (2). In: Partridge, C.J. (Ed.), Bases of evidence for practice: neurological physiotherapy. Whurr, London, pp. 92–106.

Multi-Society Task Force, 1994. Medical aspects of the persistent vegetative state. N. Engl. J. Med. 330, 1499–1508.

Narayan, R.K., Gokaslan, Z.L., Bontke, C.F., Berrol, S., 1990. Neurologic Sequelae of Head Injury. In: Rosenthal, M., Griffith, E.R., Bond, M.R., Miller, J.D. (Eds.), Rehabilitation of the Adult and Child with Traumatic Brain Injury. F A Davis, Philadelphia, pp. 94–106.

National Institute for Health and Clinical Excellence, 2006. Improving outcomes for people with brain and other CNS tumours. Available: http://www.nice.org.uk/nicemedia/pdf/csg_brain_manual.pdf.

National Institute for Health and Clinical Excellence, 2007. Head injury: triage, assessment, investigation and early management of head injury in infants, children and adults. Available: http://www.nice.org.uk/nicemedia/pdf/CG56NICEGuideline.pdf.

New Zealand National Health Committee, 1998. Traumatic Brain Injury Rehabilitation Guidelines. .

Nolte, J., 2001a. Introduction to the nervous system. In: Nolte, J. (Ed.), The Human Brain: an introduction to its functional anatomy. Mosby, St Louis, pp. 1–36.

Nolte, J., 2001b. Meningeal coverings of the brain and spinal cord. In: Nolte, J. (Ed.), The human brain: an introduction to its functional anatomy. Mosby, St. Louis, pp. 80–98.

Oddy, M., Bonham, E., Mc Millan, T.M., Stroud, A., Rickard, S., 1989. A comprehensive service for the rehabilitation and long-term care of head injury survivors. Clin. Rehabil. 3, 253–259.

Parker, J. (Ed.), 2006. Good Practice in Brain Injury Case Management. Jessica Kingsley, London & Philadelphia.

Pickard, J.D., Czosnyka, M., 2000. Raised intracranial pressure. In: Hughes, R.A.C. (Ed.), Neurological Emergencies. BMJ Publishing Group, London, pp. 173–218.

Pile-Spellman, J., 1996. Endovascular therapeutic neuroradiology. In: Tavernas, J.M. (Ed.), Neuroradiology. Williams & Wilkins, Baltimore, pp. 1045–1179.

Pollock, B.E., 2002. Contemporary Stereotactic Neurosurgery. Futura, New York.

Ponsford, J., 1995. Working With Families. In: Ponsford, J., Sloan, S., Snow, P. (Eds.), Traumatic Brain Injury: Rehabilitation for Everyday Adaptive Living. Lawrence Erlbaum, Hove, pp. 265–294.

Pope, P.M., 2002. Postural management and special seating. In: Edwards, S. (Ed.), Neurological Physiotherapy: a problem solving approach. Churchill Livingtone, London, pp. 189–217.

Povlishock, J.T., Becker, D.M.P., Cheng, C.L.Y., et al., 1983. Axonal change in minor head injury. J. Neuropathol. Exp. Neurol. 42, 225–242.

Powell, T., Partridge, T., Nicholls, T., Wright, L., Mould, H., Cook, C., et al., 1994. An interdisciplinary approach to the rehabilitation of people with brain injury. British Journal of Therapy and Rehabilitation 1, 8–13.

Quinn, B., Sullivan, S.J., 2000. The identification by physiotherapists of the physical problems resulting from a mild traumatic brain injury. Brain Inj. 14, 1063–1076.

Roberts, S., 2002. Respiratory Management of Patient with Traumatic Head Injury. In: Partridge, C.J. (Ed.), Bases of evidence for practice: neurological physiotherapy. Whurr, London, pp. 63–76.

Romano, M.D., 1974. Family response to traumatic head injury. Scand. J. Rehabil. Med. 6, 1–4.

Rosenbaum, M., Najenson, T., 1976. Changes in life patterns and symptoms of low mood as reported by wives of severely brain injured soldiers. J. Consult. Clin. Psychol. 44, 881–888.

Rosner, M.J., Colley, I.B., 1986. Cerebral perfusion pressure, intracranial pressure and head elevation. J. Neurosurg. 65, 636–641.

Rusk, H.A., Block, J.M., Loman, E.W., 1969. Rehabilitation following traumatic brain damage. Med. Clin. North Am. 52, 677–684.

Rusk, H.A., Loman, E.W., Block, J.M., 1966. Rehabilitation of the patient with head injury. Clin. Neurosurg. 12, 312–323.

Russell, W., 1932. Cerebral involvement in head injury. Brain 55, 549–603.

Scottish Intercollegiate Guideline Network, 2009. Early Management of Patients with a Head Injury (110). Scottish Intercollegiate Guideline Network. May.

Shafi, S., Diaz-Arrastia, R., Madden, C., Gentilello, L., 2008. Intracranial pressure monitoring in brain-injured patients is associated with worsening survival. J. Trauma 64, 335–340.

Sheil, A., Horn, S.A., Wilson, B., Watson, M.J., Campbell, M.J., McLellan, D.L., 2000. The Wessex Head Injury Matrix (WHIM) main scale: a preliminary report on a scale to assess and monitor patient recovery after severe head injury. Clin. Rehabil. 14, 408–416.

Smith, M., 2008. Monitoring intracranial pressure in traumatic brain injury. Anesth. Anal. 106, 240–248.

Sorenson, S.B., Kraus, J.F., 1991. Occurrence, severity, and outcomes of brain injury. J. Head Trauma Rehabil. 6, 1–10.

Sprogoe-Jakobsen, S., Falk, E., 1990. Fatal thrombosis of the basilar artery due to minor head injury. Forensic Sci. Int. 45, 239–245.

Stegmayr, B., Eriksson, M., Asplund, K., 2004. Declining mortality from subarachnoid haemorrhage: changes in incidence and case fatality from 1985 through 2000. Stroke 35, 2059–2063.

Stein, J., 1995. The posterior parietal cortex, the cerebellum and the visual guidance of movement. In: Cody, F.W.J. (Ed.), Neural Control of Skilled Human Movement. Portland Press, Chichester, pp. 31–49.

Tate, R.L., Pfaff, A., Jurjevic, L., 2000. Resolution of disorientation and amnesia during post-traumatic amnesia. J. Neurol. Neurosurg. Psychiatry 68, 178–185.

Tavernas, J.M., 1996. Angiography. In: Tavernas, J.M. (Ed.), Neuroradiology. Williams & Wilkins, Baltimore, pp. 909–1043.

Taylor, S.J., Fettes, S.B., 1998. Enhanced enteral nutrition in head injury: effect on the efficacy of nutritional delivery, nitrogen balance, gastric residuals and risk of pneumonia. J. Hum. Nut. Diet. 11, 391–401.

Teasdale, G.M., Drake, C.G., Hunt, W., Kassell, N., Sano, K., Pertuiset, B., et al., 1988. A universal subaraachoid hemorrhage scale: report of a committee of the World Federation of Neurosurgical Societies. J. Neurol. Neurosurg. Psychiatry 51 (11), 1457.

Teasdale, G., Jennett, B., 1974. Assessment of coma and impaired consciousness: a practical scale. Lancet 2, 81–84.

Teasdale, G., Jennett, B., 1976. Assessment and prognosis of coma after head injury. Acta Neurochir. (Wien) 34, 45–55.

Tennant, A., 2005. Admission to hospital following head injury in England: Incidence and socio-economic associations. Biomed Central, BMC Public Health 5, 1–8.

Thomas, D.G.T. (Ed.), 1990. Neuro-oncology:Primary Malignant Brain Tumours. Edward Arnold, London.

Thompson, R.S., Rivara, F.P., Thompson, D.C., 1989. A case control study of the effectiveness of bicycle safety helmets. N. Engl. J. Med. 32, 1361–1367.

Tresch, D.D., Farrol, H.S., Duthie, E.H., et al., 1991. Clinical characteristics of patients in the persistent vegetative state. Arch. Intern. Med. 151, 930–932.

Turnbull, A.P., Turnbull, H.R., 1991. Understanding families from a systems perspective. In: Williams, J.M., Kay, T. (Eds.), Head Injury : A Family Matter. Paul H Brooks, Baltimore, pp. 37–63.

Vickery, C.D., Sherer, M., Nick, T.G., Nakase-Richardson, R., Corrigan, J.D., Hammond, F., et al., 2008. Relationships among premorbid alcohol use, acute intoxication, and early functional status after traumatic brain injury. Arch. Phys. Med. Rehabil. 89, 48–55.

Watson, M., 1997. Evidence for 'significant' late stage motor recovery in patients with severe traumatic brain injury: a literature review with relevance to neurological physiotherapy. Phys. Ther. Rev. 2, 93–106.

Winqvist, S., Luukinen, H., Jokelainen, J., Lehtilahti, M., Näyhä, S., Hillbom, M., 2008. Recurrent traumatic brain injury is predicted by the index injury occurring under the influence of alcohol. Brain Inj. 22 (10), 780–785.

Wood, R.L., 1991. Critical analysis of the concept of sensory stimulation for patients in vegetative states. Brain Inj. 5, 401–409.

Yokota, H., Kurokawa, A., Otsuka, T., et al., 1991. Significance of magnetic resonance imaging in acute head injury. J. Trauma 31, 351–357.

Chapter | 4 |

Spinal cord injury

Sue Paddison, Frederick Middleton

CONTENTS

INTRODUCTION

Traumatic spinal cord injury (SCI) is a life-transforming condition of sudden onset that can have devastating consequences. Clinical management involves the acute phase, rehabilitation to restore potential and subsequent interventions to restore function. The objectives of management are to produce a healthy person who can choose his or her own destiny.

Current research gives rise to the hope that in the near future clinicians will be actively intervening in an attempt to alter and augment natural recovery. As this comes to fruition, functional outcomes and quality of life for SCI patients should improve.

INCIDENCE AND AETIOLOGY

Data detailed are taken from the summary in De Vivo (2007). The ratio of male to female cases is approximately 3:1, with greater male preponderance in young age groups. Spinal cord damage can be traumatic or non-traumatic. The main causes of traumatic injury are shown in Figure 4.1. Gunshots and stabbings also make small but increasing contributions (Harrison, 2000; Whalley Hammell, 1995). A significant number of patients with mental health problems will sustain injury from jumping from a height. The level of injury at the time of discharge from hospital is illustrated in Figure 4.2.

The American Spinal Injury Association (ASIA) has produced a classification system for SCI, which is explained below and the classification of injury at discharge is also detailed below (see 'Diagnosis').

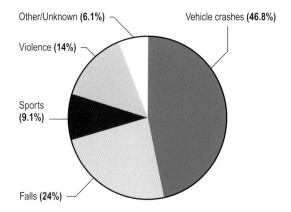

Figure 4.1 Causes of traumatic spinal cord injury. The percentages illustrated were obtained from the references cited in the text.

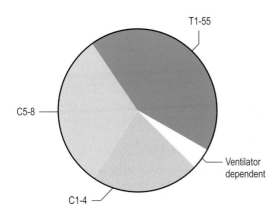

Figure 4.2 Spinal cord injury level at discharge from hospital. C, cervical; T, thoracic.

Non-traumatic aetiology is more common than traumatic. Reported incidence of nontraumatic SCI varies depending on which conditions are included in the study population. Non-traumatic most commonly result from degenerative disc disease and spinal canal stenosis, developmental anomalies (e.g. spina bifida) and congenital anomalies (e.g. angiomatous malformations); inflammation (e.g. multiple sclerosis); ischaemia (e.g. cord stroke); pressure on the cord due to expanding lesions (e.g. abcess or tumour extrinsic or intrinsic to the spinal cord) (New & Sundrajan, 2008). Each condition has distinct management needs and features. Their management will benefit from the knowledge and skills derived from an understanding of traumatic SCI, which is the focus of this chapter.

TERMINOLOGY

Terms used to describe these patients indicate the general level of the spinal injury listing body functions and structure and a list of domains of activity and participation (*International Classification of Functioning, Disability and Health*; World Health Organization, 2001).

Paraplegia

Paraplegia refers to the impairment or loss of motor, sensory and/or autonomic function in thoracic, lumbar or sacral segments of the spinal cord. Upper-limb function is spared but the trunk, legs and pelvic organs may be involved.

Tetraplegia

Tetraplegic patients have impairment or loss of motor, sensory and/or autonomic function in cervical segments of the spinal cord. The upper-limbs are affected as well

as the trunk, legs and pelvic organs. In high cervical injuries the function of respiration will be affected. The term does not include the brachial plexus or injury to peripheral nerves. 'Quadraparesis' and 'paraparesis' were terms used previously to describe incomplete lesions and are now discouraged.

TYPES OF SPINAL CORD INJURY

SCI damages a complex neural network involved in transmitting, modifying and coordinating motor, sensory and autonomic control of organ systems. This dysfunction of the spinal cord causes variable loss of homeostatic and adaptive mechanisms which keep people naturally healthy. Any damage to the spinal cord results in deficits that can only be partly predicted, as described below. The pathology of the cord will influence the presenting impairment and the resulting prognosis. It can be precisely correlated with the neurological picture because of the segmental nature of the spinal cord (Kakulas, 2004). Complete transection of the cord is uncommon. It is useful to note that whilst the incidence of SCI in the population as a whole has largely remained the same, the overall prevelence is increasing. There are an increasing number of older people with SCI, reflecting the increasing ageing of the general population, in addition there are more people surviving with SCI into old age (Box 4.1 & Box 4.2).

Over the years there has been a significant reduction in mortality and preservation of neurology in new lesions (Grundy & Swain, 2002; Whalley Hammell, 1995). There are many reasons accounting for this, including:

* changes in vehicle design and usage, as well as greater public knowledge and awareness of the dangers of moving an injured person

---

Box 4.1 Trends

* Increasing age at time of incidence onset
* Increasing survival of those with high tetraplegia
* Falls increasing as a percentage of the overall aetiology due to the increase in ageing population

---

Box 4.2 Basic facts and figures

* Mean age 37 years
* 13% over 60 years old
* Small increase in percentage of females over last 10 years

(Data from De Vivo, 2007.)

- improved medical interventions: broad-spectrum antibiotics, neuroprotective agents and advances in respiratory care
- better paramedical retrieval: improved accident and emergency resuscitation procedures and medical interventions to maintain blood pressure and oxygenation.

A previous trend towards increasing incomplete lesions has now lessened. Recent incidence at time of injury has moved closer to equal numbers of incomplete and complete lesions. It is suggested that people with the more serious injuries are surviving, including a higher number of long-term ventilator-dependant patients. It is thought that the accumulative benefits of improved advanced life support and early interventions have now become fully established. It appears that there are no further influences currently increasing the trend towards an incomplete presentation, although the outcomes of new early restorative interventions will be eagerly awaited. There is a significant trend in the reduction in length of stay in the American Model Managed Care Systems, which also reflects a lower Functional Independence Measure (FIM) score at time of discharge and an increase in complications during the first year post discharge (De Vivo, 2007).

PATHOGENESIS

A brief outline of the pathological changes that occur with SCI is now given; further details can be found in other texts such as Tator (1998).

Immediate/primary damage

Most traumatic injuries involve contusion or tearing of the underlying cord by displaced bony fragments, disc or ligaments. This results primarily in loss of axons due to damage of the white matter.

Secondary damage

Secondary damage, particularly loss of cells in the grey matter, results from a secondary process comprising changes in the cell membrane permeability, leakage of cell contents, release of chemical factors and arrival of blood cells and agents involved in the response to injury and subsequent repair. This process leads to swelling and increasing cord pressure, affecting the venous and arterial supply, and results in ischaemia, lack of necessary proteins and failure to remove the debris of injury.

Later problems

After some weeks, there is evidence of astroglial scarring with cyst formation producing distorted neural architecture. In some cases, months or years later, a syrinx, an expanding cavity within the spinal cord probably associated with disordered cerebrospinal fluid (CSF) flow, may extend rostrally to produce further spinal cord damage. This posttraumatic syringomyelia may require drainage by shunt to prevent further extension. In view of this possibility, the neurological status should be reassessed periodically (Illis, 1988) and appropriate magnetic resonance imaging (MRI) scanning performed at intervals to minimize further neurological loss.

Spinal cord plasticity

When peripheral nerve is damaged, repair can lead to significant return of function (Battiston et al., 2009; Dahlin, 2008). It has been demonstrated that the central nervous system (CNS) has the capacity to regenerate and recover. It has similarly been hypothesized that there is capacity within the spinal cord to regenerate through a number of mechanisms. Research is ongoing to identify axonal budding, unmasking and interspinal spinal circuits (central pattern generators). For further reading on neuroplasticity see Chapter 11, Adkins et al. (2006), Kleim (2009), and Schwartz and Begley (2003). A summary of research aiming to establish new treatments in the management of spinal cord damage is discussed briefly below.

Treatment approaches in immediate post-injury management

There are four main approaches currently being considered to develop treatments for SCI (Ronsyn et al., 2008):

1. Cell and tissue culture and transplantation, which includes adult and embryonic stem cells, schwann cells and olfactory ensheathing cells
2. Production and provision of nerve growth stimulating factors
3. Elimination of blocking factors which inhibit neuroregeneration
4. Techniques aimed at modifying the inflammatory response, minimizing neuronal death and scar formation.

Understanding axonal guidance systems that will be required for directed outgrowth and functional reconnection will be essential if useful functional activity is to be regained. Although much progress has been made in the laboratory setting, no techniques applied to humans, despite having been through well researched trials (Fawcett et al., 2007; Lammertse et al., 2007; Steeves et al., 2007; Tuszynski et al., 2007) have yet to emerge showing any consistent results (Johnston, 2001; Ramer et al., 2000; Ronsyn et al., 2008; Tator, 1998). Claims for successful regeneration of the chronically injured spinal cord through late repair, remain contentious. Most studies lack robust pre- and post-intervention measures with many appearing to rely on associated intensive rehabilitation to demonstrate small functional improvements.

DIAGNOSIS

Incomplete versus complete injury classification

It is important to clarify these terms, depending on the context in which they are used. From a therapeutic point of view, a patient can be called functionally incomplete when he or she presents with some motor or sensory sparing below the level of the cord lesion. The therapist should acknowledge such sparing as potential activity, which may offer important functional benefits to the patient.

ASIA Impairment Scale

In terms of diagnosis and prognosis, the classification of SCI has important ramifications. The ASIA Impairment Scale (ASIA, 2008) is the latest updated criteria for assessing and classifying functional levels of SCI, including the definitions of complete and incomplete lesions. The assessment is completed with the patient in supine, to enable testing in the acutely unstable injured person. The assessment comprises of 10 key myotomes and 28

dermatomes (Figure 4.3). Each dermatome is tested for light touch and pin prick sensation. The full description for these classifications will not be detailed here and it is available at www.asia-spinalinjury.org, with the impairment scale and classification outlined in Figure 4.4.

The ASIA system defines that a patient can have neurological sparing below the injury level, but in the absence of the sacral sparing, this is classified as a complete lesion, ASIA A, with zones of partial preservation. Where there is sensory preservation of S4–S5, the patient is classified sensory incomplete, ASIA B. This implies the preservation of the long tracts through the lesion. The classification of incomplete versus complete lesions indicates the presence of sensation in the lower sacral segments S4-S5, which implies significant prognostic indication of potential for neurological improvement. To be classified ASIA C, the patient must be assessed to have preserved S4-S5 sensation and voluntary anal sphincter motor activity. If the voluntary anal activity is absent then there must be preservation of motor function in some muscles innervated more than three levels below the motor classification level. In addition, more than half the key muscles below the neurological level must be grade 1-2/5. Similarly if half the key muscles are grade 3-5/5 then the classification

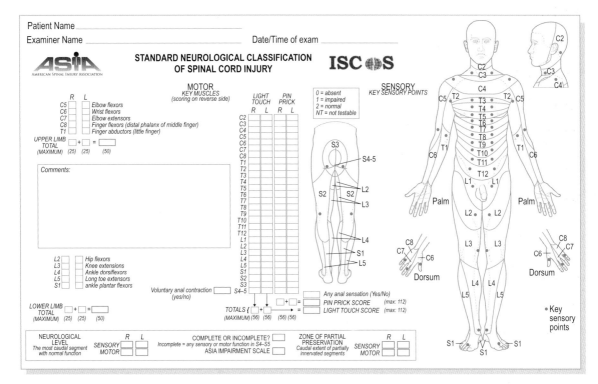

Figure 4.3 The American Spinal Injury Association (ASIA) Dermatome Chart and Impairment Scale. (American Spinal Injury Association: International Standards for Neurological Classification of Spinal Cord Injury, reprint 2008; Chicage, Il. Reprinted with permission.)

Muscle Grading	Asia Impairment Scale	Steps in Classification

Muscle Grading

0   Total paralysis

1   Palpable or visible contraction

2   Active movement, full range of motion, gravity eliminated

3   Active movement, full range of motion, against gravity

4   Active movement, full range of motion, against gravity and provides some resistance

5   Active movement, full range of motion, against gravity and provides normal resistance

5* Muscle able to exert, in examiner's judgement, sufficient resistance to be considered normal if identifiable inhibiting factors were not present

NT not testable. Patient unable to reliably exert effort or muscle unavailable for testing due to factors such as immobilization, pain on effort or contracture

Asia Impairment Scale

☐ A = **Complete:** No motor or sensory function is preserved in the sacral segments S4-S5

☐ B = **Incomplete:** Sensory but not motor function is preserved below the neurological level and includes the sacral segments S4-S5

☐ C = **Incomplete:** Motor function is preserved below the neurological level, and more than half of key muscles below the neurological level have a muscle grade less than 3

☐ D = **Incomplete:** Motor function is preserved below the neurological level, and at least half of key muscles below the neurological level have a muscle grade of 3 or more

☐ E = **Normal:** Motor and sensory function are normal

Clinical syndromes (optional)

☐ Central Cord
☐ Brown-Sequard
☐ Anterior Cord
☐ Conus Medullaris
☐ Cauda Equina

Steps in Classification

The following order is recommended in determining the classification of individuals with SCI

1   Determine sensory levels for right and left sides

2   Determine motor levels for right and left sides
    Note: in regions where there is no myotome to test, the motor level is presumed to be the same as the sensory level

3   Determine the single neurological level
    This is the lowest segment where motor and sensory function is normal on both sides, and is the most cephalad of the sensory and motor levels determined in steps 1 and 2

4   Determine whether the injury is Complete or Incomplete (sacral sparing)
    *If voluntary anal contraction = **No** AND all S4-5 sensory scores = **0** AND and any anal sensation = **No**, then injury is COMPLETE. Otherwise injury is incomplete*

5   Determine ASIA Impairment Scale (AIS) Grade:

If **Yes**, AIS=A Record ZPP (For ZPP record lowest dermatome or myotome on each side with some (non-zero score) preservation)

Is injury complete? → No

If **No**, AIS=B (Yes=voluntary anal contraction OR motor function more than three levels below the motor level on a given side)

Is Injury motor incomplete? → Yes

Are at least half of the key muscles below the (single) neurological level graded 3 or better?

No → AIS=C   Yes → AIS=D

If sensation and motor function is normal in all segments, **AIS=E.** *Note: AIS E is used in follow up testing when an individual with a documented SCI has recovered normal function. If at initial testing no deficits are found, the individual is neurologically intact; the ASIA Impairment Scale does not apply*

Figure 4.4 ASIA classification guide. (American Spinal Injury Association: International Standards for Neurological Classification of Spinal Cord Injury, reprint 2008; Chicage, Il. Reprinted with permission.)

will be ASIA D. The classification of SCI on discharge from hospital is shown in Figure 4.5.

From a prognostic point of view, research suggests that 72 hours post injury (Brown, 1994; Maynard et al., 1979), and 1 month post injury are good time points for this classification (Waters et al., 1994a, 1994b). Further assessment is advised at 3 months post injury. All patients are assessed immediately on hospital admission, to gain baseline data. The wealth of prognostic statistics is based on data obtained using these time periods.

Incomplete lesions and prognostic indicators

There are recognized patterns of incomplete cord injury which tend to present clinically as combinations of syndromes rather than in isolation. The signs and symptoms are related to the anatomical areas of the cord affected (Figures 4.6 & 4.7). Clinically, patterns of incomplete lesions are referred to as a syndrome.

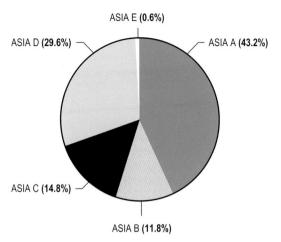

Figure 4.5 American Spinal Injury Association (ASIA) classification at discharge from hospital. (American Spinal Injury Association: International Standards for Neurological Classification of Spinal Cord Injury, reprint 2008; Chicage, Il. Reprinted with permission.)

Recent statistics show the common patterns of incomplete lesions to be the following:

- Central cord syndrome (44%)
- Cauda equina (25%)
- Brown–Séquard syndrome (17%)
- Anterior cord syndrome around 10%
- Pure posterior cord syndrome being very rare

(McKinley et al., 2007).

Anterior cord syndrome

Anterior cord syndrome describes the effects of ventral cord damage affecting spinothalamic and corticospinal tracts; there is complete motor loss caudal to the lesion, and loss of pain and temperature sensation as these sensory tracts are located anterolaterally in the spinal cord. Preservation of the posterior columns means that perception of vibration and proprioception on the ipsilateral side are intact. This syndrome can arise from anterior spinal artery embolization. Motor recovery is thought to be less in these patients in comparison with other incomplete lesions (Crozier et al, 1991; Foo, 1986).

Brown–Séquard syndrome

Originally described by Galen, this syndrome describes sagittal hemicord damage with ipsilateral (same side) paralysis and dorsal column interruption, leading to loss of proprioception, in addition to contralateral (opposite side) loss of temperature and pain sensation. The relatively normal pain and temperature sensation on the ipsilateral side is due to the spinothalamic tract crossing over to the opposite side of the cord, at the level they enter the cord. This hemisection injury of the cord is classically caused by stabbing. This syndrome has a favourable prognosis, with almost all patients ambulating successfully (Johnston, 2001). The theory for this is that, despite the loss of pinprick on the one side of the cord, axons in the contralateral cord may facilitate recovery (Little & Habur, 1985).

Figure 4.6 Cross-section of the spinal cord illustrating the main ascending and descending nerve tracts. The functions affected by damage to these tracts are indicated.

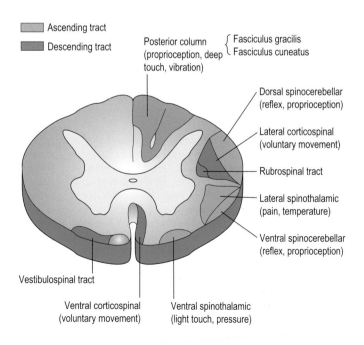

Ascending tract
Descending tract

Posterior column (proprioception, deep touch, vibration) { Fasciculus gracilis / Fasciculus cuneatus

Dorsal spinocerebellar (reflex, proprioception)

Lateral corticospinal (voluntary movement)

Rubrospinal tract

Lateral spinothalamic (pain, temperature)

Ventral spinocerebellar (reflex, proprioception)

Vestibulospinal tract

Ventral corticospinal (voluntary movement)

Ventral spinothalamic (light touch, pressure)

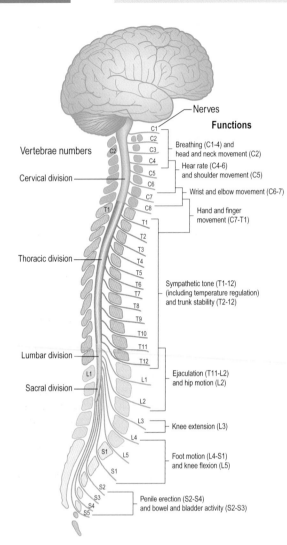

Figure 4.7 Spinal column with spinal nerve levels.

Labels within figure:
- Nerves
- Functions
- Vertebrae numbers
- Cervical division
- Thoracic division
- Lumbar division
- Sacral division
- Breathing (C1-4) and head and neck movement (C2)
- Hear rate (C4-6) and shoulder movement (C5)
- Wrist and elbow movement (C6-7)
- Hand and finger movement (C7-T1)
- Sympathetic tone (T1-12) (including temperature regulation) and trunk stability (T2-12)
- Ejaculation (T11-L2) and hip motion (L2)
- Knee extension (L3)
- Foot motion (L4-S1) and knee flexion (L5)
- Penile erection (S2-S4) and bowel and bladder activity (S2-S3)

Central cord lesion

The upper-limbs are more profoundly affected than the lower limbs and the condition is typically seen in older patients with cervical spondylosis. Due to degenerative changes in the spinal column, there are osteophytes and possible disc bulges, combined with spondylitic joint changes in the anterior part of the vertebral column. Posteriorly, the ligamentum flavum is thickened. A hyperextension injury compresses the cord in the narrowed canal and leads to interference of the blood supply. This may be already compromised in an older person and so has less potential for recovery. The central cervical tracts are predominantly affected. There is often flaccid weakness of the arms, due to lower motor neurone (LMN) lesions, and spastic patterning in the arms and legs due

to upper motor neurone (UMN) injury. Bowel and bladder dysfunctions are common, but only partial. Research findings vary, showing that 57–86% patients will ambulate, although 97% of younger patients less than 50 years ambulate compared with 41% over 50 years (Foo, 1986).

Conus medullaris

Conus medullaris presents as either UMN or LMN lesions, with or without the sacral reflexes (anal/bulbocavernus), depending on the injury. There may be avulsion of the lumbar or sacral roots from the terminal part of the cord. Bladder and bowel dysfunctions occur with variable symmetrical lower-limb defects.

Cauda equina lesion

This produces flaccid paralysis as there is peripheral nerve damage at this level of the spine, usually affecting several levels with variable sacral root interruption.

Posterior cord lesion

This rare condition produces damage to the dorsal columns (sensation of light touch, proprioception and vibration) with preservation of motor function and pain and temperature pathways. However, the patient presents with profound ataxia due to loss of proprioception.

PROGNOSIS

Recovery of the incomplete spinal cord injury

It is essential to refer to the evidence of ongoing recovery in SCI and to bear this in mind when treating these patients. Recovery will be at the forefront of a patient's mind when participating in rehabilitation.

Ninety per cent of incomplete SCI patients have some recovery of a motor level in their upper-limbs, compared to 70–85% of the complete injuries (Ditunno et al., 2000). Pinprick sparing in a dermatome is an excellent indicator of increased recovery of motor strength (Poynton et al., 1997) and it has been found that pinprick preservation below the level of the injury to the sacral dermatomes is the best indicator of useful recovery, with 75% of patients regaining the ability to walk. Fifty per cent of patients who had no sacral sparing regained some motor recovery but not of functional use (Katoh & El Masry, 1995).

Studies have found that incomplete SCI patients showed ongoing improvement in their motor activity, although this tended to slow during the second year post injury, with the exception of incomplete tetraplegics who lacked sharp/blunt discrimination and failed to demonstrate any lower-limb motor recovery. In incomplete paraplegics, there was evidence of 85% of the muscles recovering from a flicker to an antigravity grade within the first year, but if there was no activity initially, only 26% gained an antigravity grade (Waters et al., 1994a, 1994b).

It is widely accepted that incomplete SCI patients will only make useful recovery within the first 2 years post injury, but from the authors' experiential observation, recovery can continue to occur slowly for at least 5 years or more, particularly in incomplete tetraplegics.

Ambulation recovery

Between 44 and 76% of people with incomplete SCI, with preserved sensation but no motor function, have been reported to achieve ambulation (Maynard et al., 1979; Waters et al., 1994a, 1994b).

Crozier et al. (1991) reported, using ASIA assessment at 72 hours, that 89% of ASIA B–E patients with pinprick preservation went on to ambulate, compared with 11% having preserved light touch but not pinprick.

- The theory behind the significance of sacral preservation is the proximity of the spinothalamic tracts that mediate pinprick to the lateral corticospinal tracts and their shared blood supply. At 1 year post injury, 76% incomplete paraplegics (ASIA B–E) become community ambulators by 2 years, compared to 46% of incomplete tetraplegics who ambulate, probably due to upper-extremity weakness compromising the ability to perform gait (Waters et al., 1994a, 1994b). Age is a significant factor in indication of outcome (Burns & Ditunno, 2001; Ditunno et al., 1994).

Summary of changes in ASIA impairment scale from admission to discharge

- From the number of patients assessed at the time of injury found to be classified as an ASIA A, 8.5 /10 remain ASIA A at time of discharge.
- From the same ASIA A group, only 2 /100 go on to become a functional ASIA D.
- From the group of ASIA B patients, 40 /100 become ASIA C.
- From the group of ASIA C patients, more than 60 /100 become grade D.
- From the group of ASIA B patients, 20 /100 remain grade B but 1 in 5 become grade D at time of discharge

(De Vivo, 2007).

ACUTE GENERAL MANAGEMENT

Although the primary damage is to the spinal cord, every organ system can be affected. Antecedent and posttraumatic psychological and social conditions must also be given full consideration as they play their inevitable parts in the success or failure of rehabilitation. Acute and rehabilitation specialties and disciplines are necessary to provide a holistic approach, in which all team members work towards common goals, agreed between the patient and team.

Trauma management

SCI presentation remains a key issue for all professionals, who should be vigilant about the risks of activities in which they may be involved, such as on rugby fields or at swimming pools.

Immediate management

When an accident occurs involving a SCI, other injuries should be suspected and the incident history recorded; pain, bruising and/or palpable spinal deformity are likely features. This is a crucial time for appropriate management to ensure the best chances possible for survival of the spinal cord fibres.

Proper handling will avoid unnecessary further damage, and the following simple advice can be immensely valuable:

- The patient should be advised not to move.
- The airway and breathing should be checked.
- If removal to another site is necessary, the transfer should be gentle, avoiding any twisting. Lifting should be performed by at least four people, with one acting as leader to coordinate the team.
- The patient should be placed in a supine position with the head and body kept strictly in alignment.
- If unconscious, the patient should be strapped to, and supported on, a board to allow tilt and avoid aspiration.
- Normal spinal curvature should be supported by a rolled-up cloth.
- The skin should be protected from pressure and ulceration by removing objects from pockets or by removing clothes.
- Point pressure from heels on hard surfaces, or 'knocking knees', should be avoided.
- Various spinal immobilization boards, e.g. the scoop stretcher, and collars are available in ambulances for moving patients.
- Maintenance of oxygenation and blood pressure is essential.
- If possible, a motor and sensory charting should be performed for a baseline neuroassessment with diagrammatic recording.

Continuity of care

It is crucially important that continuity it maintained from site of injury, immediate first aid through ambulance/ helicopter retrieval, to A&E/trauma unit, resuscitation, investigation and stabilization, with appropriate surgical/ non-surgical interventions, then onto admission to specialist continuing care.

Admission to hospital

Currently in the UK, after sustaining an SCI the person is admitted to the local A&E or trauma unit. A full physical and neurological assessment is carried out and a decision is made about referral to a specialist unit. Spinal imaging can provide reliable evidence of stability (X-ray, MRI and/or computed tomography (CT)). The decision for management (conservative or surgical) is made after the appropriate diagnostic testing.

Summary of immediate management

- Immobilization
- Advanced trauma life support
- Decompressive and stabilizing surgery if necessary
- Recent introduction of membrane-stabilizing agents and neuroprotective agents, including steroids. Naloxone and Tirilazad have been investigated. Most recently, ganglioside GM 1 has appeared to be partly helpful, but none have yet achieved the outcome hoped for (McDonald et al., 2002).

Acute hospital management

Acute trauma management guidelines are well established (Moore et al., 1991). Management of the patient with an SCI has special features resulting from spinal cord shock. Full details are described by Grundy and Swain (2002).

Breathing

Paralysis of respiratory muscles may be a feature. Patients with acute cervical cord injuries can fatigue in their breathing. Pulse oximetry is a crude indicator of respiratory distress because it measures only haemoglobin saturation and not partial pressure of oxygen (Po_2) (Hough, 2001). Any evidence of desaturation or of falling saturation should be proactively addressed by the critical care team to maintain oxygenation and prevent further cord damage. Monitoring patients' breathing rate, pattern and colour, and noting agitation, drowsiness or distressed behaviour, is vital. Arterial blood-gas analysis may be the critical factor in deciding whether to provide ventilatory support. Respiratory failure remains one of the main causes of death in acute tetraplegia, whilst pneumonia is the leading cause of death in all persons with SCI (Jackson et al., 1994). The principles of respiratory management are covered in Chapter 15.

Circulation

The sympathetic nerve supply to the heart is via cervical, cervical thoracic and upper thoracic branches of the sympathetic trunk. Cervical and upper thoracic injuries may produce sympathetic disruption, with impairment of tachycardia response. Therefore, pulse rate may mislead in the presence of circulatory shock. There is skin vasodilation within the dermatomes caudal to the injury. This causes a lowering of blood pressure. Injudicious fluid replacement to augment the blood pressure can cause pulmonary oedema. Pharyngeal suction, urethral catheterization or simply repositioning of the patient can produce vagal overstimulation and lead to bradycardia; intravenous atropine may be required to restore normal heart rate. Tetraplegic patients are unable to maintain their body temperature due to the autonomic disruption, resulting in them taking up the surrounding temperature. This is known as a poikilothermic reaction.

Spinal cord shock

This is the phenomenon of cessation of nervous system function below the level of damage to the cord and may be due to the loss of descending neural influences. It is usually expected that after several seconds to months, the flaccid paralysis and areflexia of spinal shock are replaced by hyperexcitability, seen clinically as hyperreflexia, spasticity and spasms. More recently this has been identified as a critical period when the timing of potential interventions can influence recovering neurological systems. Studies have shown that there is competetive synaptic growth into the synaptic spaces that have been vacated. These transient vacant sites become open to repopulation by spared axons. It is at this moment that interventions should ideally target synapse growth mediating voluntary movement rather than local segmental neurons mediating spasticity and hyperreflexia (Ditunno et al., 2004; McDonald et al., 2002).

Stauffer (1983) noted that it is rare to see patients in total spinal shock and totally areflexic. Strong spasticity almost immediately post injury is indicative of an incomplete SCI. In these patients assessment of voluntary movement requires careful differentiation. In the authors' experience, development of increased muscle tone and involuntary movements may mislead patients to believe they have functional return of activity. It is important for the therapist to anticipate such reactions and to assess carefully in order to avoid confusion and disappointment.

Skin care

Denervated skin is at risk from pressure damage within 20–30 minutes of injury. If this occurs, it can cause distress and delay in the rehabilitation process. Clinical staff attending should be vigilant in monitoring the skin and should report red marks.

Gastrointestinal tract

SCI can produce ileus and gastric distension that can restrict movement of the diaphragm, further compromising breathing. A nasogastric tube should be placed for decompression if bowel sounds are absent. Gastric stress ulcers can occur and prophylactic treatment with mucosal protectors is recommended.

Bladder

Spinal shock causes retention of urine; the bladder should, therefore, be catheterized routinely in order to monitor fluid output and to protect it from overdistension damage.

Spinal stabilization versus conservative management

Spinal fractures may be classified as stable, unstable or quasistable (i.e. currently stable but likely to become unstable in the course of everyday activity). Disagreement continues between protagonists and antagonists of surgical stabilization of the spine, but surgery is increasingly used (Collins, 1995).

Definition of instability or stability of a spinal lesion has now achieved substantial agreement based on the three column principles (Dennis, 1983). There is general agreement that restoration of the anatomy of the canal is sensible in terms of giving the cord the best opportunity for recovery.

It is debated whether neurological recovery or degree of spinal stability in the long term differs with surgical or conservative management. Surgery aims to minimize neurological deterioration, restore alignment and stabilization, facilitate early mobilization, reduce pain, minimize hospital stay and prevent secondary complications (Johnston, 2001). Review of evidence over the last decade does not identify any specific timing or role for early surgical decompression. Surgical intervention within the first 72 hours after injury has been shown to be safe and a role for urgent decompression has been identified in certain circumstances and may improve neurological outcomes (Fehlings & Perrin, 2006).

From a physiotherapy and psychological point of view, the ability to mobilize a patient against gravity early seems to be a desirable outcome from surgery. This can be achieved by 7–10 days after surgery and results in a shorter inpatient stay.

Management of acute lesions at T4 and above

Surgical stabilization may be achieved by anterior or posterior fixation, or a combination of the two (e.g. Collins, 1995). Patients managed conservatively are immobilized with bed rest; depending on the degree of instability, they may have to be maintained in spinal alignment by skull traction. Traction is applied usually by halo traction, Gardner–Wells or cone calipers (Grundy & Swain, 2002).

Early mobilization may be indicated and can be achieved using a halo brace (Hossain et al., 2004). Care in handling and positioning during physiotherapy is discussed below (see 'Acute physical management').

Length of immobilization will vary depending on the extent of bony injury and ligamentous instability, in addition to whether surgery has been performed. There may be several spinal segments affected and this will also influence the length of bed rest. Multiple-level fractures in the cervical spine are usually treated conservatively by halo traction and a period of immobilization in a hard collar. Bed rest is usually for 3 months. On starting mobilization, patients with all levels of injury will usually wear a collar of some type, depending on their stability.

Management of acute lesions at T4 and below

Thoracolumbar fractures are most common at the L1 level, this being the level of greatest mobility. Patients with unstable lesions at T9 and below must not have their hips flexed greater than 30° in order to avoid lumbar flexion (CSP, 1997).

Stable wedge fractures are usually treated conservatively with a brace or plaster of Paris (or similar) jacket. Unstable burst fractures, with cord compression, will justify surgical decompression and fixation. Generally, an anterior and posterior fixation technique will require a brace to be worn for 3 months postoperatively. If the spine is stable anteriorly, it may be sufficient to stabilize posteriorly. In this situation, a brace will be recommended for 6 months.

Bracing techniques vary greatly between institutions. A moulded hard plastic (subortholen) jacket can be made from an individual casting of plaster. Many braces are commercially available 'off the shelf' or other materials are used to form a brace, e.g. leather jackets.

Special problems in spinal cord injury

Osteoporosis

Osteoporosis is a loss in bone mass without any alteration of the ratio between mineral and the organic matrix. A text by (Jiang et al., 2006) provides a comprehensive overview of osteoporosis. It is thought that immobilization for long periods and a sedentary life lead to an increase in bone reabsorption, thus causing osteoporosis.

Rapid loss of bone minerals occurs during the first 4 months following SCI. A range of data available from studies include: at 1 year bone mass density reduces in the femoral neck by 27%, mid femoral shaft by 25% and distal femur by 43%. The reduction continues in the pelvis and lower limbs over the 10 years after injury and can reduce by 50%. Tetraplegics can lose up to 16% on their bone mass density in their upper limbs. The osteoporosis may cause fractures of long bones during relatively simple manoeuvres, such as transfer or passive movements (Belanger et al., 2000). The rate of incidence of fractures has been documented to be 1% in the first year post injury, 1.3% per year at 1–9 years, 3.4% per year at 10–19 years, 4.6% per year at 20–29 years (Jiang et al., 2006).

It has been shown that early mobilization with weight bearing might prevent or slow bone-mineral loss (De Bruin et al., 1999). Bone mineral density can be preserved in bones below the level of the lesion (Frey-Rindova et al., 2000). The question is frequently asked whether a patient who has not stood for several years should recommence standing. There is a variety of opinion on how to proceed, either returning straight to standing or commencing a weight-bearing programme using a tilt table, usually combined with bone-enhancing agents, and monitoring using bone densitometry, before returning to standing in a frame. Such advice is empirical and, as yet, despite many studies, no clear guidance has been produced.

Heterotopic ossification

Calcification in denervated or UMN-disordered muscle remains an ill-understood process and commonly occurs in patients with SCI (David et al., 1993). It may be confused in the early stages with deep venous thrombosis, when it presents as swelling, alteration in skin colour and increased heat, usually in relation to a joint. During the active process, analysis of plasma biochemistry shows a raised alkaline phosphatase. It can result in loss of range of movement (ROM) and difficulty in sitting. If ossification occurs around the hips it may lead to further skin pressure problems. Treatment of this condition is discussed by David et al. (1993). It must be emphasized that stretching should be gentle, as overstretching may be a predisposing factor for this condition.

The bladder

Urological complications of SCI are major mortal and morbid risks and the reader is referred to Fowler and Fowler (1993) for a review. Spinal cord damage disrupts the neural controls of bladder function. The objectives of bladder management are to provide a system ensuring safety, continence and least social disruption.

In the acute stage the bladder is catheterized to allow free drainage, to accommodate any fluid input and output fluctuations and to avoid bladder distension. Intermittent catheterization is then established. After spinal shock passes, urodynamic studies are used to identify the emergent bladder behaviour.

Anterior sacral root electrical stimulation may be used, primarily for controlling urinary voiding, but it may also facilitate defecation and penile erection separately. Reflex micturition (by tapping the abdominal wall or stroking the medial thigh) is not favoured because the bladder is unprotected from hyperreflexic complications.

The bowel

Although morbid complications rarely arise in the bowel, social embarrassment is common and often perceived by patients as more devastating than limb paralysis. Laxatives can achieve a bowel frequency within the normal range. For intractable constipation, occasional enemas can be useful. Increasing use of anterior sacral root stimulators and other surgical techniques may be beneficial. The mainstay of bowel care is to produce a predictable pattern, to minimize incontinence, impaction and interference with activities of daily living.

Fertility

Fertility is usually maintained in women, with the ovulatory cycle being normal within 9 months after injury. Fertility in men is, however, a problem (Brindley, 1984). Improvements in fertility rates for men after SCI have been made due to several important technical advances. These include improved methods in the retrieval and enhancement of sperm, such as electroejaculation, and improved means of achieving fertilization with limited sperm quality and numbers through in vitro techniques.

Autonomic dysreflexia

Autonomic dysreflexia can be described as a sympathetic nervous system dysfunction producing hypertension, bradycardia and headache with piloerection and capillary dilation and sweating, above the level of the lesion. Some or all of these can result from any noxious stimulus such as bladder or rectal distension. If it occurs, the patient should be sat up, given appropriate medication and the underlying cause treated. Patients and therapists should be aware that the hypertension can rise sufficiently to induce cerebral haemorrhage, so this should be treated as an emergency. Mild autonomic dysreflexic symptoms act as signals to patients for toileting and induction of symptoms has been used foolishly, in the authors' view, to enhance sporting performance.

ACUTE PHYSICAL MANAGEMENT

In the early post-injury phase, physical management will mainly involve prevention of respiratory and circulatory complications, and care of pressure areas. As spinal shock starts to resolve, other physical sequelae must be addressed, such as pain, weakness and hyperreflexia leading to hypertonus and contracture.

Principles of impairment assessment

Assessment must be carried out as soon after admission as possible to obtain an objective baseline measurement of function, to identify where specific problems are likely to develop and to instigate prophylactic treatment. History of the injury is taken, including the results of relevant tests, e.g. lung function. Medical history is also noted. It is important to be aware of associated injuries, as these may influence management. The principles of assessment are discussed in Chapter 1 and a physiotheray assessment database is shown in Table 4.1.

Easy mistakes in sensory assessment

When assessing sensation of a patient with a cervical lesion, sensory levels are tested down the anterior aspect of the trunk. The patient could confirm some sensation over the front of the chest above the nipple line. This has commonly been mistaken for T1-2 sensory preservation but is actually C3/4 innervation of the "bib" area by the supraclavicular nerve.

Table 4.1 Physiotherapy assessment database

Database	• Spinal fractures • Spinal level of lesion • Spinal stability • Associated injuries • Respiratory status • Spinal shock – absent reflexes
Subjective	• Pre morbid musculo-skeletal problems • PMH: relevant respiratory factors
Objective	• Respiratory status (including FVC and cough) (Hough, 2001) • Passive range of movement of all joints • Active movement • Muscle strength: standard muscle chart (MRC, 1978) (Oxford grading scale and ASIA Chart (2002)) • Tone: modified Ashworth scale (Bohannon & Smith, 1987) • Sensory especially pin prick sensation (ASIA, 2002). • Joint range • Other injuries
Commonly used measurement tools	• ASIA (2002) • FVC (Pryor & Webber, 1998) • Modified Ashworth Scale (Bohannon & Smith, 1987) • Oxford Muscle Chart (MRC, 1978)

FVC, forced vital capacity.

Treatment objectives in the acute phase

The main objectives are:

- to institute a prophylactic respiratory regimen and treat any complications
- to achieve independent respiratory status where possible
- to maintain full ROM of all joints within the limitations determined by fracture stability
- to monitor and manage neurological status as appropriate
- to maintain/strengthen all innervated muscle groups and facilitate functional patterns of activity to assist in restoration of function where possible
- to support/educate the patient, carers, family and colleagues.

Spasticity: a reminder!

Since the spinal cord is shorter than the vertebral column, lower-vertebral injuries will not involve damage to the cord, but there will be nerve root damage which will determine the presence of spasticity. The spinal cord usually extends to the first or second lumbar vertebra (Williams, 1995). Below this level, the nerve roots descend as the cauda equina and emerge from their respective vertebral levels. Injuries at these lower levels, therefore, are peripheral nerve (LMN) injuries.

A patient with a lesion at the conus or above i.e. an upper motor neuron (UMN) injury, may present with a varied amount of spasticity. Partial or total weakness occurs, but there may be preservation of muscle bulk to some extent due to the increased tone. A patient with an LMN injury, i.e. below the level of T12, will present with flaccid paralysis or weakness only. Obviously, this cut-off level of T12 is a general rule, as an individual's anatomy may vary from the usual.

Cervical injuries and potential for brachial plexus lesions

In the immediate period of patient assessment, after an admission following a SCI, it is very difficult to determine the pathology causing the resulting loss of movement. This is especially difficult in cervical lesions where there is a reasonable possibility of brachial plexus involvement. On assessment, muscles of the upper limb could be weak or flaccid and may be presumed to result from spinal shock. If the mechanism of injury or MRI scans suggest more extensive tissue damage, it would be highly advisable to assess for a LMN injury. This can be done extensively using nerve conduction studies but may be difficult to obtain in the acute/intensive therapy unit (ITU) setting. A more rapid and broad test is to apply neurotrophic electrical stimulation to the muscles innervated by the injured nerve roots. Only an intact peripheral nerve will conduct and produce a muscle contraction. Hence this is a useful diagnostic tool in determining a brachial plexus lesion. It is most important to identify such an injury at the earliest opportunity in order to facilitate a primary repair of the brachial plexus (Birch, 1993).

Respiratory management

Effect of cord injury on the respiratory system

Respiration is a complex motor activity using muscles at various levels (see below). Patients with lesions of T1 and above will lose some 40–50% of their respiratory function, but most patients with cervical injuries have an initial vital lung capacity of only 1.5 litres or less. Thus, all patients with cervical injuries should be fully evaluated for respiratory efficiency by monitoring spirometry and P_{O_2} in the initial weeks after injury. For an overview of respiratory physiology with an explanation of the tests mentioned here and normal values, the reader is referred to relevant textbooks (e.g. Hough, 2001; Smith & Ball, 1998).

Given the aetiology of SCI, many patients sustain associated injuries affecting respiration. Lung contusion or pneumo- or haemopneumothorax is common in patients with thoracic lesions, often associated with steering-wheel impact. They present at 24–48 hours post injury with deteriorating respiratory function, with a falling P_{O_2} and rising P_{CO_2}. This is a serious development and mechanical ventilation may be required, occasionally for a number of weeks.

In other patients, deterioration of respiratory function in the first days after injury may be associated with an ascending cord lesion of two to three spinal levels, due to oedema or extending hypoxia in the cord or possibly due to fatigue. This again may lead to the need for mechanical ventilation for a period and then subsequent weaning from the ventilator as cord function returns. Occasionally the higher ascended level may become the permanent level. If significant hypoxia persists, particularly with associated low blood pressure, further damage to the cord may occur. These patients do improve their respiratory capacity with respiratory training (see below).

Atelectasis is common in patients with SCI. Subsequent infection and pneumonia still account for considerable morbidity and some mortality in tetraplegics. Prophylactic tracheostomy is often advised to assist in effective clearance of secretions. High cervical injuries are prone to bronchospasm and bronchial hypersecretion due to disrupted sympathetic response. Appropriate treatment with bronchodilators in conjunction with manual techniques will be required to maintain adequate ventilation (see Ch. 15). Chest and head injuries are commonly associated with spinal injury and provide their own respiratory problems, which must also be assessed and treated appropriately (see Ch. 3).

Muscles affecting respiratory function

The abdominal muscles are essential for forced expiration and effective coughing. They also stabilize the lower ribs and assist the function of the diaphragm. The intercostal muscles have a predominantly inspiratory function as prime movers but also as fixators for the diaphragm. These muscle groups comprise about 40% of respiratory motor effort.

The diaphragm is the main inspiratory muscle but relies on other muscles to maximize efficiency. The accessory muscles (innervated by C1–C8 nerves and cranial nerve XI) include the trapezius, sternomastoid, levator scapulae and scalenii muscles; they can act as sole muscles of inspiration for short periods, but if the diaphragm is paralysed they cannot maintain prolonged adequate ventilation unassisted (see inspiratory muscle training in sections 'Acute respiratory care and management of complications' and 'Rehabilitation: ongoing respiratory management', below) (see Box 4.3).

Chest movement

The use of accessory muscles and diaphragm function can be assessed by palpation at the lower costal border. Muscle paralysis results in altered mechanics of respiration. Studies have shown chest wall compliance in tetraplegic patients can be reduced by more than 50% of the normal value (De Troyer & Estenne, 1995). In lesions involving paralysis of the abdominal and intercostal muscles, the lower ribs will be drawn in on inspiration in a paradoxical movement (Pryor & Webber, 1998). These abnormalities reduce the efficiency of the diaphragm in producing negative intrathoracic pressure, hence causing reductions in lung volume and efficiency of ventilation. On assessment any asymmetry of chest wall movement and respiratory rate is noted.

Extreme ventilatory compromise in spinal injury is caused by one or more of the complications listed in Table 4.2.

Routine auscultation

Techniques are the same as for any other patient. The assessment can be hindered by the inability to move the patient easily to assess all lung regions. Timing of the assessment should be coordinated with the patients turning routine wherever possible.

Box 4.3 **Respiratory muscles and nerve innervation**	
Accessory muscles	C1 – C8
Diaphragm	C3 – C5
Intercostal muscles	T1 – T11
Abdominal muscles	T6 – L1

Table 4.2 Spinal cord lesions and the effects on forced vital capacity

SPINAL CORD LESION	COMPLICATION	FVC % OF NORMAL
Lumbar and low thoracic	• Able to cough • Some decreased chest wall compliance	100–70%
High thoracic	• Loss of effective cough • Further decrease in chest wall compliance • Basal collapse • Atelectasis • Increased work of breathing and paradoxical chest wall movement • Reduced expansion • Autonomic dysfunction	30–50%
Low cervical	• Diaphragm plus accessory • Inspiratory and expiratory muscle paralysis leading to decreased lung volume • Respiratory muscle fatigue • Reduced chest wall mobility • Sputum retention – infection • Collapse/consolidation • Autonomic dysfunction	20%
Upper cervical	• Accessory only – ventilated	5–10%

FVC, forced vital capacity.

Forced vital capacity

The forced vital capacity (FVC) is a readily available objective measurement of respiratory muscle function, as is peak expiratory flow rate. As mentioned earlier, it is used acutely to monitor respiratory status. If the FVC is less than 1 L, the therapist may choose to instigate either intermittent positive-pressure breathing (IPPB), e.g. the Bird respirator, or bilevel intermittent positive airway pressure (BIPAP), as discussed by Hough (2001). This assisted ventilation can be used prophylactically to maintain and increase inspiratory volume and aid clearance of secretions. It is a useful adjunct to active manual techniques for patients with sputum retention and lung collapse, and can be used to administer bronchodilators (Pryor & Webber, 1998). Elective ventilation is normally undertaken if the FVC falls below 500 ml but may be considered in some patients if FVC is around 1 L, depending on other complications that can impair the active cycle of breathing.

In cases of severe pain from rib fractures and associated soft-tissue injuries, a mixture of nitrous oxide and oxygen (Entonox) may be used and, if applicable, entrained into the IPPB circuit. Trancutaneous electrical nerve stimulation (TENS) has also been found to be effective in assisting pain management (see Ch. 12).

Breathing exercises and respiratory muscle training may also include the use of IPPB and incentive spirometry in the acute phase. Evidence to support the use of these modalities is inconclusive; however, from the experience of the authors they have been found to be beneficial adjuncts to manual treatments.

Cough

A patient with a lesion above T6 will not have an effective cough as he or she will have lost the action of the abdominal muscles. The physiotherapist can compensate for this loss by the use of assisted coughing, in order that the patient can clear secretions (Bromley, 2006). The Emerson Cough Assist Insufflator-Exsufflator is used to produce a cough by introduction of positive pressure then withdrawing negative pressure via a facemask, in order to assist secretion clearance.

Precautions in treating unstable spinal cord injury

These precautions in treating unstable SCI are outlined in Box 4.4 (CSP, 1997) and are for guidance only. They are widely accepted in many centres, but the point 2 lacks clear evidence to support this guidance. In a recent informal survey there was no agreement nationally or internationally, amongst the spinal surgeons questioned, to determine whether it is necessary to hold down the

---

Box 4.4 Precautions in treating unstable spinal cord injury

1. Unstable paraplegic SCIs: T9 and below–limit hip flexion to 30° (tailor position)
2. Unstable tetraplegic SCIs: Shoulder hold for lesions at the level of T4 and above during lower limb movements and upper limb movements above 90° glenohumeral flexion and abduction
3. Severe spasms during limb movements may cause loss of spinal alignment. Recommend shoulder hold
4. Respiratory techniques should be applied bilaterally and with a shoulder hold
5. Extreme range of movement must be avoided

---

patient's shoulder (termed a shoulder hold) during some treatment techniques. There are some centres that advocate that the patient's head is stabilized and their shoulders held down onto the bed, whilst leg movements are performed and during chest physiotherapy. This stabilization is also recommended when moving the shoulders above 90°, particularly if the patient has high levels of spasticity.

Acute respiratory care and management of complications

If no other respiratory complications are present, the physiotherapist will teach prophylactic breathing exercises to encourage chest expansion and improve ventilation. Incentive spirometry is useful for patients with mid thoracic lesions and above, to give the patient and family positive feedback during breathing exercises. Care is necessary to maintain the stability of the spine. It is advised that shoulders are held for patients with unstable lesions of T4 and above when performing an assisted cough. In these circumstances, bilateral techniques should always be used in order to maintain spinal alignment. Adapted postural drainage for an unstable lesion is performed using specialized turning beds that maintain spinal alignment.

Ventilation

Assisted ventilation may be necessary. Proactive intervention before the patient becomes exhausted will make subsequent management easier. Elective intubation is potentially less damaging to the spinal cord than intubation following cardiac arrest. Respiratory therapy for the spinally injured ventilated patient is similar to that for other ventilated patients (Hough, 2001; Smith & Ball, 1998), apart from added vigilance to protect the fracture site.

Weaning from the ventilator should start as soon as the patient's condition stabilizes. It is important to avoid fatigue whilst weaning, so careful monitoring ensures that FVC does not fall by more than 20%, or respiratory rate rise above 25–30 breaths/minute. Patients who fail to wean – usually those with a greater degree of diaphragm paralysis – require long-term ventilation (see 'The long-term ventilated patient', below).

Suctioning

This should always be undertaken with care in patients with SCI and is not recommended in the cervical non-intubated patient, as the neck cannot be extended to open the airway. It is important to assist the cough when stimulating the cough reflex, as merely stimulating the reflex will not produce an effective cough.

In patients with lesions above T6, the thoracolumbar sympathetic outflow is interrupted. During suction the vagus nerve is unopposed and the patient may become hypotensive and bradycardiac, possibly resulting in cardiac arrest. Endotracheal intubation may produce a similar response. Suction causes vagal stimulation via the carotid bodies, which pass impulses to the brain via the glossopharyngeal nerves and are sensitive to lack of oxygen (Williams, 1995). It is, therefore, wise to preoxygenate the patient, monitor heart rate and have atropine on standby.

Active assisted facilitation of movement and passive movements

As the majority of SCI patients have an incomplete injury, it is important to facilitate and utilize any active movement available. During the acute phase, whilst the patient is immobilized in bed, the physiotherapist can assist in exploiting the potential for functional return. Where patients have any active movement they should be encouraged to participate in activity and it should be purposeful if possible.

In order to produce a remembered coordinated movement pattern during assisted movements, attempts should be made to position joint girdles in functional alignment, prior to moving the limbs. During a period of sustained bed rest, an SCI individual's body schema, the internal three-dimensional, dynamic representation of the spatial and biomechanical properties of one's body, is lost from the parietal area of the brain. This means that the different joints of the body are not clearly identified during movement. On attempting a functional activity, the individual cannot differentiate the different parts of a movement resulting in an abnormal mass pattern. Care should be taken to activate each joint movement to achieve the maximum outcome possible and feed into the preparation of the body for the changes in postural adjustments resulting from voluntary movement (Mouchnino et al., 1992; Schepens et al., 2008).

Cortical mapping has demonstrated change, by the performance of passive movements with the patient visualizing the movement and in the presence of some sensory feedback (Reddy et al., 2001).

Splints may be used to provide joint support and maintain joint range of movement and muscle length. This may be essential in reducing joint pain, providing stability during movement and preventing contracture. It can also be argued that splinting may hinder activity by 'dulling' afferent input due to blanket sensation and restriction of movement.

Functional electrical stimulation (FES) is a useful adjunct to improve a movement where only a flicker is first available (see Ch. 12). Similarly, electromyographic (EMG) biofeedback can assist the patient to move in the absence of full sensation (see Ch. 12). The aims of all such movements are to:

- assist circulation
- maintain muscle length, preventing soft-tissue shortening and contracture
- maintain full ROM of all joints
- maintain and remember movement patterns.

Movements are commenced immediately after injury and features specifically important for SCI patients are now discussed. Shoulder movements are usually performed at least twice a day and leg movements once a day, in order to monitor any return of movement. For lumbar and low thoracic fractures, hip flexion should be kept to below 30°, to avoid lumbar flexion, until stability is established. Knee flexion must, therefore, be performed in Tailor's position, i.e. 'frogging' (Figure 4.8).

Special emphasis should be put on the following:

- Stretching the finger flexors with wrist in neutral to preserve tenodesis grip (Bromley, 2006)
- Ensuring a full fist can be attained with wrist extension
- Pronation and supination in elbow flexion and extension
- Full elevation and lateral rotation of the shoulder from day 1
- Stretching the long head of the triceps – arm in elevation with elbow flexion
- Stretch the rhomboids bilaterally – avoid twisting cervical spine
- Stretching the upper fibres of the trapezius muscle.

Where there is no active flexion of the fingers and thumb, it is appropriate to allow shortening of the long flexors. The ROM of individual joints at the wrist, fingers and thumb must be maintained. When the wrist is actively extended, the fingers and thumb are pulled into flexion to produce a functional 'key-type' grip, the tenodesis grip. If this contracture does not occur naturally, it can be encouraged by splinting whilst in the acute phase.

During recovery, the handling principles apply to facilitate normal movement and not to elicit spasm and reinforce the spastic pattern. Extreme ROM must be avoided, especially at the hip and knee, as microtrauma may be a predisposing factor in the formation of periarticular

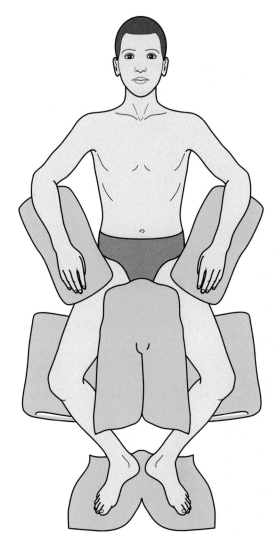

Figure 4.8 The 'frogging' or Tailor's position. This position is used to prevent movement of the lumbar spine during passive movements of the knees. It is also used to prevent mass extensor tone.

ossification (see above). Passive movements of paralysed limbs are continued until the patient is mobile and thus capable of ensuring full mobility through his or her own activities, unless there are complications, such as excessive spasm or stiffness. See Box 4.5 for key points in acute management.

A complication that may occur over the few days after injury and remain a risk for some months is the development of pulmonary emboli associated with deep venous thrombosis (DVT). Prophylactic measures, including frequent passive movement, wearing pressure stockings and early mobilization, are important. The use of antithrombolytic agents has become mandatory. Extreme vigilance with regard to leg size and other signs

Movements commence from the first day after injury:
- To monitor any return of movement
- Shoulder movements performed at least twice a day
- Leg movements performed once a day
- For lumbar and low thoracic fractures (prestabilization)
  - ☐ Hip flexion maintained below 30°
  - ☐ Knee flexion performed in Tailor's 'frogging' position
- Special emphasis placed on specific stretches to tissues of upper-limbs (see text)
- Extreme range of movement must be avoided

of DVT by all team members is important, as there is a 1–2% incidence of mortality from massive pulmonary embolus each year.

Turning and positioning/tone management

Whilst managed on bed rest patients will require frequent turning. Turning charts can be used to assist staff with a regimen over each 24-hour period, to avoid pressure-marking of anaesthetic skin and offering an opportunity to check skin tolerance. This regimen can be used in conjunction with postural drainage positions. Turning beds can be used to reposition a patient, and the choice of bed depends on the individual unit's policy.

Upper-limb positioning of the tetraplegic patient is very important during bed rest. Incomplete cervical lesions are particularly prone to shortening of soft tissues due to muscle imbalance, resulting in partial shoulder subluxation and pain.

Waring and Maynard (1991) reported that 75% of tetraplegics had shoulder pain, 60% lasting 2 weeks or more. Of the patients with pain, 39% had unilateral and 61% bilateral symptoms. In over one-third, onset was within the first 3 days postinjury and 52% within the first 2 weeks postinjury. Pain may result from muscle imbalance, spasticity, and direct trauma to the shoulder girdle, combined with the joint immobilization, central and peripheral sources of nerve pain.

Patients who are delayed in the initiation of shoulder exercises beyond 2 weeks post injury are significantly at risk of shoulder pain.

Scott and Donovan (1981) described special positioning to prevent loss of range: 90° abduction, combined with other positioning techniques, leads to decreased frequency and severity of shoulder pain.

Positioning is used to minimize spasticity similarly to patients with other conditions. When the patient is exhibiting mass muscle tone in flexion or extension, the limbs and trunk may be placed into reflex-inhibiting positions. Some examples of positioning are shown in Figures 4.8 and 4.9. Positioning is also discussed in Chapter 14 and by Pope (2002).

Antispasmodic agents may be prescribed at this stage to assist in the management of high tone and reduce the

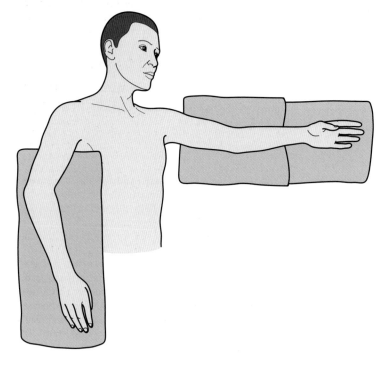

Figure 4.9 Side-lying. This position provides a comfortable resting position for the shoulders in side-lying, whilst still maintaining abduction of the shoulder and a supported biceps stretch.

complications of contracture. Botulinum toxin can be injected into specific muscles to offer the opportunity to gain muscle length, reduce pain and improve joint range of movement. This is particularly useful in the management of shoulders, as they are vulnerable to problems of pain and impingement, resulting from muscle imbalance and hypertonicity in the shoulder girdle musculature.

Preparation for and initiation of mobilization

Patient education should be intergrated into acute management, with the explanation of treatment interventions and jointly developed goals. Rehabilitation should start as soon as patients are well enough and should be encouraged to lead their goal planning.

Once radiographs have confirmed spinal stability, mobilization is initiated by progressively sitting the patient up in bed. Postural hypotension will be the main problem and patients with lesions at T6 and above will require an elasticated abdominal binder. This helps to maintain intrathoracic pressure and reduce pooling of the blood resulting from lack of abdominal tone. Once the patient starts to sit up he or she will be supported in a hard or soft collar, or a brace. Antithrombotic stockings will still be worn. Special adaptations to wheelchairs can help to reduce hypotensive fainting, e.g. reclining back and raised-leg supports. When patients can sit up for an hour they can initiate the more active phase of rehabilitation working towards the restoration of functional activities.

Pressure lifting

This is a technique in which patients lift themselves in their wheelchairs to relieve pressure. It is recommended that they lift every half-hour, for approximately 30 seconds. Where a patient cannot lift, a modified position in forward-leaning or side-to-side tilt is used.

REHABILITATION

The following section outlines management from the start of the mobilization phase through to discharge. Much of this information has been gained from the authors' experience; procedures may vary between centres but the principles are similar (Bromley, 2006; Whalley Hammell, 1995).

Aims of rehabilitation

- To establish an interdisciplinary process which is patient-focused, comprehensive and coordinated
- Physical motor functional activities with early intervention and prophylaxis to prevent further complications

- To learn new information to equip the individual with knowledge to achieve independence
- To achieve functional independence, whether physical or verbal, and equipment provision in order to facilitate this independence
- To achieve and maintain successful reintegration into the community.
- To achieve psychological adaptation to the newly acquired physical condition.

Goal-planning and outcome measures

Evaluation of progress by review of goal achievement is advised. The goals can be divided into achievable targets and should be patient-focused, appropriate and objective. It is recommended that they are created in a team environment, led by the patient, with interdisciplinary cooperation. It is at this point that patients are fully encouraged to take the locus of control for their rehabilitation. This theme is extended into the philosophy of their future reintegration. Chapter 11 discusses the issues of patient-centred practice in goal-setting and treatment, using a problem-solving approach.

There are several measures used to evaluate patient progress, applicable to an intervention or management technique. In general the World Health Organization recognizes Functional Independence Measures (FIM; Hamilton & Granger, 1991), Spinal Cord Independance Measure (SCIM: Catz A et al., 2007) and Craig Handicap Assessment and Reporting Technique (CHART; Whiteneck et al., 1992) as appropriate validated measures. Other outcome measures are discussed by Stokes (2009).

Objectives of rehabilitation

The progression of objectives as the patient gains more ability is outlined below. These objectives need to be set in relation to the level of spinal injury and the appropriate functional goals (Table 4.3). These expectations for function, depending on level of SCI, can only be a guide, especially in the light of the prevalence of incomplete lesions.

Key elements of the rehabilitation process are considered below.

Psychological aspects

Management of psychological and social issues must take place in parallel with early medical and rehabilitation aspects. It is recognized that patients will experience symptoms of stress and anxiety, and these should be treated specifically. In the early weeks and months after injury, the patient may present with rapid and dramatic changes in mood state and may express denial of his or her situation, anger at what has happened and depression, which may include stating the desire to die.

Table 4.3 Functional goals of rehabilitation in relation to the level of the spinal cord lesion

LEVEL	KEY MUSCLE CONTROL	MOVEMENT	FUNCTIONAL GOALS
C1–C3	Sternocleidomastoid Upper trapezius Levator	Neck control	Ventilator-dependent Electric wheelchair Verbally independent
C4	C3 plus diaphragm	Shoulder shrug Verbally independent	Electric wheelchair
C5	Biceps Deltoid Rotator cuff Supinator	Elbow flexion, supination Shoulder flexion, abduction	Manual wheelchair with capstans Electric wheelchair for long distance Independent brushing Teeth/hair/feeding with feeding strap
C6	Extensor carpi radialis longus, extensor carpi radialis brevis Pronator teres	Wrist extension, pronation	Tenodesis grip Manual wheelchair (capstans) Independent feeding, grooming, dressing top half, simple cooking Same-height transfers
C7	Triceps Latissimus dorsi Flexor digitorum, flexor carpi radialis, extensor digitorum	Elbow extension Finger flexion/extension	Manual wheelchair Independent activities of daily living, simple transfers, i.e. bed, car, toilet, may drive with hand controls
C8	All upper-limbs except lumbricals, interossei	Limited fine finger movements	Manual wheelchair Full dexterity
T1–T5	Varying intercostals and back muscles	Trunk support No lower-limb movements	Full wheelchair independence Orthotic ambulation
T6–T12	Abdominals	Trunk control	Orthotic/caliper ambulation
L1–L2	Psoas major Iliacus	Hip flexion	Caliper ambulation
L3–L4	Quadriceps Tibialis anterior	Knee extension Ankle dorsiflexion	Ambulation with orthoses and crutches/sticks
L5	Peronei	Eversion	Ambulation with relevant orthoses
S1–S5	Glutei, gastrocnemius Bladder, bowel, sexual function	Hip extension Ankle plantarflexion	Normal gait

Although all the members of the MDT will play a role in supporting a patient, advice and guidance from a qualified psychologist are essential and, at times, one-to-one direct patient therapy by the psychologist is necessary. The process of adaptation to spinal paralysis, reflected as integration back into the community, is a gradual one. Maintaining a positive approach with realistic expectations is essential for the patient's wellbeing (see Ch. 17).

Breaking bad news

It is important that all members of the MDT understand the implications of breaking bad news when undertaking the assessment of a new SCI patient. Often, the physiotherapist is one of the first professionals to compile a thorough physical examination and will be asked for information by the patient. It is an inevitable part of each team member's role to contribute to discussions of prognosis. A planned team approach is the best way to manage such conversations within the context of the process of information giving. This may not always be possible during a treatment session when the patient may ask about 'hopeful signs'. In this case any discussion should be based on accurate assessment with evidence-based reasoning where possible. It is unlikely that an exact answer can be given, in which case a positive emphasis on progressive goals will help the patient to focus on each phase of their rehabilitation.

Pain management

Pain can be a problem initially during movements, notably due to neurodynamics, which is impairment of movement and/or elasticity of the nervous system (Shacklock, 2005). Chronic pain is a common problem in SCI. Between 65 and 85% of patients will experience significant pain and one-third of these will be classified as severe. A modern classification of pain following spinal cord injury has been proposed by Siddall (2009). This divides pain into nociceptive and neuropathic. Nociceptive is subdivided into musculoskeletal and visceral, whilst neuropathic is divided into above, at level and below level. The comprehensive review paper by Siddall (2009) goes on to describe the mechanisms of neuropathic pain and its management with sections on general principles, surgical approaches, pharmacological options, neurostimulation, and psychological and environmental management. With such a wide range of approaches it is clear that none are uniformly successful in pain control. Further research into management systems, with particular emphasis on cognitive systems, is proceeding.

Skin care

Common sites of pressure sores are ischial (from prolonged sitting), sacral (from sheer loading), trochanteric, malleolar, calcaneal and plantar surfaces (from prolonged loading or direct trauma). Spasticity producing contractures and postural deformity are potential risk factors. Although poor nutrition, ageing, incontinence and comorbid factors increase the risk of decubitus ulceration, without ischaemia the ulcers do not arise. Therefore, patients are taught about risk management and provided with pressure redistributing mattresses and cushions.

Spasticity

SCI patients presenting with an upper motor neurone syndrome will exhibit both negative and positive symptoms. Spasticity will be a feature in this patient group, presenting a challenge in all aspects of patient management (Satkunam, 2003). It is a very large subject and requires more consideration than this chapter allows (see Ch. 14). Spasticity is difficult to define and more recently is described as a sensori-motor phenomenon related to the integration of the nervous system motor responses to sensory input. It is related to the hypersensitivity of the reflex arc resulting from the loss of descending inhibition (Ivanhoe & Reistetter, 2004). A further definition states that the disordered sensory-motor control presents as intermittent or sustained involuntary activation of muscles (Pandyan et al., 2005).

In incomplete cord lesions, depending on the pattern, spasticity tends to occur earlier and may present immediately. When severe, it will inhibit any underlying voluntary movement and create 'wrong' synaptic connections in the recovering nervous system. In complete spinal cord lesions, it most commonly becomes apparent about 3 months after the injury. It tends to reach a maximum between 6 and 12 months after injury and then diminishes, becoming more manageable. However, in a minority it remains at a high level and presents a major problem affecting function, posture and joint movement (Sheean, 1998).

A moderate amount of spasticity will assist with standing transfers, maintain muscle bulk, protect the skin to some extent and may contribute to prevention of osteoporosis. It is when the spasticity is excessive that problems occur.

Spasticity management

The management of spasticity should be undertaken by a coordinated multidisciplinary team rather than by clinicians in isolation (Barnes et al., 2001). Spinal cord spasticity presents in different patterns to that usually seen in stroke patients (Ch. 2).

The best management is prevention in the first few months after injury (Ditunno et al., 2004). Essentially in the first few days the opportunities for functional connections should be maximized.

It is also important to avoid triggering factors, such as urinary tract infection, constipation or skin breakdown. A collaborative assessment and evaluation tool to determine the best management of spasticity in SCI patients is currently being developed to accompany the document by Barnes et al. (2001).

The main medical approach is through pharmacology, although none of the drugs commonly used (baclofen, dantrolene and tizanidine) is universally effective or indeed predictable in its effect. Nerve blocks have been used for many years, usually using either phenol or alcohol. All of the above drugs have significant and numerous side-effects (see Martindale, 2007). An Intra thecal baclofen pump system can be used to deliver the baclofen directly into the spinal fluid. A small refillable pump is inserted under the skin delivering a regular treatment dose to maintain reduced levels of spasticity. As the use of intramuscular botulinum toxin increases, the use of other nerve blocks will diminish.

Surgery has some place in treatment, in the form of tendon release and nerve divisions, e.g. obturator neurectomy. These techniques can be successful, particularly where the procedure has been carried out for hygiene and posture reasons.

Functional mobility

Bed mobility

Rolling from side to side is taught first, then lying to sitting, and sitting to lying. Function is dependent upon the level of the lesion, e.g. C5, rolling side to side; C6, rolling, lying to sitting and sitting to lying; C7, independent in all aspects of bed mobility.

Sitting balance

Sitting supported in the wheelchair is progressed to sitting on a plinth supported, unsupported, static and then dynamic. Balance is practised in short and long sitting, hamstring length determining the ability to long sit independently.

Lifting

Lifting starts with partial pressure lifts in the wheelchair, and progresses to lifts on blocks on a plinth and then unaided without blocks.

Wheelchair mobility

Experience in using a variety of wheelchairs is helpful when a patient is developing their confidence in wheelchair mobility. Essential principles of safety and wheelchair skills are taught. As the patient progresses they should be given the opportunity to develop advanced skills, such as varied height kerbs, slopes, uneven terrain, tight corners and, if possible, stairs and escalater techniques. Adaptations, such as extended brakes and a modular supportive backrest, are required for higher lesions. Skills in powered chairs are based around safe use of the chair functions, manouvering and experience of outdoor terrain. These chairs may have kerb climbing functions and standing systems.

Transfers

Depending on the level of the lesion and functional ability, a sliding board may be used for legs-up and legs-down transfers on to the bed. This is progressed without a board where possible. Transfers then progress to lifting from various levels for functional activities: high to low; low to high; between two plinths; floor to plinth; floor to chair; chair to car, bath and to easy chair.

Standing programme

Care must be taken when initiating standing. The autonomic disturbance present in patients with cervical and thoracic injuries can result in significant problems with hypotension which in the early stages may affect cord perfusion. Blood pressure studies and monitoring of pressures in sitting and gradual tilt table standing have been suggested (Kassioukov et al., 2009). These problems will usually resolve as the venous return improves.

Bone loss after SCI is greatest in the lower limbs. There is some evidence, although limited, to support standing by any means can improve preservation of bone mass density in the femoral shaft and proximal femur of complete SCI individuals (Goemaere et al., 1994). However the early weight-bearing mobilization of patients might be important in preventing or slowing the bone mineral loss after injury (de Bruin et al., 1999). In practice tilt table standing is commenced as soon as possible. This has many other benefits: respiratory psychological and improved systemic body functions. Standing is of great value in retaining neuromuscular flexibility and in reduction of spasticity (Bohannon & Larkin, 1985; Eng et al., 2001; Goemaere et al., 1994; Golding, 1994).

An abdominal binder and compression stockings are recommended for patients with lesions of T6 and above. Once the patient can stand with no ill effect, progression is made to a standing frame, e.g. Oswestry Standing Frame (OSF), working up to standing for 1 hour, three times a week. Patients with lesions of C5 and below should be capable of standing into a hoist-assisted OSF. There are many standing systems commercially available which will lift the patient into a standing posture. Some wheelchairs also offer this facility. Whilst standing, trunk balance work can be re-educated, for example, removing hand support, throwing and catching a ball. Once good balance is achieved, the paraplegic patient may go on to develop gait with orthoses or actively.

There has been a variety of studies to identify the time and regularity necessary for a patient to stand. It is suggested that the amount of time will influence the reduction in spasticity and at least half an hour every day is recommended (Walter et al., 1999).

Upper-limb management

This activity is continued from the acute phase using a variety of techniques (see Chs 12 & 18). Once the patient has begun to mobilize in the wheelchair there are many options for strengthening during functional activities.

The evidence of shoulder pain in wheelchair users is undeniable – 78% of tetraplegics and 59% of paraplegics, although studies vary in numbers. Specific exercises to address muscle imbalance and maintenance of full range have been shown to reduce this incidence (Curtis et al., 1999).

Other specific exercises can be useful, e.g. assisted/resisted arm bike, resistance circuits and sporting activities. This is an enjoyable adjunct to rehabilitation and encourages reintegration.

Hydrotherapy is used for strengthening and as preparation for swimming. Patients are taught how to roll in the water and to swim. If the patient is wearing a brace, this will limit activities in the water. Anyone with an FVC of less than 1 L will need careful consideration before swimming is introduced.

Strengthening and cardiovascular fitness

The rehabilitation process incorporates components of strengthening and fitness, as part of restoration of function. An average SCI patient is eight times less active than a middle-aged sedentry man. Wheelchair users have an increased risk of secondary disabilities such as coronary heart disease, obesity, hypertension and diabetes (Finley et al., 2002). The changes in muscle function resulting from SCI lead to reduced energy expenditure and decreased strength.

Patients are motivated to achieve their physical goals in a variety of ways. Fitness training using adapted equipment is useful, e.g. an arm-powered ergonomic bike may be used for endurance. Wheelchair circuits and advanced skills are encouraged. Hydrotherapy can lead on to swimming, an enjoyable activity that can improve cardiovascular fitness. The emphasis on education for patients and the establishment of an ongoing fitness programme for SCI individuals has become a priority within the Spinal Cord Injury Centres.

The value of sports activities cannot be underestimated, even for those people who did not enjoy sports previously. The known benefits of group or sports activities translate into the rehabilitation process. Patients will often sustain an activity for much longer when engaged in a sport.

There are many charities and organizations available to promote these opportunities and to support equipment funding for SCI individuals. Activities can eventually progress to more competitive sports and clubs, as well as encouraging attendance at the many fully integrated fitness centres available. Cardiovascular fitness after SCI has been reviewed (Finley et al., 2002; Jacobs & Nash, 2001) and in general for neurological conditions in Chapter 18.

Functional electrical stimulation effects on muscle and fitness

Many studies have investigated the effects of using FES to support exercise in SCI individuals. The positive effects of FES exercise are well established, although intensity, duration and frequency of these interventions all vary (Giangregorio & McCartney, 2006). FES exercise can produce isometric contractions resulting in an increase in muscle cross-sectional area. FES cycle ergonometry (Figure 4.10) has demonstrated increases in muscle fibre area and capillary bed (Belanger et al., 2000) in addition to increasing whole body metabolism and cardiovascular fitness (Davis et al., 2008).

Functional electrical stimulation in restoration of function and gait

Research and technologies have influenced our clinical practice, e.g. body weight support treadmill gait training (Figure 4.11) is based around the central pattern generator (CPG) theory (see below). Research to incorporate FES with this training is underway. In the future methods that use the concept of activity-dependent neuroplasticity will most likely play an increasing role in the rehabilitation of SCI.

FES and its role in functional activities and gait requires further evaluation. A comprehensive review by Ragnarsson (2008) identifies the current state-of-the-art and future therapeutic potential. It has been used as a neuroprosthesis in activities of daily living (ADL) to restore upper-limb function. Surface FES systems that aim to assist paraplegic patients to walk are already approved in the USA – Parastep System (Sigmedics, Inc., IL, USA) and for incomplete injuries the Odstock Drop Foot Stimulator is widely used. The implanted devices for foot drop have been developed and are curently being used in clinical practice (Chae et al., 2000).

Despite promising advances in technology, the physiological limitations of the neuromuscular system prohibit the clinical use of FES alone to achieve a realistic and

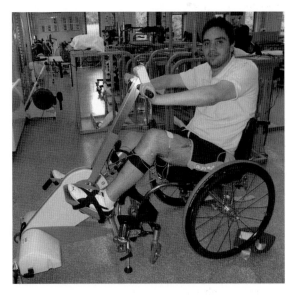

Figure 4.10 Patient using functional electrical stimulation (FES) a leg cycle ergometer.

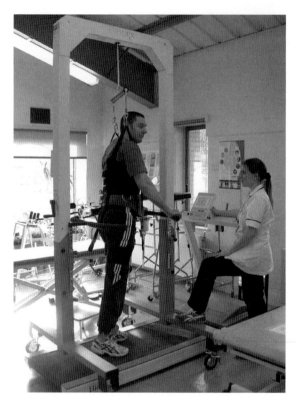

Figure 4.11 Patient using body weight support gantry and treadmill.

successful functional outcome. Gait remains inefficient, needing high energy levels. It has been demonstrated that function achieved through an external locus of control will always be of limited value to patients (Bradley, 1994). The recent research is seeking to provide cortical patterns of activity to trigger the stimulation for movement (Grill et al., 2001).

Some patients choose to use FES to maintain muscle bulk for cosmesis and others to maintain bulk or leg circulation for reduction of pressure over bony areas. Patients who are very slim with bony prominences are predisposed to pressure marking and the maintenance of muscle bulk by FES can help to reduce this problem and allow them to sit for longer in their wheelchair.

Ongoing respiratory management

Tetraplegic and some high thoracic paraplegic patients will benefit from ongoing respiratory monitoring and from respiratory training. Respiratory capacity is impaired by motor weakness, spasticity and pain. Inspiratory muscle-training devices provide resistance through a variety of devices or valves. Some studies have demonstrated some limited benefit for improving FVC (Hough, 2001; Van Houtte et al., 2006). More recently devices have been developed to produce training through the Test of Incremental Respiratory Endurance (TIRE) protocol. This system produces inspiratory muscle training working at 80% of the maximum performance (Figure 4.12). The visual display provides a goal-orientated programme for the individual to try to beat during each exercise session (www.trainair.co.uk).

Education/advice to carers/family

Carers are actively involved in the rehabilitation process and are taught how to assist with normal daily activities, to support the patient in independent living. Assisted exercises, standing programme and chest care are taught in addition to moving and handling the patient, whilst paying attention to skin care and their own safety and back care. This support is within a holistic educational advocacy provided by case mangers during rehabilitation.

Wheelchairs

The variety of wheelchairs available increases each year, including some that enable the patient to rise into standing. Initially, patients are mobilized in a standard wheelchair offering greatest support and stability, following a comprehensive assessment to ensure it is correctly fitted and adjusted. Adaptations are made to provide a well-supported, evenly balanced seating position (Harvey, 2008; Pope, 2002). Tension adjustable canvas systems and modular backrests are all valuable in producing postural control.

The key to good stability is achieved by support and alignment at the pelvis. The cushion is equally important and should be assessed in a similar way, also taking into account the need for protection of pressure areas. Various pressure assessment tools are used to evaluate skin viability when sitting and these aid cushion prescription (Barbenel et al., 1983). Later in rehabilitation, it will be appropriate to try a variety of wheelchairs to offer greater mobility and independence according to an individual's needs. In view of the incidence of shoulder pain in wheelchair users (Ballinger et al., 2000), it is appropriate to consider adaptations and weight of the wheelchairs. There are many light-weight wheelchairs available and the use of assisted wheeling systems can ease the effort of wheeling. A battery-powered third wheel or trike adaptation can be fitted onto the front of a light weight manual wheelchair to provide assisted mobility outdoors.

Powered chairs

All tetraplegic patients should always be provided with a powered chair, even if they chose a manual light-weight chair initially. This should also be considered for some

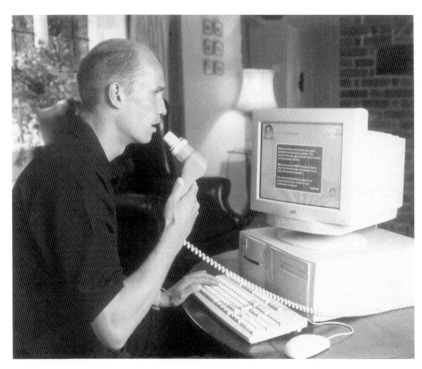

Figure 4.12 Respiratory Training Device. (From TRAINAIR, Inspiratory Muscle Training, with permission.)

paraplegics, depending on their age and expected functional activities.

Rehabilitation of incomplete lesions

The management of the incomplete patient presents many challenges, not least because experience has shown that the expected outcomes are unknown. This can affect the psychological adjustment of the patient and, as physical changes extend over many years, may delay patients in moving on with their life.

Emphasis is placed on managing muscle imbalance, spasticity and tone, and sensory loss. As incomplete lesions present with a wide range of loss of functional activity, treatment will depend on the level of disability and specific physical problems.

Treatment may include: facilitation of normal movement patterns; muscle strengthening (see Ch. 18); addressing muscle imbalance and compensations; and inhibition of spasticity (see Ch. 14). Balance re-education, gait re-education, wheelchair skills and functional activities are performed as appropriate to the patient's level of ability.

Research suggests that patterned neural activity may be an important mechanism for developing and maintaining inhibitory circuitry (McDonald et al., 2002). There

have been many studies exploring gait facilitation using a partial weight-bearing system on the treadmill. This approach is based on the principles of CPGs and repeated exercise of gait motion to increase strength, coordination and endurance (Ladouceur et al., 1997). There is evidence from animal studies that neural networks in the isolated spinal cord are capable of generating rhythmic output (reciprocally organized between agonists and antagonists) in the absence of efferent descending and movement-related afferent sources (Duysens & Van de Crommert, 1998). This is postulated to be similar in humans. Spinal systems contribute to the control of locomotion by local segmental and intersegmental spinal circuits (Grillner & Wallen, 1985).

In normal walking, it has been shown that muscle activity patterns are not centrally generated by reflex-induced activity, e.g. through stretch reflexes (Prochazka et al., 1979). The gait facilitation on the treadmill system is thought to be influenced by three main sensory sources acting on the CPGs:

1. Load/proprioceptive feedback from the extensor muscles
2. Exteroceptive afferents from the mechanreceptors of the foot
3. Joint position and muscle stretch from the hip flexors and ankle plantarflexors.

Some outcome measures being assessed as evaluation tools for this work in the national spinal injuries centres are: Walking Index for Spinal Cord Injury (WISCI; Ditunno et al., 2000) and WISCI II (Ditunno et al., 2001).

There have been concerns from physiotherapists against gait exercise too early, causing the development of 'wrong patterns'. The motion of the hip is helped by the harness so as to move almost entirely within normal range limits. Therapists helping to guide foot placement manually found this an effective way of controlling motion and blocking abnormal harmful patterns. FES has been introduced as an adjunct to assist with the gait pattern (see Ch. 12). The advantages of this gait training would be to improve systemic functions and stimulate the vegetative nervous sequelae. Early training with some weight-bearing may help reduce osteoporosis and patients have been shown to need less support after training (Abel et al., 2002).

Questions remain if this treatment is effective: is progress due to other factors, e.g. muscle plasticity or spontaneous recovery, or can the cord learn from the increased demands of loading the limbs? The supraspinal and afferent influences on the cord are not yet understood in humans.

Patients with LMN damage require early diagnosis and may benefit from acute surgical and later restorative interventions, and also provision of orthoses to accommodate for the weakness.

Assisted gait, calipers and orthoses

During rehabilitation, the patient may be assessed for suitability for walking with orthoses. Depending on the fracture, gait training will normally commence about a year after surgery, or earlier if no fixation surgery was indicated or if the patient is incomplete. There should be surgical review on an individual basis. Some patients may require a temporary orthosis during their recovery.

It should be recognized that, even if a patient has the ability to walk with calipers, he or she may not choose to or may be advised not to try. Techniques used for gait training have been discussed in detail by Bromley (2006) and an outline of the progression of training is given below.

The gait-training process is physically demanding and requires commitment. Criteria which should be considered include:

- appropriate risk assessment
- sufficient upper-limb strength to lift body weight
- full ROM of hips and knees, and no contracture
- cardiovascular fitness sufficient to sustain walking activity
- assessment of spinal deformity, e.g. scoliosis, that may hinder standing balance
- motivation of the patient
- assessment of spasticity that may make walking unsafe.

Experience has shown that many patients complete their training with calipers, only to discard them a few months or years later as walking has become too much effort. Wheelchair use may be preferable, as the hands are free for functional activities whereas they are not when walking with calipers.

Orthoses

The ability to walk with calipers and the degree of support required depend on the functional level of injury. The following are examples of orthoses used for different levels of injury:

- C7–L1: hip guidance orthosis (HGO), advanced reciprocal gait orthosis (ARGO), RGO, Walkabout
- T6–T12: caliper walk/Walkabout with rollator; progress to crutches depends on patient's function
- T9–L3: caliper walk with comfortable handle crutches
- L3 and below: appropriate orthoses or walking aid.

Initial gait work

Caliper training is commenced in backslabs of fibreglass (Dynacast) or similar light-weight casting material. The backslabs are bandaged on and toe springs applied. For all orthotic gait training adjustable training orthoses are used. Standing balance is achieved in the parallel bars, in front of a mirror, by standing in extension and resting back on the tension of the iliofemoral ligaments. The lifting technique is taught in the standing position, lifting the whole body weight with full control. Lift from sitting to standing and back to sitting is also taught.

Once the patient has achieved standing balance and the appropriate degree of support required, dynamic balance work is started. This includes turning safely, swing-to and swing-through gait patterns, and the four-point gait technique for stepping practice.

Transfers

Transferring in backslabs is then practised, from plinth to chair, chair to plinth, and from chair to standing.

Middle stage of gait work

Progression to a rollator or crutches is begun at this stage. Balance is achieved using one parallel bar and one crutch, or with a rollator and one person to assist. Gait patterns and transfers (described above) are then practised. Depending on the functional level, four-point gait with crutches is taught, then kerbs, slopes and stairs. Video assessment for problem-solving and improvement of gait techniques may be useful at this stage.

Late stage of gait work

On completion of training, the patient is measured for the definitive othoses. For patients using reciprocal gait orthoses, gait re-education is practised in the parallel bars then progressed to a rollator and possibly crutches, as outlined above.

A home standing programme for caliper patients is devised to improve confidence. This entails using backslabs daily to maintain strength and cardiovascular fitness and to improve mobility. Goals are decided mutually as to how calipers and walking aids will be used at home and at work, to achieve optimum function.

The long-term ventilated patient

Increased survival of patients with high lesions is now expected, especially in the young. Resettlement into the community requires domiciliary ventilation and a complex care package.

Once past the acute phase, their individual needs are ascertained. Specialized wheelchairs are available which can be mouth- or head-controlled. Prophylactic chest management is vital, with tracheostomy, regular bagging and suction to reduce atelectasis and prevent infection (see Ch. 15). FES for the abdominal muscles has been evaluated as a method to assist coughing (Linder, 1993).

Non-invasive ventilation may be appropriate for some patients and some others may be candidates for diaphragmatic pacing. Usually those with lesions above C3 are most successful. Lesions of C4 segmental level tend to have involvement of the anterior horn and cannot be stimulated, as stimulation relies on an intact lower motor neuron system.

Assessment involves nerve conduction studies and may include fluoroscopic examination to visualize diaphragmatic excursion (Zejdlik, 1992). Electrodes are placed around the phrenic nerve either in the thorax or neck. An external pacing box is attached to external transmitter antennae; these are placed over the implanted receivers and when stimulated provide diaphragmatic contraction (Buchanan & Nawoezenski, 1987). There is no set regime for training but some patients have managed to achieve 24-hour pacing. Others use the ventilator part-time.

Initially, physiotherapy will aim to maximize strength in all innervated muscles to assist in head control and strengthen accessory respiratory muscles. Glossopharyngeal breathing techniques and use of a biofeedback training system can allow the patient to manage for short periods off the ventilator. Regular tilt table standing is recommended in addition to passive movements. Management of spasticity is also an important consideration (see Ch. 14) and may involve medication.

The aim for these patients is to achieve verbal independence and control of their environment. Technology offers systems linked to computerized environmental controls, operated by a head or mouth control, or voice-activated.

Children with spinal cord injury

The number of children with spinal cord damage which is non-congenital is thankfully quite low. Numbers vary between studies but a study gives an example that less than 2% of children admitted with all forms of traumatic injury have an SCI (Brown et al., 2001). Traumatic causes are mostly traffic accidents and falls.

In very young children, the head is proportionally larger and heavier and, therefore, injuries are commonly cervical. The range of maximum flexion of the cervical spine tends to move lower as the child gets older (Grundy & Swain, 2002). The review provided by Vogel and Anderson (2003) offers a comprehensive overview of the management of children with SCI. Other texts include Osenback and Menezes (1992) and Short et al. (1992).

Special considerations for children with SCI include the following:

- Children are very sensitive to hypotension, autonomic dysfunction and thermoregulatory dysfunction. There is potential for damage of the immature brain from chronic hypotension when first mobilizing.
- Children have a high metabolism and therefore have high calorific needs for healing and recovery.
- Paralytic ileus is a very common problem in cervical and thoracic lesions.
- Standing is a priority in rehabilitating children. It is important for social skills and development of curiosity, is essential in preventing osteoporosis and facilitates the development of the epiphyseal growth plates. A number of methods can be employed to maintain standing using many mobile standing systems. Spinal support braces, calipers or other orthotic supports are used to allow supported standing and walking. The child can stay in the brace for 90% of the day and remain ambulant for 80% of the day, although realisitically this can be very difficult to achieve.
- The child must be closely monitored during growth spurts for the development of spinal deformity, e.g. scoliosis. Soft-tissue shortening is caused by altered posture and muscle imbalance, leading to further deformity.
- Support and education of the parents about the implications of the SCI will enable them to educate their child and family, and monitor the child for any complications. Schooling should be continued during rehabilitation, in liaison with the education authorities. Ongoing communication with the local education teams will ensure a smooth discharge and aid reintegration.
- Transitioning of adolescents into adult services requires a greater amount of support and planning from the professionals involved in the individual's care.

Discharge plan, reintegration and follow-up

The process of rehabilitation and reintegration is complex, involving many agencies and resources. The development of the case management process has helped to coordinate the complex process of discharge into the community. The patient thus has an advocate to complement the core rehabilitation team, providing support in overcoming functional difficulties and liaise with the various organizations and authorities throughout rehabilitation.

In the UK 74% of patients are discharged to their own home, the remainder to an interim placement, residential or nursing care or a local hospital (SIA, 2009).

On discharge all patients will require further close follow-up and reassessment, which may involve the community teams. Ideally this will be a multidisciplinary review to maintain continued support, monitor physical wellbeing and facilitate reintegration. During rehabilitation, patients are introduced to groups and organizations, such as SIA and Back Up, who can offer social and peer support and leisure activities, whilst also providing advisory role, to assist in the reintegration process.

A home visit is made by the occupational therapist and community team and may include school or workplace. The physiotherapist may be involved to assess mobility issues. If home adaptations or rehousing are not completed but the patient is ready for discharge, transfer to an interim placement may be necessary.

Preparation for discharge begins at the beginning of rehabilitation, in order to facilitate a supported process. From the authors' experience, we know that many incomplete patients with UMN and LMN lesions go on to make functional recovery past the quoted time of 2 years. As physiotherapists, we can ensure this opportunity is not lost and real qualitative changes can be made. The economic implications are strongly argued when someone can be kept mobile and carer input reduced. We must encourage utilization of all treatment modalities and equipment available.

Patients will need ongoing follow-up and may require later-stage interventions, such as tendon transfer and implant surgery to restore function (mentioned previously). The spinal injuries unit should be available as a resource back-up when any complications or problems arise.

CONCLUSION

The management of the person with SCI is complex and lifelong. A functional, goal-oriented, interdisciplinary, rehabilitation programme should enable the patient with SCI to live as full and independent a life as possible. Evidence-based therapeutic interventions are already altering our expectations and the development of technology and pharmacology offers exciting prospects for the management of SCI individuals. Current research gives rise to the hope that in the near future clinicians will be actively intervening in an attempt to alter and augment natural recovery. As this comes to fruition, functional outcomes and quality of life for SCI patients should improve.

CASE STUDY

Clinical reasoning in a case for later intervention more than 2 years post spinal cord lesion.

Patient: JG (date of birth 1975)

Pathology

- **1998** – headed a ball playing football, aged 23 years. Onset of upper anterior chest pain and altered sensation. Patient reported a tight sensation around his upper chest. After various musculoskeletal treatments the patient sought a surgical opinion. He was initially misdiagnosed with a possible lymphoma and underwent three operative procedures
- **Isotope imaging** later revealed osteoblastoma
- **2000** – further operative procedures to remove the osteoblastoma and provide internal fixation via metalwork and bone grafting, resulting in an incomplete spinal cord lesion at T2/3. Later in 2000 a further operation was required to revise the fixation and provide longer fixation from C7 to T6
- **Seven operative procedures** with associated scarring and soft-tissue damage
- **Hypertonus** – presents with increased tone in both lower limbs; extensor greater than flexor. Patient reports variable abdominal spasms
- **Weakness** – initially complete loss of motor and sensory function below T3 postoperatively. From 2000 the gradual return of motor and sensory function. He was finally able to stand and take his first steps after 3 months
- **Initial management** as an inpatient in acute and rehabilitation units for more than 7 months. Further outpatient treatment in neuro-physiotherapy department
- **SCIC** – refer to the Spinal Cord Injury Centre for rehabilitation; 24 months later (total of 4+ years postoperative episode of SCI)
- **ASIA Impairment Classification** – on initial assessment ASIA C. Sensory T3 and motor S2 (S3-5 not tested) on the right. Sensory T3 and motor L2 on the left
- **Brown Séquard** incomplete SCI presentation.

Previous medical history

- No history of previous illnesses or injuries.

Social history

- Returned to full time employment. Working in a mostly sedentary profession but is required to undertake international travel
- Prior to the SCI, he enjoyed football, swimming, golf and tennis
- He reports that when he feels under duress he notices his tone increases.

Body structure and function (impairments)

- Asymmetrical head alignment
- Compensatory increased muscle activity in neck and shoulder girdle
- Loss of normal body image
- Altered mid-line orientation
- Associated movements in left upper limb to augment trunk stability
- Reduced selective activity of trunk and shoulder girdle L>R
- Weakness/low tone of trunk left >right
- Sensory deficit T3 to S2 (S3-5 not tested) loss of pin prick and temperature sensation on right side
- Proprioceptive deficit affecting both ankles and feet
- Hypertonia of left adductors, knee extensors, posterior crural muscles (neural and non-neural components)
- Weakness/reduced pelvic stability (left glutei and trunk extensors)
- Contracture and loss of range/stiffness around left foot and ankle
- Autonomic dysfunction – sweating down left side of trunk and lateral half of left hand
- Altered balance systems and compensatory strategies
- Soft tissue damage and scarring around T3 with resulting muscle damage and dysfunction.

Activity limitations

- Inconsistent and unstable gait pattern
- Poor left foot clearance in stepping, relies on a stick to assist gait
- Requires upper limb assistance to move from sitting to standing
- Sleep disturbance due to involuntary lower limb spasms
- Unable to walk and carry anything in his upper limbs
- Requires a stick to mobilize.

Participation restrictions

- Reduced efficiency of gait means he tires quickly
- Difficulty walking outdoors on windy days, in busy environments and on uneven surfaces

- Limited ability to participate in sports
- Unable to manage some ADLs independently, such as lifting heavy items, carrying hot food, reaching up to cupboards.
- Unable to manage home and garden maintenance.

Main problem

- Weakness around left trunk from T3 to lower limb (see Table 4.4 for muscle charts on initial assessment and changes after treatment)
- Sensory deficits
- Hypertonia most dominant in left lower limb extensors
- Low tone in left trunk.

Compensations

- Postural asymmetry deviated to right from mid-line to augment postural control
- Postural scoliosis leading to neck and shoulder pain (see Figure 4.13)
- Reduced knee flexion in gait
- Contracture of left gastrocnemius and soleus muscles with structural soft tissue changes in the left foot
- Altered balance strategies favouring the right side of the body and relying on the right upper limb finger touch to enhance balance by direct feedback into the vestibular systems.

Patient's perception of main problems

- Effortful gait pattern
- Weakness in stomach muscles

Table 4.4 Muscle chart at initial assessment and at review following treatment

KEY ASIA MUSCLE	INITIALLY		3 YEARS LATER	
	Left	Right	Left	Right
T1	5	5	5	5
L2	3	5	4	5
L3	4 sp	5	4 sp	5
L4	1	5	2	5
L5	3	5	4	5
S1	4 sp	5	4 sp	5

ASIA, American Spinal Injury Association; Sp – denotes spasticity present during movement.

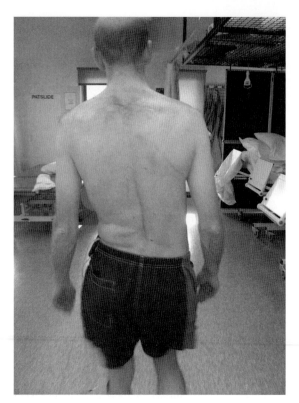

Figure 4.13 Postural imbalance during gait on left leg weight bearing.

- Stiffness in the left leg
- Neck and shoulder locks up and is painful.

Hypothesis

- Address established altered biomechanical issues
- Facilitate selective activity around the pelvis and trunk to stabilize the body over the left pelvis and lower limb
- Improve left ankle range of movement
- Provide feedback to augment carry over where sensory deficit hinders movement and motor learning
- Enhance activity and maintain posture and soft tissue length by use of orthotics and FES so as to provide a 'remembered' joint posture and movement sequencing in a functional activity
- Use improved functions as unique 'carry over' checks to enhance the individual's motivation to engage in treatment strategies.

Outcome measures

Related to impairment

- ASIA Impairment scale
- Photographs of standing alignment.

Related to activity and participation

- Video analysis/motion analysis
- 10 m walk test
- Physiological Cost Index (PCI) – A gait efficiency measure of energy cost per distance travelled
- Berg Balance Scale
- Active left knee raise in standing (centimetres).

Treatment progression summary

- Initial treatment set out to evaluate various off the shelf orthotics to improve left foot lift. A Foot Up splint was helpful but caused skin marking. Referral to the orthotics team provided a Neurodyn splint; a soft splint that maintains ankle dorsiflexion and provides some eversion
- Soft tissue techniques combined with inhibitory mobilizations in weight bearing, to produce eccentric lengthening of the extensors of the left lower limb (see Figure 4.14)

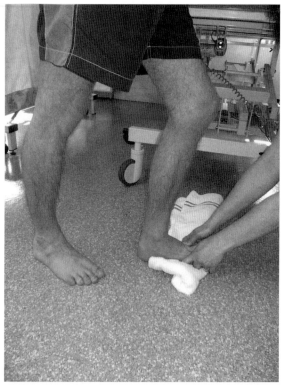

Figure 4.14 Therapist using manual techniques to gain soft tissue length and facilitate acceptance of base of support in weight bearing over the left foot. A towel wedge provides lengthening of the plantar aspect of the foot and calf muscle complex.

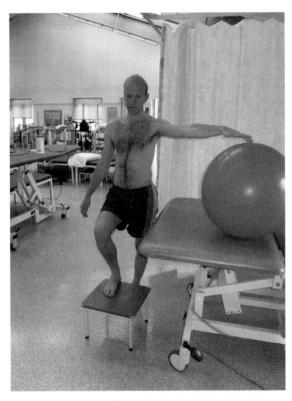

Figure 4.15 Achieving standing stability over the left leg to step up onto stool with the right leg. Sensory input from finger touch augments postural control systems.

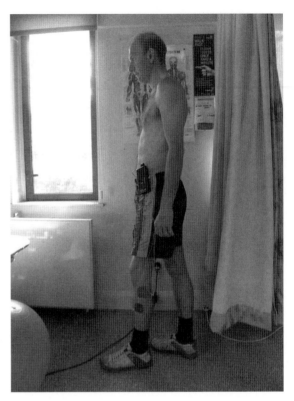

Figure 4.16 Patient stands with an Odstock Drop Foot Stimulator (ODFS) set up to provide ankle dorsiflexion. A second channel can be added to provide gluteal stimulation in stance phase or knee flexion in swing phase.

- Facilitation of left-sided stability in functional movements, to improve trunk control. Working towards maintaining this control during left leg weight-bearing activities (see Figure 4.15)
- A key activity found to provide effective carry over – step down on the stairs with the facilitation around the foot and knee, produced improved active release of the leg in standing and enabled the leg to be flexed up to step over a threshold. This was previously unachievable
- A home exercise programme was developed to improve and then maintain increased functional range of movement in the left foot and ankle. Further exercises focused on improvement of dynamic trunk stability moving over the left leg
- Assessment of Odstock Drop Foot Stimulator (ODFS) using single channel stimulator to provide foot clearance with eversion in gait. The dual channel stimulator was assessed to provide foot clearance and knee flexion in swing phase. FES augmented strengthening of the improved ankle

range and assisted in maintaining this range (see Figure 4.16)
- Treatment aimed to improve trunk symmetry and balance. Facilitation of balance systems through the left trunk and pelvis in perch sitting and progressing to standing (see Figure 4.17)
- Progress to add rotation into dynamic movements and challenge ankle strategies. Gradual reduction in extensor spasms offered opportunity to improve freedom of movement in the left leg
- Improved confidence in trunk control and balance resulted in reduced dependence on a walking stick. Only using when walking outdoors for longer distances
- Facilitation of alignment of shoulder girdles to address shoulder pain and radiating pain from T3
- Progress to reduce compensations and release left upper limb from the trunk
- Improved activity in left ankle evertors and dorsiflexors augmented by ODFS.

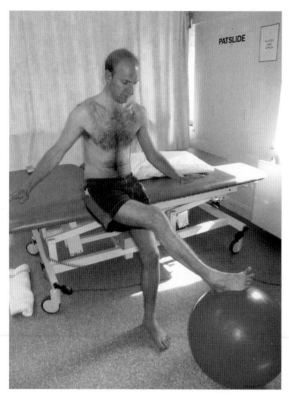

PATSLIDE

Figure 4.17 Dynamic postural control from sitting, incorporating limb rotation combined with ankle control. Progressed into standing.

Outcome summary

Berg scores

First assessment = 52/56
Reassessment 3 years later = 56/56

10 m walk scores

First assessment: 17 steps in 10 seconds using ODFS and one stick
Assessment 3 years later: 14 steps in 5.35 seconds with ODFS

PCI scores

Without ODFS over 10 m = 0.04
With ODFS over 10 m = 0.02

JG is demonstrating improved efficiency in gait when using the FES.

Activities

JG is now able to gradually return to golf, improving endurance to walk further and requiring less rests. His forthcoming goal is to carry his eagerly awaited baby twins.

REFERENCES

Abel, R., Schablowski, M., Rupp, R., Gemer, H.J., 2002. Gait analysis on the treadmill – monitoring exercise in the treatment of paraplegia. Spinal Cord 40, 17–22.

Adkins, D.L., Boychuk, J., Remple, M.S., et al., 2006. Motor training induces experience-specific patterns of plasticity across motor cortex and spinal cord. J. Appl. Physiol. 101 (6), 1776–1782.

American Spinal Injuries Association (ASIA) 2008. International Standards for Neurological and Functional Classification of Spinal Cord Injury, reprint 2008. American Spinal Injuries Association, Chicago, IL.

Ballinger, D.A., Rintala, D.H., Hart, K.A., 2000. The relation of shoulder pain and range of motion problems to functional limitations, disability and perceived health of men with spinal cord injury: a multifaceted longitudinal study. Arch. Phys. Med. Rehabil. 81, 1575–1581.

Barbenel, J.C., Forbes, C.D., Lowe, G.D.O., 1983. Pressure Sores. Macmillan Press, London.

Barnes, M., Bhakta, B., Moore, P., et al., 2001. The Management of Adults with Spasticity using Botulinum Toxin. A Guide to Clinical Practice. Harvard Health, Byfleet.

Battiston, B., Papalia, I., Tos, P., Geuna, S., 2009. Peripheral nerve repair and regeneration research. Int. Rev. Neurobiol. 87, 1–7.

Belanger, M., Stein, R.B., Wheeler, G.D., et al., 2000. Electrical stimulation: can it increase muscle strength and reverse osteopenia in spinal cord individuals? Arch. Phys. Med. Rehabil. 81 (8), 1090–1098.

Birch, R., 1993. Management of brachial plexus injuries. In: Greenwood, R., Barnes, M.P., McMillan, T.M. et al., (Eds.), Neurological Rehabilitation. Churchill Livingstone, London, pp. 587–606.

Bohannon, R.W., Larkin, P.A., 1985. Passive ankle dorsiflexion increases in patients after a regime of tilt table-wedge board standing. A clinical report. Phys. Ther. 65, 1676–1678.

Bohannon, R.W., Smith, M.B., 1987. Interrater reliability of a modified Ashworth scale of muscle spasticity. Phys. Ther. 67, 206–207.

Bradley, M., 1994. The effects of participating in a functional electrical stimulation exercise programme on affect in people with FES. Arch. Phys. Med. Rehabil. 75, 676–679.

Brindley, G.S., 1984. The fertility of men with spinal injury. Paraplegia 22, 337–348.

Bromley, I., 2006. Tetraplegia and Paraplegia, sixth ed. Churchill Livingstone, London.

Brown, P., 1994. Pathophysiology of spasticity. J. Neurol. Neurosurg. Psychiatry 57, 773–777.

Brown, R.L., Brunn, M.A., Garcia, V.F., 2001. Cervical spine injuries in children: a review of 103 patients treated consecutively at a level 1 pediatric trauma center. J. Pediatr. Surg. 36, 1107–1114.

Buchanan, L.E., Nawoezenski, D.A., 1987. Spinal Cord Injury Concepts and Management Approaches. Williams & Wilkins, London.

Burns, A.S., Ditunno, J.F., 2001. Establishing prognosis and maximizing functional outcomes after spinal cord injury. Spine 26, S137–S145.

Catz, A., Itzkovich, M., Tesio, L., et al., 2007. A Multicentre international study on the Spinal Cord Independence Measure, version III: Rasch psychometric validation. Spinal Cord 45, 275–291.

Chae, J., Kilgore, K., Triolo, R., et al., 2000. Functional neuromuscular stimulation in spinal cord injury. Phys. Med. Rehabil. Clin. N. Am. 11, 209–226.

Chartered Society of Physiotherapy (CSP), 1997. Standards of Physiotherapy Practice for People with Spinal Cord Lesions. CSP, London.

Crozier, K.S., Groziani, V., Ditunno, J.F., et al., 1991. Spinal cord injury, prognosis for ambulation based on sensory examination in patients who are initially motor complete. Arch. Phys. Med. Rehabil. 72, 119–121.

Collins, W., 1995. Surgery in the acute treatment of spinal cord injury: a review of the past forty years. J. Spinal Cord Med. 18, 3–8.

Curtis, K.A., Tyner, T.M., Zachary, L., et al., 1999. Effect of a standard exercise protocol on shoulder pain in long term wheelchair users. Spinal Cord 37, 421–429.

Dahlin, L.B., 2008. Techniques of peripheral nerve repair. Scand. J. Surg. 97 (4), 310–316.

David, O., Sett, P., Burr, R.G., et al., 1993. The relationship of heterotopic ossification to passive movements in paraplegic patients. Disabil. Rehabil. 15, 114–118.

Davis, G.M., Hamzaid, N.A., Fornusek, C., 2008. Cardiorespiratory, metabolic and biomechanical responses during functional electrical stimulation leg exercise: health and fitness benefits. Artif. Organs. 32 (8), 625–629.

Dennis, F., 1983. Three column spine and its significance in the classification of acute thoracolumbar spinal injuries. Spine 8, 817–831.

De Bruin, E.D., Frey-Rindova, P., Herzog, R.E., Dietz, V., Dambacher, M.A., Stussi, E., 1999. Changes of tibia bone properties after spinal cord injury: effects of early intervention. Arch. Phys. Med. Rehabil. 80 (Suppl. 2), 214–220.

De Troyer, A., Estenne, M., 1995. The Respiratory System in Neuromuscular Disorders. In: Roussos, C. (Ed.), The Thorax: Disease Edition: Part C. Marcel Dekker, pp. 2177–2317.

De Vivo, M.J., 2007. Trends in spinal cord injury rehabilitation outcomes from Model systems in the United States; 1973-2006. Spinal Cord 45, 713–721.

Ditunno, J.F., Young, W., Donovan, W.H., 1994. The International Standards booklet for neurological and functional classification of spinal cord injury. Paraplegia 32, 70–80.

Ditunno, J.F., Ditunno, P.L., Graziani, V., et al., 2000. Walking index for spinal cord injury (WISCI). An international multi centre validity and reliability study. Spinal Cord 38, 234–243. Revision: (WISCI II), 2001. Spinal Cord 39, 654–656.

Ditunno, J.F., Little, J.W., Tessler, A., et al., 2004. Spinal shock revisited: a four-phase model. Spinal Cord 42, 383–395.

Duysens, J., Van de Crommert, H.W.A. A., 1998. Neural control of locomotion: Part 1: The central pattern generator from cats to humans. Gait Posture 131–141.

Eng, J.J., Levins, S.M., Townson, A.F., et al., 2001. Use of prolonged standing for individuals with spinal cord injuries. Phys. Ther. 81 (8), 1392–1399.

Fawcett, J.W., Curt, A., Steeves, J.D., et al., 2007. Guidelines for the conduct of clinical trials for spinal cord injury as developed by the ICCP panel: spontaneous recovery after spinal cord injury and statistical power needed for therapeutic clinical trials. Spinal Cord 45 (3), 190–205. Epub 2006 Dec 19 (Review).

Fehlings, M.G., Perrin, R.G., 2006. The timing of sugical intervention the treatment of acute spinal cord injury: a systematic review of clinical evidence. Spine 31 (Suppl. 11), S28–S35.

Finley, M.A., Rodgers, M.M., Keyser, R., 2002. Impact of physical exercise on controlling secondary conditions associated with spinal cord injury. Neurology Report.

Foo, D., 1986. Spinal cord injury in forty four patients with cervical spondylosis. Paraplegia 24, 301–306.

Fowler, C.J., Fowler, C.G., 1993. Neurogenic bladder dysfunction and its management. In: Greenwood, R., Barnes, M.P., McMillian, T.M. et al., (Eds.), Neurological Rehabilitation. Churchill Livingstone, London, pp. 269–277.

Frey-Rindova, P., de Bruin, E.D., Stussi, E., et al., 2000. Bone Moneral density in Upper and Lower Extremities during 12 months after spinal cord injury measured by peripheral quantitative computed tomography. Spinal Cord 38 (Suppl. 1), 26–32.

Giangregorio, L., McCartney, N., 2006. Bone Loss and Muscle Atrophy in Spinal Cord Injury: Epidemiology, Fracture Prediction and Rehabilitation Strategies. J. Spinal Cord Med. 29 (5), 489–500.

Goemaere, S., Van Laere, M., De Nerve, P., et al., 1994. Bone mineral status in paraplegics patients who do not perform standing. Osteoporos. Int. 4, 138–143.

Golding, J.S., 1994. The mechanical factors which influence bone growth.

Eur. J. Clin. Nutr. 48 (Suppl. 1), S178–S185.

Grill, W.M., McDonald, J.W., Peckham, P.H., et al., 2001. At the interface: convergence of neural regeneration and neuroprostheses for restoration of function. J. Rehabil. Res. Dev. 38, 633–639.

Grillner, S., Wallen, P., 1985. Central pattern generators for locomotion, with special reference to vertebrates. Annu. Rev. Neurosci. 8, 233–261.

Grundy, D., Swain, A., 2002. ABC of Spinal Cord Injury, fourth ed. British Medical Journal Publications, London.

Hamilton, B.B., Granger, C.V., 1991. A Rehabilitation Uniform Data System. Buffalo Publications, New York.

Harrison, P., 2000. The First 48 Hours. Spinal Injuries Association, London.

Harvey, L., 2008. Management of Spinal Cord Injuries. Churchill Livingstone, Edinburgh.

Hough, A., 2001. Physiotherapy in Respiratory Care: An Evidence Based Approach to Respiratory Management and Cardiac Conditions, third ed. Nelson Thornes, Cheltenham.

Hossain, M., McLean, A., Fraser, M.H., 2004. Outcome of halo immobilisation of 104 cases of cervical spine injury. Scott. Med. J. 49 (3), 90–92.

Illis, L.S., 1988. Spinal Cord Dysfunction Assessment. Oxford University Press, Oxford.

Ivanhoe, C.B., Reistetter, T.A., 2004. Spasticity: The misunderstood part of the upper motor neuron syndrome. Am. J. Phys. Med. Rehabil. 83 (Suppl.), S3–S9.

Jackson, A.B., Groomes, T.E., 1994. Incidence of respiratory complications following spinal cord injury. Arch. Phys. Med. Rehabil. 75 (3), 270–275.

Jacobs, P.L., Nash, M.S., 2001. Modes, benefits and risks of voluntary and electrically induced exercise in persons with spinal cord injury. J. Spinal Cord Med. 24, 10–18.

Jiang, S.-D., Dai, L.-Y., Jiang, L.-S., 2006. Osteoporosis after a spinal cord injury. Osteoporos. Int. 17, 180–190.

Johnston, L., 2001. Human spinal cord injury: new and emerging approaches

to treatment. Spinal Cord 39, 609–613.

Kakulas, B.A., 2004. Neuropathology: the foundation for new treatments in spinal cord injury. Spinal Cord 42 (10), 549–563.

Kassioukov, A., Eng, J.J., Warburton, D., Teasell, R., 2009. A Systematic Review of the Management of Orthostatic Hypotension after Spinal Cord Injury. Arch. Phys. Med. Rehabil. 90 (5), 876–885.

Katoh, S., El Masry, W.S., 1995. Motor recovery of patients presenting with motor paralysis and sensory sparing following cervical spinal cord injury. Paraplegia 33, 506–509.

Kleim, J.A., 2009. Lennon, S., Stokes, M. (Eds.), Pocketbook of Neurological Physiotherapy. Churchill Livingstone, Edinburgh, pp. 41–50.

Ladouceur, M., Pepin, A., Norman, K.E., et al., 1997. Recovery of walking after spinal cord injury. Adv. Neurol. 72, 249–255.

Lammertse, D., Tuszynski, M.H., Steeves, J.D., et al., 2007. International Campaign for Cures of Spinal Cord Injury Paralysis. Guidelines for the conduct of clinical trials for spinal cord injury as developed by the ICCP panel: clinical trial design. Spinal Cord 45 (3), 232–242. Epub 2006 Dec 19 (Review).

Linder, S.H., 1993. Functional electrical stimulation to enhance cough in spinal cord injury. Chest 103, 166–169.

Little, J.W., Habur, E., 1985. Temporal course of motor recovery after Brown Séquard spinal cord injury. Paraplegia 23, 39–46.

Martindale: the complete drug reference, thirtyfifth ed 2007. Pharmaceutical Press, London.

Mc Donald, J.W., Becker, D., Sadowsky, M.D., et al., 2002. Late recovery following spinal cord injury. J. Neurosurg. (Spine2) 97, 252–265.

McKinley, W., Santos, K., Meade, M., et al., 2007. Incidence and outcomes of spinal cord injury clinical syndromes. J. Spinal Cord Med. 30 (3), 215–224.

Maynard, F.M., Reynolds, G.G., Fountain, S., et al., 1979. Neurological prognosis after traumatic quadraplegia, three years experience of California Regional Spinal Cord

Injury Care System. J. Neurosurg. 50, 611–616.

Medical Research Council (MRC) of the United Kingdom, 1978. Aids to Examination of the Peripheral Nervous System. Memorandum No 45. Palo Alto, Calif: Pedragon House.

Moore, E.E., Mattox, K.L., Feliciano, D.V., 1991. Trauma, second ed. Appleton & Lange, Connecticut.

Mouchnino, L., Aurenty, R., Massion, J., et al., 1992. Coordination between equilibrium and head-trunk orientation during leg movement: a new strategy build up by training. J. Neurophysiol. 67 (6), 1587–1598.

New, P.W., Sundrajan, V., 2008. Spinal Cord 46, 406–411.

Osenback, R.K., Menezes, A.M., 1992. Paediatric spinal cord and vertebral column injury. Neurosurgery 30, 385–390.

Pandyan, A.D., Gregoric, M., Barnes, M.P., Wood, D., Van Wijck, F., Burridge, J., Hermens, H., Johnson, G.R., 2005. Spasticity: clinical perceptions, neurological realities and meaningful measurement. Disabil. Rehabil. 27, 2–6.

Pope, P.M., 2002. Postural management and special seating. In: Edwards, S. (Ed.), Neurological Physiotherapy: A Problem Solving Approach. second ed. Churchill Livingstone, London, pp. 189–217.

Poynton, A.R., O'Farrel, D.A., Shannon, F., et al., 1997. Sparing of sensation to pinprick predicts motor recovery of a motor segment after injury to the spinal cord. J. Bone Joint Surg. Br. 79, 952–954.

Prochazka, A., Stephens, J.A., Wand, P., 1979. Muscle spindle discharge in normal and obstructed movements. J. Physiol. 287, 57–66.

Pryor, J.A., Webber, B.A., 1998. Physiotherapy for Respiratory and Cardiac Problems, second ed. Churchill Livingstone, Edinburgh.

Ragnarsson, K.T., 2008. Functional Electrical stimulation after spinal cord injury; current use, therapeutic effects and future direction. Spinal Cord 46, 255–274.

Ramer, M.S., Harper, G.P., Bradbury, E.J., 2000. Progress in spinal cord research. A refined strategy for the

International Spinal Research Trust. Spinal Cord 38, 449–472.

Reddy, H., Floyer, A., Donaghy, M., et al., 2001. Altered cortical activation with finger movements after peripheral denervation: comparison of active and passive tasks. Exp. Brain Res. 138 (4), 484–491.

Ronsyn, M.W., Berneman, Z.N., Van Tendeloo, V.F.I., et al., 2008. Can cell therapy heal a spinal cord injury. Spinal Cord 46, 532–539.

Satkunam, L.E., 2003. Rehabilitation medicine: 3. Management of adult spasticity. Can. Med. Assoc. J. 169 Review (11), 1173–1179.

Scott, J.A., Donovan, W.H., 1981. The prevention of shoulder pain and contracture in the acute tetraplegia patient. Paraplegia 19, 313–319.

Schepens, B., Stapley, P., Drew, T., 2008. Neurons in the pontomedullary reticular formation signal posture and movement both as an integrated behavior and independently. J. Neurophysiol. 100 (4), 2235–2253.

Schwartz, J.M., Begley, S., 2003. The Mind and the Brain: Neuroplasticity and the Power of Mental Force. Harper Collins, New York.

Shacklock, M., 2005. Clinical Neurodynamics: a new system of musculoskeletal treatment. Elsevier Health, London.

Sheean, G. (Ed.), 1998. Sasticity Rehabilitation. Churchill Communications Europe, London.

Short, D.J., Frankel, H.L., Bergström, E.M.K., 1992. Injuries of the Spinal Cord in Children. Elsevier Science, London.

Siddall, P.J., 2009. Management of neuropathic pain following spinal cord injury; now and in the future. Spinal Cord 47, 352–359.

Spinal Injuries Association (SIA), 2009. Preserving and developing the national spinal cord injury service. Research report May 2009. Spinal Injuries Association, London.

Smith, M., Ball, V., 1998. Cardiovascular/Respiratory Physiotherapy. Mosby, London.

Stauffer, E.S., 1983. Rehabilitation of posttraumatic cervical spinal cord quadraplegia and pentaplegia. In: The Cervical Spine. Lippincott, Philadelphia.

Steeves, J.D., Lammertse, D., Curt, A., et al., 2007. International Campaign for Cures of Spinal Cord Injury Paralysis. Guidelines for the conduct of clinical trials for spinal cord injury (SCI) as developed by the ICCP panel: clinical trial outcome measures. Spinal Cord 45 (3), 206–221. Epub 2006 Dec 19 (Review).

Stokes, E.K., 2009. Outcome measurement. In: Lennon, S., Stokes, M. (Eds.), Pocketbook of Neurological Physiotherapy. Churchill Livingstone, Edinburgh, pp. 192–201.

Tator, C.H., 1998. Biology of neurological recovery and functional restoration after spinal cord injury. Neurosurgery 42, 696–707.

Tuszynski, M.H., Steeves, J.D., Fawcett, J. W., et al., 2007. International Campaign for Cures of Spinal Cord Injury Paralysis. Guidelines for the conduct of clinical trials for spinal cord injury as developed by the ICCP Panel: clinical trial inclusion/exclusion criteria and ethics. Spinal Cord 45 (3), 222–231. Epub 2006 Dec 19 (Review).

Van Houtte, S., Vanlandewijke, Y., Gosselink, R., 2006. Respiratory muscle training in persons with spinal cord injury: a systematic review. Respir. Med.

Vogel, L.C., Anderson, C.J., 2003. Spinal Cord Injury in children and adolescents: a review. Spinal Cord Med. 26 (3), 193–203.

Waring, W.P., Maynard, F.M., 1991. Shoulder pain in acute traumatic quadraplegia. Paraplegia 29, 37–42.

Waters, R.L., Adkins, R.H., Yakura, J.S., et al., 1994a. Motor and sensory recovery following incomplete paraplegia. Arch. Phys. Med. Rehabil. 75, 67–72.

Waters, R.L., Adkins, R.H., Yakura, J.S., et al., 1994b. Motor and sensory recovery following incomplete tetraplegia. Arch. Phys. Med. Rehabil. 75, 306–311.

Walter, J.S., Sola, P.G., Sacks, J., et al., 1999. Indications for a home standing program for individuals with spinal cord injury. J. Spinal Cord Med. 22 (3), 152–158.

Whalley Hammell, K., 1995. Spinal Cord Injury Rehabilitation. Chapman & Hall, Canada.

Whiteneck, G.G., Charlifue, S.W., Gerhart, K.A., et al., 1992. Quantifying handicap: a new measure of long-term rehabilitation outcomes. Arch. Phys. Med. Rehabil. 73, 519–526.

Williams, P., 1995. Gray's anatomy, thirtyeighth ed. Churchill Livingstone, Edinburgh.

World Health Organization, 2001. International Classification of Functioning, Disability and Health. World Health Organization, Geneva. Available online at: http://www.who.int/classification/icf.

Zejdlik, C.P., 1992. Management of Spinal Cord Injury, second ed. Jones & Bartlett, Boston.

USEFUL WEBSITES

www.net.edu/nscisc.
www.asia-spinalinjury.org.
www.spinal.co.uk.
www.backuptrust.org.uk.

Chapter | 5 |

Multiple sclerosis

Lorraine De Souza, David Bates

CONTENTS

INTRODUCTION

Multiple sclerosis (MS) is the major cause of neurological disability in young and middle-aged adults. It is almost twice as common in women as in men, and though it can present at any age from childhood to the elderly, it has a peak incidence between the ages of 25 and 35 years. The impact of MS upon the lives of those affected can be enormous, partly because the course of the illness is unpredictable and partly because its effects and symptoms are so protean.

The course of the disease ranges from a single transient neurological deficit with full recovery to, in its most severe form, permanent disability being established within weeks or months of onset. Many people remain mobile and can live a near-normal life, but physiotherapists tend to see those whose lives are more seriously affected.

PATHOLOGY

MS is the principal member of a group of disorders known as 'demyelinating diseases'. Many conditions involve the process of demyelination as part of their disease pathology but the term 'demyelinating disease' is reserved for those conditions which have the immune-mediated destruction of myelin as the primary pathological finding, with relative sparing of other elements of central nervous system (CNS) tissue.

The other conditions that are part of this group are rare and may be variants of MS. They include:

- diffuse cerebral sclerosis of Schilder
- concentric sclerosis of Balo
- neuromyelitis optica of Devic
- the acute disseminated encephalomyelitides (ADEM), which may be postinfective or postvaccinal
- acute necrotizing haemorrhagic encephalomyelitis, which is probably due to herpes infection
- other demyelinating diseases with a known underlying infective or metabolic cause are now classified according to their specific pathology (Scolding, 2001).

The demonstration that a serum autoantibody present in neuromyelitis optic (Lennon et al., 2004), subsequently shown to be an IgG antibody binding to the aquaporin-4 water channel (Lennon et al., 2005), allows a clear distinction to be made between most people with MS and the majority of those whose clinical pattern involves the optic nerves and spinal cord. It is possible that better understanding of the pathology and immunology of the demyelinating diseases will result in the recognition and identification of other clinical sub-types of the disease.

Demyelination of nerve fibres

In the CNS, myelin is produced by oligodendrocytes (Shepherd, 1994). Each oligodendrocyte gives off a number of processes to ensheath surrounding axons. These processes, which envelope the axon, form a specialized membranous organelle – the myelin segment. A myelinated nerve fibre has many such myelin segments, all of

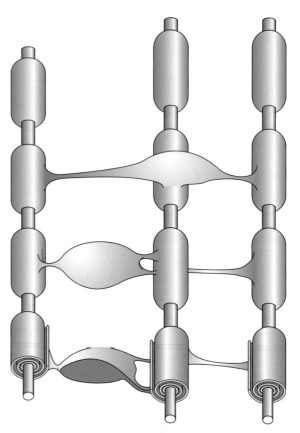

Figure 5.1 Myelinated nerve fibres in the central nervous system.

a similar size, arranged along its length. Between the myelinated segments there is an area of exposed axon known as the node of Ranvier. The myelin segment is termed the 'internode' (Figure 5.1). When an action potential is conducted along the axon, ionic transfer predominantly occurs across the axonal membrane at the node of Ranvier. The lipid-rich myelin of the internode insulates the axon and inhibits ionic transfer at the internode. This arrangement of segmental myelination allows rapid and efficient axonal conduction by the process of saltatory conduction where the signal spreads rapidly from one node of Ranvier to the next.

When myelin is lost the insulation fails and the action potential cannot be conducted normally and at speed along the nerve, the function of which thereby effectively ceases, even though the axon remains intact.

Distribution of plaques

Pathological examination of the brain and spinal cord reveals characteristic plaques of MS which are predominantly, though not exclusively, in the white matter where most myelin is deposited around the axons of the fibre tracts.

The lesions are random throughout the cerebral hemispheres, the brainstem, the cerebellum and the spinal cord, but there is a proponderance of lesions in the periventricular white matter, particularly at the anterior and posterior horns of the lateral ventricles, within the optic nerves and chiasm and in the long tracts of the spinal cord.

The microscopic appearance of a plaque depends upon its age. An acute lesion consists of a marked inflammatory reaction with perivenous infiltration of mononuclear cells and lymphocytes (Lucchinetti et al., 1996). There is destruction of myelin and degeneration of oligodendrocytes with relative sparing of the nerve cell body (neurone) and the axon. Axonal integrity may be disrupted early in the inflammatory process and may be the most important determinant of residual damage and disability (Trapp et al., 1998). In older lesions there is infiltration with macrophages (microglial phagocytes), proliferation of astrocytes and laying down of fibrous tissue. Ultimately this results in the production of an acellular scar of fibrosis which has no potential for remyelination or recovery.

It is suggested by some pathologists that the variation seen in the appearance of individual plaques indicates hetrogeneity in the underlying pathology and differing immunological causes of MS (Lucchinetti et al., 2000). Others, however, feel that the variability in lesions may represent only a temporal progression of the pathology and that varying lesions are within the same individual (Prineas et al., 2001). It is evident that the pathology in people with primary progressive MS (PPMS) differs from that seen in relapsing remitting disease (RRMS) (Bruck et al., 2003).

Remyelination

Remyelination can occur following an acute inflammatory demyelinating episode. There are, within the brain, oligodendroglial precursors which can mature into oligodendrocytes, infiltrate the demyelinated area and provide partial remyelination of axons (Prineas & Connell, 1978). This can be demonstrated in postmortem tissue and, though remyelination always appears thinner than the original myelin, it may allow functional recovery.

Axonal damage

It is now recognized that during the acute inflammatory phase of the disease axonal transection and damage occurs in the demyelinating plaque (Trapp et al., 1998). In the later stages of the disease, and in addition to the scarring which develops at the site of the inflammatory plaques, there is increasing damage to the axons which can be seen both at the site of the original inflammation and distant from the areas involved in the original inflammation. It is likely that this axonal damage is an important part of the pathology of MS and, though less well recognized and researched than demyelination, is probably responsible for the more progressive and chronic forms of the illness. This axonal loss can be demonstrated on magnetic resonance imaging (MRI) scans as atrophy of the brain white matter, ventricular dilatation, 'black holes' and degeneration of the long ascending and descending tracts of the brainstem and spinal cord. Brain atrophy is also the main morphological counterpart of psychological deficits and dementia occurring in people with MS (Loseff et al., 1996).

AETIOLOGY AND EPIDEMIOLOGY

Geographical prevalence

Epidemiological research into MS has been bedevilled by problems with ascertainment, identification of the baseline population to estimate prevalence, and the difficulty in interpreting minor changes in the small numbers of patients identified. Nonetheless, there appears to be a reproducible finding that the prevalence of MS varies with latitude (see Langton Hewer, 1993, for a review). In equatorial regions the disease is rare, with a prevalence of less than 1 per 100 000, whereas in the temperate climates of northern Europe and North America this figure increases to about 120 per 100 000 and in some areas as high as 200 per 100 000. In the UK it has a prevalence of about 80 000, affecting approximately 120 in every 100 000 of the population (O'Brien, 1987).

There is a similar, but less clearly defined relationship of increasing prevalence with latitude in the southern hemisphere. Some regions with the same latitude have widely differing prevalence of MS; Japan has a relatively lower incidence, whereas Israel has an unexpectedly high level; the two Mediterranean islands of Malta and Sicily have a 10-fold difference in prevalence. Studies within the USA appear to confirm this variation with latitude but may in part reflect genetic differences in the origin of the populations, predominantly derived from European Caucasians (Page et al., 1993).

Genetic influences

A familial tendency towards MS is now well established but no clear pattern of Mendelian inheritance has been found. Between 10 and 15% of people with MS have an affected relative, which is higher than expected from population prevalence. The highest concordance rate is for identical twins – about 30%; non-identical twins and siblings are affected in 3–5% of cases. Children of people with MS are affected in about 0.5% of cases (Ebers et al., 1986).

A genetic factor is supported by the excess of certain major histocompatibility (MHC) antigens in people with MS. Human leukocyte antigen (HLA) A_3 and B_7 are over-represented in people with MS and the HLA complex on chromosome 6 has been considered as the possible site of an MS 'susceptibility gene'. Systematic genome screening to attempt to define the number and location of susceptibility genes has been undertaken (Sawcer & Compston, 2003) and the most obvious candidates are DR(2)15 and DQ6, the former genotype is now defined as DRB1*1501, DRB5*0101 and the latter DQA1*0102, DQB2*0602. More recently assocation has been suggested with genes encoding the cytokines IL2 (Matesanz et al., 2004) and IL7 (Lundmark et al., 2007); almost all genes so far identified affect the immune system. Recently an axonal gene, KIF1B, has been identified to carry a susceptibility risk (Aulchenko et al., 2008). The probability is that, as in the case of diabetes mellitus, any genetic factor in MS is likely to involve several different genes and be complex (Compston, 2000).

Viral 'epidemic' theory

One other intriguing aspect of epidemiology of MS is the so-called 'epidemics' of MS occurring in the Faroes, the Orkney and Shetland Islands, and Iceland in the decades following the Second World War (Kurtzke & Hyllested, 1986). It was suggested that the occupation troops may have introduced an infective agent which, with an assumed incubation period of 2–20 years, resulted in the postwar 'epidemic'. It should be emphasized that despite extensive research no such infective agent has ever been isolated. Several factors influence the accuracy of such research and one or two errors in the numerator, when defining the base population, would make huge differences in the interpretation of the data.

Migration studies have lent support to the possibility of incomers adopting the risk and prevalence of MS closer to their host population. Studies have suggested that when migration occurs in childhood, the child assumes the risk of the country of destination, but these studies rely upon relatively small numbers of defined cases and interpretation is difficult (Dean & Kurtzke, 1971).

Summary

It is highly likely that MS is the product of both environmental and genetic factors. Exposure to some external agent, possibly viral, during childhood in those who are genetically susceptible results in the development of an autoimmune response against native myelin. When the blood–brain barrier is subsequently injured, often in the context of an infective illness, the autoimmunity can manifest, the myelin is attacked and the symptoms develop. Many autoimmune diseases are more common in women than men but whereas some commonly coexist, there is no evidence that other autoimmune diseases are more prevalent in people with MS than in the general population.

CLINICAL MANIFESTATIONS

There are different types of MS, which are classified in Table 5.1. The disease can run a benign course with many people able to lead a near-normal life with either mild or moderate disability.

The fundamental clinical characteristic of MS is that episodes of acute neurological disturbance, affecting non-contiguous parts of the CNS, are separated by periods of remission; attacks are disseminated in time and place. The disease can be progressive in nature and initially, resolution following a relapse is usually complete. Some attacks, however, do not recover completely, there remains some continuing disability and further attacks can leave the individual with increasing and permanent neurological disability.

The disease can enter a phase of secondary progression, in which deterioration occurs without evident exacerbations.

Rarely, particularly with the presentation of paraparesis in older males, the disease may be steadily progressive from the outset. This is termed 'primary progressive' multiple sclerosis.

Table 5.1 Classification of multiple sclerosis	
CLASSIFICATION	**DEFINITION**
Benign MS	One or two relapses, separated by some considerable time, allowing full recovery and not resulting in any disability
Relapsing remitting MS	Characterized by a course of recurrent discrete relapses, interspersed by periods of remission when recovery is either complete or partial
Secondary progressive MS	Having begun with relapses and remissions, the disease enters a phase of progressive deterioration, with or without identifiable relapses, where disability increases even when no relapse is apparent
Primary progressive MS	Typified by progressive and cumulative neurological deficit without remission or evident exacerbation
MS, multiple sclerosis.	

Table 5.2 Classification of multiple sclerosis according to certainty of diagnosis

Clinically definite MS	Two attacks and clinical evidence of two separate lesions Two attacks; clinical evidence of one lesion and paraclinical evidence of another separate lesion
Laboratory-supported definite MS	Two attacks; either clinical or paraclinical evidence of one lesion and CSF oligoclonal bands One attack; clinical evidence of two separate lesions and CSF oligoclonal bands One attack; clinical evidence of one lesion and paraclinical evidence of another, separate lesion and CSF oligoclonal bands
Clinically probable MS	Two attacks and clinical evidence of one lesion One attack and clinical evidence of two separate lesions One attack; clinical evidence of one lesion and paraclinical evidence of another, separate lesion
Laboratory-supported probable MS	Two attacks and CSF oligoclonal bands

Paraclinical evidence is derived from magnetic resonance imaging, computed tomographic scanning or evoked potentials measurement. CSF, cerebrospinal fluid; MS, multiple sclerosis.

MS can also be classified according to the certainty of diagnosis (Table 5.2). It should always be remembered that the diagnosis is one of exclusion; haematological and biochemical investigations are essential to rule out other confounding diseases and, during the course of the disease, the physician must always be willing to reconsider the possibility of differential diagnosis. The classification of disease by the certainty of the diagnosis is of predominant importance for the inclusion of patients into drug trials and for epidemiological studies (McDonald et al., 2001; Poser et al., 1983). Recently an updated classification of diagnostic criteria has been produced (Polman et al., 2005) and this is currently being assessed.

Early signs and symptoms

It is a common misconception that the first attack of MS strikes as a 'bolt out of the blue', in a young adult previously in good health. In fact, a careful history will often reveal vague feelings of ill health over the preceding months or years, often taking the form of sensory disturbances, aches, pains and lethargy. Not uncommonly there is a history which clearly suggests a previous episode of demyelination, such as the symptom of double vision, blurring of vision or blindness, rotational vertigo or weakness. Such episodes have often been dismissed as trivial by the patient and, as such, are poorly remembered and may not have caused the person to seek advice from the general practitioner. Demyelination can occur anywhere throughout the white matter of the CNS and, therefore, the initial presentation of MS is extremely variable.

Visual symptoms

- Visual loss
- Double vision.

The most common single symptom in presentation is of acute or subacute visual loss in one, or rarely both, eyes. Twenty-five per cent of patients will present in this way, often with pain or discomfort in the eye and the classical symptom of a lesion in an optic nerve (optic neuritis or retrobulbar neuritis) is of loss of colour vision of the eye followed by blurring and ultimately by a central scotoma (blind spot) and visual loss. Improvement usually begins spontaneously within days to weeks; in about 30% of cases recovery will be complete but the remainder will be aware of some reduction in visual acuity or of the brightness of their vision. Following an episode of optic neuritis, the optic disc becomes pale and atrophic (optic atrophy). More than one-half of those presenting with optic neuritis will go on to develop other signs of MS. Those who do not may have had a single episode of inflammatory demyelination or they may have some other disease entity.

Double vision (diplopia) is a particularly common presenting complaint and may be due to weakness of muscles innervated by the third, fourth or sixth cranial nerves, or the connections between their nuclei in the brainstem. A very characteristic abnormality is an internuclear ophthalmoplegia due to a lesion of the medial longitudinal fasciculus, in which there is failure of adduction of the adducting eye on lateral gaze with nystagmus in the abducting eye. When a bilateral internuclear ophthalmoplegia is seen in the young adult this is virtually diagnostic of MS.

Neurological deficit

The second most common presenting symptom is a clearly defined episode of neurological deficit, that may occur alone or with others, such as:

- weakness
- numbness
- unsteadiness, imbalance, clumsiness
- slurred speech
- nystagmus

- intention tremor
- trigeminal neuralgia.

Weakness, numbness or tingling can affect one or more limbs. Symptoms may develop acutely over minutes or chronically over weeks to months, but more typically they evolve over hours or days. Such a presentation, with or without sphincter involvement, usually indicates an area of spinal demyelination. Lhermitte's phenomenon, which is the sensation of shooting, electric-shock-like sensations radiating down the back and into the legs when the neck is flexed, is a symptom of cervical cord irritation and is commonly described when there is demyelination within the cervical spinal cord.

Not infrequently the disease may begin with the signs and symptoms of cerebellar dysfunction causing unsteadiness, imbalance, clumsiness and dysarthria (slurring of speech). Examination may reveal the patient to have nystagmus (a jerky movement of the eyes), an intention tremor (see Ch. 4) and a cerebellar dysarthria, the combination of which is termed Charcot's triad and is one of the classical features of MS. These symptoms are due to demyelination occurring within the brainstem and there are a wide variety of brainstem syndromes causing cranial nerve disturbances and long tract signs. Other clues are the development of trigeminal neuralgia, or tic douloureux (sharp facial pains), in young adults suggesting the presence of a lesion within the brainstem.

Possible signs and symptoms in the course of multiple sclerosis

A number of symptoms and signs can become established and can be severe, although many can occur at any stage of the disease. These include:

- fatigue
- optic atrophy – with associated visual symptoms
- ophthalmoplegia – with facial sensory and motor symptoms
- cerebellar disease causing nystagmus, ataxia and tremor
- muscle hypertonia
- muscle weakness
- brisk reflexes
- impaired walking ability
- sphincter disturbances
- sexual dysfunction
- psychiatric and psychological disturbances
- symptoms being exacerbated by heat and cold.

General weakness and fatigue are almost invariable symptoms, and fatigue may indeed be the presenting symptom in people with MS. There is often optic atrophy with associated decreased visual acuity, a central scotoma or large blind spot and pupillary abnormalities. There may be bilateral internuclear ophthalmoplegia with facial sensory disturbance, or weakness, and a brisk jaw jerk,

with slurring speech. There is usually evidence of cerebellar disease with nystagmus, ataxia and tremor which, in its most severe form (dentatorubral) can be incapacitating such that any attempt to move the limbs precipitates violent uncontrollable movements and prevents mobility and feeding. In the limbs there is usually increased tone and weakness in a pyramidal distribution. The reflexes are pathologically brisk; the plantar responses are extensor. Walking is usually affected due to progressive weakness, spasticity and ataxia, and the combination of spasticity and ataxia is suggestive of inflammatory demyelination. Many people will rely on walking aids and a significant proportion will need a wheelchair.

When there is disease affecting the spinal cord, symptoms of sphincter disturbances are common. These range from mild urgency and frequency of micturition to acute retention of urine, constipation and incontinence. Sexual dysfunction is common with erectile and ejaculatory difficulties in men and loss of libido in women. Modern prospective studies of the effect of pregnancy in MS are reassuring and there is no reason to suggest that families should be limited. During pregnancy, the patient has a statistically lower likelihood of relapse, though this may be counterbalanced by a slight increase early in the puerperium.

Psychiatric and psychological disturbances are common (see Ch. 17). Depression is the most common affective disturbance in MS and may compound the underlying physical problems, exaggerating symptoms of lethargy and reduced mobility. With diffuse disease some people develop frank dementia, a few become psychotic and epileptic seizures are seen in 2–3% of cases, an increase of four to five times over that of the normal population. Patients can show evidence of emotional instability or affective disturbance. Euphoria, or inappropriate cheerfulness, was said to be a classical feature of the disease but this is now considered a myth. It is, in practice, quite rare and probably occurs when lesions affect the subcortical white matter of the frontal lobes, resulting in an effective leucotomy.

Patients will frequently record an increase in their symptoms with exercise and with a rise in body temperature. The physiology behind these symptoms is probably the same, due to the fact that the propagation of an action potential along a neurone is greatly affected by temperature. Nerve conduction in an area of demyelination can be critical and paradoxically an increase in temperature, which normally improves conduction, may, in the demyelinated axon, result in a complete conduction block. This phenomenon of worsening of symptoms with exercise and increased temperature is Uhthoff's phenomenon and is most dramatically manifest when patients describe how they are able to get into a hot bath but not able to extricate themselves. Patients should be warned to avoid extremes of temperature and overexertion to avoid this increase in symptoms (Costello et al., 1996).

DIAGNOSIS

To make a clinical definitive diagnosis of MS there has to be a history of two attacks and evidence, clinically, of two separate lesions (Poser et al., 1983). It is also important to remember that other diagnoses should be excluded and, since at presentation all these criteria may not be fulfilled, corroborative paraclinical, laboratory and radiological evidence is usually sought (see O'Connor, 2002, for a review).

Magnetic resonance imaging

MRI of the head and spinal cord is extremely useful in demonstrating the lesions of MS (see Figure 2.2 in Ch. 2). Typically, high signal lesions on T2-weighted sequences are seen throughout the white matter. Gadolinium enhancement demonstrates areas of active inflammation with breakdown in the blood–brain barrier, which are associated with an acute relapse (Paty et al., 1988). In particular circumstances, as with acute optic neuritis or cervical myelopathy, the demonstration on an MRI scan of disseminated asymptomatic lesions is particularly helpful in confirming the diagnosis and there are rigid criteria for interpreting the MRI scan changes. Newer techniques, such as fluid-attentuated inversion recovery (FLAIR) and magnetization transfer imaging (MTI), improve the sensitivity and selectivity of MRI in MS (Filippi et al., 1998).

Lumbar puncture

Analysis of the cerebrospinal fluid (CSF) in a patient suspected of having MS is valuable diagnostically. There is production of immunoglobulin (mainly IgG) within the CNS and these antibodies are detected by biochemical analysis of the CSF. Electrophoresis of the CSF allows the immunoglobulin fraction to separate into a few discrete bands (oligoclonal bands) and simultaneous analysis of the immunoglobulin from the blood can demonstrate that these antibodies are confined to the CNS and, therefore, provide confirmatory evidence of inflammatory CNS disease (Tourtellotte & Booe, 1978).

The antigens that provoke this antibody response have not been identified, nor is it known whether the response is integral to the underlying pathogenic process or a 'bystander reaction'. The CSF normally contains very few cells but during an acute exacerbation of MS there may be an increase in the lymphocytes in the CSF. The level of protein in the CSF is slightly raised but the level of sugar is normal. CSF examination is important in helping to differentiate other diseases from MS and is one of the prerequisites to making a diagnosis of primary progressive MS.

Evoked potentials

A typical history, the signs of more than one lesion affecting the CNS, together with disseminated white-matter lesions shown on MRI and the presence of unmatched oligoclonal bands in the CSF, puts the diagnosis beyond reasonable doubt. However, when one or more of these findings are inconclusive further support for the diagnosis may be obtained by evoked potential (EP) testing (Misulis, 1993) (Figure 5.2). These tests, which include visual, brainstem auditory and somatosensory evoked potentials (VEP, BAEP, SSEP) may provide evidence of a subclinical lesion, which has previously been undetected (Halliday & McDonald, 1977). For example, the finding of abnormal SSEPs from both legs, in a patient presenting with blindness in an eye, strongly suggests a lesion in the spinal cord and raises the possibility of MS. The demonstration of more than one lesion is essential in making a secure diagnosis of MS.

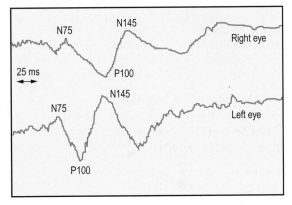

Figure 5.2 Evoked potentials (EP). A visual EP: study showing the typical prolonged latency and poor waveform in a lesion of the right optic nerve, such as potic neuritis, in a patient with multiple sclerosis.

THE MANAGEMENT OF MULTIPLE SCLEROSIS

Not all MS patients require active intervention but even those with mild symptoms should be given support and advice from appropriate professionals, relevant to the patient's condition and circumstances. Interventions available for those with moderate to severe disabilities mainly involve drug therapy and physiotherapy. For a recent review of the management of MS, see O'Connor (2002).

There is no proven benefit from any dietary restrictions, though there is suggestive evidence that diets low in animal fat and high in vegetable oil and fish-body oil have potential benefits (Klaus, 1997; Payne, 2001).

Breaking the news

The neurology outpatient clinic is full of people with a history of episodic neurological symptoms, particularly sensory disturbances. The decision to investigate depends upon the individual presentation, consideration of the evidence for relapses, the clinical and objective evidence for multiple sites of disease, and the suspicion of the physician. Anxious, polysymptomatic patients with normal neurological examination would not usually be investigated for the possibility of MS and, although the symptom of fatigue is common in MS, it may also be a physiological symptom which is heightened by the presence of depression.

At present many neurologists, jointly with their patients, prefer not to investigate a single resolved attack, especially when there are no objective signs. However, if early treatment with disease-modifying therapies can reduce long-term disability, then the threshold for investigating such patients will be lowered.

The diagnosis of MS is in part the exclusion of other diagnoses, but when the clinical conditions and the laboratory and imaging tests support the diagnosis, then such should be discussed with the patient with the aim of reducing the initial shock and giving an optimistic picture of the prognosis. Once the diagnosis of MS has been intimated, it is important that individuals have time to ask questions and be given the necessary information, often in the form of literature or videos, to enable them to formulate their questions. It is here that the role of an MS specialist nurse is so vital; he or she can visit the patient at home, provide more time than is possible for the physician and hopefully answer many of the relevant questions.

Drug therapy

Many patients with MS do not require drug therapy but when they do, there are three treatment options (see Ch. 28):

1. Drug management of an acute exacerbation, e.g. steroids
2. Symptomatic drug therapy to alleviate individual problems, e.g. antispasticity drugs
3. Use of disease-modifying therapies to reduce the underlying pathological process, e.g. interferons.

Since MS is an incurable condition, drug treatments aim primarily to manage acute episodes and specific symptoms. The disease-modifying therapies are, at best, only partially effective to date.

The management of the acute exacerbation

Corticosteroids hasten recovery from an acute exacerbation of MS and improve rehabilitation. The most commonly used agent is intravenous methylprednisolone (Martindale, 2007).

Steroids have many significant and potentially serious side-effects, including aseptic necrosis of the femoral head, immunosuppression, sugar intolerance, osteoporosis, weakness of muscles and even psychosis, all of which may be deleterious to the patient with MS. The most important side-effects are dose-related and guidelines for frequency should be followed.

There is some evidence that the use of steroids in early acute symptoms of MS, specifically optic neuritis, may retard the development of MS during the next 2 years (Beck et al., 1993). However, the use of long-term steroids has no effect on the natural history of the disease and the risks outweigh any benefit.

Symptomatic drug therapy

The effective use of symptomatic agents is intended to make the life of the person with MS more tolerable (Thompson, 2001).

Spasticity

One of the most common symptoms of MS is spasticity, often in association with painful cramps and spasms. There are a number of effective agents available, some working at a central level, others peripherally. Baclofen is a GABA-receptor agonist and acts centrally by inhibiting transmission at the spinal level. It reduces tone but may thereby reveal weakness and always needs to be titrated in the individual patient. Its most common side-effects are those of more widespread depression of the CNS, such as drowsiness and sedation. It should always be remembered that legs with hypertonic muscles are weak and a degree of spasticity may have a beneficial splinting action, which aids mobility. The use of baclofen, together with physiotherapy, is often most beneficial. When more intractable spasticity is present, baclofen may be given intrathecally via an implanted subcutaneous pump and the smaller dose thereby required has the advantage of reducing side-effects.

Tizanidine (Zanaflex) is another centrally acting agent which is less sedating and has less of an underlying effect on muscle than baclofen but is potentially hepatotoxic (Martindale, 2007). Again it must be used by titration against the symptoms and spasticity in the individual patient and is used together with physiotherapy to improve mobility.

Dantrolene sodium reduces contraction of skeletal muscles by a direct action on excitation–contraction coupling, decreasing the amount of calcium released from the sarcoplasmic reticulum. Its action is more pronounced on the fast fibres in the muscle, which results in a diminution of reflex activity and spasticity rather than voluntary contraction. It is therefore theoretically less likely to cause the side-effect of weakness but its major side-effect is of generalized fatigue.

Benzodiazepines, such as diazepam and clonazepam, may have a role to play in the management of spasticity, though they are more likely than other agents to result in drowsiness and are therefore most useful for night-time spasms and cramps when their sedation is advantageous.

In severe painful spasticity, where the aim is to alleviate the distressing symptoms or to aid nursing care rather than to restore function, there are a number of more invasive procedures which may be useful. Local injection of botulinum toxin causes a flaccid paralysis in the muscles injected, with minimal systemic side-effects. The effect usually lasts for 3 months and may be repeated indefinitely (Snow et al., 1990). More graduated doses of the toxin can improve mobility in people with less severe spasticity. The more destructive techniques of intrathecal or peripheral nerve chemical blocks, or surgery are now rarely required.

When treating the symptom of spasticity it is important to remember that it may often be worsened by triggers such as constipation or underlying infection, particularly urinary tract infection or decubitus ulceration. Infective causes should be sought and treated whenever spasticity appears unexpectedly or worsens.

Pain

People with MS develop pain for a variety of reasons, some of which are central and some peripheral. Plaques affecting the ascending sensory pathways frequently cause unpleasant dysaesthesiae, or allodynia, on the skin, often with paraesthesiae. Such central pain is most responsive to centrally acting analgesics, such as the antiepileptics carbamazepine, sodium valproate or gabapentin. It may also respond to tricyclic antidepressants, such as amitriptyline or dothiepin. Alternatively, electrostimulation with cutaneous nerve stimulation (see Ch. 12) or dorsal column stimulation (Tallis et al., 1983) can be effective.

The second cause of pain is the spasms described as part of spasticity in the previous section. The third is that the abnormal posture, so often adopted by people using walking aids or in wheelchairs, itself results in pain and discomfort in the back and limbs. These symptoms are often best helped with physiotherapy and simple analgesics.

The lancinating neuralgic pains, such as trigeminal neuralgia, may respond to antiepileptic therapy with carbamazepine or gabapentin but they can also be helped by steroids, particularly if occurring in the course of an acute exacerbation. If these agents are not effective, then trigeminal neuralgia may respond to surgical intervention; a lesion is placed within the Gasserian ganglion.

Cannabis is thought to be helpful for MS patients but is not used widely and is currently under investigation. Principles of pain management are discussed in Chapter 16.

Bladder, bowel and sexual dysfunction

These symptoms, which often occur in combination, are due to spinal cord disease and have a major impact upon the patient (see Barnes, 1993, for a review).

Bladder disturbance

Pelvic floor exercises may help in women and the combination of clean intermittent self-catheterization (CISC) and the use of anticholinergic agents, such as oxybutinin or tolterodine, usually helps to overcome the problem of incomplete emptying and hyperreflexia, which are the common causes of this syndrome. The most appropriate approach to bladder management is to recognize the common symptoms of urgency and frequency, and to measure residual urine by ultrasound after the patient has passed urine and if this is greater than 100 ml, educate the patient in CISC and prescribe a bladder relaxant. If there is less than 100 ml residual then the use of a bladder relaxant alone is probably sufficient.

When nocturnal frequency and enuresis cause a problem, the synthetic diuretic desmopressin (DDAVP) may be used but care should be taken to avoid hyponatraemia (low serum sodium), particularly in the elderly.

When there is severe bladder spasticity, the intravesical installation of the neurotoxic agent botulinum toxin may reduce detrusor hyperreflexia.

It is rare now to require permanent catheterization but, when necessary, this is better provided by the suprapubic route and ultimately urinary diversion may be necessary.

Bowel disturbances

Constipation is the most common symptom but it may be complicated by faecal incontinence intermittently. A bowel-training programme is usually most successful with the use of iso-osmotic laxatives and ensuring adequate fibre intake.

Sexual dysfunction

Erectile dysfunction in men is a common problem and is now helped by the use of sildenafil, which has been demonstrated, in a randomized placebo controlled trial, to be effective (DasGupta & Fowler, 2003). Alternative methods are still available, but the use of intracorporeal papaverine has now been replaced by prostaglandin.

In women there are many factors which may affect the expression of sexuality, including neurological symptoms from sacral segments, such as diminished genital sensitivity, reduced orgasmic capacity and decreased lubrication (Hulter & Lundberg, 1995).

Both sexes are affected by leg spasticity, ataxia, vertigo and fatigue. Counselling may be appropriate in some cases and referral to a specialist counselling service, such as SPOD, may be useful (see Appendix 2 'Associations & Support Groups').

Fatigue

Almost all patients with MS will, at some time, complain of fatigue and in the majority of cases it is regarded as being the most disabling symptom. Pharmacological treatment is disappointing, though amantidine and pemoline have been suggested to be beneficial. Other agents used in the past have now been replaced by the less addictive modafinil. Reassurance and graded exercise programmes are considered to be at least as effective (see 'Physical management', below). There has been the recent suggestion that use of a long acting form of 4 aminopyridine, a sodium channel blocker, has a benefit in reducing fatigue (Goodman et al., 2008).

Tremor

The treatment of tremor in MS, as in most other situations, is difficult (see Ch. 14). Minor action tremors may be helped by the use of beta-blockers, such as propranolol, or low-dose barbiturates such as primidone. The more disabling intention tremor of cerebellar disease and the most disabling dentatorubral thalamic tremor, which prevents any form of movement or activity, is refractory to treatment. There have been reports of agents such as clonazepam, carbamazepine and choline chloride helping individuals, and by serendipity, the antituberculous agent isoniazid has been shown to be effective but should be given with a vitamin B_6 supplement. None of these treatments are particularly effective and the possibility of deep brain stimulation is now being increasingly considered. Surgical treatments are most effective for unilateral tremor; bilateral treatment is associated with significant morbidity and mortality.

Psychological symptoms

Depression is the most common symptom and, if clinically significant, requires treatment with antidepressant medication, either a tricyclic agent or a selective serotonin reuptake inhibitor (Martindale, 2007). Cognitive dysfunction is reported to occur in up to 60% of patients. Psychological issues and behavioural management are discussed in Chapter 17.

Epilepsy

Epilepsy is rare in MS but more common than in a peer group. It is treated with anticonvulsants. Electroencephalography (EEG) will identify unrelated primary generalized epilepsy, but most seizures in MS are focal and may cause secondary generalization.

Disease-modifying therapies

Three forms of immunomodulatory therapy, beta-interferon, glatiramer acetate and natalizumab, are licensed and have been shown in large controlled, randomized clinical trials to be effective in reducing the frequency and severity of relapses and delaying the development of disability in people with relapsing remitting MS. Immunosuppressive therapy has also received much attention. For a review of disease-modifying therapies, see Corboy et al. (2003).

Interferon-β

Interferons are naturally occurring polypeptides produced by the body in response to viral infection and inflammation. There are three types, alpha (α), beta (β) and gamma (γ), all of which have antiviral, antiproliferative and immunomodulatory properties. All have been tried in MS because of the postulation that the disease might have a viral origin. Interferon α may have some effect, but requires further study; interferon γ has been shown to be deleterious. Interferon β, however, has been shown to be beneficial.

An initial trial, giving interferon β by intrathecal route, showed a reduction in attack rate and was followed by a large trial in North America using the bacterially derived product interferon β-1b (IFBN Multiple Sclerosis Study Group, 1993). This showed that high doses of interferon β-1b, given subcutaneously on alternate days, reduced clinical relapses by one-third over 2 years as compared to placebo. There was a dramatic reduction in the changes seen on the MRI scans in the treated group but the study was not powered to show an effect upon progression of disability (Paty & Li, 1993).

Subsequent studies using a mammalian cell-line-derived interferon β-1a have shown benefit, in both frequency of attack and in development of disability (Jacobs et al., 1996; PRISMS Study Group, 1998), and three agents are now available:

1. The original interferon β-1b (Betaferon)
2. The subcutaneous interferon β-1a given thrice-weekly (Rebif)
3. The intramuscular form of interferon β-1a (Avonex), given once-weekly

These agents are licensed for use in relapsing remitting MS and a national trial is underway in the UK to compare the different agents in a novel 'risk-sharing scheme', in which the proof of efficiency in reducing attack rate and disability, as well as in cost-effectiveness, is being studied.

There are common side-effects of injection site reactions and flu-like symptoms; the latter are ameliorated by the use of non-steroidal anti-inflammatory agents. A variable number of patients, between 4 and 40%, may develop antibodies to the interferon, though the effect of these antibodies is still under review.

The effect of the agents in people with secondary progressive disease only appears to be beneficial in those who have acute exacerbations occurring in addition to their progressing disease (European Study Group on Interferon β-1b in Secondary Progressive Multiple Sclerosis, 1998) and to date there has been no benefit shown in people with primary progressive illness. The use of these immunosuppressive agents may be effective only in that phase of the disease proven to be inflammatory and immune-mediated, and not in the phase of more prolonged axonal injury to the CNS.

Glatiramer acetate

The synthetic polypeptide glatiramer acetate made to imitate part of the antigenic area of myelin basic protein, and therefore to block the effect of putative antibodies upon the disease process, has been shown to be effective in reducing relapse rate and improving disability in a randomized controlled clinical trial (Johnson et al., 1995). It has to be taken parenterally (Martindale, 2007). It is well tolerated, freer from side-effects than the interferons and is now widely licensed for use in relapsing remitting MS. There is less evidence about its effectiveness in secondary progressive disease and a trial in primary progressive disease showed it was without effect.

Natalizumab

The monoclonal antibody natalizumab, which blocks adhesion molecules on the endothelial surface of blood vessels, thereby preventing the ingress of activated T-cells to the central nervous system, has been shown to be more effective than the standard disease modifying therapies (Polman et al., 2006). Shortly after the agent was first licensed, two patients who had taken part in a study in North America, in which natalizumab and interferon ß1a was compared with interferon ß-1a alone, were reported to have developed the opportunistic infection progressive multi-focal leukoencephalopathy (PML) due to JC virus which is present in more than 80% of normal individuals. The drug was therefore withdrawn for a time, but has been re-launched since 2007 and there have been three further reports of PML. The regulatory authorities currently limit the use of this monoclonal antibody to patients with rapidly evolving, severe relapsing remitting MS or those who have failed to respond to a full and adequate course of ß interferon.

Immunosuppression

Despite our incomplete understanding of the pathogenesis of MS, there is strong circumstantial evidence of an autoimmune process. There is increasing interest in treating MS with immunosuppression and cytotoxic agents ranging from azathioprine, methotrexate and cyclophosphamide to cyclosporin A and total lymphoid irradiation. There is even a trial of bone marrow transplantation, but it remains a research tool (Fassas et al., 2002). With each of these agents, some claims of initial success have been encouraging but have not generally stood up to more rigorous trials. A great difficulty in assessing the effectiveness of such treatments in MS is the unpredictable progression of the disease and the possibility of a placebo effect (Goodin et al., 2002).

Despite such reservations, immunosuppressive agents are used worldwide and a recent meta-analysis suggested that the use of azathioprine shows a modest reduction in both attack rate and in the rate of progression of the disease (Yudkin et al., 1991). It is recognized that 6 months is necessary for the agent to show its therapeutic effect. These agents are usually reserved for patients with a particularly malignant form of MS and in whom other treatments have not prevented relentless progression.

Cyclophosphamide has been commonly used in some parts of Europe and North America but it is difficult to evaluate in a double-blind fashion because of its marked side-effects (Weiner et al., 1993) and it is not used widely in the UK because of its toxicity.

Methotrexate has also been used and shown to have some effect on retarding the rate of progression in patients with progressive disease (Goodkin et al., 1995), but further corroborative evidence should be obtained.

The most recent arrival in the field of treatment of progressing disease is mitoxantrone (Hartung et al., 2002). This potentially cardiotoxic drug (Ghalie et al., 2002a) is given in boluses at intervals over a period of years. Again, it is necessary to monitor carefully white cells, since it significantly suppresses the T cells (Ghalie et al., 2002b), but it does have some beneficial effect and despite a risk of acute leukaemia it is widely used.

New therapies

Apart from the monoclonal antibodies, several agents are now in phase III trials and will be expected to produce results from 2010 onwards. They include: the sphingosine-1-phosphate receptor agonist fingolimod, which sequestrates lymphocytes in the peripheral lymphoid tissues; the dihydro-orotate dehydrogonase inhibitor teriflunomide, which is an immunomodulator shown to be effective in experimental allergic encephalomyelitis; the synthetic purine nucleoside analogue cladribine which depletes T-cells; and fumaric acid (BG12). There are also drugs under earlier study including lacquinomod which is cytotoxic, and firategrast and UCB232, both of which block adhesion molecules with an action similar to natalizumab. All of these agents have the advantage that they can be taken orally.

Studies are underway with other monoclonal antibodies, alemtuzumab directed against the receptor CD52, which depletes all white blood cells; daclizumab directed against the IL2 receptor which suppresses T-cell replication; and Rituximab directed against CD20 which depletes B-cells. All of these agents show promise; all appear to have greater effects on the immune system than current therapies and therefore potential complications with intercurrent infections, opportunistic infections and possibly other and far reaching immune effects, will need careful study and monitoring. The advantage of these agents, which have to be given parenterally, is that they are effective for a relatively long time and infusions may be as infrequent as once a year. All carry the possibility of antibody formation and the risk of infusion reactions.

All currently licensed therapies and most in trial are directed toward the initial inflammatory phase of the disease and are most effective in RRMS. There is little therapeutic benefit for those with SPMS and no treatment has been shown to affect PPMS. In future it is possible the most effective immunomodulating agents used early in the disease may have a neuroprotective effect, and specific neuroprotective agents will be sought. In addition new processes using stem cells and directed monoclonal antibodies and small molecules may encourage or permit remyelination and repair.

PHYSICAL MANAGEMENT

People with MS are often referred for physiotherapy, or request it for themselves, when they experience loss of movement skill or the ability to perform functional activities. Not all patients deteriorate to this degree but if they reach this stage, the disease has caused irreversible damage to the CNS and created a level of impairment which results in noticeable and persistent disability. This section focuses on progressive conditions but the MS Healthcare Standards (Freeman et al., 1997a, 2001) recommend early intervention for those with mild impairment (see below).

The attitude of the physiotherapist towards the person with MS during their initial encounters is crucial, as it will set the scene for the therapist–patient relationship and any ensuing programme of physiotherapy. The patient may fear that the therapist could expose further physical weaknesses and insufficiencies. Physiotherapists need to be aware that the same professional skills that can help the patient can also undermine self-confidence.

The success of treatment should not be determined by whether or not the patient improves, but rather by whether he or she achieves the best level of activity, relevant to lifestyle, at each stage of the disease (De Souza, 1990) and whether the patient's own goals have been reached. In order to achieve this, the treatment of those with MS is best approached with a philosophy of care (Ashburn & De Souza, 1988).

Approaches to physiotherapy

Physiotherapy for those with MS acts mainly at the level of function and activity and is unlikely to modify the lesions or change the progression of the disease. For the majority of people with MS, it is likely that physiotherapy will be one of several treatments and should, therefore, address the issues of disability within the context of the aims of other treatments and the needs of the individual. In addition, people with MS are likely to be engaged in several self-help activities they value and therapy should build on this motivation (O'Hara et al., 2000).

An approach to physiotherapy that views the individual in his or her social, family, work and cultural roles informs the physiotherapist about the impact of disablement on the individual's lifestyle. This is important in the case of MS as it mostly affects young adults who, when diagnosed, will face an average of 35–42 years living with this disease (Poser et al., 1989). A shift in focus away from problems and towards a more positive attitude, which considers disablement as just one of a variety of ways in which a normal life may be pursued, has been called for (Oliver, 1983). An understanding of the priorities of individuals with disability, the value they attach to different activities and their choices for conducting their lives should have a profound influence on the physiotherapy provided (Williams, 1987).

The approach to physiotherapy should therefore be patient-centred, with the patient taking an active participatory role in treatment. This will include consultation for joint decision-making and goal-setting, the opportunity to exercise choice and the provision of information so that the patient has feedback on progress and knowledge of his or her level of ability.

Principles of physiotherapy

Treatment plans should be flexible and responsive to the needs of the patient as they change over time. Although each patient should be considered as an individual, Ingle et al. (2002) have determined what deterioration might be expected over a 2-year period in progressive MS, in terms of the Kurtzke Scale (Kurtzke, 1983), walking ability (10-m timed walk), and upper-limb ability (nine-hole peg-test). Therapy should encompass not only the changes due to progression of MS, but also life changes such as employment, pregnancy and childbirth, parenthood and ageing. The principles of physiotherapy have been described by Ashburn and De Souza (1988) and further by De Souza (1990). These include:

- encourage development of strategies of movement
- encourage learning of motor skills
- improve the quality of patterns of movement
- minimize abnormalities of muscle tone
- emphasize the functional application of physiotherapy
- provide support to maintain motivation and cooperation, and reinforce therapy
- implement preventive therapy
- educate the person towards a greater understanding of the symptoms of MS and how they affect daily living.

Four primary aims of physiotherapy were also identified:

1. Maintain and increase range of movement (ROM)
2. Encourage postural stability
3. Prevent contractures
4. Maintain and encourage weight-bearing.

The underlying principle for all the above is one of building on, and extending, the patient's abilities. Emphasis during assessment and treatment should be on what the individual can and does achieve, rather than on what he or she fails to achieve.

Assessment

Assessment is discussed in Chapter 3 but aspects of specific importance to MS will be addressed here.

Fatigue

As mentioned above, fatigue is a well-documented symptom of MS; it is reported to occur in 78% of patients (Freal et al., 1984). It is related to neither the amount of disability nor to mood state (Krupp et al., 1988). The assessment of fatigue should include:

- the daily pattern of fatigue
- times of the day when energy is high, reasonable and low
- activities or occurrences (e.g. hot weather) which worsen or alleviate fatigue
- the functional impact of fatigue on everyday activities
- whether fatigue is localized to specific muscle groups (e.g. ankle dorsiflexors), a body part (e.g. hand or leg), or functional system (e.g. vision or speech)
- whether central fatigue is causing overall excessive tiredness.

Formal, standardized assessment of fatigue can be carried out, if appropriate, for reports, audit or research, using the Fatigue Severity Scale (Krupp et al., 1989). The results of any physical assessments carried out on people with MS can easily be influenced by their fatigue. It is not unusual for MS patients to have a worse outcome when undergoing a battery of tests and a better one when tests are distributed over time or rest periods are given. Excessive fatigue, in association with poor physical fitness, has a deleterious effect on activities of daily living (ADL: Fisk et al., 1994).

Activities of daily living

It is important to know exactly what information is required from an assessment of ADL. If the information needed concerns what the MS person can do overall, then the assessment requirement is one of the physical capacity of the individual to complete the tasks in the ADL instrument. However, if the information needed is about what the person does on a daily basis, it will require an exploration of the person's social, family and cultural roles. Once again, the effects of fatigue may have a profound influence on how choices are made. For example, a person may choose to have help to wash and dress in the morning in order to save energy for the journey to work,

or may elect to have shopping done so as to have sufficient time and energy to collect the children from school.

It should be noted that many of the domestic (e.g. changing and bathing the baby, or playing with children) and social (e.g. talking on the telephone, or surfing the internet) activities carried out by young adults are not reflected in the available standardized ADL assessments.

Cognitive assessment

The importance of cognitive dysfunction and its assessment in MS has been brought to the attention of research and clinical readership (Rao, 1990). Detailed cognitive assessment is best carried out by a health-care professional with expertise in the field (e.g. clinical psychologist). The physiotherapist should ensure that he or she accesses such assessments when available, as limitations identified will inform the provision of therapy (see Ch. 17). Where expert cognitive assessment and diagnosis is unavailable, the physiotherapist may find simple, generic assessments for memory, mood and visuomotor action helpful. Often the person with MS or their family members will recount cognitive problems as part of the difficulties they cope with in everyday life.

Patient self-assessment

Participation of the patient in assessment should be encouraged by the physiotherapist so that self-evaluation is instrumental to the process. This evaluation should address the following issues:

- The individual's perception of his or her abilities and limitations
- Ability to cope
- Willingness to change
- Personal priorities and expectations of physiotherapy.

The self-assessment should be formally documented, dated, and form part of the assessment record in the physiotherapy and/or medical notes.

Planning treatment

The assessment forms the basis for developing a plan of treatment, deciding the goals and priorities and formulating a process which will put the plan into action. All these issues must be negotiated with the patient, who provides the context within which physiotherapy must operate from his or her experience of living with the disease and preferred lifestyle. A scheme for negotiating a goal-directed plan of physiotherapy has been suggested by De Souza (1997). It highlights the active roles played by both the physiotherapist and the patient and advocates shared responsibility for the actions to be taken in order for the plan to be operational.

A guided self-care programme suitable for people with MS living in the community has recently been demonstrated to have beneficial effects (O'Hara et al., 2002). It facilitates the priorities of the MS person to be central to the planning and execution of the programme, and promotes client empowerment to help those with MS pursue strategies which are beneficial to their health.

In order to have a good chance of succeeding, a plan of physiotherapy should have the following features:

- Meets the patient's needs
- Provides a focus on agreed goals
- Is a feasible and negotiated plan of action
- Is progressive in nature
- Harmonizes with other concurrent treatments
- Is acceptable to the individual and carers, as appropriate
- Is flexible to changing circumstances.

The need for good communication and interpersonal skills employed throughout the process of therapy cannot be overemphasized.

The physiotherapist needs to reflect on the long-term nature of the disease and the longer lasting effects of health care. A health promotion approach is helpful to those experiencing limitations and challenges due to the MS. Promoting a self-help model of care places the person with MS and their carers at the centre of decision-making and in the context of managing change due to MS, to develop expertise in living successfully with this unpredictable and distressing condition (see De Souza et al., 2005)

Physiotherapy interventions

Physiotherapy is a widely used treatment for MS patients, who often demand it and have high expectations of its value. As Matthews (1985) stated: 'Every account of the rehabilitation of patients with multiple sclerosis includes physiotherapy and every physician uses it.' However, research evidence of the specific benefits of physiotherapy is scarce despite widespread recommendations for its use. This is not surprising as the majority of physiotherapy treatments for a wide range of conditions, including MS, have developed ad hoc from an empirical base rather than from a scientific research base. Nonetheless, all have the underlying aim of reducing disability and increasing ability. Two issues are pertinent in planning physiotherapy:

1. Timing – when should therapy be given?
2. Content – what therapy should be given?

Timing of intervention

The issues concerning therapy are:

- when it should be given in the course of the disease
- how long it should continue
- how often it should be given.

Early intervention was seen by some authors as desirable, though not always possible (Ashburn & De Souza, 1988;

Todd, 1986). However, there were few suggestions advocating therapy on the basis of disease duration; rather, patients are referred for physiotherapy, or seek it for themselves, when MS has resulted in a noticeable disability rather than at the time of diagnosis (De Souza, 1990).

The National Institute for Health and Clincial Effectiveness (NICE) published guidelines for the management of MS at all stages (NICE, 2003). Although specific physiotherapy treatment is not recommended at this early stage, the physiotherapist should be appraised of the recommendations and be able to participate as part of the care team. A small trial compared 12 people with mild MS undertaking exercise classes twice weekly, with a control group of a similar 12 people receiving advice once a month. This study found that the exercise group had improvements in exercise capacity, quality of life and fatigue, and that quality of life and fatigue improvements carried over after the 3-month intervention was finished (McCullagh et al., 2008). General exercises, tone management, posture and fatigue management are recommended for those with minimal impairment (Freeman et al., 1997a, 2001), while, based on research evidence, inpatient and outpatient rehabilitation is recommended for those with moderate disability (Di Fabio et al., 1997, 1998; Freeman et al., 1997b, 1999; Solari et al., 1999; Wiles et al., 2001).

It is not known whether rest or exercise is more appropriate during a relapse and the lack of research in this area may be due to the random nature of attacks and the wide fluctuations in symptoms seen in relapsing patients. Despite this, some authors have recommended therapy during recovery from relapse and considered it effective (Alexander & Costello, 1987), but evidence of effectiveness was not provided. Another argument could be that maintenance of ability during relapse might enable the patient to maximize the benefit of remission. However, it is recommended that every person experiencing decrease in function or increased dependency due to a relapse of MS be referred to a specialist rehabilitation service for assessment and support (NICE, 2003).

Several authors have favoured long-term intervention (Ashburn & De Souza, 1988; Greenspun et al., 1987; Sibley, 1988) but optimum frequency of treatment was not examined. One study reported significant benefits of long-term intervention in a prospective group study of non-relapsing MS subjects (De Souza & Worthington, 1987). Those gaining benefit received on average 8 hours of physiotherapy a month for 18 consecutive months. Patients receiving less physiotherapy did not show significant improvements in function. A systematic review of exercise therapy for MS concluded that exercise therapy can be beneficial for people with MS not experiencing an exacerbation (Reitberg et al., 2006). On the basis of the scant information available, the issue remains open regarding frequency and timing of treatment.

Type of intervention

Very little research is available to indicate what type of physiotherapy should constitute the content of a treatment programme, although many opinions have been expressed.

Stretching

A clear consensus, and some experimental evidence, exists in favour of muscle stretching (see Ch. 14). Research on a small number of patients has shown that muscle hypertonus can be reduced, and voluntary range of lower-limb movement increased, by muscle stretching (Odeen, 1981). In addition, muscle stretching was considered valuable by many authors (e.g. Alexander & Costello, 1987; Arndt et al., 1991; De Souza, 1990; Sibley, 1988) and no reports have so far come to light which counsel against its use.

Active exercise

Active exercises have been advocated in the treatment of MS but for varying reasons. They have been suggested for retraining function (De Souza, 1984), muscle strengthening (Alexander & Costello, 1987), retraining of balance and coordination (Arndt et al., 1991; De Souza, 1990) and maintaining ROM (Ashburn & De Souza, 1988).

Despite the support for active exercises for MS, only a few studies have investigated their use. One reason for such general agreement may be the predilection of physiotherapists for exercise regimens for a wide variety of conditions. However, it has been shown that chronic disuse of muscles in MS causes not only weakness but also extreme fatiguability (Lenman et al., 1989) as it does in normal muscle. This could imply that active exercises are beneficial for maintaining and increasing strength and endurance, but this implication needs to be examined in MS patients.

A physiotherapy programme utilizing both muscle stretching and free active exercise was evaluated in a prospective long-term study of MS patients (De Souza & Worthington, 1987) which showed that, whilst the motor impairments worsened, subjects who had an intensive physiotherapy programme deteriorated significantly less than those who had had less treatment. In addition, functional, balance and daily living activities were also significantly improved in the group receiving more treatment. This study is one of the few which has provided research-based evidence for the efficacy of a long-term physiotherapy programme for MS. The efficacy of short-term intervention for improving disability was found in a trial providing individualized outpatient rehabilitation over 6 weeks (Patti et al., 2002). On the basis of evidence from nine randomized controlled trials systematically reviewed by Reitberg et al. (2005), exercise therapy is considered beneficial for increasing activity and participation.

In addition, a meta-analysis of 13 research articles provided cumulative evidence that exercise training is associated with improvement in quality of life in people with MS (Motl & Gosney, 2008).

Therapeutic exercises causing fatigue were widely thought to be damaging and the consensus is that moderate exercise is appropriate but that too much, which precipitates fatigue, is inappropriate. However, few studies have been carried out to determine the appropriate quantities of active exercises (see 'Aerobic exercises', below), and fatigue thresholds may differ between individuals. Some evidence exists that feelings of increasing fatigue are not reflected in concurrent objective measures of gait performance, implying that different neural pathways may underlie the two aspects in this disease (Morris et al., 2002). However, exercise classes, using simple exercise equipment, for those with mild MS have been found to improve fatigue (McCullagh et al., 2008).

Weight-resisted exercises

Weight-resisted exercises were advocated by Alexander and Costello (1987) for MS, despite an earlier finding that a large proportion of patients deteriorated (Russell & Palfrey, 1969). This type of treatment would seem to be inappropriate for inclusion in a physiotherapy programme.

Aerobic exercises

Aerobic exercise is a relatively new approach to treatment for MS, as it is for other neurological disorders (see Ch. 18 for a review). Current available evidence indicates that there are benefits for patients, particularly those with mild disability. This approach to treatment aims to increase overall physical activity and cardiovascular effort, prevent general muscular weakness and reduce health risks due to deconditioning and disuse.

Aerobic exercise programmes for MS of up to 6 months have been shown significantly to increase physical fitness, improve mood and enhance cardiovascular demand (Petajan et al., 1996; Ponichtera-Mulcare et al., 1997; Tantacci et al., 1996). Benefits to gait have also been reported (Rodgers et al., 1999). Increases in activity level, reduced fatigue and improvement in health perception have recently been reported for an aerobic exercise training programme (5 × 30 min per week of bicycle exercise) for people with mild to moderate MS (Kurtzke scores 2.5–6.5; mean 4.6, SD 1.2) over a period of only 4 weeks (Mostert & Kesselring, 2002). Adverse reactions to aerobic exercises are reported to be low in the above studies. For example, Mostert and Kesselring (2002) reported symptom exacerbations in the form of increased spasticity, paraesthesia and vertigo in 10% of 63 graded maximal exercise tests, and in only 6% of 180 training sessions. Such effects were not reported for other conditions and could have been due to heat sensitivity (Ch. 18).

Walking aids

Physiotherapy to maintain ambulation has been considered beneficial by many authors (e.g. Burnfield & Frank, 1988) but no agreement on the use of lower-limb bracing could be determined (Alexander & Costello, 1987; Arndt et al., 1991). Walking aids were also widely recommended by the above authors but care must be taken to avoid postural instability and deformity with long-term use (Todd, 1982). It would seem, therefore, that opinion is generally in favour of patients using aids if required, but warns against overreliance. Walking aids are discussed further below.

Hydrotherapy, heat and cold

Many anecdotal reports exist as to the usefulness or otherwise of hydrotherapy and heat or cold therapy. Burnfield (1985), as both a doctor and an MS patient, recommended avoiding hydrotherapy as 'it may make things worse and bring on fatigue'. Conversely, Alexander and Costello (1987) stated that exercises in a pool could be beneficial. However, these reports lack specificity as they do not refer to any particular symptoms or signs being affected by the treatment.

With respect to heat and cold, Forsythe (1988), another doctor with MS, reported that warm baths aided muscle-stretching exercises. Burnfield (1985), however, found that cool baths were beneficial, but also described one case where this treatment had a 'disastrous' result. Descriptions were not given as to what constituted either the benefit or the disaster, but these anecdotal reports serve to highlight the individual nature of responses to intervention experienced by some MS patients.

Clear warnings against heat therapy in MS were given by Block and Kester (1970), who thought that it caused severe exacerbation of clinical and subclinical deficits, while De Souza (1990) warned against the use of ice, or ice-cold water, in patients with compromised circulation, as this can cause vasoconstriction and further reduce the circulation.

Electrical stimulation

Low-frequency neuromuscular electrical stimulation can be beneficial for some MS patients (Worthington & De Souza, 1990), but the need for careful selection of patients for this form of treatment is emphasized as it does not benefit all MS patients. In addition, neuromuscular stimulation is recommended as an adjunct to other physiotherapy, mainly active exercise and muscle stretching (see Ch. 12).

Conclusions

In the absence of any sound evidence, and no consensus of clinical opinion regarding hydrotherapy, heat or cold therapy, and the small amount of evidence available on muscle stimulation, these treatments may not be appropriate for general application in MS, but may prove helpful to some individuals. On the basis of available evidence, the two components of physiotherapy likely to be the most useful in MS are muscle stretching and active exercises. It is further suggested that the exercises should incorporate training to improve ambulation, and also be paced so as to account for fatigue. These treatment components may be appropriate for a physiotherapy intervention programme for the majority of people with MS, and are further described by De Souza (1984, 1990), and Ashburn and De Souza (1988), and are summarised below.

A physiotherapy treatment programme

The programme proposed by Ashburn and De Souza (1988) consisted of active and active-assisted free exercises based upon 12 core exercises, and a simple muscle-stretching regimen. The emphasis of the active exercise programme was on functional activities, and the use of the exercises to achieve a functional goal was taught. For example, a sequence which incorporated knee rolling, side sitting (stretch exercise), low kneeling, high kneeling, half kneeling and standing would achieve the functional activity of rising up from the floor. Other gross body motor skills, such as transferring, may be retrained in a similar way. Benefits to MS patients from facilitation (impairment-based) and task-oriented (disability-focused) physiotherapy were observed, with no differences between the two approaches (Lord et al., 1998).

The active exercise programme could also be adjusted to emphasize balance activities. These incorporated 'hold' techniques into the basic exercise programme to encourage postural stabilization and stimulate balance reactions. Patients were required to hold certain positions and postures for a few seconds to begin with and subsequently gradually to increase the period. For example, the position of high kneeling was required to be held for a 10-second period without the patient using any upper-limb support, while an upright standing posture utilizing a narrow base of support and no upper-limb aid was required to be held for 30 seconds. Patients could self-monitor their progress and were encouraged to note their levels of achievement.

The programme may be adjusted to individual levels of ability, e.g. by diversifying exercises in a variety of sitting or kneeling positions if the individual is unable to stand. The emphasis of the different exercises may also be adjusted according to the needs of individuals. Those whose major problems are spasticity, and muscle and joint stiffness, require an emphasis on stretching and increasing active and passive ROM. Those with problems of ataxia and instability need more emphasis on the smooth coordination of movements, and on balance and postural stability. The majority of MS patients will have a combination of different motor symptoms, and a balanced programme will need to be constructed.

Management of the multiple sclerosis patient with mainly hypertonic symptoms

Physiotherapy for an MS patient with predominantly symptoms of spasticity is generally similar to that for other neurological patients with the same problem (see Ch. 14). However, some specific issues need to be attended to in MS, and the progressive nature of the disease borne in mind. Most importantly, any decision to reduce the level of muscle tone must have a clear objective, and an identifiable and achievable functional benefit. A high level of tone is useful for some MS patients, e.g. those who use their spasticity for standing, transferring or for utilizing a swing-to or swing-through gait pattern for crutch-walking (De Souza, 1990; Ko Ko, 1999). For these people, spasticity should not be reduced at the expense of their mobility.

For other MS patients, spasticity will hinder their ability, masking movement and adding to the effort of voluntary actions, so reduction of muscle tone may be appropriate for these patients. However, careful monitoring of any movement is required during the reduction of tone, as in MS the spasticity often overlies other symptoms, such as weakness or ataxia, which are more difficult for the patient to cope with than the spasticity (De Souza, 1990).

Some MS patients exhibit an extremely changeable distribution of tone in different positions, e.g. lower-limb extensor hypertonus in standing and flexor hypertonus in lying. These features are probably due to lesions disrupting CNS pathways which control limb and trunk postural responses to muscular information. Irrespective of the variability of spasticity in MS patients, there are certain muscle groups which tend to exhibit the symptom more than others. It should be recalled that, where there is a hypertonic muscle group, there is also generally another muscle group, often the antagonists, which exhibits low tone. These imbalances, if allowed to become permanent, will result in contractures and deformity. The muscle groups most often developing contracture in people with MS are:

- trunk rotators
- trunk lateral flexors
- hip flexors
- hip adductors
- knee flexors
- ankle plantarflexors
- inverters of the foot.

Spasticity in the upper limbs is less common than in the lower limbs; the muscle groups most often affected are the wrist and finger flexors, and the shoulder adductors and internal rotators. Occasionally, the forearm pronators and elbow flexors are affected, but the full flexion pattern of spasticity, as seen in the hemiplegic arm, is rare, though not unknown, in MS.

Physiotherapy for spasticity is described in Chapter 14. With MS, simple strategies to alleviate spasticity, which patients can carry out for themselves, are preferable. The techniques of choice are muscle stretching and the use of positions which retain prolonged muscle stretch (Ashburn & De Souza, 1988; De Souza, 1990).

The effectiveness of physiotherapy in reducing spasticity in MS has been demonstrated using F-wave amplitude as a measure of motor neurone excitability (Rosche et al., 1996).

Management of the multiple sclerosis patient with ataxia

Ataxia is one of the major motor symptoms affecting people with MS. It rarely occurs in isolation, and is most commonly seen with other motor symptoms, notably spasticity. It is a disturbance that, independently of motor weakness, alters the direction and extent of a voluntary movement and impairs the sustained voluntary and reflex muscle contraction necessary for maintaining posture and equilibrium.

The main problem that ataxic MS patients show is an inability to make movements which require groups of muscles to act together in varying degrees of co-contraction. The difficulty is easily observed during gait, as the single-stance phase requires the co-contraction of leg muscles in order to support body weight, whilst at the same time a coordinated change in the relative activity of the muscles is needed to move the body weight forward (e.g. from a flexed hip position at heel strike to an extended hip position at toe-off). The ataxic patient has greatest difficulty with this phase of gait and either uses the stance leg as a rigid strut, or staggers as coordination is lost. Compensation is often afforded by walking aids which reduce the need for weight support through stance, whilst providing at least two (one upper- and one lower-limb) points of support in all phases of gait. The reduction of upper-limb weight-bearing has been considered an essential component for retaining functional gait in ataxic patients (Brandt et al., 1981). Using walking aids, the ataxic patient can ambulate with the hips remaining in flexion, thus eliminating the need to effect a coordinated change from hip flexion to extension while bearing weight through the stance leg.

The aim of physiotherapy is to counteract the postural and movement adjustments made by the ataxic patient in order to encourage postural stability and dynamic weight-shifting, and to increase the smooth coordination of movement. It is also to prevent the preferred postures of ataxic patients, adopted to eliminate their instability, from becoming functional or fixed contractures (De Souza, 1990). The features of postural abnormality are:

- an exaggerated lumbar lordosis
- an anterior pelvic tilt

- flexion at the hips
- hyperextension of the knees
- weight towards the heel parts of the feet
- clawed toes (as they grip the ground).

The different types of ataxia have been reviewed by Morgan (1980) and are summarised in Table 5.3 with the main features of motor dysfunction. In MS there may be a mixture of cerebellar, vestibular and sensory components depending on the sites of the lesions.

Ataxia is a very complex movement disorder and there is little research evidence to inform the content of physiotherapy programmes to treat this symptom. However, there are some indications that physiotherapy can help (Armutlu et al., 2001; Brandt et al., 1986) and, indeed, may be essential for preventing unnecessary inactivity and dependency, and for reducing the risk of falls. The key issue in the treatment of ataxia is to identify the predominant problem to guide the primary aims of treatment. This should be achieved by careful observational assessment of the ataxic patient carrying out a range of activities. Generally, patients should progress from simple movements to more complex ones as they master the ability to coordinate muscle groups.

Table 5.3 Types of ataxia and associated motor disorders

Sensory ataxia
• A high-stepping gait pattern
• More reliance on visual or auditory information about leg or foot position

Vestibular ataxia
• Disturbed equilibrium in standing and walking
• Loss of equilibrium reactions
• A wide-based, staggering gait pattern

Cerebellar ataxia
• Disturbance in the rate, regularity and force of movement
• Loss of movement coordination
• Overshooting of target (dysmetria)
• Decomposition of movement (dyssynergia)
• Loss of speed and rhythm of alternating movements (dysdiadochokinesia)
• Incoordination of agonist–antagonist muscles and loss of the continuity of muscle contraction (tremor, e.g. intention tremor)

Assessment and treatment strategies for the ataxic MS patient are summarised in Table 5.4. There is little research evidence to indicate the most useful way forwards for treatment, however, the use of PNF, Frenkel Co-ordination Exercises and Cawthorne-Cooksey exercises, prehaps with the additional use of Johnson Pressure Slpints, may be helpful (see Armutlu et al., 2001). In the light of no clear evidence base for treatment physiotherapy for ataxia must by necessity take a pragmatic approach.

Therapy techniques that could be used to good effect include:

- weight-shifting in different positions (e.g. kneel walking, step stride and side stride standing)
- lowering and raising the centre of gravity (e.g. by knee bending and straightening in standing; or moving from high kneeling to side sitting and back to high kneeling)
- proprioceptive neuromuscular facilitation techniques (see Ch. 12)
- the use of slow reversals, rhythmic movements and stabilizations.

Whichever techniques are employed, due attention must be given to fatigue. Within a therapy session frequent periods of rest are generally required and the work performed in a session may be wasted if the patient has been exhausted by the treatment.

Aids for mobility

Mobility is perhaps the major functional disability in MS. Scheinberg (1987) stated that when patients are asked about their main problem with MS, 90% will cite a walking difficulty. In addition, those with more severe mobility problems incur a greater individual, state and health services cost burden (Holmes et al., 1995). Therefore maintaining walking ability for as long as possible is a priority and should form a primary aim of physiotherapy.

Walking may be limited by a number of problems evident in MS such as changes in muscle tone, poor balance, fatigue, lack of safety and confidence, and poor visual discrimination of the environment. Tentative evidence exists that walking practice using treadmill training improves speed and endurance, but the positive effects have limited carryover in time (van den Berg et al., 2006).

Walking aids have both advantages and disadvantages (Table 5.5) and therapists need to be aware of both in order to discuss the issues with their patients (De Souza, 1990). The main detrimental effects of using a walking aid and the ways by which physiotherapy can reduce the disadvantages have been identified by Todd (1982). Once a mobility aid has been provided, regular review is essential, as the fluctuating and progressive nature of MS may indicate a need to change the type of aid used or the type

Table 5.4 Assessment and treatment approaches for patients with ataxia

Predominant problem	Dysfunction expressed in	Primary aims of treatment
Maintaining equilibrium	Weight-bearing and weight transference	Increase postural stability
		Enhance control of the centre of gravity in weight-shifting
		Encourage maintenance of the control of the centre of gravity in movement from one position to another
		Progress from a wide to a narrow base of support
Coordination of dynamic movement	Patterns of movement	Enhance smoothness of control of movement patterns
		Progress from simple to complex patterns
		Progress from fast to slow movements
Located in body axis and trunk	Gross body movements (e.g. transfers)	Independent and free head movement
		Increase control of movement to, from and around the midline (body axis)
		Encourage movement of limb girdles in relation to body axis (especially rotation)
Located in limbs	Voluntary body movements	Enhance proximal limb stabilization
		Encourage coordinated activity of agonist and antagonist muscle groups
		Progress from large-range to small-range movements
		Reduce the requirement for visual guidance of movement

Table 5.5 Advantages and disadvantages of aids to mobility

ADVANTAGES	DISADVANTAGES
Increased safety and stability	Less lower-limb weight-bearing
Reduced risk of falls	Loss of lower-limb muscle strength
Increased walking distance	Reduced head and trunk movements
Increased walking speed	Reduction of balance reactions
Increased gait efficiency	Alteration of muscle tone
Improved quality of gait pattern	Postural abnormality (e.g. hip flexion, trunk lateral flexion)
Reduced fatigue	Upper-limb function may be compromised

of gait pattern employed. Follow-up is also essential if a mobility aid has been provided for a patient during a relapse, as any recovery of movement must be maximized and not compromised by the patient retaining an inappropriate aid or gait pattern for his or her level of recovery (De Souza, 1990).

Regular use of mobility aids may have a detrimental effect on the upper limbs and the physiotherapist should include an examination of them in the review process. The major issues to be addressed are:

- loss of upper-limb function
- injury to soft tissue, particularly of the shoulders
- joint and muscle pain, including neck pain
- loss of joint ROM
- compromised skin integrity, especially of the palmar surfaces of the hands.

This section has focused primarily on the physical aspects of walking and the need for aids. However, walking is not only a physical function but also has social, emotional and cultural meanings. For some, the personal disadvantages outweigh the physical advantages, and they decide not to use recommended mobility aids. This could be interpreted, mistakenly, as non-compliance with professional advice, or non-acceptance of the disability if the physiotherapist has not explored and understood the social, cultural and emotional needs of the patient.

Management of the immobile person with multiple sclerosis

People with MS may become immobile, either due to progression of the disease causing severe disablement or due to during a relapse. It is essential that, when immobile in relapse, the patient is managed in a way that will not disadvantage functional ability after relapse, or prolong unnecessarily the duration of immobility and dependency. Physiotherapy should provide preventive treatment, maintenance regimens and appropriate, staged active exercises when recovery first becomes apparent. Table 5.6 illustrates a typical preventive and maintenance physiotherapy programme.

Attention should also be directed to the general good health and wellbeing of the patient. For example, if immobility lasts over several days or weeks, help may be needed to retain a sound level of nutrition, a social support network or for continence management.

For those who are immobile due to the severity of the MS, a symptom management approach involving all members of the care team is advised (Cornish & Mattison, 2000). The *MS Healthcare Standards* (Freeman et al., 2001) have recommended appropriate provision under key issues, such as information access, expertise, communication and coordination, community care and mobility, respite care, and long-term and palliative care. The physiotherapist is likely to be a part of the professional care team for those with very severe MS and should be knowledgeable and fully appraised of the current recommended standards.

Helping carers

People with MS generally have a number of family members and friends who also have to learn to live with MS. As Soderburg (1992) stated, 'the diagnosis of MS will affect every aspect of family life. Its impact will extend to work roles, economic status, relationships within the family,

---

Table 5.6 Preventive and maintenance physiotherapy for immobile patients with multiple sclerosis

PREVENT	TREATMENT
Respiratory inadequacy	Establish correct breathing pattern
Partial lung collapse Chest infections	Teach deep breathing exercise in recumbent and sitting positions
Accumulation of sputum	Promote effective cough
Cyanosis	Ensure air entry to all areas of lung
Circulatory stasis	Active rhythmic contraction and relaxation of lower-limb muscles
Deep vein thrombosis*	Massage, passive movement or use of mechanical aids if no activation of muscles possible
Contractures	Ensure full passive range of movement at all joints
	Correction and support of posture in lying and sitting
	Prolonged stretch of hypertonic muscles
Pressure sores	Distribute loading over weight-bearing body surfaces
	Avoid pressure points
	Change position frequently and regularly
	Support correct posture
	Implement moving and handling techniques that protect skin integrity
Muscle atrophy	Encourage active contraction in all able muscle groups
	Use passive and assisted movements as appropriate
	Implement assisted or aided standing when safe and within patient tolerance

and relationships between the family and the larger community'. Professional carers, such as physiotherapists, have an important role in helping the informal carers. Teaching safe and efficient moving and handling techniques is a major area where direct physiotherapeutic intervention can bring substantial benefits. There are also benefits to carers' health and improvements in their social engangement due to the provision of low intensity long-term multi-disciplinary therapy to people with MS (Khan et al., 2007).

Research has found that most of the day-to-day care of people with MS is provided by family or friends in the form of personal care, help with mobility, household tasks, leisure and employment (O'Hara et al., 2004). Therefore, therapists need to be aware that any new professional engagement with those living with MS is likely to be supplementary to an existing complex care network. Professional health carers need to become aware of these existing strategies when intervening to support and enhance these practices (De Souza et al., 2005).

Carers should be valued participants of the healthcare team, and be part of the decision-making process (McQueen Davis & Niskala, 1992). Tasks that may be required of carers should not compromise their long-term support in order to achieve a short-term goal. Just as the person with MS is identified and treated as an individual with specific needs, so should the uniqueness of the carer's needs be acknowledged. Physiotherapists need to provide professional input to safeguard carers' wellbeing and promote their continued health (De Souza et al., 2005). Recognition must also be given to the social and family role of the carer, and the environmental and emotional settings within which caring takes place. It should be remembered that care-giving takes place throughout the day and night (Spackman et al., 1989).

The cooperation of carers cannot be assumed, but must be negotiated. When a carer consents to carry out a task, it is inappropriate to assume that a blanket consent has been obtained for all tasks. The carer should have the opportunity to exercise choice, discretion and judgement about what is best for him or her. Even in situations where carers consent, their willingness to help must be consonant with their apparent physical, psychological and emotional abilities to do so. This issue deserves particular attention where the main carer is an elderly parent, and even more so when the carer is a child (Blackford, 1992; Segal & Simpkins, 1993). Physiotherapists must be aware of the current local and national recommendations, and demonstrate that they have executed their duty of care to both patient and carer.

CONCLUSION

MS is probably one of the most complex and variable conditions encountered by physiotherapists. There is no 'typical' MS patient or presentation of the disease. People with MS require comprehensive management that incorporates the expertise appropriate to their symptoms, yet is flexible and able to respond rapidly to their changing pattern of need.

An interdisciplinary team approach to the management of MS will improve the quality, continuity and comprehensiveness of care, with the patient and carer being integral to the team. Patients require information and support to enable their own involvement in the management of the condition, retain a sense of control and achieve maximal independence. A systematic review of multidisciplinary rehabilitation for people with MS concluded that there was good evidence for intensive inpatient therapy leading to improvement in activity (disability), but that this pattern of treatment had little effect on impairment (Khan et al., 2007). In addition, the review reported that sufficient evidence existed that showed that low-intensity therapy over a longer term resulted in improvements in quality of life and benefits to carers in terms of better general health and more social activities (Khan et al., 2007).

As a team member, the physiotherapist will be required to have high levels of assessment, treatment and interpersonal skills, and in-depth knowledge of MS. In general terms, patients should be advised to enjoy as full and as active a life as possible. Whilst excessive exercise should probably be avoided, regular exercise is to be encouraged, though patients should be warned at times of acute infective illness that they should rest and control fever. Best practice does not consist of a series of interventions, but embodies a cohesive care plan, which allows the patient to develop skills for living.

The importance of a sympathetic and understanding medical adviser, whether physician, nurse or therapist, who has the trust and confidence of the patient cannot be overstated. There are many support groups, such as the MS Society, to which people with MS can be directed and most regional centres now run new diagnostic clinics to inform and enable people newly diagnosed with the condition.

A philosophy of care encompasses an understanding that functions such as walking and transferring reach far beyond the physical issues and extend to social, cultural, psychological and emotional effects of loss and limitation. The physiotherapist, therefore, cannot just offer treatment, but must also offer care and support to all those who need to learn to live with MS.

CASE HISTORY

Presenting history and diagnosis

Mrs H is 47 years old and experienced her first symptoms attributed to MS in 1981 at the age of 21. She suffered weakness and sensory disturbance in both legs for 2 weeks and recovered without any residual disability. In 1983, she experienced a relapse following her second pregnancy and did not recover fully, being left with some residual loss of movements in her lower limbs and intermittent spasms. Her doctor referred her for investigations. Although MS was suspected, it was not confirmed at this stage.

In 1984, Mrs H complained of generalized tiredness, closely followed by sensory deficits in both legs. She was admitted to hospital and, while under investigation, experienced a sudden onset of partial paralysis in her legs. Her history, the results of a lumbar puncture and evidence from an MRI brain scan clearly indicated that she had a definite diagnosis of relapsing remitting MS.

Once her diagnosis was made, Mrs H was treated with adrenocorticotrophic hormone (ACTH), the medication of first choice to alleviate relapses of MS. However, she was left with some residual loss of sensation and movement in her lower limbs, and was referred to a neurological rehabilitation team with special expertise in MS. Mrs H attended with her husband, who was concerned for her and supportive.

Commentary

It became clear that Mr and Mrs H were a team and had a strong relationship. As a team, they were willing to work with the professional staff, participating in decisions and in planning of treatment. With the agreement of Mrs H, both she and her husband were always seen together, and would be allowed the time and privacy within appointments with the professional care team to discuss issues between themselves.

Initial assessment by specialist team

Mrs H was judged to have mild disability due to her MS. However, her major concerns focused on her fatigue, loss of sensation and anxiety about being able to care for her new baby and meet the demands of her first child, who was 3 years old. Mr and Mrs H also wanted to know more about MS and were provided with information booklets and given the contact address and telephone number of the MS Society. Mrs H was given a simple 3-day diary to use as a self-assessment of her fatigue. She was asked to note her worst times of fatigue, the best times when fatigue was low/non-existent, and times when she needed a lot of effort to manage, or could manage with a bit of effort. Her general practitioner and health visitor were informed of her neurological management programme and asked to contact the professional care team with any queries or concerns about her progress.

Initial treatment programme

From her self-management of fatigue, a distinct pattern emerged. The physiotherapist, together with Mrs H and her health visitor, worked out a daily routine where most activity occurred in the morning. Mrs H was given a 15-minute active exercise programme to do in the morning

and a 10-minute stretching exercise programme to do mid-afternoon. She and the children would take a nap in the early afternoon. Mrs H was provided with information about how to cradle her baby in a large scarf used as a sling across her shoulder and how to breast-feed in side-lying, in order to reduce the fatigue of having to hold the baby for feeding.

Four years after diagnosis

On formal assessment in 1987, there was increasing spasticity in her legs, the left being worse than the right. She remained mobile, but began to rely on holding on to walls and furniture, and struggled to remain independent in ADL.

Treatment

Mrs H attended for 6 weeks of outpatient physiotherapy, twice a week, which focused on functional and balance activities, lower-limb ROM exercises and gait re-education. This required Mr H to drive her to the hospital 22 miles each way, and to take time off. They also had to arrange paid child care for their younger child and be back to pick up the older child from school at 3 p.m.

Mrs H gained important benefits from her treatment. She improved her mobility so that she was walking indoors without the support of walls and furniture, and chose to have a walking stick to help, should she need it. Her upper-limb function and ROM were checked during her attendance at outpatient physiotherapy and found to be functionally normal. Her home exercise regimen was updated, and it was decided to seek more local physiotherapy support from community services or MS therapy centre.

She had no further treatment for 6 months, until the local NHS community physiotherapy service was able to offer 1 month's (once a week) treatment at home. The community physiotherapist continued the functional activities and gait re-education programme, and carried out a reassessment.

Reassessment

The reassessment demonstrated that Mrs H had lost some voluntary ROM in her left lower limb, but could walk 12 m unaided at a rate of 1.2 m/s. Thereafter, she needed to use her walking stick, and could then manage another 15 m. She had full function and range of movement in her upper limbs and continued to be independent in ADL. The community physiotherapy services agreed to continue to see Mrs H once a month.

11 years after diagnosis

In 1995, Mrs H suffered a significant relapse of MS, lasting 1 month. Initially, her legs 'gave way' and she was admitted to hospital with sudden onset of flaccid paralysis of her lower limbs and urinary incontinence. She received intravenous steroids, and was referred for urodynamic tests to assess her bladder dysfunction. The consultant neurourologist decided that adequate bladder management should be achieved with medication (desmopressin), but would review Mrs H on a 3-monthly basis.

Mrs H was anxious, depressed and tearful about her condition and requested help. She was referred to a counsellor specializing in MS, and provided with the number of the MS Society's 24-hour counselling helpline service, which she reported that she and her husband had subsequently used.

Commentary

Relapses of MS are unpredictable, and people with the disease and their family are, understandably, completely unprepared for what might happen due to a relapse.

The counsellor helped Mrs H refocus on what she could do, rather than what she could not do, and, following counselling, Mr and Mrs H were motivated to attend again for further physiotherapy assessment and treatment.

On physiotherapy assessment, Mrs H was found to have severe loss of ROM in the lower limbs with hypertonus in the extensor muscle groups. She could stand independently, but needed upper-limb support to walk. Her posture and balance were abnormal, which caused problems with transfers. However, she retained independent transferring ability and had bladder control with the help of medication. Her walking ability had been reduced to 15 m with the aid of a triwheel delta walker. She was referred to a local MS therapy centre for physiotherapy which comprised:

- free active exercises, or active-assisted exercises for the lower limbs, aimed at reducing tone and increasing voluntary range of movement
- stretching regimen, aimed at maintaining muscle and joint flexibility and reducing tone
- static and dynamic muscle contractions of the lower-limb muscle groups aimed at preventing disuse atrophy
- weight-bearing, standing and gait re-education, aimed to facilitate transfers and mobility
- postural re-education, aimed at normalizing tone and strengthening trunk muscles

- upper-limb and respiratory exercises, aimed at maintaining arm/hand function and lung capacity
- information and advice about aids and appliances to help with everyday tasks
- options for referral to community occupational therapy services, counselling, the disablement assessment centre, aimed at opening up the network of care available to people with MS
- reassessment at 6-monthly intervals, aimed at retaining contact with Mrs H, monitoring progress, and continuing to provide advice and support.

18 years after diagnosis

Mrs H made progress since her major relapse. She regained the ability to walk 20 m with a triwheel delta walker, was independent in transfers and retained upper-trunk and upper-limb strength and function. She elected to use a wheelchair for outings. On assessment by the community occupational therapist, Mrs H now uses a perching stool in the kitchen, a seat in the shower and has taken up embroidery, which she used to do before she had her first child. She is also learning computer skills alongside her elder child, and has just set up the family's first web-page.

Commentary

The case of Mrs H illustrates the ups and downs of living with MS. She shows great determination to do her best to live with MS. It is thought that Mrs H has now reached the secondary progressive stage of the disease. Although the absence of relapses cannot be guaranteed, further deterioration is likely to be slowly progressive. Mrs H has taken up activities which use her upper-limb functions, and which she enjoys. She considers that her quality of life is 'quite good – all things considered'.

The case of Mrs H illustrates that the role of the physiotherapist includes, not only one of providing assessment and treatment, but also of supporting people and their families, providing information, and referring on to allow access to the network of care. It also illustrates that successful management of MS focuses not only on the physical impact of the disease, but also on the whole person and context of his or her personal and family life.

REFERENCES

Alexander, J., Costello, E., 1987. Physical and surgical therapy. In: Scheinberg, L.C., Holland, N.J. (Eds.), Multiple Sclerosis: A Guide for Patients and their Families. second ed. Raven Press, New York, pp. 79–107.

Armutlu, K., Karabudak, R., Nurlu, G., 2001. Physiotherapy approaches in the treatment of ataxic multiple sclerosis: a pilot study. Neurorehabil. Neural Repair 15, 203–211.

Arndt, J., Bhasin, C., Brar, S.P., et al., 1991. Physical therapy. In: Schapiro, R.T.

(Ed.), Multiple Sclerosis: A Rehabilitation Approach to Management. Demos, New York, pp. 17–66.

Ashburn, A., De Souza, L.H., 1988. An approach to the management of multiple sclerosis. Physiotherapy Practice 4, 139–145.

Aulchenko, Y.S., Hoppenbrouwers, I.A., Ramagopalan, S.V., et al., 2008. Genetic variation in the KIF1B locus influences susceptibility to multiple sclerosis. Nat. Genet. 40, 1402–1403.

Barnes, M., 1993. Multiple sclerosis. In: Greenwood, R., Barnes, M.P., McMillan, T.M. et al., (Eds.), Neurological Rehabilitation. Churchill Livingstone, London, pp. 485–504.

Beck, R.W., Cleary, P.A., Trobe, J.D., et al., 1993. The effect of corticosteroids for acute optic neuritis on the subsequent development of multiple sclerosis. N. Engl. J. Med. 329, 1764–1769.

Blackford, K.A., 1992. Strategies for intervention and research with children or adolescents who have a parent with multiple sclerosis. Axon Dec, 50–55.

Block, J.M., Kester, N.C., 1970. The role of rehabilitation in the management of multiple sclerosis. Mod. Treat. 7 (5).

Brandt, T., Krafczyk, S., Malsbenden, J., 1981. Postural imbalance with head extension: improvement by training as a model for ataxia therapy. Ann. N. Y. Acad. Sci. 374, 636–649.

Brandt, T., Buchele, W., Krafczyk, S., 1986. Training effects on experimental postural instability: a model for clinical ataxia therapy. In: Bles, W., Brandt, T. (Eds.), Disorders of Posture and Gait. Elsevier, Amsterdam, pp. 353–365.

Bruck, W., Lucchineti, C.F., Lassman, H., 2003. The pathology of primary progressive multiple sclerosis. Mult. Scler. 8, 93–97.

Burnfield, A., 1985. Multiple Sclerosis: A Personal Exploration. Souvenir Press, London.

Burnfield, A., Frank, A., 1988. Multiple sclerosis. In: Frank, A., Maguire, P. (Eds.), Disabling Diseases – Physical, Environmental and Psychosocial Management. Heinemann Medical, London.

Compston, D.A.S., 2000. Distribution of multiple sclerosis. In: Compston, A., Ebers, G., Lussmann, H. et al., (Eds.), McAlpine's Multiple Sclerosis. third ed. Churchill Livingstone, New York, pp. 63–100.

Corboy, J.R., Goodin, D.S., Frohman, E.M., 2003. Disease-modifying therapies for multiple sclerosis. Current Treatment Options in Neurology 5, 35–54.

Cornish, C.J., Mattision, P.G., 2000. Symptom management in advanced multiple sclerosis. CME Bulletin Palliative Medicine 2, 11–16.

Costello, E., Curtis, C.L., Sandel, I.B., et al., 1996. Exercise prescription for individuals with multiple sclerosis. Neurology Report 20, 24–30.

DasGupta, R., Fowler, C.J., 2003. Bladder, bowel and sexual dysfunction in multiple sclerosis: management strategies. Drugs 63, 153–166.

De Souza, L.H., 1984. A different approach to physiotherapy for multiple sclerosis patients. Physiotherapy 70, 429–432.

De Souza, L.H., 1990. Multiple Sclerosis: Approaches to Management. Chapman & Hall, London.

De Souza, L.H., 1997. Physiotherapy. In: Goodwill, J., Chamberlain, M.A., Evans, C. (Eds.), Rehabilitation of the Physically Disabled Adult. second ed. Chapman & Hall, London, pp. 560–575.

De Souza, L.H., Worthington, J.A., 1987. The effect of long-term physiotherapy on disability in multiple sclerosis patients. In: Clifford Rose, F., Jones, R. (Eds.), Multiple Sclerosis: Immunological, Diagnostic and Therapeutic Aspects. John Libbey, London, pp. 155–164.

De Souza, L.H., Ide, L., Neophytou, C., 2005. Promoting a self-help care model for the management of multiple sclerosis. Chapter 15 In: Scriven, A. (Ed.), Health Promoting Practice: The contribution of Nurses and Allied Health Professions. Palgrave Press, pp. 195–208.

Dean, G., Kurtzke, J.F., 1971. On the risk of multiple sclerosis according to the age at immigration to South Africa. Br. Med. J. 3, 725–729.

Di Fabio, R.P., Choi, T., Soderberg, J., et al., 1997. Health related quality of life for patients with progressive multiple sclerosis: influence of rehabilitation. Phys. Ther. 77, 1704–1716.

Di Fabio, R.P., Soderberg, J., Choi, T., et al., 1998. Extended outpatient rehabilitation: its influence on symptoms frequency, fatigue and functional status for persons with progressive multiple sclerosis. Arch. Phys. Med. Rehabil. 79, 141–146.

Ebers, G.C., Bulman, D.E., Sadovnick, A. D., 1986. A population-based study of multiple sclerosis in twins. N. Engl. J. Med. 315, 1638–1642.

European Study Group on Interferon β-1b in Secondary Progressive Multiple Sclerosis, 1998. Placebo controlled multi-centre randomised trial of interferon β-1b in the treatment of secondary progressive multiple sclerosis. Lancet 352, 1491–1497.

Fassas, A., Deconinck, E., Musso, M., et al., 2002. Haematopoietic stem cell transplantation for multiple sclerosis; a retrospective multi centre study. J. Neurol. 249, 1088–1094.

Filippi, M., Horsefield, M.A., Ader, H.J., et al., 1998. Guidelines for using quantitative measures of brain magnetic resonance imaging abnormalities in monitoring the treatment of multiple sclerosis. Ann. Neurol. 43, 499–506.

Fisk, J.D., Pontefract, A., Ritvo, P.G., et al., 1994. The impact of fatigue on multiple sclerosis. Can. J. Neurol. Sci. 21, 9–14.

Forsythe, E., 1988. Multiple Sclerosis: Exploring Sickness and Health. Faber & Faber, London.

Freal, J.E., Kraft, G.H., Coryell, J.K., 1984. Symptomatic fatigue in multiple sclerosis. Arch. Phys. Med. Rehabil. 65, 135–138.

Freeman, J., Johnson, J., Rollinson, S. et al., (Eds.), 1997a. Standards of Healthcare for People with MS. Multiple Sclerosis Society, London.

Freeman, J.A., Lagndon, D.W., Hobart, J.C., et al., 1997b. The impact of inpatient rehabilitation on progressive multiple sclerosis. Ann. Neurol. 42, 236–244.

Freeman, J.A., Lagndon, D.W., Hobart, J.C., et al., 1999. Inpatient rehabilitation: do the benefits carry over into the community? Neurology 52, 50–56.

Freeman, J., Ford, H., Mattison, P. et al., (Eds.), 2001. Developing MS Healthcare Standards. Multiple Sclerosis Society, The MS Society, London.

Ghalie, R.G., Edan, G., Laurent, M., et al., 2002a. Cardiac adverse effects associated with mitoxantrone (Novantrone) therapy in patients with MS. Neurology 59, 909–913.

Ghalie, R.G., Mauch, E., Edan, G., et al., 2002b. A study of therapy-related acute leukaemia after mitoxantrone therapy for multiple sclerosis. Mult. Scler. 8, 441–445.

Goodin, D.S., Frohman, E.M., Garmany, G.P., 2002. Disease modifying therapies in multiple sclerosis: report of the therapeutics and technology assessments sub-committee of the American Academy of Neurology and the MS Council for Clinical Practice Guidelines. Neurology 58, 169–178.

Goodkin, D.E., Rudick, P.S., Vanderbrug Medendorp, S., et al., 1995. Low dose (7.5 mg) oral methotrexate reduces the rate of progression of chronic progressive multiple sclerosis. Ann. Neurol. 37, 30–40.

Goodman, A.D., Brown, T.R., Cohen, J.A., et al., 2008. Dose comparison trial of sustained-release fampridine in multiple sclerosis. Neurology 71, 1134–1141.

Greenspun, B., Stineman, M., Agri, R., 1987. Multiple sclerosis and rehabilitation outcome. Arch. Phys. Med. Rehabil. 68, 434–437.

Halliday, A.M., McDonald, W.I., 1977. Pathophysiology of demyelinating disease. Br. Med. Bull. 33, 21–27.

Hartung, H.P., Gonsette, R., Konig, N., et al., 2002. Mitoxantrone in progressive multiple sclerosis: a placebo-controlled, double-blind, randomised, multicentre trial. Lancet 360, 2018–2025.

Holmes, J., Madgwick, T., Bates, D., 1995. The cost of multiple sclerosis. British Journal of Medical Economics 8, 181–193.

Hulter, B.M., Lundberg, O.L., 1995. Sexual function in women with advanced multiple sclerosis. J. Neurol. Neurosurg. Psychiatry 59, 83–86.

IFBN Multiple Sclerosis Study Group, 1993. Interferon β-1b is effective in relapsing-remitting multiple sclerosis. I. Clinical results of multicentre, randomised, double-blind, placebo-controlled trial. Neurology 43, 655–661.

Ingle, G.T., Stevenson, V.L., Miller, D.H., et al., 2002. Two year follow-up study of primary and transitional progressive multiple sclerosis. Mult. Scler. 8, 108–114.

Jacobs, L.D., Cookfair, D.L., Rudick, R.A., et al., 1996. Intramuscular interferon β-1a for disease progression in relapsing multiple sclerosis. Ann. Neurol. 39, 285–294.

Johnson, K.P., Brooks, B.R., Cohen, J.A., et al., 1995. Copolymer-1 reduces relapse rate and improves disability in relapsing-remitting multiple sclerosis: results of a phase III multicentre, double blind, placebo controlled trial. Neurology 45, 1268–1276.

Khan, F., Turner-Stokes, L., Ng, L., et al., 2007. Multidisciplinary rehabilitation for adults with multiple sclerosis. Cochrane Database Syst. Rev. (2) CD006036; doi: 10.1002/14651858. CD006036.pub2.

Klaus, L., 1997. Diet and multiple sclerosis. Neurology 49 (Suppl. 2), S55–S61.

Ko Ko, C., 1999. Effectiveness of rehabilitation for multiple sclerosis. Clin. Rehabil. 13 (Suppl. 1), 33–41.

Krupp, L.B., Alvarez, L.A., LaRocca, N.G., et al., 1988. Fatigue in multiple sclerosis. Arch. Neurol. 45, 435–437.

Krupp, L.B., La Rocca, N.G., Muir-Nash, J., et al., 1989. The fatigue severity scale. Application to patients with multiple sclerosis and systemic lupus erythematosus. Arch. Neurol. 46, 1121–1123.

Kurtzke, J.F., 1983. Rating neurological impairment in multiple sclerosis: an expanded disability scale (EDSS). Neurology 33, 1444–1452.

Kurtzke, J.F., Hyllested, K., 1986. Multiple sclerosis in the Faroe Islands: II. Clinical update, transmission and the nature of MS. Neurology 36, 307–312.

Langton Hewer, R., 1993. The epidemiology of disabling neurological disorders. In: Greenwood, R., Barnes, M.P., McMillan, T.M. et al., (Eds.), Neurological Rehabilitation. Churchill Livingstone, London, pp. 3–12.

Lenman, J.A.R., Tulley, F.M., Vrbová, G., et al., 1989. Muscle fatigue in some neurological conditions. Muscle Nerve 12, 938–942.

Lennon, V.A., Wingerchuck, D.M., Kryzer, T.J., et al., 2004. A serum antibody marker of neuromyelitis optica: distinction from multiple sclerosis. Lancet 364, 2106–2112.

Lennon, V.A., Kryzer, T.J., Pittock, S.J., et al., 2005. IgG marker of optic-spinal multiple sclerosis binds to the aquaporin-4 water channel. J. Exp. Med. 202, 473–477.

Lord, S.E., Wade, D.T., Halligan, P.W., 1998. A comparison of two physiotherapy treatment approaches to improve walking in multiple sclerosis: a pilot randomised controlled study. Clin. Rehabil. 12, 477–486.

Loseff, N.A., Wang, L., Lai, H.M., et al., 1996. Progressive cerebral atrophy in multiple sclerosis. A serial MRI study. Brain 19, 2009–2019.

Lucchinetti, C.F., Bruek, W., Rodriguez, M., et al., 1996. Distinct patterns of multiple sclerosis pathology indicates heterogeneity in pathogenesis. Brain Pathol. 66, 259–274.

Lucchinetti, C.F., Bruck, W., Parisi, J., et al., 2000. Hetrogeneity of multiple sclerosis lesions:implications for the pathogenesis of demyelination. Ann. Neurol. 47, 707–717.

Lundmark, F., Duvefelt, K., Hillert, J., 2007. Genetic association analysis of the interleukin 7 gene (IL7) in multiple sclerosis. J. Neuroimmunol. 192, 171–173.

Martindale: the complete drug reference, thirtyfifth ed. 2007. Pharmaceutical Press, London.

Matthews, W.B., 1985. Symptoms and signs in multiple sclerosis. In: Matthews, W.B., Acheson, E.D., Batchelor, J.R., Weller, R.O. (Eds.), McAlpine's Multiple Sclerosis. Edinburgh, Churchill Livingstone.

Matthews, W.B., Acheson, E.D., Batchelor,, J.R., et al., 1991. McAlpine's Multiple Sclerosis, second ed. Churchill Livingstone, Edinburgh.

McCullagh, R., Fitzgerald, A.P., Murphy, R.P., et al., 2008. Long-term benefits of excercising on quality of life and fatigue in multiple sclerosis patients with mild disability: a pilot study. Clin. Rehabil. 22, 206–214.

McDonald, W.I., Compston, A., Edan, G., et al., 2001. Recommended diagnostic criteria for multiple sclerosis: guidelines from the International Panel for the Diagnosis of Multiple Sclerosis. Ann. Neurol. 50, 121–127.

McQueen Davis, M.E., Niskala, H., 1992. Nurturing a valuable resource: family caregivers in multiple sclerosis. Axon March, 87–91.

Matesanz, F., Fedetz, M., Leyva, L., et al., 2004. Effects of the multiple sclerosis associated -330 promoter polymorphism in IL2 allelic expression. J. Neuroimmunol. 148, 212–217.

Misulis, K.E., 1993. Essentials of Clinical Neurophysiology. Butterworth Heinemann, London.

Morgan, M.H., 1980. Ataxia – its causes, measurement and management. Int. Rehabil. Med. 2, 126–132.

Morris, M.E., Cantwell, C., Vowles, L., et al., 2002. Changes in gait and fatigue from morning to afternoon in people with multiple sclerosis. J. Neurol. Neurosurg. Psychiatry 72, 361–365.

Mostert, S., Kesselring, J., 2002. Effects of a short-term exercise training program on aerobic fitness, fatigue, health perception and activity level of subjects with multiple sclerosis. Mult. Scler. 8, 161–168.

Motl, R.G., Gosney, J.L., 2008. Effect fo exercise training on quality of life in multiple sclerosis a meta-analysis. Mult. Scler. 14, 129–135.

National Institute for Health and Clinical Effectiveness, 2003. Multiple Sclerosis. National clinical guideline for diagnosis and management in primary and secondary care. Clinical Guideline 8. Issue date 23 November 2003.

O'Brien, B., 1987. Multiple Sclerosis. Office of Health Economics Publications no 87, London.

O'Connor, P., 2002. Key issues in the diagnosis and treatment of multiple sclerosis. An overview. Neurology 59 (Suppl. 3), S1–S33.

Odeen, I., 1981. Reduction of muscular hypertonus by long-term muscle stretch. Scand. J. Rehabil. Med. 13, 93–99.

O'Hara, L., De Souza, L.H., Ide, L., 2000. A delphi study of self-care in a community population of people with multiple sclerosis. Clin. Rehabil. 14, 62–71.

O'Hara, L., Cadbury, H., De Souza, L., et al., 2002. Evaluation of the effectiveness of professionally guided self-care for people with multiple sclerosis living in the community: a randomised controlled trial. Clin. Rehabil. 16, 119–128.

O'Hara, De Souza, L.H., Ide, L., 2004. The nature of care giving in a community sample of people with multiple sclerosis. Disabil. Rehabil. 26 (24), 1401–1410.

Oliver, M.J., 1983. Social Work with Disabled People. Macmillan Press, London.

Page, W.F., Kurtzke, J.F., Murphy, F.M., et al., 1993. Epidemiology of multiple sclerosis in US veterans: ancestry and the risk of multiple sclerosis. Ann. Neurol. 33, 632–639.

Patti, F., Ciancio, M.R., Cacopardo, M., et al., 2002. Effects of a short outpatient rehabilitation treatment on disability of multiple sclerosis: a randomised controlled trial. J. Neurol. 250, 861–866.

Paty, D.W., Li, D.K.B., 1993. The UCB MS/MRI study group and the IFNB multiple sclerosis study group. Interferon β-1b is effective in relapsing remitting multiple sclerosis II MRI results in a multi-centre randomised, double blind, placebo controlled trial. Neurology 43, 663–667.

Paty, D.W., Oger, J.J.F., Kastrukoff, L.F., et al., 1988. MRI in the diagnosis of MS: a prospective study with comparison of clinical evaluation, evoked potentials, oligoclonal banding and CT. Neurology 38, 180–185.

Payne, A., 2001. Nutrition and diet in the clinical management of multiple sclerosis. J. Hum. Nutr. Diet. 14, 349–357.

Petajan, J.H., Gappmaier, E., White, A.T., et al., 1996. Impact of aerobic fitness and quality of life in multiple sclerosis. Ann. Neurol. 39, 432–441.

Polman, C.H., Reingold, S.C., Edan, G., et al., 2005. Diagnostic criteria for multiple sclerosis: 2005 revisions to the "McDonald Criteria" Ann. Neurol. 58, 840–846.

Polman, C.H., O'Connor, P.W., Havrdova, E., et al., 2006. A randomized, placebo-controlled trial of natalizumab for relapsing multiple sclerosis. N. Engl. J. Med. 354 (9), 899–910.

Ponichtera-Mulcare, J.A., Matthews, T., Barrett, G., et al., 1997. Change in aerobic fitness of patients with multiple sclerosis during 6-month training program. Sports Medicine, Training and Rehabilitation 7, 265–272.

Poser, C.M., Paty, D.W., Scheinberg, L., et al., 1983. New diagnostic criteria for multiple sclerosis: guidelines for research protocos. Ann. Neurol. 13, 227–231.

Poser, S., Kurtzke, J.F., Schaff, G., 1989. Survival in multiple sclerosis. J. Clin. Epidemiol. 42, 159–168.

Prineas, J.W., Connell, F., 1978. The fine structure of chronically active multiple sclerosis plaques. Neurology 28, 68–75.

Prineas, J.W., Kwon, E.E., Chow, E.S., et al., 2001. Immunopathology of secondary-progressive multiple sclerosis. Ann. Neurol. 50, 646–657.

PRISMS study group, 1998. Randomised double blind, placebo controlled study of interferon β-1a in relapsing/remitting multiple sclerosis. Lancet 352, 1498–1504.

Rao, S.M., Cognitive Function Study Group, 1990. A Manual for the Brief Repeatable Battery of Neuropsychological Tests in Multiple Sclerosis. National MS Society, New York.

Reitberg, M.B., Brooks, D., Uitdehaag, B.M.J., et al., 2005. Exercise therapy for multiple sclerosis (Cochrane Review). In: The Cochrane Library. Issue 1. Oxford.

Rodgers, M.M., Mulcare, J.A., King, D.L., et al., 1999. Gait characteristics of individuals with multiple sclerosis before and after a 6-month aerobic training program. J. Rehabil. Res. Dev. 36, 183–188.

Rosche, J., Rub, K., Niemann-Delius, B., et al., 1996. Effects of physiotherapy on F-wave amplitudes in spasticity. Electromyogr. Clin. Neurophysiol. 36, 509–511.

Russell, W.R., Palfrey, G., 1969. Disseminated sclerosis: rest-exercise therapy – a progress report. Physiotherapy 55, 306–310.

Sawcer, S., Compston, A., 2003. The genetic analysis of multiple sclerosis in Europeans: concepts and design. J. Neuroimmunol. 143, 13–16.

Scheinberg, L.C., 1987. Introduction. In: Scheinberg, L.C., Holland, N.J. (Eds.), Multiple Sclerosis: A Guide for Patients and their Families. second ed. Raven Press, New York, pp. 1–2.

Scolding, N., 2001. The differential diagnosis of multiple sclerosis. J. Neurol. Neurosurg. Psychiatry 71 (Suppl.), 9–15.

Segal, J., Simpkins, J., 1993. 'My Mum Needs Me': Helping Children with Ill or Disabled Parents. Penguin Books, London.

Shepherd, G.M., 1994. Neurobiology. Oxford University Press, New York.

Sibley, W., 1988. Therapeutic Claims in Multiple Sclerosis. Demos, New York, p. 104.

Snow, B.J., Tsui, J.K.C., Bhatt, M.H., et al., 1990. Treatment of spasticity with botulinum toxin: a double blind study. Ann. Neurol. 28, 512–515.

Soderberg, J., 1992. MS and the family system. In: Kalb, R., Scheinberg, L.C. (Eds.), Multiple Sclerosis and the Family. Demos, New York, pp. 1–7.

Solari, A., Filipini, G., Gasro, P., et al., 1999. Physical rehabilitation has a positive effect on disability in multiple sclerosis patients. Neurology 52, 57–69.

Spackman, A.J., Doulton, D.C., Roberts, M.H.W., et al., 1989. Caring at night for people with multiple sclerosis. Br. Med. J. 299, 1433.

Tallis, R.C., Illis, L.S., Sedgwick, E.M., 1983. The quantitative assessment of the influence of spinal cord stimulation on motor function in patients with multiple sclerosis. International Journal of Rehabilitation Medicine 5, 10–16.

Tantacci, G., Massucci, M., Piperno, R., et al., 1996. Energy cost of exercise in multiple sclerosis patients with low degree of disability. Mult. Scler. 2, 161–167.

Thompson, A.J., 2001. Symptomatic management and rehabilitation in multiple sclerosis. J. Neurol. Neurosurg. Psychiatry 71 (Suppl. 2), ii22–ii27.

Todd, J., 1982. Physiotherapy in multiple sclerosis. In: Capildeo, R., Maxwell, A. (Eds.), Progress in Rehabilitation: Multiple Sclerosis. Macmillan Press, London, pp. 31–44.

Todd, J., 1986. Multiple sclerosis – management. In: Downie, P.A. (Ed.), Cash's Textbook of Neurology for Physiotherapists. fourth ed. Faber & Faber, London, pp. 398–416.

Tourtellotte, W.W., Booe, I.M., 1978. Multiple sclerosis: the blood–brain barrier and the measurement of *de novo* central nervous system IgG synthesis. Neurology 28 (Suppl.), 76–82.

Trapp, P.D., Peterson, J., Ransohoff, R. M., et al., 1998. Axonal transection in the lesions of multiple sclerosis. N. Engl. J. Med. 338, 278–285.

van den Berg, M., Dawes, H., Wade, D.T., et al., 2006. Treadmill training for individuals with multiple sclerosis: a pilot randomised trial. J. Neurol. Neurosurg. Psychiatry 77, 531–533.

Weiner, H.L., Mackin, G.A., Orav, E.J., et al., 1993. Intermittent cyclophosphamide pulse therapy in progressive multiple sclerosis: final report of the Northeast Cooperative Multiple Sclerosis Treatment Group. Neurology 43 (5), 910–918.

Wiles, C., Newcombe, R.G., Fuller, K.J., et al., 2001. A controlled randomised crossover trial of the effects of physiotherapy on mobility in chronic multiple sclerosis. J. Neurol. Neurosurg. Psychiatry 70, 174–179.

Williams, G., 1987. Disablement and the social context of daily activity. Int. Disabil. Stud. 9, 97–102.

Worthington, J.A., De Souza, L.H., 1990. The use of clinical measures in the evaluation of neuromuscular stimulation in multiple sclerosis patients. In: Wientholter, H., Dichgans, J., Mertin, J. (Eds.), Current Concepts in Multiple Sclerosis. Elsevier, London, pp. 213–218.

Yudkin, P.L., Ellison, G.W., Ghezzi, A., et al., 1991. Overview of azathioprine treatment in multiple sclerosis. Lancet. 338, 1051–1055.

FURTHER READING

Compston, A., Ebers, G., Lassman, H., et al., (Eds.), 1998. McAlpine's Multiple Sclerosis. third ed. Churchill Livingstone, London.

Paty, D.W., Ebers, G.C. (Eds.), 1997. Multiple Sclerosis. EA Davis, Philadelphia.

Chapter | 6 |

Parkinson's disease

Diana Jones, Jeremy Playfer

CONTENTS

INTRODUCTION

Parkinson's disease (PD) is a chronic progressive neurodegenerative disorder and an important cause of disability especially in older people. Although PD is usually classified as a movement disorder, it also causes a range of non-motor disorders including cognitive and mood dysfunction, difficulties in communication and autonomic dysfunction. While the cause of PD remains unknown, the description of the pathological features of the condition has become much more complete over the last decade. The loss of neurones which produce the neurotransmitter dopamine in the substantia nigra in the mid-brain explains many of the motor features and this understanding has led to effective drug therapy with dopaminergic drugs. The death of these neurones is associated with the presence of Lewy body inclusions in the surviving cells which contain an accumulation of an abnormal synaptic protein alpha-synuclein. There is also evidence of mitochondrial dysfunction and oxidative stress causing damage to these neurones. The better understanding of the pathophysiology raises hopes for improved treatment in the future.

Idiopathic PD (IPD) accounts for over 70% of all cases of the more general syndrome of parkinsonism (Macphee, 2001). Rare monogenetic variants are important for understanding pathophysiology but account for less than 10% of cases. Secondary parkinsonism may result from a variety of pathological processes including drugs, toxins, trauma and vascular disease. Parkinsonism is a clinical syndrome characterized by slowness of movement (brady-kinesia) accompanied by increased muscle tone (rigidity) and resting tremor (Calne et al., 1992). Later in the disease, postural instability and problems with gait, balance and falls become prominent problems (Bloem et al., 2004). Management requires a multi-disciplinary approach with physiotherapists, occupational therapists and speech thera-pists as vital members in the team (NICE, 2006).

KEY POINTS

♦ PD is a progressive neurodegenerative disorder causing motor and non-motor symptoms.
♦ The cause remains unknown, although the pathology is increasingly understood, including importantly, the loss of dopaminergic neurones in the substantia nigra.
♦ IPD accounts for most parkinsonism (slow movement, increased tone, resting tremor and postural instability, requiring multi-disciplinary management).

Epidemiology

The incidence of PD in the UK is 18 per 100 000 of pop-ulation per year, amounting to approximately 10 000 new cases per year. The prevalence of the disease, the total number of cases in the population, is 164 per 100 000 of population. There are approximately 140 000 people with PD in the UK (Meara & Hobson, 2000).

PD becomes more common with increasing age (1% of the population over 65 have PD). Although PD is more likely to occur in males, because females survive longer, there is a fairly even distribution of overall cases between the sexes. PD is age-related with the commonest onset in the seventh decade. Age is the strongest risk factor for developing PD. Onset at a younger age, especially below the age of 35, always raises the possibility of genetic var-iants of PD (De Lau & Bretele, 2006).

Studies of mortality in PD are limited by the accuracy of death certification and diagnostic confusion between PD and other neurodegenerative conditions. Most studies suggest that PD reduces life expectancy with overall stan-dardized mortality ratios between 1.5 and 2.7 (Louis et al., 1997). Patients with PD are less likely to die of car-diovascular disease or cancer than the general population, but have an increased risk of dying of chest infections (Fall et al., 2003). Cognitive impairment increases mortal-ity significantly (Aarsland, 2008). Patients with PD have a higher risk of hospital and nursing home admissions with consequent ecconomic impact (Vossius et al., 2009).

KEY POINTS

♦ In the UK, approximately 140 000 people have PD (including 1% of the over 65s).
♦ IPD is age-related with the commonest onset in the seventh decade. Onset before the age of 35 suggests a genetic variant of PD.

Aetiology

The causes of sporadic PD are unknown; however, it is likely that the disease results from a combination of fac-tors such as ageing, environmental toxins and genetic sus-ceptibility, resulting in convergent mechanisms causing cell death in vulnerable dopaminergic neurones (Greena-myre & Hastings, 2004).

A variety of environmental factors have been implicated in the development of PD. The most dramatic example is the neurotoxin N-methyl-4-phenyl-1,2,3,6-tetrahydropyri-dine (MPTP). This substance is chemically related to com-mon pesticides such as paraquat. It was a contaminant of illicit recreational drugs, which led to a mini-epidemic of drug-induced parkinsonism in the early 1980s in Califor-nia. Patients exposed to MPTP presented with a sudden dramatic onset of PD features and were particularly liable to develop complications such as dyskinesias and cogni-tive failure (Langston et al., 1983, 1999).

MPTP when given to primates produced a valuable experimental model of PD, although the pathology in the basal ganglia was distinctive, without the characteristic Lewy bodies of the naturally occurring disease. Experi-ments demonstrate damage to mitochondrial function from free radicals produced as a result of oxidation of MPTP catalysed by the enzyme monoamino oxidase type B. Similar changes in mitochondrial function are present in the natural disease. Some speculate that IPD results from chronic damage to mitochondrial function due to expo-sure to toxins in the environment, resulting in oxidative stress in dopamine-producing neurones (Schapira, 2008). Potential environmental toxins include pesticides, manga-nese and copper. Cigarette smoking and drinking large amounts of caffeine have weak protective effects, reducing the risks of PD (De Lau & Bretele, 2006).

Increased familial association in PD was postulated over 100 years ago by Sir William Gowers. Mjones (1949), in a study of Scandinavian families, inferred autosomal domi-nant inheritance with partial penetration. In a study of a set of twins using the technique of PET scanning, preclini-cal changes were found which when analysed showed her-editability was 20% (Burn et al., 1992; Ward et al., 1983). The younger the age at onset of the disease, the more likely genetic factors play a role in aetiology.

Genetic studies are reinforcing the impression that PD does not have a single cause. To date, twelve genes associated with rare forms of the disease have been identified. The first Park gene to be discovered (a gene in which an abnormality may cause some cases of PD) was determined in the Italian–American Contursi kindred and was a point mutation in a gene that produces a protein called alpha-synuclein (Polymeropoulos et al., 1996). This protein accumulated in the Lewy body (the hallmark pathological sign of PD). The gene demonstrates autosomal dominance.

A rare form of juvenile PD found in Japan was associated with a mutation in the parkin gene (Lansbury & Brice, 2002). This gene codes for an enzyme associated with the protein ubiquitin found in the Lewy body. Both the abnormalities in the alpha-synuclein and parkin genes affect the ability of the neurone to destroy abnormal proteins. Accumulation of abnormal proteins is a feature of many neurodegenerative conditions, including, most notably, Alzheimer's disease. The regulation of protein quality within cells by the ubiquitin proteosome system appears compromised in the neurones affected in PD. There are other biochemical abnormalities which indicate that mitochondria are susceptible to damage caused by oxidative stress and that this can trigger cell death. Proteins which are products of other genetic mutations associated with familial PD (PINK1, DJ-1, LAARK2) are allowing scientists to increasingly understand the molecular pathways involved in neurodegeneration and hold out the hope of more effective future treatments (Wood-Kaczmar et al., 2006).

KEY POINTS

- PD is likely to result from a combination of ageing, exposure to toxins and genetic susceptibility causing neuronal death, possibly following chronic mitochondrial damage.
- Genetic factors are most likely to play a role in the aetiology of earlier onset PD. To date, twelve genes associated with rare forms of the disease have been identified.

Pathophysiology

The pathology responsible for PD occurs in a group of grey matter structures in the subcortical region of the cerebrum and in the ventral midbrain, the basal ganglia (Flaherty & Grabiel, 1994). They consist of the striatum (caudate nucleus and putamen), the globus pallidus (internal and external parts), the subthalamic nucleus and the substantia nigra (compact and reticular parts). Neurodegeneration occurs most importantly in the pars compacta of the substantia nigra. This area is rich in neuromelanin-containing cells, which give the region its characteristic pigmented appearance. In PD there is less of the pigment as a result of the loss of more than 70% of the neuromelanin-containing neurones. The death of these cells appears to result from programmed cell death (apoptosis) as opposed to necrosis (accidental cell death). Apoptosis is a sequential process initiated by the cell itself in which the genetic material of the cell is enzymatically degraded. Immune cells remove the dying cells. Destruction of this population of cells results in neurochemical changes, the most important of which is dopamine depletion. The substantia nigra is the main source of the neurotransmitter dopamine and projects on to the striatal region. Dopamine is synthesized from the amino acid L-tyrosine. In PD, as the amount of dopamine available falls, compensatory changes occur in the circuitry of the basal ganglia, and these changes are responsible for most of the features we observe in PD.

In the last decade the development of immunostaining for ubiquitin has created a better picture of the distribution of Lewy bodies. Using these techniques, Braak et al. (2006) produced a model of the stages of development of the disease suggesting that the initial pathology is not in the substantia nigra but in the lower brain stem and the olfactory bulb. At the later stages Lewy bodies become plentiful in the cerebral cortex. This model explains many of the clinical features of PD, in particular why patients should have loss of smell as an early feature and why so many patients develop dementia later in the disease (Braak et al., 2006). The extranigral pathology, including non-dopaminergic pathways in the limbic system and cortex, also explains the non-motor features of PD such as autonomic dysfunction, sleep disorders, sensory changes and psychiatric disorders (Lim et al., 2009).

The basal ganglia are part of a series of parallel loops linking with the thalamus and the cerebral cortex (particularly the motor cortex and frontal cortex). Whilst there is considerable debate about the circuitry of the basal ganglia, the classic model proposes two principal pathways concerned with movement – the direct and the indirect pathways (Flaherty & Grabiel, 1994) (Figure 6.1). The direct pathway flows from the putamen and inhibits the internal part of the global pallidus (GPi) and the substantia nigra reticulata (SNr). These two nuclei project to the thalamus. The indirect pathway, as its name suggests, is longer and links the putamen and the external segment of the global pallidus (GPe) via the subthalamic nucleus (STN) to the GPi and the SNr. The two pathways have opposite effects on basal ganglia output to the thalamus. In PD, the decreased production of dopamine leads to an increased inhibitory output to the thalamus so that the rest of the circuit from the thalamus to the cortex suppresses movement, causing bradykinesia. Dopamine is a modulatory neurotransmitter and its deficiency results in a change in background tone, resulting in rigidity and releasing the inhibition of tremor. The medical

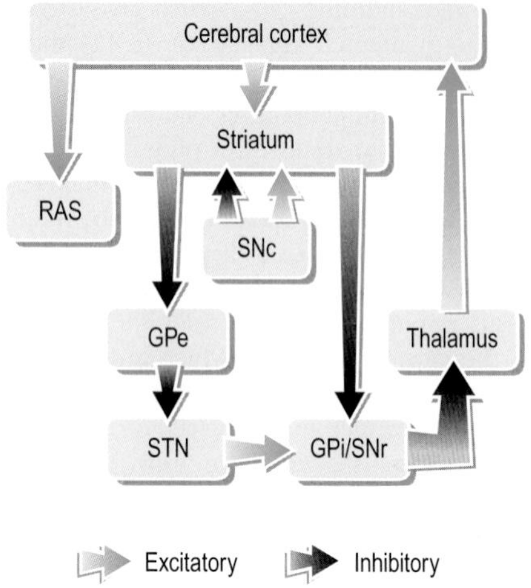

Figure 6.1 Neural circuit in Parkinson's disease. RAS, reticular activating system in spinal cord and brain stem; SNc, substantia nigra pars compacta; GPe, globus pallidus externa; STN, subthalamic nucleus; GPi, globus pallidus interna; SNr, substantia nigra pars reticulata

treatment of PD is concentrated on replacing the deficient dopamine.

Dopamine is stored in presynaptic vesicles. Action potentials release dopamine across the synaptic cleft. The action on the postsynaptic cell depends on the interaction with dopamine receptors. There are at least six different types of dopamine receptors. These consist of two families, D1-like and D2-like (Strange, 1992). The distribution of dopamine receptors varies throughout the brain depending on the functions undertaken. D2 receptors are most important in mediating motor effects. Both levodopa and dopamine agonists used in the treatment of PD are capable of increasing the stimulation of D2 receptors.

KEY POINTS

- Pathology occurs in the basal ganglia (i.e. the striatum, globus pallidus, subthalamic nucleus and, most importantly, in the pars compacta of the substantia nigra).
- Programmed cell death (apoptosis) results in neurochemical changes, most importantly depletion of the modulatory neurotransmitter dopamine.
- As the available dopamine falls, compensatory changes in the basal ganglia arise: the circuit from thalamus to cortex suppresses movement, causing bradykinesia, while a change in background tone results in rigidity and the released inhibition of tremor.
- The medical treatment of PD is concentrated on replacing the deficient dopamine.

Clinical features

The diagnosis of PD depends on the recognition of characteristic clinical signs. At least two of three cardinal features need to be present to make the diagnosis. These are bradykinesia, rigidity and tremor at rest.

Bradykinesia (also termed akinesia or hypokinesia) is a poverty of voluntary movement, with a slower initiation of movement and a progressive reduction in the speed and amplitude of repetitive actions. Bradykinesia is a mandatory sign; the diagnosis of PD cannot be made in its absence. The sign is established firstly by general observation, notably the lack or slowness of spontaneous facial expression and absent arm swing on walking, and then by watching the patient undertake a repetitive opposition with the thumb and each of the other fingers in turn. This is the sign which most improves on treatment.

Rigidity is experienced by the patient as stiffness, and sometimes muscular pain. The physical sign of rigidity is an experience of resistance to passive movement, usually tested by flexion and extension of the wrist or elbow. It can be equally elicited in the lower limbs and trunk. The distribution and severity of rigidity vary between patients and at different times in the same patient. There is a background increase in tone, which gives rise to constant resistance throughout the whole range of movement; this is termed 'lead pipe' rigidity. Most characteristically, PD patients exhibit 'cog-wheel' rigidity where the resistance has a ratchet quality. This is due to the combination of increased background tone and tremor and is pathognomonic of parkinsonism.

Tremor is the presenting sign in 70% of patients with PD. PD tremor is defined as an alternating movement most commonly seen in the upper limb as a reciprocal movement of thumb and forefinger, so-called 'pill-rolling' tremor. The frequency is 4–6Hz. Importantly, PD tremor is present at rest and diminishes or is abolished by active movement. The tremor is asymmetrical at the onset of PD, spreading to the other limb later in the disease.

Postural instability, the fourth cardinal sign of PD, develops later in the disease. The characteristic stooped posture is the result of a dominance of flexor tone over extensor tone. Patients may fall backwards (retropulsion) or forwards (propulsion) on examination. Shuffling gait is in part a compensatory change, with the shortening of the stride reducing postural instability. Patients' ability to initiate or sustain movement may be affected by transient loss of voluntary movement of the feet. Such freezing episodes usually occur late in the disease and are often related to 'off' periods, when medication is failing. Freezing and festination (increased step frequency with very small step amplitude), often occur together during specific activities, such as making a turn, or in specific locations, such as narrow spaces (Giladi et al., 2001). Most falls in PD arise from intrinsic (mainly balance disorders) rather than extrinsic (environmental) factors (Bloem et al., 2004).

Non-motor features

The importance of non-motor features of PD which have adverse effects on quality of life is increasingly recognized (NICE, 2006). Mental health problems, difficulties in communication, sleep disorders, falls and autonomic and sensory disturbance (especially pain) comprise the most important of these (Chaudhury et al., 2004). Speech is affected, with the voice becoming monotonous, exhibiting reduced volume and a lack of rhythm and variety of emphasis, with marked psychosocial implications (Miller et al., 2006). Speech impairment is often associated with problems of swallowing. Drooling occurs despite indications of decreased salivary production in PD (Proulx et al., 2005). It is not unusual for patients to complain of muscle pain and this can be due to dystonia, which is an abnormal pattern of muscle contraction, most characteristically toe curling, associated with the wearing off of drug effects.

Autonomic nervous system signs include an increased tendency to bladder hyperreflexia, postural hypotension and sexual dysfunction. Gastro-intestinal manifestations include dysphagia, drooling, weight loss and constipation. Sleep disorders are increasingly recognized as a feature of PD. Daytime hypersomnolence can disrupt rehabilitation. Rapid eye movement sleep disorder, restless legs syndrome, inverted sleep–wake cycle and nocturnal akinesia afflict patients with PD and are often not recognized (Barone et al., 2004). The lack of movement and ability to turn at night can adversely affect sleep (Stack & Ashburn, 2006).

Mental problems complicate the latter stages of PD. Subtle cognitive changes occur early in the disease, particularly frontal lobe executive dysfunction. As the disease develops, other psychiatric problems emerge. Depression, dementia and psychosis are the most common of these (Hindle, 2001). Recognition and active management of these problems is essential as the symptoms can often be improved by drug therapy (Chaudhury & Schapira, 2009).

KEY POINTS

♦ Diagnosis depends on recognizing characteristic signs: bradykinesia, rigidity and tremor.

♦ Bradykinesia (poor voluntary movement with slow initiation and progressive reduction in speed and amplitude) must be present for PD to be diagnosed.

♦ Rigidity (resistance to passive movement) brings stiffness and/or pain. Increased tone gives rise to constant resistance ('lead pipe' rigidity). Increased tone plus tremor gives ratchet-like 'cogwheel' rigidity.

♦ Tremor (most commonly seen as 'pill-rolling') is the presenting sign in most cases, present at rest, diminished by movement and asymmetrical at onset, spreading later.

♦ Postural instability, a fourth cardinal sign, develops later in the disease.

♦ Non-motor features (such as mental health problems, communication difficulties, sleep disorders, falls and autonomic and sensory disturbance) also affect quality of life in PD.

Making a clinical diagnosis

The diagnosis of PD is based on clinical criteria based on the UK Parkinson's Disease Society (PDS) Brain Bank Criteria (Gibb & Lees, 1988). Correlation of the clinical diagnosis of PD in practice with postmortem findings in PD brain-bank studies revealed a 25% diagnostic error rate (Hughes et al., 1992a, b). This is very significant as all the patients had been seen by either neurologists or geriatricians who are experts in the field of PD and applied the strictest diagnostic criteria. This research was repeated 10 years later and the error rate had gone down to 10% (Hughes et al., 2001). Nevertheless, in ordinary practice it is likely that some of the patients who have been labelled with PD actually have other related conditions. The commonest differential diagnoses are essential tremor; drug-induced PD; PD plus syndromes such as multiple system atrophy (MSA), progressive supranuclear palsy (PSP); arteriosclerotic parkinsonism; viral infections such as postencephalic parkinsonism; repeated head trauma as experienced by sportsmen such as boxers (dementia pugilistica); rare metabolic diseases such as Wilson's disease; rare genetic disorders such as Hallervorden–Spatz syndrome; normal-pressure hydrocephalus; diffuse Lewy body disease; cortical basal ganglionic degeneration; and tumours as rare causes of misdiagnosis (Lennox & Lowe, 1997; Litvan, 1997; Quinn, 1989, 1995). The NICE guidelines recommend that anyone suspected to have PD should be referred before treatment has started to a specialist with expertise in the differential diagnosis of the condition and that the diagnosis be regularly reviewed (NICE, 2006).

Therapists must always be alert for atypical cases of PD. In particular, patients who present with symmetrical bilateral signs or who have a disproportionate amount of postural instability at an early stage in the disease should be suspected of having atypical parkinsonism and their diagnosis reviewed. Single photon emission computed tomograhpy (SPECT) can be used to differentiate essential tremor and PD, but imaging is not essential to make the diagnosis of PD (NICE, 2006). Techniques such as positron emission tomography, magnetic resonance spectroscopy and transcranial sonography are used in research and not in routine practice.

PHARMACOLOGICAL MANAGEMENT

Two crucial areas of decision-making in relation to medication can be identified:

• Which treatment to initiate in the early stages of the disease?
• How to prevent or reduce the motor complications of drug treatment (abnormal involuntary movements, dyskinesias and dystonias)?

Patients often need complex combinations of drugs (Bhatia et al., 1998; Olanow & Koller, 1998). Apart from anticholinergic drugs (benzhexol, procyclidine), the symptoms of PD are treated by replacing lost dopaminergic function. The anticholinergic drugs are now only used in younger patients with tremulous disease, as in the longer term they can affect cognitive function and are best avoided in the older patient. They have a range of unpleasant side-effects including dry mouth, postural hypotension and bladder problems, and have low efficacy (Playfer, 2001).

Levodopa (Madopar or Sinemet) is the most widely used drug for Parkinson's patients. In these drugs levodopa is combined with a decarboxylase inhibitor which prevents peripheral metabolism of levodopa to dopamine. Levodopa is the most effective drug at relieving parkinsonian symptoms; however, its use is associated with two major long-term complications – fluctuations in motor performance and abnormal involuntary movements. Levodopa has a short half-life and its effects can wear off. Once this occurs, increasing dosage of drugs causes involuntary movements affecting the face and tongue or choreoathetoid movements of the limbs. The response to levodopa can become unpredictable and patients can exhibit rapid switches from being 'on', where motor performance is well maintained, to being 'off', where they are immobile or frozen. Moments of freezing (gait blocks), which are more common in the later stages and after long-term levodopa treatment, can occur in both the 'on' and 'off' state (Nieuwboer et al., 1997). On–off syndrome

becomes so unpredictable that it is extremely disabling to patients and drug strategies are needed to cope with this problem (Clarke & Sampaio, 1997).

The half-life of levodopa can be increased by the use of adjunct therapy. These are enzyme inhibitors which slow the breakdown of levodopa. Catechol-*O*-methyltransferase (COMT) inhibitors inhibit the enzyme catechol-*O*-methyltransferase, which is responsible for inactivating levodopa by methylation. One such agent, Entacapone, a reversible peripheral COMT inhibitor, is given together with each dose of levodopa. The drug is well tolerated and has been shown effectively to increase 'on' time and reduce wearing-off (Poewe & Granata, 1997). A second agent, tolcapone, has been withdrawn in Europe because of liver toxicity.

Monoamine oxidase type B inhibitors, exemplified by selegiline, inhibit the oxidative metabolism of dopamine. In addition to making levodopa more efficient, selegiline may be neuroprotective. The DATATOP study in the USA showed that use of selegiline before the introduction of levodopa delayed the necessity to start levodopa therapy (Parkinson Study Group, 1989). Although these results were originally interpreted as the drug being neuroprotective, the debate continues. A larger study on this drug, undertaken by the UK Parkinson's Disease Research Group, indicated that the side-effects of levodopa were increased and that there was increased mortality (Lees, 1995). Since this finding selegiline has been much less widely used. Selegiline has a mild antidepressant and mood-elevating effect. However, it also tends to increase hallucinations and other psychiatric problems.

An alternative to initial therapy with levodopa is to use dopamine agonists. These drugs act directly on the post-synaptic receptor and, unlike levodopa, are not dependent on the dopaminergic neurones. Use of these drugs has increased because they have fewer long-term motor complications. In addition it is recognized that, if the turnover of dopamine is reduced, there is the potential to protect neurones from oxidative stress. Continuous stimulation of the dopamine receptor is considered desirable pharmacologically: the short half-life of levodopa gives rise to a pulsatile stimulation, which may be responsible for dyskinesias.

Many of the dopamine agonists have long half-lives and therefore can approach continuous dopaminergic stimulation. There are currently six available orally acting dopamine agonists and one parenteral drug. Two of these drugs are now not widely used: bromocriptine (because of poor patient tolerance) and lisuride (because of psychiatric side-effects). Pergolide, ropinirole, cabergoline and pramipexole have all been shown to reduce long-term motor complications and are selected for individual patient use on varying pharmacological characteristics (Clarke, 2001).

Apomorphine is possibly the most potent and effective dopamine agonist in the treatment of PD but can only be used parenterally together with a drug blocking its major side-effect of nausea. Apomorphine can be used by means of a pen injection to rescue patients in an 'off' state. Continuous subcutaneous infusion of apomorphine has proved an effective treatment for patients with severe motor complications. Use of such drugs depends on availability of PD nurse specialists. A preparation of L-Dopa in a gel (Duo-dopa) that can be infused to achieve continuous dopamine stimulation has recently had success in difficult cases but it is expensive and requires expert support (Poewe, 2009). The dopamine agonist rotigitine is available as a transdermal patch.

The NICE guidelines (2006) conclude that there is no universal first choice drug therapy for either the early or late phases of PD. They also found no strong evidence that any current medication is neuroprotective.

KEY POINTS

- Important considerations are (1) which treatment to initiate in early PD and (2) how to minimize the motor complications of drug treatment?
- Symptoms are treated by replacing lost dopaminergic function. Anticholinergic drugs are now only used in younger patients with tremor.
- Levodopa is most widely used but associated with motor fluctuations and abnormal movements: patients can switch rapidly from being 'on' to being 'off'.
- Monoamine oxidase type B inhibitors inhibit the oxidative metabolism of dopamine.
- Dopamine agonists are an alternative initial therapy, with fewer long-term motor complications. Many approach continuous dopaminergic stimulation.
- As yet, there is no universal first choice drug therapy for PD.

SURGICAL APPROACHES

With the introduction of levodopa, the need for surgery, widely used prior to the 1970s, diminished but the emergence of long-term complications has led to renewed interest. The success of surgery depends on carefully defined indications and patient selection. Surgery is most suitable for physically fit younger patients who have motor complications refactory to medical treatment but who have previously responded to levodopa and do not have significant mental ill health (NICE, 2006). Two types of surgical approaches are available.

Implantation of fetal cells

Transplanted fetal mesoencephalic cells harvested from aborted fetuses, grown in cell culture and injected into the brain in a form of cell suspension, have been shown to survive in the brain and replace the production of dopamine (Hauser et al., 1999). This type of surgery remains experimental and controversial, and disabling dyskinetic movements following such transplants have been reported in the USA. Fetal transplants were pioneered in Sweden where successful long-term follow-up has been demonstrated (Lindvall, 1998). Manipulation of the patient's own cells by genetic therapy is an active area of research. The number of transplants undertaken is minuscule compared with the number of patients with PD and the procedure is never likely to be a mass treatment. Cell implants are currently suspended because of complications (severe involuntary movements) associated with the technique (Snyder & Olanow, 2005).

Stereotactic surgery and implantation of stimulators

Better understanding of the pathophysiology of PD has helped to identify areas in the brain that may be targets for stereotactic surgery or the implantation of stimulators. The original target for such surgery was the thalamus. This has been replaced in recent years by targeting either the globus pallidus or, more recently, the STN. The target area of the brain may be lesioned to reduce its output (to benefit the movement disorder) or it may be stimulated (to inhibit output with similar effect). Use of stimulators to the STN can demonstrate dramatic improvements in patients' motor abilities; however, these procedures are still awaiting the outcome of large prospective double blind controlled trials. Improvement in clinical symptoms after surgery is not reflected in increases in habitual physical activity, and addressing behavioural change through rehabilitation may be warranted (Rochester et al., 2009). Unfortunately, cognitive and psychiatric problems in PD can be worsened by surgery and great caution has to be applied to the selection of patients (Limousin et al., 1998).

KEY POINTS

- Surgery is most suitable for fit young patients with motor complications who have previously responded to levodopa and do not have significant mental health problems.
- Implantation is experimental and controversial: disabling dyskinesia has been reported. Injected fetal cells have survived in the brain and replaced dopamine production.
- Brain areas may be targets for stereotactic surgery or stimulator implant. STN stimulation can bring dramatic improvement in motor ability; however, these procedures await the outcome of large trials. Surgery can worsen cognitive and psychiatric problems.

TEAM MANAGEMENT OF PARKINSON'S DISEASE

Key priorities for implementation of best practice in PD over the course of the condition are referral to an expert for accurate diagnosis; expert review; regular access to a PD nurse specialist; access to physiotherapy, occupational therapy and speech and language therapy; and consideration of palliative care needs (NICE, 2006). Also relevant to PD service development are the quality requirements, supported by evidence-based markers of good practice, articulated within the National Service Frameworks (NSF), particularly the NSF for Long Term Conditions (LTC) (Department of Health (DH), 2005). The NSF for LTC (DH, 2005) underlines the need for access to the full range of rehabilitation professionals to provide timely, on-going and comprehensive specialist rehabilitation in hospital, in specialist settings and in the community for people with long-term neurological conditions.

The evidence reviewed by NICE (2006) highlighted the key role for the PD nurse specialist in clinical monitoring and medication management and in providing a continuing point of contact for support and information. Occupational therapy was recommended with particular reference to the maintenance of social function and self care, and to environmental and cognitive assessment and intervention. Speech therapy was recognized as valuable in improving quality of speech and communication, including the use of the Lee Silverman Voice Treatment (LSVT). The profession also had a role in the review and management of the safety and efficiency of swallowing and minimizing the risk of aspiration. The NICE (2006) PD guideline reported that there was encouraging high-quality evidence of the effectiveness for some physiotherapy interventions for people with PD. Physiotherapy should be available to people with PD with particular reference to gait re-education, improvement of balance and flexibility; enhancement of aerobic capacity; improvement of movement initiation; improvement of functional independence, including mobility and activities of daily living; and provision of advice regarding safety in the home environment. NICE (2006) also recognized that there was positive evidence of the value of the Alexander technique. A pragmatic phase III randomized controlled trial investigating the clinical and cost effectiveness of physiotherapy and occupational therapy in people with PD (PD REHAB) is currently being undertaken (National Institute for Health Research, 2009). Further trials to investigate the components of physiotherapy (and their effect in the earlier stages of the disease) were recommended (NICE, 2006).

The Primary Care Task Force for the PDS (UK), in their guide for primary care teams (PDS, 1999), highlights the input of the full PD team, including GPs, therapists, social workers, dieticians, as well as experts in neuropsychiatry, neurosurgery and palliative care, in the management of PD in the diagnostic, maintenance, complex and palliative clinical disease stages. However, many patients could not access physiotherapy due to lack of provision (NICE, 2006), a fact underlined by the results of the latest survey of the membership of the PDS in the UK (PDS, 2008), which reported that almost half of respondents had never had a physiotherapy assessment or course of treatment.

KEY POINTS

- Best practice entails referral to an expert for diagnosis; expert review; regular access to a PD nurse specialist; access to physiotherapy, occupational therapy and speech and language therapy; and consideration of palliative care needs.
- The National Service Framework for Long Term Conditions is also relevant, underlining the need for access to timely, on-going and comprehensive specialist rehabilitation.

MODEL OF PHYSIOTHERAPY MANAGEMENT

Morris (2000) underlines the importance of a multidisciplinary approach and good communication between team members, patients and carers in her seminal model for physical therapy in PD. The basic assumption of the model is that normal movement can be promoted by utilizing treatment strategies that bypass the defective basal ganglia, with the rationale for therapy interventions based on a comprehensive understanding of the pathophysiology and resultant clinical features of the condition (see earlier sections). This knowledge underpins approaches using external (e.g. auditory and visual) and internal (e.g. attentional) cues, which address the size and timing of movements; task-specific training, which addresses difficulties with long sequences of well-learned, automatic movements and performance of multiple tasks; and the environment of therapy to maximize learning, i.e. ideally where the difficulty is most problematic. A sound knowledge of PD medication or surgery and their effect on function is important, together with the effects of ageing, any concurrent pathology, and existing long-term secondary effects of PD and other conditions on the musculoskeletal and cardiovascular systems (Morris, 2000).

The physiotherapy treatment paradigm is likely to evolve in future to take cognizance of recent work in animal models. Morris (2006) cites work on pharmacological, learning and exercise approaches which point to the possibility of neuroprotection and neuroplasticity in neurodegenerative disorders. The link between rehabilitation and neural adaptation is likely to be an increasing focus of research.

KEY POINTS

- Movement may be promoted by strategies that bypass the defective basal ganglia, with the rationale based on understanding the pathophysiology and clinical features of PD.
- This knowledge underpins approaches using cues to address the size and timing of movements; task-specific training, which addresses difficulties with movement sequences and performance of multiple tasks; and the environment of therapy to maximize learning.
- The link between rehabilitation and neural adaptation is an increasing focus of research.

GUIDELINES FOR PHYSIOTHERAPY FOR PEOPLE WITH PARKINSON'S DISEASE

Physiotherapy guidelines have been developed in the UK (Ashburn et al., 2004; Plant et al., 2001) and more recently in the Netherlands in 2004 (Keus et al., 2004b, 2007), published on line in English in 2006 (Centre for Evidence Based Physiotherapy, 2009). The Dutch guideline synthesized evidence up to October 2003. The team have subsequently looked at the evidence for the period October 2003 to December 2007 and concluded that the guideline recommendations stand with some updated details in relation to cueing and lower-limb strength training (Keus et al., 2009a).

The Dutch Guidelines include four evidence-based Quick Reference Cards (QRCs). These are designed to directly support clinical practice, particularly physiotherapists who do not treat large numbers of PD patients, in the full range of hospital- or community-based practice contexts. The QRCs can be downloaded, as part of the guidelines, from the Centre for Evidence Based Physiotherapy website (2009). A group of UK clinical and research physiotherapists have worked together to review the four QRCs to ensure contextual and cultural relevance in relation to UK physiotherapy practice in PD (Ramaswamy et al., 2009). The sections on the physiotherapy diagnostic and therapeutic process in PD below will broadly map onto the Dutch QRCs and include the modifications for UK practice. The evidence base for physiotherapy will be reviewed briefly within each section. A case study will highlight the use of the QRCs with a person with PD in the maintenance/complex phase of the condition.

KEY POINTS

- UK and Dutch physiotherapy guidelines have been developed. The latter (published online in English) include evidence-based Quick Reference Cards to support therapists.

PHYSIOTHERAPY DIAGNOSTIC PROCESS

Referral to physiotherapy

Whilst many patients who require physiotherapy are not being referred (NICE, 2006; PDS, 2008), studies in the Netherlands have concluded that others may be receiving care inappropriately or are being treated over unsuitably long time periods (Keus et al., 2004a; Nijkrake et al., 2006). Referrers require a strong evidence base and confidence in the PD specific expertise within available services to refer (Keus et al., 2009a). Box 6.1 sets out the indications for referral to physiotherapy, incorporating recommendations from the Dutch guidelines (Keus et al., 2004b) and areas of strength of evidence highlighted in the NICE guidelines (2006). Morris (2006) argues strongly for routine early referral to physiotherapy prior to the commencement of medication to enable baseline levels of impairments, activity limitation and participation restrictions to be assessed for later evaluation of disease progression. Referral at this stage would also allow the teaching of strategies for moving with large amplitude movements for building on later in the disease process (Morris, 2006). Investigation of the effectiveness of early referral is a recommendation of the NICE PD guideline (2006). Note that PD tremor is not amenable to physiotherapy, although it may be decreased by relaxation methods (Keus et al., 2004b).

Physiotherapy history taking

Physiotherapy history taking must start with an understanding of issues from the patient (and carer) perspective, together with their aspirations for the episode of care (Table 6.1). Where possible, to minimize fatigue especially when clear speech may be difficult to produce, information should be obtained from existing sources and verified with the patient. The International Classification of Functioning, Disability and Health (ICF) (WHO, 2002) domains can be used to structure questioning, focusing initially on participation

Box 6.1 **Indications for referral to physiotherapy in Parkinson's disease**

Activity limitations and impairments of function especially with respect to:

Transfers

Body posture

Reaching and grasping

Balance (including flexibility)

Gait (including movement initiation)

Inactivity or a decreased physical capacity

Increased risk of falling or fear of falling

Activity limitations and impairment of function as a result of neck and shoulder complaints

Need for information about the consequences of Parkinson's disease, especially regarding those activity limitations relating to posture or movement affecting mobility and activities of daily living

Need for provision of advice regarding safety in the home environment

Carer's need for information and advice, e.g. aiding mobility and transfers

Increased risk of pressure sores.

(Based on Keus et al., 2004; NICE, 2006.)

commitment. Information prescriptions will direct people with long-term conditions and professionals to targeted sources of information on both disease-specific and generic issues such as employment, driving, finances and support groups that have been verified as reliable and relevant. Professionals can prescribe information on PD, or patients and carers can self-prescribe via the developing NHS Choices (2009) website.

Physical examination

History taking provides the basis for the subsequent focusing of the physical examination on specific areas of functioning related to core areas of physiotherapy, namely physical capacity, transfers, body posture, reaching and grasping, balance and gait (Keus et al., 2004b). Reported or detected sensory alterations should be noted and described. Assessing physical capacity will include focusing on the mobility of cervical, thoracic and other joints, length of muscles, and strength of major muscle groups. Problems with key transfers, such as stand to sit and sit to stand, getting into and out of bed as well as rolling in bed, car transfers and getting off the floor, will be evaluated. A focus on posture, reaching and grasping will include assessment of posture in sitting, walking and lying and the ability to actively correct posture and manipulate objects. The locus of pain and its origin, e.g. musculoskeletal, dystonic, central, should be determined. Balance will be evaluated in a range of conditions including standing with eyes open and closed, sit to stand, turning, walking, reaching, and multi-tasking with combinations of motor and cognitive tasks. Falls history will be followed-up (see Ch. 20). Gait assessment will include evaluation of starting, stopping, stride length, walking speed, festination and freezing; in addition to this arm swing under a range of conditions (e.g. clear and wide, narrow and congested environment; single, dual and multiple tasks) and trunk rotation will be analysed.

The Dutch Guidelines QRC 2 (Keus et al., 2004b) directs physiotherapists to standardized outcome measures in core areas of physiotherapy which have been agreed as optimal via consensus methods, and these have recently been reviewed for cultural relevance in the UK. Measures can be used to gauge health status in two domains: overall health status and status in highly specific areas (see Table 6.2 for suggested measures in specific areas). Recommended outcome measures in relation to overall health status in PD will be described initially, followed by a description of measures for specific areas.

The Patient Specific Complaints Questionnaire (Beurskens et al., 1996; Keus et al., 2004b) lists activity limitations and participation restrictions that can be experienced as a result of PD. Individuals are asked to identify the five most important activities and indicate how difficult it was to perform the activity in the past week on a visual analogue scale. The three most difficult activities

restrictions in relation to roles and relationships, and progressively focusing on related activity limitations and impairments to body structures and functions in relation to the core areas of physiotherapy – transfers, body posture, balance, reaching and grasping, and gait (Keus et al., 2004b). The influence of time of day, medication, fatigue and tremor on activities should be noted. Questioning about physical activity levels and falls will highlight the need to undertake more detailed assessment in the physical examination phase. Treatment for PD and other conditions will be noted. It is important to explore both environmental and personal contextual factors (WHO, 2002) with a potential to influence treatment outcome. These include the attitudinal and physical environment at home, at work and within the health-care system; the individual's own attitude to living with their condition; and cognitive and emotional factors.

Information to enable people to make informed decisions and contribute to the management of their condition themselves in partnership with professionals is seen as a key component of a person-centred service for people with long-term neurological conditions (DH, 2005). The UK NHS Constitution (DH, 2009) makes information a right and is backed up by legislation for the first time. Web-based information prescriptions have been developed to contribute to this

Table 6.1 Diagnostic process. Quick reference card 1: History-taking

Patient perceived problems		
Course of the disease and current status	Onset of complaints; how long since the diagnosis; result of earlier diagnostics; severity and nature of the condition	
Participation problems	Problems with relationships; profession and work; social life including leisure activities	
Impairments in functions and limitations in activities	Transfers	Sit down; rise from floor or chair; get in or out of bed; roll over in bed (sleeping problems); get in or out of a car
	Body posture	Ability to actively correct posture; pain due to postural problems; problems with reaching, grasping, and moving objects
	Balance	Feeling of impaired balance while standing and during activities; orthostatic hypotension; difficulty with dual tasking (motor activity, cognitive)
	Reaching and grasping	Household activities (small repairs, clean, cook, slice food, hold a glass or cup without spilling); personal care (bath, get dressed/undressed, button up, lace up shoes)
	Gait	Use of aids; walk in the house; climb the stairs, walk short distances outside (100 m); walk long distances outside (>1 km); start; stop; turn; speed; onset of festination; onset of freezing (use the Freezing of Gait Questionnaire); relation to falls and the use of cues
	Influence of tiredness, the time of the day and medication on the performance of activities; influence of tremor on the performance of activities	
Physical activity	Frequency and duration per week compared to the Department of Health's recommendation of at least 30 min/day for 5 days a week; if unsure, use Phone FITT or General Practice Physical Activity Questionnaire (GPPAQ) depending on your patient	
Falls risk	For recording fall incidents and near fall incidents, use the questionnaire 'History of Falling' For fear of falling, if patient has had near misses this past year, use the International Falls Efficacy Scale (FES-I)	
Co-morbidity	Pressure sores; osteoporosis and mobility-limiting disorders such as arthrosis, rheumatoid arthritis, heart failure and chronic obstructive pulmonary disease (COPD)	
Treatment	Current treatment (e.g. medication and outcome) and earlier medical and allied health therapy treatment type and outcome	
Other factors	Mental factors	Ability to concentrate; memory; depression; feeling isolated and lonely; being tearful; anger; concern for the future
	Personal factors	Insight into the disease; socio-cultural background; attitude (e.g. with regard to work); coping (e.g. the perception of the limitations and possibilities, the patient's solutions with regard to the limitations)
	External factors	Attitudes, support and relations (e.g. with partner, primary care physician, employer); accommodation (e.g. interior, kind of home); work (content, circumstances, conditions, and relations)
Expectations	Expectations of the patient with regard to prognosis; goal and course of the treatment; treatment outcome; need for information, advice and coaching	

(Reproduced with permission of Royal Dutch Society of Physiotherapy. Keus S H J, Hendriks H J M, Bloem B R et al 2004 KNGF Guidelines for physical therapy in Parkinson's disease. Dutch Journal of Physiotherapy 114(supplement 3) 1-86. (English translation 2006) Modified for UK context (with permission) by Ramaswamy et al., 2009.)

can be evaluated at the beginning and at the end of treatment. The Parkinson's Disease Questionnaire 39 (PDQ-39) is a PD-specific measure of health status (Jenkinson et al., 1995). The 39-item questionnaire generates a score in eight domains of quality of life: mobility, activities of daily living, emotions, stigma, social support, cognitions, communication and bodily discomfort. A short form of the questionnaire (PDQ-8) based on eight items from the longer version generates a single index score, performs similarly to the longer version (Jenkinson et al., 1997) and may, therefore, be more suitable for clinical practice. In contrast to the PDQ-39 the EQ-5D is a generic measure of health outcome applicable to a wide range of conditions, providing a single index value for health status. Individuals indicate their level of health by ticking one of three levels of difficulty in relation to mobility, self-care, usual activity, pain and anxiety/depression. The EQ-5D (EuroQol, 2009) has been adopted as a key patient reported outcome measure within the NHS (DH, 2008) and has been validated in the PD population (Schrag et al., 2000).

Measurement in PD is complicated by clinical fluctuations (Morris et al., 1998); however, recording current medication, the time of day, time since last dose, and 'on' or 'off' status can guide the taking of comparable measurements in relation to specific areas of the physical examination (Table 6.2). Three measures are suggested as potentially appropriate for the evaluation of physical activity. The Phone-FITT (Gill et al., 2008) is a brief interview of older adults designed to measure frequency, intensity, time and type of physical activity undertaken by older people with potentially lower levels of activity. Summary scores are derived for household, recreational and total physical activity. The measure can be telephone- or self-completed. The General Practice Physical Activity Questionnaire (GPPAQ) (DH, 2006) is a validated screening tool for use in primary care to help inform a practitioner when a brief intervention to increase physical activity is appropriate in adults (16–74 years of age). It provides a 4-level physical activity index, categorizing patients as active, moderately active, moderately inactive and inactive. The 6-minute walk test (Guyatt et al., 1985), a measure of how far a patient can walk in 6 minutes, can be used with patients who are not experiencing freezing to evaluate physical capacity. Footwear and level of encouragement should remain consistent in any follow-up testing (Arnadottir & Mercer, 2000; Enright et al., 2003). The Modified Parkinson's Activity Scale (Keus et al., 2009b; Nieuwboer et al., 2000), a comprehensive practical test of gait (including dual tasking) and transfers (including rolling over in bed), taking about 15 minutes to complete, can be used to assess functional mobility. The tragus to wall measurement is recommended to evaluate body posture. A measurement of the horizontal distance between the right tragus and the wall is made with the person instructed to stand with their heels and buttocks against the wall, knees extended, shoulders back and chin tucked in. The distance has been correlated with radiographic change in the cervical spine (Haywood et al., 2004).

A range of balance outcome measures are suggested to cover the spectrum of potential deficits. The Timed Up and Go (TUG) test (Morris et al., 2001; Podsialdo & Richardson, 1991) measures how quickly an individual can rise from a chair, walk 3 metres, turn round, walk back to the chair and sit down. The retropulsion test evaluates the response to an unexpected, quick and firm backwards pull on the shoulder (Visser et al., 2003), where the normal reaction is to take two quick, large steps back with no requirement for the assessor to catch the individual. The History of Falls 10 question checklist (Stack & Ashburn, 1999) helps people recount falls and near-misses (fall events) and to identify the surrounding circumstances. An initial unspecific question, 'Have you fallen or ended-up on the ground for any reason?' is posed, and if a positive response is gained 10 questions are worked through. The number of falls is ascertained, and for each fall the location; activity at the time; possible

Table 6.2 Outcome measurement in physiotherapy for Parkinson's disease

PHYSICAL CAPACITY	TRANSFERS	BODY POSTURE/ REACHING AND GRASPING	BALANCE	GAIT
Phone FITT General Practice Physical Activity Questionnaire Six-minute walk test	Parkinson Activity Scale Timed Up and Go test	Tragus to wall measures either side combined with height	Timed Up and Go test Retropulsion test Falls Efficacy Scale Falls diary Questionnaire History of Falling	Parkinson Activity Scale Timed Up and Go test Freezing of Gait questionnaire Ten-meter walk test Dual task, e.g. walk and carry

(Based on Keus et al., 2004, and Ramaswamy et al., 2009)

cause; how the individual landed; number of near-misses in a specified time period; frequency of near-misses; activity during near-falls; individual's own theory about why they nearly fell; and how they saved themselves are explored (Stack & Ashburn, 1999).

It is also important to gauge fear of falling and the International Falls Efficacy Scale (FES-I) (Yardley et al., 2005), developed under the auspices of the Prevention of Falls Network Europe (ProFaNE, 2009), can capture which tasks increase a person's fear of falling, the likelihood of increasing falls risk and if patients have had near-misses in the past year. A short version of the full 16 item FES-I is recommended for use in clinical practice.

The Ten-meter walk test is a reliable instrument to identify the comfortable walking speed of PD patients (Schenkman et al., 1998). This can provide information for auditory cueing of gait at, above or below baseline, and the basis for calculating stride length for visual cueing (see Cueing section). Patients may report problems with freezing, feeling their feet are glued to the floor, and yet be unable to demonstrate it in the clinic (Nieuwboer et al., 1998). The Freezing of Gait Questionnaire (FOG-Q) is a six–item scale (range 0–24) consisting of four items which assess severity of freezing and two items which assess gait difficulties in general (Giladi et al., 2000). Item three of the six item FOG-Q has recently been identified as an effective screening question for the presence of freezing (Giladi et al., 2009).

KEY POINTS

- Early referral to physiotherapy allows the teaching of strategies for building on later.
- History taking starts with understanding patients' (and carers') issues and aspirations, before focusing on core activity limitations which will focus the physical examination.
- Providing information to enable people to make informed decisions about their management in partnership with professionals is a key component of a person-centred service for people with long-term neurological conditions.
- Balance and gait need evaluation under multiple conditions, using a battery of measures.

THERAPEUTIC PROCESS

Treatment goals

Dutch guidelines QRC 3 (Figure 6.2) displays a time line for an individual with PD, identifying early, middle and late stages, and their relationship to the Hoehn and Yahr

(1967) stages and the clinical staging proposed by the Primary Care Task Force for PDS (UK) (PDS, 1999). Goals of physiotherapy are articulated for each stage. Goals reflect health gain and health maintenance in the early and middle stages, and comfort in the later stages (PDS, 1999).

Issues of location, format, intensity and duration of therapy are closely related to goals. Keus et al. (2004b) reviewed available evidence to propose recommendations. Improvements in physical capacity are likely to require exercise equipment and space. Fitness activity should take place in a gym or a therapy environment with appropriate equipment, potentially at a low treatment frequency (e.g. once a week) and a duration of 8 weeks. In the middle phase, when activity limitations are paramount, the home setting where those activities are proving problematic will be the preferred treatment context; a treatment frequency of several times per week over a 4 week period is likely to be required.

Individual sessions supplemented by group work comprised the model of service delivery favoured by specialist physiotherapists in an evaluation of best practice in the UK (Ashburn et al., 2004). Most groups were run on a multidisciplinary basis with monitoring, exercise, advice, the sharing of information and an emphasis on self-management as the key components. In the same study, people with PD identified having their personal needs met as the main benefit of individual sessions, whilst the social contact and motivation provided by group work were also valued (Ashburn et al., 2004). Ellis et al. (2005) evaluated a 6-week group programme which focused on gait training, simulation of everyday activities, general physical activity and relaxation. Results showed that people with PD gained short-term benefits in relation to quality of life related to mobility, comfortable walking speed and activities of daily living from group treatment in addition to their medication therapy.

The importance of context of therapy was highlighted in a study of a home physiotherapy programme undertaken by Nieuwboer et al (2001). Functional activity was measured in both the hospital and home contexts, with improvement of functional activity scores assessed at home more than twice those observed in hospital. The researchers postulate that this was due to better retention of treatment strategies within the actual learning context. Morris et al. (2009) conducted a trial of movement strategies versus musculoskeletal exercises during 2 weeks of inpatient stay. Both approaches, but particularly movement strategy training, were associated with short-term improvements in disability and quality of life with some loss of performance at 3 month follow-up. There is a need to research how best to support inpatient and group therapy gains over time in the community, in the context of a degenerative condition.

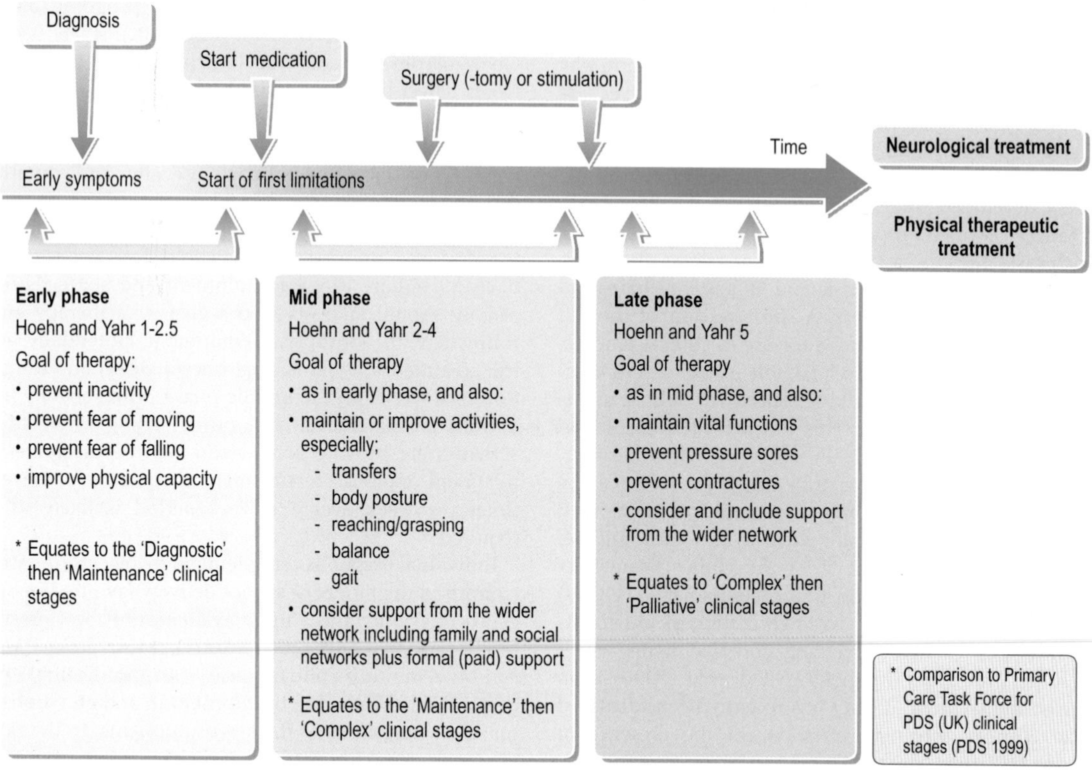

Figure 6.2 Therapeutic process. Quick Reference Card 3: Specific treatment goals. (Reproduced with permission of Royal Dutch Society of Physiotherapy. Keus S H J, Hendriks H J M, Bloem B R et al. 2004 KNGF Guidelines for physical therapy in Parkinson's disease. Dutch Journal of Physiotherapy 114(supplement 3) 1-86. (English translation 2006) Modified for UK context (with permission) by Ramaswamy et al., 2009.)

A comprehensive understanding of both the home environment and support mechanisms is particularly important when assessment and treatment are taking place in hospital (Morris, 2006). As with assessment, treatment in both the 'on' and 'off' stages of the medication cycle is advisable. Teaching movement strategies will be undertaken in the 'on' phase, with the efficacy of, for instance, cognitive movement and cueing strategies monitored in the 'off' phase (Keus et al., 2004b). Involvement of the carer is important, but particularly if the patient has psychological or cognitive impairment, such as depression or dementia, affecting attention or memory. The physical, emotional and cognitive status of carers also needs to be taken into account (see Case study). Special information for carers to support them and help them reinforce the messages from therapy sessions is useful. The RESCUE project, a trial of cueing therapy in the home (Nieuwboer et al., 2007), made patient and carer information sheets about cueing downloadable from the project website and CD Rom (see Resources).

KEY POINTS

- Physiotherapy goals differ as Parkinson's disease progresses.
- Location, format, intensity and duration of therapy are closely related to goals.
- UK specialists favour individual treatment sessions supplemented by groups.
- Training at home and in movement strategies enhance functional gains.
- Provide treatment in the 'on' and 'off' stages; consider and involve the carers.

Treatment strategies

A summary of the treatment strategies that can be employed for different treatment goals is provided in the Dutch guidelines QRC 4 (Keus et al., 2004b). The following section reviews the rationale behind, and the principal uses of, the main treatment strategies in PD.

Cognitive movement strategies

The basal ganglia play a pivotal role in running complex motor sequences that make up skilled, largely automatic, movement such as walking and turning in bed. Phasic neural activity acts as a cue to initiate movement and release linked submovements of a movement sequence (Iansek et al., 1997). Basal ganglia deficit means that the rehabilitation of gross motor skills in PD prioritizes compensatory as opposed to normal movement strategies (Kamsma et al., 1995). Compensatory strategies are atypical approaches to meeting the sensory and motor requirements of a task (Shumway-Cook & Woollacott, 1995). In PD compensatory cognitive movement strategies are used to address ongoing motor control difficulties, such as processing sequential tasks and undertaking motor and cognitive tasks concurrently (Kamsma et al., 1995; Müller et al., 1997; Nieuwboer et al., 2001). Box 6.2 highlights the principles underlying the development of compensatory movement strategies, which can be applied to activities such as getting out of a chair, turning in bed and getting into a car. These centre on breaking down complex tasks into their component parts and undertaking single aspects of the task in appropriate order under conscious control without other distractions.

Box 6.2 **Principles underlying compensatory movement strategies**

Break down complex movement sequences into simple component parts

Arrange parts in a logical, sequential order

Utilize prior mental rehearsal of the whole movement sequence

Perform each part separately, ideally ending in a stable resting position from which the next step can be initiated

Execute each part under conscious control

Avoid simultaneous motor or cognitive tasks

Use appropriate visual, auditory and somatosensory cues to initiate and maintain movement.

(Based on Kamsma et al., 1995; Morris, 2000.)

Cueing

Failure to maintain automatically the appropriate scale and timing of sequential movements is a key motor problem experienced with basal ganglia disorder. The medial basal ganglia and supplementary motor area pathways are consistently hypoactive in neuroimaging work investigating internally generated, automatic movements in people with PD; these pathways are relatively over-activated in normal individuals. When a movement is externally generated using cues, the lateral (superior) parietal, thalamus, and premotor areas are relatively more activated (Debaere et al., 2003; Samuel et al., 1997). Although there are many other complex circuits involved (Nieuwboer et al., 2008), this account can be helpful in understanding the basis of therapy which aims to help patients employ alternative routes to bypass the faulty basal ganglia.

Therapeutic cueing uses external temporal or spatial stimuli to facilitate movement initiation and continuation (Nieuwboer et al., 2007). In relation to gait, in the early stages of the condition cues can be used to maintain quality and help training to avoid deconditioning, while in the later stages they can help compensate for reduction of automaticity (Nieuwboer et al., 2008). Systematic reviews have reported marked immediate effects of cues on gait parameters (walking speed, step length and step frequency) (Deane et al., 2001a, 2001b; Lim et al., 2005; Rubenstein et al., 2002). Carryover to uncued performance and generalization to activities of daily living is limited in laboratory studies (e.g. Morris et al., 1996) and was not found either in the largest home-based trial of cueing, the RESCUE trial, although improved walking confidence did carryover (Nieuwboer et al., 2007). The RESCUE trial, which reported small, specific improvements in gait and freezing after intervention, measured outcomes with cues absent. This might be an underestimation of the real effect when using cues (Keus et al., 2009a) and warrants further study.

Cues are chosen for their specific outcomes according to modality (mode of delivery – auditory, visual or other) and parameter (specificity of information provided – spatial or temporal, and amplitude or frequency settings). Cues that focus on step amplitude (visual markers or attentional strategies) primarily affect step size (e.g. Canning, 2005); stripes 50–60 cm apart can be used as a starting point. Cues that focus on step frequency (rhythm) primarily affect number of steps (e.g. Rochester et al., 2005); baseline stepping frequency during straight-line walking can be used as a starting point. Attentional strategies can be used discretely (Behrman et al., 1998), but can be difficult to sustain especially in the later stages of the condition. Laboratory work has shown that an associate cue strategy, combining a metronome beat with an attentional strategy to increase step size, is effective, including during a functional task (Baker et al., 2007). Table 6.3 provides examples of cueing for different problems, including turning and performing dual tasks. Auditory cues reduce step variability during turning (Willems et al., 2007) and cues help dual task interference, potentially by reducing the attention needed for gait (Rochester et al., 2007). Evaluation of cognitive status is important, especially when working on cueing for dual tasks. Training is progressed from simple to more complex tasks, first in the open and then in more complex environments, in 'on' and 'off' medication phases as appropriate (Nieuwboer et al., 2008).

Table 6.3 Examples of cueing for different gait problems

PROBLEM	CUE MODALITY	CUE PARAMETER
Freezing	Auditory Associate strategy Visual	Step frequency – 10% below baseline just maintaining rhythm Below baseline auditory rhythm paired with 'taking a big step' instruction Stripes on the floor at freezing of gait-provoking 'hot spots' around the house
Gait initiation	Auditory Visual (line on floor)	Weight transfer in time to a slow beat and then instruction to 'step out' Step over line to start
Step size	Visual Attention Associate strategy	Lines on floor or on pavement, carpets Concentrate on taking big steps or active heel strike Auditory rhythm paired with 'taking a big step'
Turning	Auditory Visual	Step in time to the beat through turn, maintain stepping rhythm Mark lines on floor in turning space, i.e. toilet floor
Dual tasks	Auditory Somatosensory Associate cue (auditory and attention)	Practice simple task, straight-line walk with cue. Reduce frequency of cue by 10–15% Build up task difficulty to incorporate additional tasks Practice with cue in home and outdoor environments. Reduce frequency of cue by 10–15%

(Reproduced with permission of Wolters Kluwer Health/Lippincott Williams & Wilkins. Nieuwboer A, Rochester L, Jones D 2008 Cueing gait and gait-related mobility in patients with Parkinson's disease. Developing a therapeutic method based on the International Classification of Functioning, Disability, and Health. Topics in Geriatric Rehabilitation 24:151-165, p. 160.)

The rationale for cueing can be employed to address a range of issues such as posture, reaching and speech. The tendency to flexion in PD can be corrected by verbal and visual feedback (Weissenborn, 1993), however this requires constant reinforcement. The Dutch physiotherapy guideline has been updated (Keus et al., 2009a) to include a recommendation that audiovisual cues enhance the performance of sit to stand based on the work of Mak and Hui-Chan (2007). The team that developed LSVT, an amplitude-based speech and voice training approach incorporating internally cued focused attention to loudness, suggests that the intensive practice of amplitude should be undertaken across disciplines with individual patients, promoting speech, locomotion and reaching, and they hypothesize that this would have the potential for promoting disease modification in relation to neuroplasticity (Farley et al., 2008).

Exercise

Muscle weakness in PD is both a consequence of ageing and reduced activity, and a result of reduced basal ganglia output leading to lower levels of cortical and spinal motor activation (Glendenning & Enoka, 1994). Goodwin et al., (2008) highlights evidence in animal models of PD which indicate the benefits of exercise in relation to neuroplasticity and the stimulation of dopamine synthesis in remaining dopaminergic cells. A systematic review and meta-analysis of randomized controlled trials of exercise interventions for people with PD, with exercise defined as 'a planned, structured physical activity which aims to improve one or more aspects of physical fitness', was undertaken (Goodwin et al., 2008). The types of exercise interventions employed in the included trials, mainly undertaken in outpatient settings, included stretching; progressive exercise training; aerobic exercise; strengthening exercises; balance training; relaxation and muscle activation; body weight supported, weighted and unweighted treadmill training; and Qigong. Fourteen randomized controlled trials of mostly moderate quality contributed to the results of the systematic review, which found evidence to support exercise as beneficial with regards to physical functioning, health-related quality of life, strength, balance and gait speed for people with PD. There was insufficient evidence to support or refute the value of exercise in reducing falls or depression.

Posture and coordination exercise programmes

A trial based on a 12-week Alexander technique programme (Stallibrass et al., 2002) reported improved coordination and greater ease of performance of everyday activities. Teaching patients to move in a relaxed, coordinated manner, focusing on exercising axial structures, in 30 individual sessions over 10 weeks resulted in improved mobility and coordination (Schenkman et al., 1998). Whilst breathing exercises might be incorporated into rehabilitation programmes (Schenkman et al., 1998), there is a need for further research on the specific effects of pulmonary rehabilitation in PD given the range of pulmonary function abnormalities and their contribution to mortality (Polatli et al., 2001).

Joint mobility and muscle strength training

Joint mobility is regularly included with gait and balance training in the protocols of exercise programmes for people with PD tested in trials. Such programmes have reported improvements in motor skills, activities of daily living and mental functioning (e.g. Comella et al., 1994; Patti et al., 1996). Likewise strength training, in tandem with, for example, balance training or aerobic training, has proved effective at increasing strength in patients in early to middle phase PD (e.g. Bridgewater & Sharpe, 1996; Hirsch et al 2003). Updated Dutch guideline work (Keus et al., 2009a) report that a high-force, eccentric resistance training of the lower extremities improved stair descent, the six-minute walk test and muscle volume (Dibble et al., 2006). The Dutch guidelines recommend that hydrotherapy for patients with PD should involve individual supervision (Keus et al., 2004b).

Balance training

Problems with balance may develop about 5 years after initial symptoms, although problems may not appear until much later (Müller et al., 2000). People with PD can take advantage of programmes designed to help balance in healthy older people provided their specific problems are taken into consideration (Keus et al., 2004b). A 10-week programme of balance and strength training (an hour a week, 3 times a week, using visual and vestibular feedback and training lower limb muscles at 60% of maximum strength resistance) improved balance (Hirsch et al., 2003; Toole et al., 2000).

Falls prevention

On average, recurrent falling can become problematic 10 years after initial symptoms (Wenning et al., 1999). In a prospective study of 109 subjects with IPD designed to establish incidence of falls, 70% fell during a 1-year follow-up, and recurrent falls occurred in approximately 50% of patients during the same period (Wood et al., 2002). Teaching patients how to get up off the floor many help reduce fear of falling and attention to footwear is important (Keus et al., 2004b); see also Chapter 20. Ashburn et al. (2007) undertook a randomized controlled trial of a home-based exercise programme designed to prevent the risk of falls in people with PD. A significant effect in favour of exercise was not reported. The trial included the maintenance of a falls diary over a 6-month period and a set of questions about every recorded fall (Ashburn et al., 2008). On analysis, six activity-cause combinations which are likely to challenge most people with PD accounted for over half of the described falls. The six combinations from most to least common were: tripping; freezing, festination and retropulsion; postural instability when bending or reaching; transferring; walking; and washing and dressing. The authors found individuals fell at home in 80% of cases, and were ambulant on 45% of occasions, standing in 32% and transferring in 21%. The key recommendations for therapy practice from this study complement those of QRC 4 (Keus et al., 2004b):

- Find ways to make standing tasks safer or prepare patients to manage them better
- Ask specifically about key activity-cause combinations
- Incorporate outdoor observation in assessment
- Consider environmental adaptation
- Teach cognitive strategies to manage (or avoid) situations that challenge balance
- Optimize motor skills (Ashburn et al., 2008).

Aids

Working closely with occupational therapy colleagues is important when considering aids and adaptations. Walking aids require careful assessment, training and monitoring. A walking stick ('laser cane') and a walking frame ('USTEP'), both equipped with a laser beam to provide a visual cue, have been designed to aid people with PD who experience freezing (Lindop, 2009). Working with both family and formal carers in the community, residential or nursing home settings to assess support for transfers to chairs, toilets, baths and beds may highlight the need for appropriately positioned rails, raised or rising seats, sliding boards, hoists and wheelchairs. Specialist cushions may be required to promote skin care, in tandem with good positioning and weight relief management. Hip protectors may be appropriate for people who are at risk of falling.

Electrotherapy

Therapists must note that deep brain stimulators are a contraindication for any form of diathermy. Subcutaneous nodules are a common side-effect of the administration of the dopamine agonist apomorphine hydrochloride via infusion in the complex phase of the condition. A pilot study to assess the effectiveness of ultrasound in the treatment of nodules compared real versus sham ultrasound and found no significant difference in hardness and tenderness of tissue (Poltawski et al., 2009). Sample size was, however, determined for a larger scale trial, and user opinion on the treated area's suitability for injection established as a meaningful outcome.

Patients and carers should always be informed of follow-up activity after a course of therapy. The referrer should be updated on progress, a point of contact established for future reference, a review appointment set if appropriate, and information provided to support the strategies and activities promoted during the course of therapy.

KEY POINTS

- Multiple treatment strategies warrant consideration.
- Compensatory cognitive movement strategies address difficulty processing sequential tasks and undertaking concurrent tasks.
- Cueing impacts on movement (e.g. gait, speech) by bypassing the faulty basal ganglia, using external temporal or spatial stimuli and/or attentional strategies.
- A variety of exercise types appear to benefit function, quality of life, strength, balance and gait in PD; effects on depression and falls are uncertain.
- If their specific requirements are taken into consideration, people with PD can participate in balance programmes designed for healthy elderly people.
- Falls prevention strategies include identifying challenging activities and tasks and making them safer; to reduce fear, teach people how to get up after a fall.
- If providing walking aids, assess, train and monitor the patient carefully.
- Deep brain stimulators are a contraindication for any form of diathermy.
- After treatment, update the referrer, schedule a review and plan follow-up and support.

USING THE DUTCH PHYSIOTHERAPY GUIDELINES QUICK REFERENCE CARDS IN PRACTICE – A CASE EXAMPLE

This section highlights how the Dutch physiotherapy guidelines QRCs (Keus et al., 2004b) can be used in practice. It will focus on QRC 1 (Table 6.1) to illustrate history-taking during a follow-up review with a male PD patient (Mr M), aged 76, in the maintenance/complex

phase of the condition (see Table 6.4). Brief details will be given of the potential use of QRCs 2, 3 and 4 in this case.

QRC 2: Physical Examination

This will include assessment of: physical capacity – focusing on mobility of thoracic spinal joints; transfers – focusing on car, but including chair and bed transfers; body posture – focusing on increased flexion when standing and walking; balance – focusing on multi-tasking, near falls; gait – focusing on decreased stride length, speed, arm swing, and freezing in doorways, with obstacles, when multi-tasking and with unexpected interruptions. Observation of difficulties of bus travel will be made in the community. Outcome measures for body posture, balance and gait (see Table 6.3) will be undertaken.

QRC 3: Therapeutic Process: Specific Treatment Goals

This highlights the fact that some early phase goals are still relevant, e.g. prevention of fear of falling, but that middle phase goals of addressing problems with transfers, posture, balance and gait are paramount, with consideration of the role and health of the spouse.

QRC4: Treatment Strategies

This would point to a focus on cognitive movement strategies for transfers; cueing for gait and posture problems; together with muscle strength and trunk mobility training for gait, balance, posture and falls prevention. The physiotherapy service could consider an approach to local bus and taxi services about contributing to training sessions for their personnel on the mobility needs of older and disabled people using public transport and taxis.

ACKNOWLEDGEMENTS

Royal Dutch Society for Physiotherapy and Wolters Kluwer Health/Linnincott Williams & Wilkins for permission to reproduce material.

Thanks to Bhanu Ramaswamy and PD contact and spouse for case study.

Table 6.4 Diagnostic process QRC 1: history-taking

Patient's perceived problems	Would like to be more confident at using the bus, and wife feels he would benefit from feeling more confident when getting into and out of taxis	
Course of the disease and current status	PD for 28 years. In maintenance/complex, middle phase of condition.	
Participation problems	Poor mobility outdoors, including using transport, starting to make going out problematic. Wife thinks he is self-conscious about his mobility problems (and that that contributes to his reluctance to use taxis, although he is happy to go out with family or friends to familiar places).	
Impairments in functions and limitations in activities	Transfers	Getting in and out of cars, especially taxis, when people don't know how he likes to do things and tend to pull and push him; can still get on/off the floor; bed transfers problematic now if medication levels low even with the addition of a bed lever
	Body posture	Noticing an increase in forward flexed posture that is becoming more difficult to correct; no pain
	Balance	Impaired balance, particularly during bus travel
	Reaching and grasping	More difficulty with small items requiring dexterity, plus now has to have morning help for personal care from Social Services
	Gait	Walking outside the home poses less challenges than indoors, where doorways cause him to experience the feeling of his feet being stuck to the floor (freezing): he has, however, flagged up outside mobility as his main perceived problem. He holds on to furniture for balance indoors and uses a stick on bad days, at night and always outside. Uses stair lift. Often when walking back from the local supermarket Mrs M has to alter her pace as Mr M, having walked one way with relative ease, struggles to walk home.
	Definite patterns of decreased ability after evening tea nearing bedtime.	
Physical activity	Mr M does a weekly exercise class with other people with PD and his walking is better after the class. He enjoys outdoor bowling and fishing, and tries to keep himself generally fit, and has recently joined a gym.	
Falls risk	When asked about his feelings about falling and his concerns, he responded that there was hardly anything he did these days that did not cause him to worry that he might fall. This subjective account was confirmed by completion of the 7 items of the FES-I short form which showed him to be 'very concerned' taking bath or shower, going up or down stairs, reaching up or down, walking up or down a slope; 'fairly concerned' about getting in or out of a chair, going out to a social event, and 'somewhat concerned' about getting dressed and undressed.	
Co-morbidity	Restrictive pulmonary disease (drug related fibrosis secondary to bromocriptine use).	
Treatment	Experiencing a significant loss of mobility following the removal of one of his PD drugs from the market; gradual improvement as new medications are tried and titrated up.	
Other factors	Mental factors	Tries to remain cheerful and accepting, but does experience episodes of frustration and low mood
	Personal factors	Engaged in self-management through weekly exercise group
	External factors	Lives in a terraced house with wife aged 74, who has been experiencing increasing pain and disability from osteoarthritis for last 9 years. She has recently fallen and is experiencing dizzy spells. Mr M has supportive friends too, is still picked up to go bowling and is in a League Team.
Expectations	Hopes for advice on how to move about in the community with more confidence to prevent social withdrawal; expects to be kept on review at the local hospital by the Neurology Team as well as to attend the Day Hospital for review if and when he requires a course of therapy.	

REFERENCES

Aarsland, D., Beye, M.E., Kreuz, M.W., 2008. Dementia in Parkinson's Disease. Curr. Opin. Neurol. 21, 676–682.

Arnadottir, S.A., Mercer, V.S., 2000. Effects of footwear on measurements of balance and gait in women between the ages of 65 and 93 years. Phys. Ther. 80, 17–27.

Ashburn, A., Fazakarley, L., Ballinger, C., et al., 2007. A randomised controlled trial of a home-based exercise programme to reduce risk of falling among people with Parkinson's disease. J. Neurol. Neurosurg. Psychiatry 78, 678–684.

Ashburn, A., Jones, D., Plant, R., et al., 2004. Physiotherapy for people with Parkinson's disease in the UK: an exploration of practice. International Journal of Therapy and Rehabilitation 11, 160–166.

Ashburn, A., Stack, E., Ballinger, C., et al., 2008. The circumstances of falls among people with Parkinson's disease and the use of falls diaries to facilitate reporting. Disabil. Rehabil. 30, 1205–1212.

Baker, K., Rochester, L., Nieuwboer, A., 2007. The immediate effect of attentional, auditory, and a combined cue strategy on gait during single and dual tasks in Parkinson's disease. Arch. Phys. Med. Rehabil. 88, 1593–1600.

Barone, P., Amboni, M., Viyale, C., 2004. Treatment of nocturnal disturbances and excess daytime sleepiness in Parkinson's disease. Neurology 63, S35–S38.

Behrman, A., Teitelbaum, P., Cauraugh, J.H., 1998. Verbal instructional sets to normalise the temporal and spatial gait variables in Parkinson's disease. J. Neurol. Neurosurg. Psychiatry 65, 580–582.

Beurskens, A.J., de Vet, H.C., Koke, A.J., 1996. Responsiveness of functional status in low back pain: a comparison of different instruments. Pain 65, 71–76.

Bhatia, K., Brooks, D., Burn, D., et al., 1998. Guidelines for the management of Parkinson's disease. Hosp. Med. 59, 469–480.

Bloem, B.R., Hausdorff, J.M., Visser, J.E., et al., 2004. Falls and freezing of gait in Parkinson's disease: a review of two interconnected, episodic phenomena. Mov. Disord. 19, 871–884.

Braak, H., Bohl, J.R., Muller, C.M., et al., 2006. Stanley Fahn Lecture 2005: The staging procedure for the inclusion body pathology associated with sporadic Parkinson's disease reconsidered. Mov. Disord. 21, 2042–2051.

Bridgewater, K.J., Sharpe, M.H., 1996. Aerobic exercise and early Parkinson's disease. J. Neurol. Rehabil. 10, 233–241.

Burn, D.J., Mark, M.H., Playford, E.D., et al., 1992. Parkinson's disease in twin studies with 18F-DOPA and positron emission tomography. Neurology 42, 1094–1900.

Calne, D., Snow, B.J., Lee, C., 1992. Criteria for diagnosing Parkinson's disease. Ann. Neurol. 32, 125–127.

Canning, C., 2005. The effect of directing attention during walking under dual-task conditions in Parkinson's disease. Parkinsonism Relat. Disord. 11, 95–99.

Centre for Evidence Based Physiotherapy, 2009. English translation of KNGH Guidelines for physical therapy in patients with Parkinson's disease. https://www.cebp.nl/?NODE=69.

Chaudhury, K.R., Schapira, A., Martinez-Martin, P., 2004. The holistic management of Parkinson's disease using a novel non motor symptom scale and questionnaire. Adv. Clin. Neurosci. Rehabil. 4, 20–24.

Chaudhury, R.K., Shapira, A., 2009. Non-motor symptoms of Parkinson's disease: dopaminergic pathophysiology and treatment. Lancet Neurol. 8, 464–474.

Clarke, C., 2001. Medical management – dopamine agents. In: Clarke, C. (Ed.), Parkinson's Disease in Practice. Royal Society of Medicine, London, pp. 51–60.

Clarke, C.E., Sampaio, C., 1997. Movement Disorders Cochrane Collaborative Review Group. Mov. Disord. 12, 477–482.

Comella, C.L., Stebbins, G.T., Brown-Toms, N., et al., 1994. Physical therapy and Parkinson's disease: a controlled clinical trial. Neurology 44, 376–378.

Debaere, F., Wenderoth, N., Sunaert, S., et al., 2003. Internal vs external generation of movements: differential neural pathways involved in bimanual coordination performed in the presence or absence of augmented visual feedback. Neuroimage 19, 764–776.

De Lau, L.M., Bretele, M.M., 2006. Epidemiology in Parkinson's disease. Lancet Neurol. 5, 525–535.

Deane, K., Jones, D.E., Ellis-Hill, C., et al., 2001a. Physiotherapy for Parkinson's disease: a comparison of techniques. Cochrane Database Syst. Rev. 1, CD002815.

Deane, K., Jones, D.E., Playford, E.D., et al., 2001b. Physiotherapy versus placebo or no intervention in Parkinson's disease. Cochrane Database Syst. Rev. 3, CD002817.

Department of Health, 2005. The National Service Framework For long-term conditions. Crown Copyright, London.

Department of Health, 2006. The General Practice Physical Activity Questionnaire (GPPAQ). Crown Copyright, London.http://www.dh. gov.uk/en/Publicationsandstatistics/Publications/PublicationsPolicyAndGuidance/DH_063812.

Department of Health, 2008. Guidance on the routine collection of patient reported outcome measures (PROMS). Crown Copyright, London.http://www.dh.gov.uk/en/Publicationsandstatistics/Publications/PublicationsPolicyAndGuidance/DH_092647.

Department of Health, 2009. The NHS Constitution. Crown Copyright, London.

Dibble, L.E., Hale, T.F., Marcus, R.L., et al., 2006. High-intensity resistance training amplified muscle hypertrophy and functional gains in persons with Parkinson's disease. Mov. Disord. 21, 1444–1452.

Ellis, T., De Goede, C.J., Feldman, R.G., 2005. Efficacy of a physical therapy program in patients with Parkinson's disease: a randomized controlled trial. Arch. Phys. Med. Rehabil. 86, 626–632.

Enright, P.L., McBurnie, M.A., Bittner, V., et al., 2003. The 6-min walk test: a quick measure of functional status in elderly adults. Chest 123, 387–398.

EuroQol Group, 2009. What is EQ-5D. http://www.euroqol.org/home.html.

Fall, P.A., Saleh, A., Fredrickson, M., et al., 2003. Survival time, mortality and cause of death in elderly patients from Parkinson's disease: a nine year follow up. Mov. Disord. 18, 1312–1316.

Farley, B.G., Fox, C.M., Ramig, L.O., et al., 2008. Intensive amplitude-specific therapeutic approaches for Parkinson disease: Toward a neuroplasticity-principled rehabilitation model. Topics in Geriatric Rehabilitation 24, 99–114.

Flaherty, A.W., Grabiel, A.M., 1994. Anatomy of the basal ganglia. In: Marsden, C.D., Fahn, S. (Eds.), Movement Disorders, 3. Butterworth-Heinemann, New York, pp. 3–27.

Gibb, W.R.G., Lees, A.J., 1988. The relevance of the Lewy body to the pathogenesis of idiopathic Parkinson's disease. J. Neurol. Neurosurg. Psychiatry 51, 745–752.

Giladi, N., Shabtai, H., Rozenburg, E., et al., 2001. Gait festination in Parkinson's disease. Parkinsonism Relat. Disord. 7, 135–138.

Giladi, N., Shabtai, H., Simon, E., et al., 2000. Construction of freezing of gait questionnaire for patients with Parkinsonism. Parkinsonism Relat. Disord. 6, 165–170.

Giladi, N., Tal, J., Azulay, T., et al., 2009. Validation of the freezing of gait questionnaire in patients with Parkinson's disease. Mov. Disord. 24, 655–661.

Gill, D., Jones, G., Zou, G.Y., Speechley, M., 2008. The Phone-FITT: a brief physical activity interview for older adults. J. Aging Phys. Act. 16, 292–315.

Glendenning, D.S., Enoka, R.M., 1994. Motor unit behaviour in Parkinson's disease. Phys. Ther. 74, 61–70.

Goodwin, V.A., Richards, S.H., Taylor, R.S., et al., 2008. The effectiveness of exercise interventions for people with Parkinson's disease: a systematic review and meta-analysis. Mov. Disord. 23, 631–640.

Greenamyre, J.T., Hastings, T.G., 2004. Biomedicine. Parkinson's – divergent causes, convergent mechanisms. Science 304, 1120–1122.

Guyatt, G.H., Sullivan, M.J., Thompson, P.J., et al., 1985. The 6-minute walk: a new measure of exercise capacity in patients with chronic heart failure. Can. Med. Assoc. J. 132, 919–923.

Hauser, R.A., Freeman, T.B., Snow, B.J., et al., 1999. Long-term evaluation of bilateral fetal nigral transplantation in Parkinson's disease. Arch. Neurol. 56, 179–187.

Haywood, K.L., Garratt, A.M., Jordan, K., et al., 2004. Spinal mobility in ankylosing spondylitis: Reliability, validity and responsiveness. Rheumatology 43, 750–757.

Hindle, J.V., 2001. Neuropsychiatry. In: Playfer, J.R., Hindle, J. (Eds.), Parkinson's Disease in the Older Patient Arnold, London, pp. 106–107.

Hirsch, M.A., Toole, T., Maitland, C.G., et al., 2003. The effects of balance training and high intensity resistance training on persons with idiopathic Parkinson's disease. Arch. Phys. Med. Rehabil. 84, 1109–1117.

Hoehn, M.M., Yahr, M.D., 1967. Parkinsonism: onset, progression and mortality. Neurology 17, 427–442.

Hughes, A.J., Daniel, S.E., Kilford, L., et al., 1992a. Accuracy of clinical diagnosis of idiopathic Parkinson's disease: a clinicopathologic study of 100 cases. J. Neurol. Neurosurg. Psychiatry 55, 181–184.

Hughes, A.J., Ben-Shlomo, Y., Daniel, S.E., et al., 1992b. What features improve the accuracy of clinical diagnosis in Parkinson's disease: a clinicopathologic study. Neurology 42, 1142–1146.

Hughes, A.J., Daniel, S.E., Lees, A.J., 2001. Improved accuracy of clinical diagnosis of Lewy body Parkinson's disease. Neurology 57, 1497–1499.

Iansek, R., Bradshaw, J., Phillips, J., et al., 1997. Basal ganglia function and Parkinson's disease. In: Morris, M., Iansek, R. (Eds.), Parkinson's Disease: a Team Approach. Southern Health Care Network. Cheltenham, Australia, pp. 173–188.

Jenkinson, C., Peto, V., Fitzpatrick, R., et al., 1995. Self reported functioning and well being in patients with Parkinson's disease: comparison of the Short Form Health Survey (SF-36) and the Parkinson's Disease Questionnaire (PDQ-39). Age Ageing 24, 505–509.

Jenkinson, C., Fitzpatrick, R., Peto, V., et al., 1997. The PDQ-8: Development and validation of a short-form Parkinson's disease questionnaire. Psychology and Health 12, 805–814.

Kamsma, Y.P.T., Brouwer, W.H., Lakke, J.P.W.F., 1995. Training of compensational strategies for impaired gross motor skills in Parkinson's disease. Physiother. Theory Pract. 11, 209–229.

Keus, S.H.J., Bloem, B.R., Hendriks, E.J., et al., 2007. Evidence-based analysis of physical therapy in Parkinson's disease with recommendations for practice and research. Mov. Disord. 22, 451–460.

Keus, S.H.J., Bloem, B.R., Verbaan, D., et al., 2004a. Physiotherapy in Parkinson's disease: utilization and patient satisfaction. J. Neurol. 251, 680–687.

Keus, S.H.J., Hendriks, H.J.M., Bloem, B.R., et al., 2004b. KNGF Guidelines for physical therapy in Parkinson's disease. Dutch Journal of Physiotherapy 114 (Suppl. 3), 1–86. (Royal Dutch Society for Physical Therapy (KNGF) 2006 English translation https://www.cebp.nl/?NODE=69).

Keus, S.H.J., Munneke, M., Nijkrake, M.J., et al., 2009a. Physical therapy in Parkinson's disease: evolution and future challenges. Mov. Disord. 24, 1–14.

Keus, S., Nieuwboer, A., Bloem, B., et al., 2009b. Clinimetric analyses of the Modified Parkinson Activity Scale. Parkinsonism Relat. Disord. 15, 263–269.

Langston, J.W., Ballard, P.A., Tetrud, J.W., et al., 1983. Chronic parkinsonism in humans due to a product of meperidine-analog synthesis. Science 219, 979–980.

Langston, J.W., Forno, L.S., Tetrud, J., et al., 1999. Evidence for active nerve cell degeneration in the substantia nigra of humans years after 1-methyl-4-phenyl-1,2,3,6-tetrahydrophyridine exposure. Ann. Neurol. 46, 598–605.

Lansbury, P., Brice, A., 2002. Genetics of Parkinson's disease and biochemical studies of implicated gene products: commentary. Curr. Opin. Cell. Biol. 14, 653.

Lees, A.J., 1995. Comparison of therapeutic effects and mortality data of levodopa and levodopa combined with selegiline in patients with early, mild Parkinson's disease. Parkinson's Disease Research Group of the United Kingdom. Br. Med. J. 311, 1602–1607.

Lennox, G.G., Lowe, J.S., 1997. Dementia with Lewy bodies. In: Quinn, N.P. (Ed.), Parkinsonism. Baillière-Tindall, London, pp. 147–166.

Lim, I., van Wegen, E., de Goede, C., et al., 2005. Effects of external rhythmical cueing on gait in patients with Parkinson's disease: a systematic review. Clin. Rehabil. 19, 695–713.

Lim, S.Y., Fox, S.H., Lang, A.E., 2009. Overview of the extranigral aspects of Parkinson disease. Arch. Neurol. 66, 167–172.

Limousin, P., Krack, P., Pollok, P., et al., 1998. Electrical stimulation of the subthalamic nucleus in advanced Parkinson's disease. N. Engl. J. Med. 339, 1105–1111.

Lindop, F., 2009. Using laser walking aids with a patient with Parkinson's disease: a case report. Agility 1, 4–7.

Lindvall, O., 1998. Update on fetal transplantation: the Swedish experience. Mov. Disord. 13 (Suppl. 1), 83–87.

Litvan, I., 1997. Progressive supranuclear palsy and corticobasal degeneration. In: Quinn, N.P. (Ed.), Parkinsonism. Baillière-Tindall, London, pp. 167–185.

Louis, E.D., Marder, K., Cote, L., et al., 1997. Mortality from Parkinson's disease. Arch. Neurol. 54, 260–264.

Macphee, G.J.A., 2001. Diagnosis and differential diagnosis of Parkinson's disease. In: Playfer, J.R., Hindle, J. (Eds.), Parkinson's Disease in the Older Patient. Arnold, London, pp. 43–77.

Mak, M.K., Hui-Chan, C.W., 2007. Cued task-specific training is better than exercise in improving sit-to-stand in patients with Parkinson's disease: a randomized controlled trial. Mov. Disord. 23, 501–509.

Meara, J., Hobson, P., 2000. Epidemiology of Parkinson's disease and parkinsonism in elderly subjects. In: Meara, J., Koller, W. (Eds.),

Parkinson's Disease and Parkinsonism in the Elderly. Cambridge University Press, Cambridge, pp. 111–122.

Miller, N., Noble, E., Jones, D., et al., 2006. Life with communication changes in Parkinson's disease. Age Ageing 35, 235–239.

Mjones, H., 1949. Paralysis agitans. A clinical genetic study. Acta Psychiatr. Neurol. 25 (Suppl. 54), 1–195.

Morris, M.E., 2000. Movement disorders in people with Parkinson disease: a model for physical therapy. Phys. Ther. 80, 578–597.

Morris, M.E., 2006. Locomotor training in people with Parkinson's disease. Phys. Ther. 86, 1426–1435.

Morris, M.E., Iansek, R., Churchyard, A., 1998. The role of the physiotherapist in quantifying movement fluctuations in Parkinson's disease. Aust. J. Physiother. 44, 105–114.

Morris, M.E., Iansek, R., Kirkwood, B., 2009. A randomized controlled trial of movement strategies compared with exercise for people with Parkinson's disease. Mov. Disord. 24, 64–71.

Morris, M.E., Iansek, R., Matyas, T.A., et al., 1996. Stride length regulation in Parkinson's disease. Normalization strategies and underlying mechanism. Brain 119, 551–568.

Morris, S., Morris, M.E., Iansek, R., 2001. Reliability of measurements obtained with the Timed "Up & Go" test in people with Parkinson disease. Phys. Ther. 81 (2), 810–818.

Müller, J., Wenning, G.K., Jellinger, K., et al., 2000. Progression of Hoehn and Yahr stages in Parkinsonian disorders: a clinicopathologic study. Neurology 55 (6), 888–891.

Müller, V., Mohr, B., Rosin, R., et al., 1997. Short-term effects of behavioural treatment on movement initiation and postural control in Parkinson's disease: a controlled clinical study. Mov. Disord. 12, 306–314.

National Institute for Health and Clinical Excellence, 2006. Parkinson's Disease. Diagnosis and management in primary and secondary care. National Institute for Health and Clinical Excellence, London.http://guidance.nice.org.uk/CG35.

National Institute for Health Research, 2009. Health Technology Assessment

programme. Randomised controlled trial to assess the clinical- and cost-effectiveness of physiotherapy and occupational therapy in Parkinson's disease (PD REHAB). http://www.ncchta.org/project/1748.asp.

NHS Choices, 2009. Parkinson's disease. http://www.nhs.uk/Conditions/Parkinsons-disease/Pages/Introduction.aspx.

Nieuwboer, A., De Weerdt, W., Dom, R., et al., 1998. A frequency and correlation analysis of motor deficits in Parkinson patients. Disabil. Rehabil. 20, 142–150.

Nieuwboer, A., De Weerdt, W., Dom, R., et al., 2000. Development of an activity scale for individuals with advanced Parkinson disease: reliability and "on-off" variability. Phys. Ther. 80, 1087–1096.

Nieuwboer, A., De Weerdt, W., Dom, R., et al., 2001. The effect of a home physiotherapy program for persons with Parkinson's disease. J. Rehabil. Med. 33, 266–272.

Nieuwboer, A., Feys, P., De Weerdt, W., et al., 1997. Is using a cue the clue to the treatment of freezing in Parkinson's disease? Physiother. Res. Int. 2, 125–134.

Nieuwboer, A., Kwakkel, G., Rochester, L., et al., 2007. Cueing training in the home improves gait-related mobility in Parkinson's disease: The RESCUE-trial. J. Neurol. Neurosurg. Psychiatry 78, 134–140.

Nieuwboer, A., Rochester, L., Jones, D., 2008. Cueing gait and gait-related mobility in patients with Parkinson's disease. Developing a therapeutic method based on the International Classification of Functioning, Disability and Health. Top. Geriatr. Rehabil. 24, 151–165.

Nijkrake, M.J., Bloem, B.R., Keus, S.H., et al., 2006. Quality of allied health care in Parkinson's disease. Mov. Disord. 21, S131.

Olanow, C.W., Koller, W.C., 1998. An algorithm (decision tree) for the management of Parkinson's disease. Neurology 50 (Suppl. 3), S1–S57.

Parkinson's Disease Society, 1999. Parkinson's Aware in Primary Care. A guide for primary care teams developed by the Primary Care Task Force for PDS (UK). Parkinsons Disease Society, London.

Parkinson's Disease Society, 2008. Life with Parkinson's today – room for improvement. Parkinson's Disease Society, London.

Parkinson Study Group, 1989. Effect of deprenyl on the progression of disability in early Parkinson's disease. N. Engl. J. Med. 321, 1364–1371.

Patti, F., Reggio, A., Nicoletti, F., et al., 1996. Effects of rehabilitation therapy on Parkinsonians' disability and functional independence. Neurorehabil. Neural Repair 10, 223–231.

Plant, R., Jones, D., Thomson, J., et al., 2001. Guidelines for Physiotherapy Practice in Parkinson's Disease. Northumbria University, Newcastle upon Tyne.

Playfer, J.R., 2001. Drug therapy. In: Playfer, J.R., Hindle, J. (Eds.), Parkinson's Disease in the Older Patient. Arnold, London, pp. 283–309.

Podsialdo, D., Richardson, S., 1991. The timed "Up & Go": a test of basic functional mobility for frail elderly persons. J. Am. Geriatr. Soc. 39, 142–148.

Poewe, W., 2009. Treatments for Parkinson's disease-past achievements and current clinical needs. Neurology 72, S65–S73.

Poewe, W., Granata, R., 1997. Pharmacological treatment of Parkinson's disease. In: Watts, R.L., Koller, W.C. (Eds.), Movement Disorders: Neurologic Principles and Practice. McGraw-Hill, New York, pp. 201–209.

Polatli, M., Akyol, A., Çildag, O., et al., 2001. Pulmonary function tests in Parkinson's disease. Eur. J. Neurol. 8, 341–345.

Poltawski, L., Edwards, H., Todd, A., et al., 2009. Ultrasound treatment of cutaneous side-effects of infused apomorphine: A randomized controlled pilot study. Mov. Disord. 24 (1), 115–118.

Polymeropoulos, M.H., Higgins, J.J., Golbe, L.I., et al., 1996. Mapping of a gene for Parkinson's disease in the Contursi kindred. Ann. Neurol. 40, 767–775.

PRoFaNE Prevention of Falls Network Europe, 2009. Find FES-I translations by country. http://www.profane.eu. org/eu_map/FESI_by_country.php.

Proulx, M., De Courval, F.P., Wiseman, M.A., et al., 2005. Salivary production in Parkinson's disease. Mov. Disord. 20, 204–207.

Quinn, N., 1989. Multiple system atrophy – the nature of the beast. J. Neurol. Neurosurg. Psychiatry 52 (suppl.), 78–89.

Quinn, N., 1995. Parkinsonism – recognition and differential diagnosis. Br. Med. J. 310, 447–452.

Ramaswamy, B., Jones, D., Goodwin, V., et al., 2009. Quick Reference Cards (UK) and Guidance Notes for physiotherapists working with people with Parkinson's disease. Parkinson's Disease Society, London. http://bgsmdslive.org/QuickReference Cards_physio.pdf.

Rochester, L., Baker, K., Jones, D., et al., 2009. Does deep brain stimulation of the STN in advanced Parkinson's disease change habitual physical activity? Mov. Disord. 24 (Suppl. 1), S472.

Rochester, L., Hetherington, V., Jones, D., et al., 2005. The effect of external rhythmic cues (auditory and visual) on walking during a functional task in homes of people with Parkinson's disease. Arch. Phys. Med. Rehabil. 86, 999–1006.

Rochester, L., Nieuwboer, A., Baker, K., et al., 2007. The attentional cost of external rhythmical cues and their impact on gait in Parkinson's disease: effect of cue modality and task complexity. J. Neural. Transm. 114 (10), 1243–1248.

Rubenstein, T., Giladi, N., Hausdorff, J., 2002. The power of cueing to circumvent dopamine deficits: a review of physical therapy treatment of gait disturbances in Parkinson's disease. Mov. Disord. 17, 1148–1160.

Samuel, M., Cabballos-Baumann, A., Blin, J., et al., 1997. Evidence for lateral premotor and parietal overactivity in Parkinson's disease during sequential and bimanual movements. A PET study. Brain 120, 963–976.

Schapira, A.H.V., 2008. Mitochondria in the aetiology and pathogenesis of Parkinson's disease. Lancet Neurol. 7, 97–109.

Schenkman, M., Cutson, T.M., Kuchibhatla, M., et al., 1998. Exercise to improve spinal flexibility and function for people with Parkinson's disease: a randomized, controlled trial. J. Am. Geriatr. Soc. 46, 1207–1216.

Schrag, A., Selai, C., Jahanshahi, M., et al., 2000. The EQ-5D - a generic quality of life measure - is a useful instrument to measure quality of life in patients with Parkinson's disease. J. Neurol. Neurosurg. Psychiatry 69, 67–73.

Shumway-Cook, A., Woollacott, M.H., 1995. Motor Control. Theory and Practical Applications. Williams & Wilkins, Baltimore.

Snyder, B., Olanow, C.W., 2005. Stem cell treatment for Parkinson's disease: an update for 2005. Curr. Opin. Neurol. 18, 376–385.

Stack, E., Ashburn, A., 1999. Fall events described by people with Parkinson's disease: implications for clinical interviewing and the research agenda. Physiother. Res. Int. 4, 190–199.

Stack, E., Ashburn, A., 2006. Impaired bed mobility and disordered sleep in Parkinson's disease. Mov. Disord. 21 (9), 1340–1342.

Stallibrass, C., Sissons, P., Chalmers, C., 2002. Randomized controlled trial of the Alexander technique for idiopathic Parkinson's disease. Clin. Rehabil. 16, 695–708.

Strange, P.C., 1992. Dopamine receptors in the basal ganglia. Mov. Disord. 8, 263–270.

Toole, T., Hirsch, M.A., Forkink, A., et al., 2000. The effects of a balance and strength training program on equilibrium in Parkinsonism: a preliminary study. Neurorehabilitation 14, 165–174.

Visser, M., Marinus, J., Bloem, B.R., et al., 2003. Clinical tests for the evaluation of postural instability in patients with Parkinson's disease. Arch. Phys. Med. Rehabil. 84, 1669–1674.

Vossius, C., Nilsen, O.D., Larsen, J.P., 2009. Parkinson's disease and nursing home placement: the economic impact of the need for care. Eur. J. Neurol. 16, 194–200.

Ward, C.D., Duvoisin, R.C., Ince, S.E., et al., 1983. Parkinson's disease in 65 pairs of twins and in a set of quadruplets. Neurology 33, 815–824.

Weissenborn, S., 1993. The effect of using a two-step verbal cue to a visual target above eye level on the parkinsonian gait: a case study. Physiotherapy 79, 26–31.

Wenning, G.K., Ebersbach, G., Verny, M., et al., 1999. Progression of falls in postmortem-confirmed parkinsonian disorders. Mov. Disord. 14, 947–950.

Willems, A., Nieuwboer, A., Chavret, F., et al., 2007. Turning in Parkinson's disease patients and controls: the effect of auditory cues. Mov. Disord. 22, 1871–1878.

Wood, B.H., Bilclough, J.A., Bowron, A., et al., 2002. Incidence and prediction of falls in Parkinson's disease: a prospective multidisciplinary study.

J. Neurol. Neurosurg. Psychiatry 72, 721–725.

Wood-Kaczmar, A., Gandhi, S., Wood, N.W., 2006. Understanding the molecular causes of Parkinson's disease. Trends Mol. Med. 12, 521–528.

World Health Organization, 2002. Towards a common language of

function, disability and health. The international classification of functioning, disability and health. World Health Organization, Geneva.

Yardley, L., Beyer, N., Hauer, K., et al., 2005. Development and initial validation of the Falls Efficacy Scale-International (FES-I). Age Ageing 34, 614–619.

RESOURCES

Association of Physiotherapists in PD Europe DVD support for the KNGF guidelines for physical therapy in patients with PD. http://www.appde.eu/EN/resources.asp.

Parkinson's Disease Society, 2007. The Professional's Guide to Parkinson's Disease. Parkinson's Disease Society, London.http://www.parkinsons.org.uk/advice/publications/booklets/healthsocialprofessionals.aspx.

Rescue Consortium, Using cueing to optimise mobility in Parkinson's disease. RESCUE project CD Rom. http://www.rescueproject.org.

Chapter | 7 |

Huntington's disease

Monica Busse, Lori Quinn, Oliver Quarrell

CONTENTS

INTRODUCTION

George Huntington gave the first clear and concise account of the condition in 1872 and the term Huntington's disease (HD) is now widely accepted as the name of the condition. HD is a progressive neurodegenerative disorder characterized as a triad of a movement disorder, often choreic in nature, an affective disturbance and a cognitive impairment. It is inherited with an autosomal dominant pattern of inheritance, so, on average, half the offspring of an affected person will develop the condition with both males and females being affected.

Inevitably, a chapter in a physiotherapy textbook will concentrate on the physical aspects of the condition, but for most families and carers a much greater problem is the behavioural change which can lead to irritability, aggression, depression or apathy. Professionals dealing with HD patients need to have an understanding of the neuropsychological and neuro-psychiatric aspects of HD which will help with their management of the patient. Over time the needs of the patient and family change, so professionals need to reassess their management. This chapter will describe the genetic and pathological features before going on to describe the stages of the condition and the associated physiotherapy management. A number of useful texts are available for a wider discussion of the condition including Bates et al. (2002), Quarrell (2009) and Walker (2007).

PREVALENCE AND ASPECTS OF NATURAL HISTORY

Most UK studies quote a prevalence of 4–10 per 100 000, with similar results from studies from Europe and the US, and low prevalence figures reported from Japan and Finland (Harper, 2002). Whilst HD may be considered a rare disorder it must be remembered that for every affected person there are approximately twice that number who have the mutation and are currently asymptomatic (Conneally, 1984). The median duration of HD is between 16 and 21 years (Foroud et al., 1999; Roos et al., 1993) so this represents a considerable demand on families and carers.

HD can develop at almost any age from under 20 years (and occasionally under 10 years) to over 75 years, but most people develop the condition between the ages of 35 and 55 years, which is after the usual years of reproduction (Harper et al., 1988). One consequence of this is that the 50% risk for an asymptomatic person does not decline appreciably until s/he is going through middle age.

Individuals with an age of onset less than 20 years are described as having the juvenile form of HD. It is difficult to know precisely how many patients have early onset, but 5% is a reasonable estimate. Young people with juvenile HD may develop problems with speech, bradykinesia and dystonic movements earlier in the course in the illness; this topic is reviewed in Quarrell et al. (2009).

KEY POINTS

Main features

- Huntington's disease affects approximately 10 people per 100 000 of the population.
- Both males and females are affected.
- Onset can be from under 10 years to over 75 years, but most people develop the condition between the ages of 35 and 55 years.
- As well as the movement disorder, which is often choreic in nature, significant cognitive and behavioural problems may occur, which may be more of a problem to the family and carers.

GENETICS

As HD is a dominant disorder; each cell contains one normal copy and one abnormal copy of the gene. The gene for HD was cloned in 1993 (Huntington's Disease Collaborative Research Group, 1993) and the protein for which it codes was named huntingtin. The first part of the HD gene has a sequence CAGCAG...CAG which is repeated a number of times. CAG codes for the amino acid

glutamine so that the huntingtin protein contains a sequence called a polyglutamine repeat. The mutation causing HD is an expansion of the number of CAG repeats in the gene and therefore the polyglutamine repeat in the protein. Up to 35 repeats would be considered normal, although there is a possibility that if a person has a repeat size at the upper end of this range it could expand into the pathological range in future generations; a result between 36 and 39 repeats is abnormal, but it is possible that a person may develop the condition late or even live a full life and not develop HD; 40 or more repeats is considered definitely abnormal (ASHG/AMCG statement, 1998). At a mathematical level, there is a correlation between the average age of onset and the CAG repeat size but there is such a wide variation that it is not possible to predict the age of onset for an individual from knowing the CAG repeat size.

An asymptomatic individual with an affected parent has a prior probability of 50% of inheriting the HD gene. Such a person could have a genetic test at this stage. This is called a predictive test. As there is no effective treatment to alter the natural history of HD such tests are used cautiously in conjunction with counselling and according to widely accepted international guidelines drawn up by an ad hoc committee of the International Huntington's Association/World Federation of Neurology Research Group on Huntington's chorea (1994). Less than 20% of adults at risk of HD choose to have a predictive test (Tassiker et al., 2009).

It is worth noting that reproductive options can be discussed with a couple where one partner has an affected parent. These could form the basis of a separate chapter but in brief the options include: not having children or to have children and accept that they will be at 25% risk. If the 'at risk partner' is shown to be gene positive (see above), the couple may consider a test in pregnancy with the implication of seriously considering termination of pregnancy. In addition to this, there is a complex genetic test which allows a couple to consider a test in pregnancy without the partner at 50% risk being tested directly. Finally, there is the possibility of pre-implantation genetic diagnosis which can be done either in the case where one partner is known to have the gene or is at risk. Discussing these options with a couple requires referral to a skilled genetic counsellor.

KEY POINTS

Genetics

- The pattern of inheritance is autosomal dominant, so half the offspring of an affected person will inherit the Huntington's disease (HD) gene.
- The mutation is an expansion of a DNA sequence which codes for the amino acid glutamine.

- The protein product is called huntingtin.
- Abnormal huntingtin contains an increased number of glutamines in the first part of the protein; a person with 36–39 repeats may develop HD during a lifetime, but a person with more than 40 repeats will definitely develop the condition.
- Less than 20% of people at risk of developing HD choose to have a predictive test.
- There are a number of reproductive options available for couples.

PATHOLOGY

The gene is widely expressed in the cells of the body but some cells within the brain are very sensitive to abnormal huntingtin and there is selective neurodegeneration. An explanation for the selective neurodegeneration characteristic of HD is unclear. The most striking cell loss occurs in the basal ganglia but other areas of the brain including the cortex are also affected. The anatomy of the basal ganglia is shown in Figure 7.1. To emphasize this point it should be noted that the brain of a patient with HD will be smaller and weigh less than that of an age-matched control. The efferent medium spiny neurons within the caudate and putamen nuclei, which are collectively called the striatum, are especially sensitive to the abnormal huntingtin protein (see Figure 7.2).

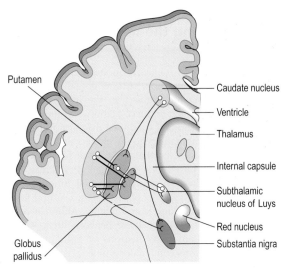

Figure 7.1 Location of the nuclei comprising the basal ganglia. This coronal section through the brain is slanted anteroposteriorly in order to show all the structure on one section. Note the two parts of the globus pallidus. The two subdivisions of the substantia nigra (pars reticulate and pars compacta) are not shown in this figure. The connections from the caudate nucleus and putamen to the substantia nigra are shown terminating in the pars reticulate. The dopaminergic connection from the pars compacta is not shown.

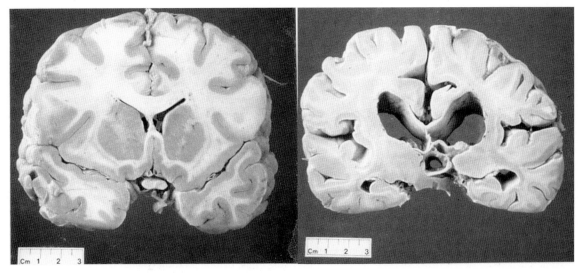

Figure 7.2 Photographs of the cut surfaces of the brain of an age-matched control (left) and a patient with Huntington's disease (right). The massive loss of the basal ganglia is apparent. (Reproduced from Harper, 1991, with permission.)

Implications of pathology for understanding the movement disorder

The striatum receives excitatory inputs from the cortex. The efferent medium spiny neurons contain inhibitory neurotransmitters which project to the internal globus pallidus via direct and indirect pathways (Albin et al., 1989). Figure 7.3 shows a simplified diagram of the process. In broad terms, damage to the indirect pathway leads to overstimulation of the thalamo-cortical feedback and chorea (random purposeless movements), whereas loss of the direct pathway results in increased inhibition of the thalamus and less activity of the thalamo-cortical feedback producing bradykinesia and rigidity. Although both pathways degenerate, the balance between them is disturbed. The medium spiny neurons of both the direct and indirect pathways contain dopamine receptors, which are consistently reduced in Huntington's disease. Conventionally, excitatory D1 receptors are on the direct and inhibitory D2 receptors are on the indirect pathway. This means that whilst it is possible to control the chorea of patients with dopa blocker and dopa depleting drugs, this may worsen the bradykinesia and dystonia.

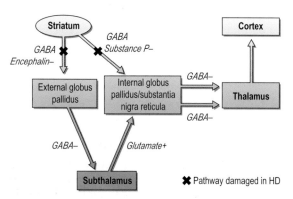

Figure 7.3 Connections of the basal ganglia, showing the pathways damaged in Huntington's disease. GABA, gamaaminobutyric acid.

Implications of pathology for understanding the behavioural problems

Of equal importance to the understanding of the condition is that there are fronto-striatal connections which are disturbed. At first this may result in a patient becoming less perceptive of the needs of others, which may be noticed by close family members. As time progresses they become less able to switch between tasks, plan ahead or change a plan in the light of new information and become increasingly self-centred. This results in patients becoming irritable and having temper outbursts much more easily. In addition, there may be problems with anxiety and depression. Family members become adept in working around these behavioural changes by minimizing provocations and allowing outbursts to blow over. As part of the fronto-striatal changes, a patient may lose interest in activities and become apathetic.

As an example, a patient with HD may decide it is time to be taken for a walk. A professional may reasonably explain that they are busy working with someone else and they will take the patient for a walk presently. This may pacify the HD patient temporarily only for that person to return a few minutes later requesting that they be taken for a walk. Knowledge of the cognitive and behavioural problems of HD may enable a professional to understand the need to explain what is going to happen to the patient and perhaps repeat the explanations.

At present, there is no treatment to delay the onset of HD or to slow down the rate of neurodegeneration. However, much can be done to educate families and professionals to work around the behavioural problems; pharmacological interventions such as antidepressants and dopa blockers should be used to manage the behavioural aspects of the condition.

Understanding pathology at the level of the cell

HD should be easy to explain because one gene is involved with one mutation that affects a single protein. Unfortunately, this is not the case because huntingtin is involved in many cellular processes. Apart from man, no natural animal develops HD. Following the identification of the gene a tremendous research effort involved developing animal models. The first of these, and most studied, was the R6 mice which contain multiple copies of the first part of the HD gene (Mangiarini et al., 1996). These mice die before they develop significant cell death. One feature of the cells is that they contain aggregates of the first part of the huntintin protein (Davies, et al., 1997). These aggregates are now recognized as occurring in human HD brains (DiFiglia et al., 1997). It is unclear as to whether these aggregates are directly related to the cellular pathology or represent a defence mechanism within the cell. There are a number of different animal models; details of their similarities and differences are not relevant to this chapter, but animal models have enabled an understanding that neuronal cells are dysfunctional ('sick') before they die which gives hope for interventions to alter the natural history of the disease. This natural history is modelled in Figure 7.4 with neuronal dysfunction preceding the onset of symptoms. In the absence of serendipity, an understanding of the pathology at the cellular level using animal and cellular models is the way forward for developing and subsequently testing new treatments for HD.

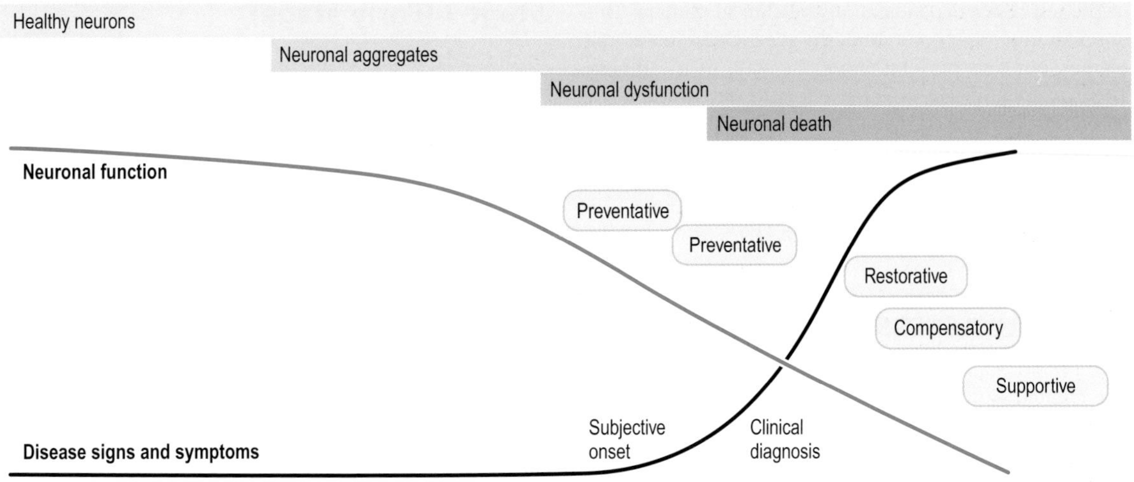

	Pre-manifest/Prodermal	Early stage	Mid-stage	Late-stage
WHO ICF classification of functioning	Pathology	Impairments	Activity restrictions	Participation restrictions
Primary physiotherapy aim	Advise on appropriate physical activities	Delay the onset of mobility restriction	Maintain function and delay further deterioration	Limit impact of complications

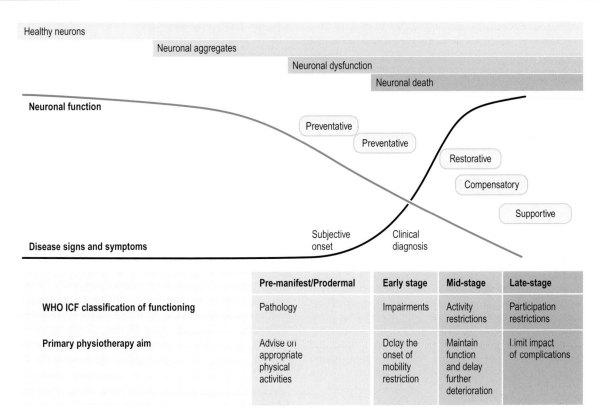

Figure 7.4 Primary physiotherapy aims and the continuum of Huntington's disease. (Modified from the Walker et al., Huntington's Disease. Lancet 2007;369 (9557): 218-28, with permission from Elsevier.)

KEY POINTS

Pathology

- Although a number of areas of the brain are affected, the most striking cell loss occurs in the basal ganglia, principally the caudate and putamen nuclei (striatum).
- Abnormal huntingtin is expressed in every cell but an explanation for the selective neurodegeneration is unclear.
- A disturbance in the balance between the direct and indirect pathways within the basal ganglia can result in chorea in the early stages of the disease, and increasing dystonia and bradykinesia later in the disease course.
- A disturbance of connections between the basal ganglia and the frontal cortex results in a range of behavioural problems, including irritability and apathy.
- Normal huntingtin is involved in a number of different cellular processes; there is incomplete understanding of how abnormal huntingtin causes some cells to be become dysfunctional and eventually die.

Life history of the disease

If a person has inherited the gene there will be a period of time where she/he is completely asymptomatic. In time, the neurones become dysfunctional. Onset of HD is insidious with non-specific problems such as mood change or being slightly forgetful, which can be attributed easily to other mundane causes. A person in this prodromal stage may become depressed, but a clinical diagnosis cannot be made confidently until motor signs, such as chorea, appear. These may be infrequent, of low amplitude and may not be noticed by the patient, family or clinician with limited experience of the condition. Indeed even at a time when the chorea is quite obvious it may be denied as a problem by the patient (Snowden et al., 1998).

If a patient is seen when there are obvious signs of HD, the CAG repeat size may be measured from a venous blood sample to confirm the clinical diagnosis. It is important to realize that the result of the genetic test will be the same whether the individual is completely asymptomatic, in the prodromal phase, or in the early, middle or later stages of HD. As with any test the interpretation of the test result depends upon the clinical context. This raises an important issue about the genetic test: it is a 'trait marker' but says nothing about the state of the illness. There is a significant research effort to determine other laboratory biomarkers ('state markers') which can track the development and progression of the disease (Henley et al., 2005). The boundaries between early, middle and late stages are ill defined, but nonetheless they form a useful way of categorizing the impact of HD.

CLINICAL ASSESSMENT

The Unified Huntington's Disease Rating Scale (UHDRS) (Huntington Study Group, 1996) is a rating system that is used to quantify the severity of Huntington's disease. It was developed as a clinical rating scale to assess four domains of clinical performance and capacity in individuals with HD: motor function, cognitive function, behavioural abnormalities, and functional capacity. These scores can be calculated by summing the various questions of each section. The UHDRS is useful for tracking changes in the clinical features of HD over time, and appears to be appropriate for repeated administration during clinical studies. Stages in Huntington's disease are traditionally defined by the Total Functional Capacity scale, developed by Shoulson and Fahn (1979), which classifies patients into one of five stages of disease progression (Marder et al., 2000). The staging evaluates patients based on functioning for ADLs, domestic chores, finances, work and overall care level. Mid-stage is typically defined as levels II-III (see Table 7.1).

Stage I (Early stage)

In the early stages of the disease, the person with HD is able to remain functional and independent, retaining their ability to work and drive (HDSA, 2000). Movement disorders include minor involuntary movements, reduced coordination and linearly progressive motor impersistence or inability to maintain a voluntary muscle contraction at a constant level (Walker, 2007). Even at this stage, it may be possible to detect some slowing of saccadic eye movements (rapidly moving the eye to a new target; this is done by asking the patient to move his/her eye to one corner in response to a cue). Voluntary motor tasks (fine and gross motor skills) may become increasingly difficult as the disease progresses (Aubeeluck & Wilson, 2008). Cognitive tasks also become more difficult with reduced ability to sequence and organize information (HDSA, 2000). Deficits in gait have been identified across the spectrum of HD (Churchyard et al., 2001; Grimbergen et al., 2008; Hausdorff et al., 1998; Koller & Trimble, 1985; Rao et al., 2008). Decreased gait velocity, stride length, and increased time in double support compared to healthy controls may occur (Rao et al., 2008). These impairments appear to worsen with increasing disease severity and can be useful markers of disease progression and treatment efficacy.

Stage II and III (Middle stage)

During the middle stages of HD, involuntary movements such as chorea increase. In the early stages of HD, this is typically seen in the fingers, hands and face muscles, but as the disease progresses, it can be seen throughout the

STAGE OF DISEASE AND ASSOCIATED TFC SCORE	CATEGORY OF TFC				
	Occupation	Finances	Domestic chores	Activities of daily living	Care level
Stage I TFC 11–13	Normal 3	Normal 3	Normal 2	Normal 3	Home 3
Stage II TFC 7–10	Reduced capacity for normal job 2	Slight assistance 2	Normal 2	Normal 3	Home 3
Stage III TFC 3–6	Marginal work only 1	Major assistance 1	Impaired 1	Minimal impairment 2	Home 3
Stage IV TFC 1–2	Unable 0	Unable 0	Unable 0	Gross tasks only 1	Home or chronic care facility 1
Stage V TFC 0	Unable 0	Unable 0	Unable 0	Total care 0	Full-time skilled nursing 0

Table 7.1 The Total Functional Capacity (TFC) Scale

(Reproduced from Shoulson I, Fahn S, 1979 Huntingdon Disease: clinical care and evaluation, Neurology, with permission).

body, including in all four extremities and the trunk. Chorea does not usually result in a direct impairment of motor function, however voluntary motor impairments may have a functional impact (Walker, 2007).

Dystonic postures (abnormal, sustained posturing) in sitting or standing (Louis et al., 1999) and in movements such as shoulder elevation, foot inversion and supination, and trunk extension might be present. People may experience frequent loss of balance and falls, which interfere with their ability to walk and maintain an upright position (Busse et al., 2009). Common tasks during which patients demonstrate balance problems include those where the base of support is decreased; tandem standing and walking, dual tasks, eyes closed and in response to external perturbations (Bilney et al., 2003b; Quinn & Rao, 2002). Falls are frequent in people with HD; 60% of people with early to mid-stage HD in two separate studies ($n=45$ & $n=24$) reported two or more falls in the previous 12 months (Busse et al., 2009; Grimbergen et al., 2008). Falls can have physical and psychological consequences (Myers et al., 1996). The fear of future falls may be a more pervasive problem than falls per se, as fear of falls may lead to people restricting their physical activities. Self-imposed restriction of daily activities leads to immobility and consequently osteoporosis, reduced fitness and social isolation (Grimbergen et al., 2004). Individuals with HD have also been found to have lower-limb muscular weakness compared to age-matched controls (Busse et al., 2008a). Strength can be measured clinically by manual muscle testing or by functional observation of strength during task performance (e.g. stair climbing or evidence of gait deviation during walking).

Stage IV and V (Late stage)

In the advanced stages of the disease motor symptoms continue to progress, severely limiting mobility. Choreic and dystonic movement may further increase (see Figure 7.4), but involuntary movements are often overshadowed by Parkinsonian symptoms (Aubeeluck & Wilson, 2008; HDSA, 2000) such as bradykinesia or slowness of movement. People with HD can also experience pain, particularly in the later stage of the disease. The source of this pain can be unknown; however, dystonia or muscle imbalances can often cause musculoskeletal pain. Excessive chorea can cause pain if people injure themselves by hitting their arm or leg into an object or hard surface.

Weight loss can occur in part due to impaired swallowing function (Aubeeluck & Wilson, 2008; HDSA, 2000). People may no longer be able to work or drive and will need assistance when performing some activities of daily living (ADL) (HDSA, 2000).

Even though people with HD appear to be in constant movement, their underlying volitional movements during task performance have been found to be slower than healthy controls for reaching (Quinn et al., 2001) and ambulation (Delval et al., 2006; Delval et al., 2007). Bradykinesia can typically be evaluated by measuring time to complete a task (movement time). Akinesia or delayed initiation of movement is also seen. In research studies, akinesia is typically measured by reaction time. In the clinical setting, it is often difficult to quantitatively evaluate akinesia, but delays in onset of movement for various tasks can be noted. Impaired speech results in difficulties communicating, and cognitive and psychiatric deterioration may continue, but it is thought that patients retain some comprehension (HDSA, 2000). At this stage most people will require assistance in all aspects of daily living, relying fully on nursing care (HDSA, 2000). Despite the severity of the neurological disorder, the primary causes of death in HD are aspiration pneumonia, cardiovascular disease and complications from falls (Sorensen & Fenger, 1992; Walker, 2007).

Physiotherapy assessment

The physiotherapy aims should be both anticipatory and responsive to the disease stage (see Figure 7.4) with interventions to assist HD patients to maintain independence, functional capacity and participation in society (Bilney et al., 2003a).

The World Health Organization International Classification of Functioning, Disability and Health (ICF) (WHO, 2001) is useful as an aid in structuring assessment of a person's functioning and participation (see Figure 7.5), and in allowing consideration of the triad of motor, cognitive and psychiatric symptoms that are often seen in HD. The ICF can be used for functional status assessment, goal setting and treatment planning, and focuses on aspects of a person's health and health-related well-being in terms of activities and participation, i.e. the description of the tasks (activities) and/or life situations (participation) in which the person wishes to engage, and the impact that impaired body function or structure is having on these aspects. The ICF further takes into consideration the contextual factors (both environmental and personal), which may impact on a person's life, and the relationships with body function/structure, activities and participation. The specific impairments and associated activities and participations that may need consideration when assessing a person with HD are listed in Table 7.2. Documentation of the impact of the noted impairments on functional abilities, activities and participation is important to help highlight specific factors that contribute to a patient's functional problems and inform the clinical reasoning process in terms of maximizing functional abilities. Qualifiers of the degree of impairment, and the performance and capacity of activities and participation enable essential documentation of disability and health status.

The subjective assessment allows the physiotherapist to evaluate the patient's presenting problem(s), in the context

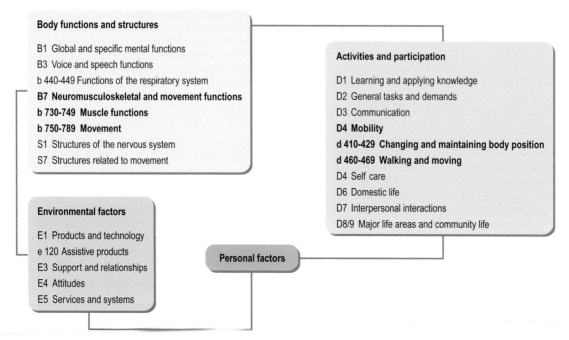

Figure 7.5 Illustration of the WHO ICF domains and coding to the Huntington's disease triad. Bold text indicates areas that are key components of the physiotherapy assessment.

Table 7.2 Specific impairments and associated activities and participations that may need consideration when assessing a person with Huntington's disease

IMPAIRMENTS IN BODY STRUCTURE AND FUNCTION	

B1 Global and specific mental functions
B3 Voice and speech functions
b 440-449 Functions of the respiratory system
B7 Neuromusculoskeletal and movement functions
b 730-749 Muscle functions
b 750-789 Movement functions
S1 Structures of the nervous system
S7 Structures related to movement
	Cognitive-perceptual:
	  Memory
	  Executive functions
	  Spatial abilities
	Neuromuscular:
	  Chorea
	  Dystonia
	  Strength
	  Flexibility

FUNCTIONAL ABILITIES	
Activities and participation	
D1 Learning and applying knowledge D2 General tasks and demands D3 Communication D4 Mobility d 410-429 Changing and maintaining body position d 460-469 Walking and moving D5 Self care D6 Domestic life D7 Interpersonal interactions D8/9 Major life areas and community life	Speech Feeding, drinking (swallowing, sucking) Bathing, toileting, dressing Household chores Cooking, cleaning Walking (distance, speed, shoes)

Continued

Table 7.2 Specific impairments and associated activities and participations that may need consideration when assessing a person with Huntington's disease—cont'd

Activities and participation—cont'd

For each functional activity, therapists should evaluate and document the level of assistance or caregiver burden needed to complete the task, and also determine the patient's skill level (e.g. time to complete task, consistency of task performance, etc).

This section can include any of the following skills, as appropriate: self-care and home management including activities of daily living (bed mobility, dressing, self care, toileting, bathing, eating, cooking, preparing meals and instrumental activities of daily living)

Listing of specific skills assessed (e.g. ambulation, sitting ability, standing ability, sit to stand, wheelchair skills, stair climbing, feeding, bed mobility). Therapists should evaluate and document the functional performance of skills that are pertinent to the person with HD's independence.

ENVIRONMENTAL FACTORS

E1 Products and technology e 120 assistive products E3 Support and relationships E4 Attitudes E5 Services and systems For each functional activity, therapists should evaluate and document the level of assistance or caregiver burden needed to complete the task, and also determine the patient's skill level (e.g. time to complete task, consistency of task performance, etc.). This section can include any of the following skills, as appropriate: Assistive and adaptive devices Environmental, home and work (job/school) barriers	Equipment: Assistive devices, feeding drinking, dressing equipment Wheelchair, brace, walker

Specific coding for the domains are shown.

of their past medical history and how this may affect their ability to live independently and within society. This also provides the opportunity to build a therapeutic, collaborative relationship, and facilitate realistic goal setting. It must be noted that the patient's caregiver(s) should be involved, particularly if the patient has difficulties communicating as a result of cognitive or physical impairment. The objective assessment should include assessment of neuromuscular, musculoskeletal (posture, range of motion, pain and muscle strength), cardio-respiratory and cardio-vascular impairments. An overview of the HD specific considerations for the physiotherapy assessment is shown in Table 7.3. These are useful to aid clinical reasoning and goal setting but are not necessarily outcomes that are sensitive to change over time. There are numerous outcome measures that have potential utility in the assessment of efficacy of physiotherapy interventions for people with HD. Measurement tools that have been used in previous HD-related studies are presented in Table 7.4 and are classified according to the WHO ICF. The Berg Balance Scale, Timed Up and Go Test and the Functional Reach Test have all been found to be valid and responsive clinical measures in HD and are considered useful to detect those at risk of falls (Busse et al., 2009; Grimbergen et al., 2008; Rao et al., 2009).

Goal setting

The physiotherapy goals should be specific and functional in nature, and should address specific problems or participation restrictions that are amenable to physiotherapy intervention. Goals should be focused on specific outcomes that are agreed upon by patient and therapist, and should be measurable and testable.

Even though HD is a degenerative disease, it is still possible for physiotherapists to set goals for improvements in functional performance. The goals should be functional and participation based and not necessarily impairment-focused. Goals to decrease chorea or dystonia are not realistic for physiotherapy. Furthermore, amelioration of any particular impairment in HD may not translate into functional improvements; therefore, therapists should focus on functional gains while attempting to ascertain the influence various impairments have on activity limitations in each person.

Table 7.3 Specific assessment points for consideration in Huntington's disease

SUBJECTIVE ASSESSMENT

Patient information and demographics
Current condition: concerns that led the patient to seek services of physiotherapist; current and prior therapeutic interventions; current stage of Huntington's disease (HD) and age of onset
Past medical history: prior hospitalizations, surgeries and pre-existing medical and other health-related conditions; family history
Medications: list any medications taken for HD symptoms as well as for other medical conditions
Home environment, i.e. living environment and community characteristics; family and living situation; family and caregiver resources; assistive devices and equipment
Employment/work, i.e. current work situation and requirements
Health status, i.e. prior functional status in self care and home management, including activities of daily living (ADLs) and instrumental activities of daily living (IADLs).
Community, leisure and social activity participation
General health perception/quality of life
Physical function (e.g. mobility, sleep patterns, restricted bed days)
Psychological function (e.g. memory, reasoning ability, depression, anxiety)
Behavioural health risks (e.g. smoking, drug abuse)
Level of physical fitness

OBJECTIVE ASSESSMENT	SPECIFIC ASSESSMENT POINTS
Posture: Head/neck/trunk, upper extremities and lower extremities	Standing and sitting
Respiratory function: Lung function tests may highlight obstructive or restrictive disorders of the respiratory system. Measurement of vital capacity in supine and upright positions can identify weakness of the diaphragm (American Thoracic Society, 2002). Forced expiratory Volume in 1 second (FEV1), Forced Vital Capacity (FVC), FEV1/FVC ratio, Peak Expiratory Flow Rate (PEFR) should also be considered using standardized spirometry techniques (Miller et al., 2005).	Ausculatation Breathing patterns Cough Exercise tolerance
Skin integrity	Decubiti, abrasions, open wounds
Pain	Location, type, pain scale rating
Sensation	Location, type
Reflexes	Clonus Babinski
Range of motion: Head/neck/trunk, upper extremities and lower extremities	Active and passive movements
Movement patterns: Chorea, dystonia, bradykinesia, tremor and rigidity	Consider all affected body segments
Mobility: Gait assessment	Base of support Tonal changes Deviations
Endurance	a. Tolerance to standing and upright position b. Tolerance to upright sitting position

Continued

Table 7.3 Specific assessment points for consideration in Huntington's disease—cont'd

ADDITIONAL CONSIDERATIONS	
Behaviour	Combative Labile Impulsive
Cooperation	Carry over of new skill from session to session; follows simple, one step directions and follows multiple step directions
Safety awareness and problem solving	

Table 7.4 Classification of outcome measures according to the WHO ICF

PARTICIPATION	ACTIVITIES	IMPAIRMENTS
The Short Form-36 (Quinn & Rao, 2002; Ware & Sherbourne, 1992)	Self paced and fast paced 10 m walk (Busse et al., 2009; Quinn & Rao, 2002; Watson, 2002)	Berg Balance scale (Berg et al., 1992; Busse et al., 2009; Grimbergen et al., 2008; Quinn & Rao, 2002)
Barthel Index (Zinzi et al., 2007)	The Timed Up & Go (TUG) Test (Busse et al., 2009; Podsiadlo & Richardson, 1991; Rao et al., 2009)	Tinetti Balance & Gait (Tinetti, 1986; Zinzi et al., 2007).
	Physical Performance Test (PPT) (Reuben & Siu, 1990; Zinzi et al., 2007)	
	Activities Specific Balance Confidence Scale (Busse et al., 2009; Grimbergen et al., 2008; Powell & Myers, 1995). Modified Falls Efficacy Scale (Quinn & Rao, 2002)	Functional Reach Test (Rao et al., 2009)
		Four square step test (Dite & Temple, 2002)

Developing and documenting a plan of care for a patient with HD should include specific physiotherapy procedures as well as the coordination and communication that needs to take place with other professionals, caregivers or family members so that the physiotherapy plan can be implemented. This may also include referrals to other professionals and additional documentation of any planned home programme and patient/caregiver education. The physiotherapy Case Histories for early, mid and late stage HD included in this chapter (see below) provide an example of the approach to physiotherapy assessment, treatment planning provision and evaluation of provided intervention according to the WHO ICF framework.

Rationale for physiotherapy intervention

Physiotherapy is recognized as a health-care profession, which utilizes 'physical approaches to promote, maintain and restore physical, psychological and social well-being' (CSP, 2002). The physiotherapist aims to promote quality of life and independence by encouraging activity and providing support within functional tasks (Royal Dutch Society for Physical Therapy (KGNF), 2004). Physiotherapy is also focused on safety and interventions may be aimed at the prevention of falls (KGNF, 2004).

The beneficial role of physiotherapy within basal ganglia disorders has been previously illustrated within Parkinson's disease (PD), with two recent systematic reviews reporting that physiotherapy can improve multiple factors including physical functioning, health-related quality of life (HR-QoL), strength, balance and gait (Goodwin et al., 2008; Nieuwboer et al., 2007). The literature in support of physiotherapy for people with HD is, however, less clear. Two systematic reviews have noted that there is a small amount of evidence supporting physiotherapy within HD, but this is somewhat overshadowed by poor methodological rigour, small sample sizes, unclear selection criteria resulting in potential heterogeneity in participant groups, and a lack of follow-up (Bilney et al., 2003b;

Busse & Rosser, 2007). More supportive evidence is continually becoming available. For example, a before-after trial with a sample size of 40 found an intensive rehabilitation programme of six sessions per week, held over 3 weeks demonstrated an improvement in motor function over a 2-year period (Zinzi et al., 2007). The positive findings from environmental enrichment studies in mice provides support for active interventions, such as physiotherapy, in people with HD. Mice with HD, placed within an environment providing physical, mental and social stimulation, have a slower disease progression, and maintain motor function for longer (Dobrossy & Dunnett, 2005; Hockly et al., 2002). Enhanced voluntary physical activity (in the pre-symptomatic stages) has also been found to contribute to positive effects of environmental stimulation (van Dellen et al., 2008).

Based on these studies and the biological rationale, there is a place for physiotherapy within the management of people with HD, although in-depth efficacy studies are still required. Small (*n*=1–10) studies imply that cognitive strategies, external cueing techniques, balance training as well as a combination of muscle strengthening, stretching and cardiovascular exercise are recommended to be appropriate interventions (Bilney et al., 2003b; Churchyard et al., 2001).

PRINCIPLES AND PRACTICE OF PHYSIOTHERAPY INTERVENTION

In terms of a general strategy for physiotherapy interventions, it is important to consider HD as a spectrum; physiotherapy management of people with HD should be modified according to individual problems and to the stage of the disease (Busse et al., 2008b).

Referral and assessment should take place early in the disease; 'or even in the pre-manifest stage (Busse et al., 2008b). Current intervention focuses on symptomatic management. However, there is increasing support for early intervention where an impact may be made on biological processes with the potential to influence the natural history of the condition. In addition, early referral to physiotherapy for people with HD may be beneficial in a number of ways. It enables practitioners to ascertain a baseline for the person with HD, supports the establishment of a therapeutic relationship between the person with HD, practitioner and caregivers, and ensures early intervention to try and maintain mobility and function for as long as possible (Busse et al., 2008b).

The main goals of physiotherapy intervention will generally change over time; interventions will initially be preventative, and gradually may become restorative (see Figure 7.4). Management during the different stages are outlined below and illustrated further by the Case Histories.

Early and middle stage management

The primary goal of patients with HD in the earlier stages of the disease who are undergoing physiotherapy is often to improve their walking ability (speed, coordination, balance) or to simply continue walking for as long as possible.

The focus of gait training should be on identifying those aspects of gait which are functionally limiting (Rao et al., 2008), and then designing an intervention plan that is aimed at ameliorating or compensating for the gait impairments, and providing training so that the patient can reach their ambulation goals. The influence of the practice environment on learning and carryover, and interaction with the environment directly affects the movement that emerges (Bassile & Bock, 1995). Structuring practice of walking within an environment that is realistic to the current life situation of the person with HD is likely to yield the best results.

Balance training and strengthening of the postural muscles (core stability) should begin in the early stage of the disease and should take place in the environment where the individual's problems are most apparent. General flexibility and strengthening programmes may also be required in line with impairments documented.

Balance activities should be task specific (Shumway-Cook & Woollacott, 2001). Progression from a wide to narrower base of support, from static to dynamic activities, from a low to high centre of gravity, and increasing the degrees of freedom that must be controlled can be considered; however, the key principle is that the balance demand of a specific task should be assessed and addressed. Task-specific training is particularly appropriate for people with movement disorders (Bilney et al., 2003a, 2003b) because motor disturbances are typically context-dependent, and are typically seen in complex, well-learned tasks such as walking and reaching. People should be taught to deliberately prepare in advance for forthcoming threats to balance, or to focus their attention on maintaining balance before a task in which equilibrium is challenged is initiated. It is thought this strategy allows people to use frontal cortical systems to regulate stability, rather than rely upon the impaired basal ganglia mechanisms (Bilney et al., 2003a). Training the person with HD to step in response to perturbations, with an emphasis on speed and accuracy of the stepping strategy, is also recommended. Balance training may be enhanced through the use of auditory and visual cueing. To address inability to attend to more than one task at a time, interventions could include instruction to attend to one task at a time (Delval et al., 2008b). People at high risk of falls should be taught to break down complex activities into simple tasks and to focus their attention on performing each task separately; alternatively, having people with HD practise doing two activities at the same time under various practice and context conditions, may be a beneficial component to balance training (Delval et al., 2008b).

A major aim for therapeutic intervention in HD is for therapists to teach people with HD how to effectively bypass damaged basal ganglia structures and use frontal neural pathways to control movement (Bilney et al., 2003a, 2003b). This involves accessing the motor system by the patient responding to a visual or auditory input (which occurs through frontal pathways), rather than self-initiating movement (which occurs through the basal ganglia-cortical pathway). Sensory cueing involves the use of augmented sensory information, typically in the form of external visual, auditory or manual cueing, to improve performance in a task. There is some controversy as to whether individuals with HD can benefit from rhythmic auditory cues to improve gait characteristics (Delval et al., 2008a; Thaut et al., 1999). Synchronizing gait to rhythmic cues from a metronome (but not music) has been shown to assist the modulation of gait speed in people with HD (Thaut et al., 1999); however, under dual task conditions metronome cues may be less helpful due to attentional deficits in people with HD (Delval et al., 2008a).

KEY POINTS

Early and middle stages

A major aim in the early and middle stages of the disease is to teach people with HD how to effectively bypass damaged basal ganglia structures and use frontal neural pathways to control movement.

Interventions in the early and middle stages should focus on:

1. restoring underlying impairments whenever possible
2. preventing secondary impairments that may affect postural stability
3. facilitating task-specific sensory and motor strategies necessary for meeting postural control demands
4. practicing the maintenance of postural control in a variety of tasks and environments.

Later stage management

As the disease progresses, compensatory strategies such as using sensory cues or attentional strategies can be implemented. Assistive devices (walker with wheels is preferred) and safety equipment, such as a helmet or elbow and knee protectors, may be recommended. Because cognitive impairments also increase in number and severity as the disease progresses, additional compensatory strategies, such as providing cues with goal-directed feedback, teaching skills using one-step commands and providing treatment in a quiet, non-distracting environment should also be considered. Practice should take place through repetition, allowing sufficient time for the person with HD to understand what is required of them and with key points continually being reinforced (Rao et al., 2005).

Assessment of the home, work and community environments in which the person with HD must function should be conducted and modifications made accordingly; in addition, prescription of assistive devices, home-adaptive equipment or modifications may be required. It is critical that the physiotherapist considers the nature of the disease process when considering devices and adaptive equipment. As functional status may be constantly changing, assessment should incorporate both the immediate and the longer-term need. It is important for the therapist to consider equipment that is adaptable to a patient's changing condition. Standard walkers and four-point canes are difficult to manoeuvre and can interfere with natural gait pattern. As balance impairments progress in the middle stages of the disease, a rollator walker with four swivel wheels, and either hand or push-down breaks is often recommended. Walking sticks can be hazardous for patients with excessive choreic movements. Specialized seating needs should be considered; this may include increased seat-back height and depth, tilt and appropriate foot support. Hard surfaces and edges of assistive devices and wheelchairs should be protected with padding where necessary. Choosing the right kind of adaptive equipment is a collaborative process. Balancing independence and safety requires special consideration for each person's individual needs (Rao et al., 2005). Use of certain devices and equipment, such as those described above, may provide the necessary support to maximize a person's functional abilities.

Protective techniques are often used for people with HD, who have an increased risk of bruising and fractures due to involuntary choreic movements. People with HD may benefit from protective padding on the elbow, forearms knees and shins to minimize injury. In order to maximize a patient's ambulatory independence, a therapist may recommend use of a helmet and other body padding as the disease progresses. A helmet may prevent serious head injury in case of a fall, and therefore allows a patient who might otherwise be considered 'unsafe' the opportunity to continue to ambulate independently. Restraint should be kept to a minimum; uncontrolled movements should be minimized as far as possible by considering posture and positional changes.

Respiratory problems may develop at any stage but are more likely to occur in the late-middle and late stages of the disease when mobility becomes more limited. Rigidity, bradykinesia and dystonia eventually lead to immobility and dependence for all care in people with HD (Ribchester et al., 2004). Immobility and postural changes may result in decreased respiratory function (Lin et al., 2006). As with many progressive neurological conditions, the major cause of death in HD is respiratory failure (Lanska et al., 1988; Sørensen & Fenger, 1992) due to factors such as weakened respiratory muscles and/or swallowing problems.

Respiratory interventions, such as deep breathing exercises, body positioning to optimize ventilation–perfusion, modified postural drainage, and airway clearance techniques may be required for specific respiratory problems (see Ch. 15). Caregivers may be taught assisted coughing techniques and a suction machine should be made available for patients who have difficulty clearing secretions. Educating caregivers regarding the signs of aspiration is also important.

Palliative care

Palliative care services have an important role in helping people with HD and their families to prepare for the later stages of HD (Moskowitz & Marder 2001; Travers et al., 2007). The ultimate aim for palliative care is to achieve the best possible quality of life for patients and their families. To this end, coordinated management of the physical and cognitive effects of disease progression is essential. The physiotherapist can advise on seating and positioning, respiratory management, as well as relaxation techniques. It should be noted that the use of feeding tubes in patients with dementia is controversial (Cervo et al., 2006); a recent report provides a comprehensive review of the issues involved in the use of feeding tubes for patients with neurological disease which should be patient centred and not based on the convenience of staff or carers (Royal College of Physicians and British Society of Gastroenterologists, 2010). Obtaining a patient's views of feeding tubes and end-stage care is better discussed and recorded at a time before they lose capacity (Simpson, 2007).

KEY POINTS

Overall physiotherapy management of the person with Huntington's disease

◆ Huntington's disease (HD) is a progressive neurodegenerative disorder; the needs of the person with HD change over time.
◆ The role of the physiotherapist develops in response to the clinical need over the prolonged course of the illness; it is important for physiotherapists to consider the cost implications of their services throughout a life-long disease.
◆ Therapists should act in an advisory capacity to patients from an early stage, and provide more intensive intervention when a change in functional status warrants this.
◆ Interventions will initially be preventative and gradually become restorative.
◆ Palliative care services have an important role in helping people with HD and their families to prepare for the later stages of HD.
◆ Early intervention is important to aid the clinical reasoning process and a collaborative partnership along the spectrum of the disease.

CASE HISTORIES

CASE HISTORY 1: Early-stage Huntington's disease

The following case history is modified with permission from Smith et al. (2007).

Subjective assessment

Patient information and demographics

Ms J. was a 50-year-old woman, referred to outpatient physiotherapy because of mild clumsiness and balance problems. Ms J. had not been formally diagnosed with HD. However, her father had died from complications of the disease 5 years previously. She chose not to be tested for the Huntington gene mutation. Through magnetic resonance imaging (MRI) examination, mild degeneration of the caudate and putamen was identified. Past medical history included treatment for depression.

Social history and participation restrictions

Ms J. was an active woman and avid bike rider. She regularly rode to work, about 7 miles, and had participated in many bike adventure trips. She was employed by a large company as an administrative assistant. She was married and had a 15-year-old son at the time of referral.

Objective assessment

Posture and range of motion – Passive and active range of motion were within normal limits. Muscle strength was generally 4/5
Cardio respiratory function – Resting heart rate 80 bpm, blood pressure 100/70
Skin integrity – Not assessed
Pain – None reported
Sensation – Sensation to light touch, pinprick and proprioception was intact; deep tendon reflexes were brisk without clonus
Reflexes – Not assessed
Movement patterns – Chorea, dystonia, bradykinesia, tremor and rigidity.

Ms J. demonstrated mild, low amplitude increasing to high amplitude (under stress) choreiform movements. Finger to thumb tapping and diadochokinesia was arrhythmic and slow. She displayed mild bilateral incoordination with finger-to-nose and finger-to-finger tests.

Impairments in body structure and function

B1 Global and specific mental functions

Ms J. was oriented to person, place and time. She did not feel that her memory or attention had diminished, nor did her family report any personality changes.

B7 Neuromusculoskeletal and movement functions

Balance. She could sit independently without any back support for an indefinite period of time. She could stand up from a sitting position without assistance but slowly. She stood independently without support. Although she could stand with her feet together, her gait was wide-based.

Functional abilities

Activities and participation

D4 Mobility. Ms J. scored 11/13 on the Huntington's Disease Functional Capacity Scale. She did not report difficulty performing her job related tasks. She did require some assistance with domestic and financial affairs due to her lack of organization. She was living at home and was independent with all self care and home management. Due to the choreiform movements, Ms J. was beginning to experience difficulty with driving, especially at night. This impacted on her ability to drive her son to his sporting events. She had been actively involved in organizing fundraisers, practices and other team-related events for her son, but was considering dropping these activities. Ms J.'s ability to cycle to work was only minimally affected at time of referral. She reported riding slowly and cautiously. Some days she had to convince herself to ride because she felt so tired. Ambulation – walking on a flat surface, ascending and descending stairs and on uneven terrain all posed no difficulty for Ms J. She had difficulty with tandem (heel-to-toe) walking.

D5 Self Care. Ms J. planned and made all family meals and completed all household tasks. Ms J. complained that she was slower performing these tasks and felt disorganized. She was independent in all her self-help skills.

Environmental factors

Her home was a large two-story house, most flooring being wood with a variety of floor coverings.

Treatment planning

At the time of writing, Ms J.'s deficits were minimal. According to the HD Functional Capacity Scale, she was at Stage 1 of the condition. She was independent with all of her ADLs. She was continuing her work as a secretary and was able to carry out her household responsibilities with minimal assistance. On some days she did not feel comfortable riding or driving to work, so she would take the bus, which required additional planning. She was especially concerned about being able to maintain her riding ability.

Therapeutic goals focused on maintaining her ability to complete all ADLs independently, preservation of present range of motion and strength, and overall preservation of her ability to move independently. To accomplish these goals, we recommended an exercise programme to help maintain her range of motion and strength. In addition, anticipatory guidance was provided to her and her family about the consequences of HD and the need to plan for eventual movement limitations. She was instructed in relaxation strategies to decrease her stress and minimize her choreic movements. We also recommended that she take mini-breaks at work, to help her to stay focused and organized.

Due to her status, ongoing intervention was not currently necessary. One to two sessions of education and anticipatory guidance were considered adequate as Ms J. and her family were knowledgeable about the consequences of the condition. Ms J. was encouraged to become involved in a 3–5 times per week community-based exercise programme. This programme consisted of a variety of aerobic activities such as stationary bike, treadmill, elliptical training and aerobic exercise classes. Additionally, a comprehensive strength training programme was designed. To maintain flexibility, Ms J. chose to participate in a flexibility and strength class and planned also to participate in a yoga programme. Because riding was of particular concern to Ms J., she engaged a personal trainer who was knowledgeable in cycling exercises.

A variety of referral sources that she might benefit from over the course of the next 6 months were presented to Ms J. These were intended to help her maintain an organized environment at home, continue with the performance of her household duties and structure management of her financial affairs. The referrals included an organization specialist, a HD support group, a physiotherapist who specialized in office ergonomics, and an occupational therapist who specialized in assistive technology.

Outcome measures and goal setting

Because Ms J. indicated that she would like to maintain an active role in decision-making regarding her condition for as long as possible, she would need to establish collaborative relationships with a variety of professionals. A 6-month re-assessment with the physiotherapist is appropriate. In addition to re-examining physical status and maintaining functional status, the therapist and Ms J. would be able to discuss the need for any additional resources.

Summary of progress

This patient was provided with a variety of strategies to maintain safe ambulation, strength and flexibility. Over the next decade, it is probable that she will become increasingly dependent on others for assistance with activities of daily living, home management and professional responsibilities. Future issues for her will include dependence related to ADLs, domestic management and ability to work. Prior to her inability to continue working, her employer may need to make adaptations to her work environment, such as changing her workstation, providing her with a time-management device, and project management software to help her stay organized.

CASE HISTORY 2: Home-based physiotherapy in mid-stage Huntington's disease

The following case history is modified from Quinn and Rao (2002).

Subjective assessment

Patient information and demographics

Male, aged 49 years; diagnosed with HD 17 years ago with gradual progression of HD symptoms since then; now referred for physiotherapy due to more rapid decline in functional abilities; numerous falls over the past 3 months. Main concern of patient and relative is to prevent further falls and injuries, and to improve balance. Wants to maintain his independence in current living situation for as long as possible.

Medications include: Clonazepam, 5 mg, b.i.d. (a benzodiazepine that facilitates the effects of the inhibitory neurotransmitter GABA, used for anxiety control); Reserpine, 25 mg b.i.d. (a dopamine depleting agent that acts to reduce the amplitude of ballistic movements); Zoloft, 50 mg 2½ q.d (a selective serotonin reuptake inhibitor whose net effect is to increase serotonin levels, used for depression).

Medical/surgical history – no significant medical history prior to diagnosis of HD.

Social history and participation restrictions

Lives alone in a flat with no steps and a lift to get to the front door. Has had assistance of a carer at home for the last 4 years, input includes preparing meals, basic housekeeping, assistance with household organization, and assistance with grocery shopping.

Not currently working; used to work as a lawyer at a law firm until 17 years ago, at which time he began having difficulty performing his job; has not worked since that time.

Functional status/activity level – Total Functional Capacity scale score of 6/13; primary form of exercising is walking with the supervision of carer. Has been going to the gym for weight-lifting and cardiovascular exercises, but stopped this about 6 months prior to this assessment because it was becoming too difficult. Enjoys spending time with family and friends, and travels by plane twice a year to visit relatives in different parts of the country.

Objective assessment

Posture and range of motion – shoulder asymmetry (right shoulder higher than left); moderate lateral trunk lean to left (indicative of dystonia)

Respiratory function – Vital signs: HR - 84 bpm; BP 140/84; RR: 14 bpm; aerobic capacity was not specifically assessed. No specific fatigue or dyspnoea reported
Skin integrity – Some bruising on anterior lower legs bilaterally, and on forearms bilaterally; skin intact
Pain – No reports of pain
Sensation – Intact sensation to light touch throughout bilateral UE and LE
Reflexes – Deep Tendon Reflex (DTR) 4+ bilateral Achilles; spasticity noted bilateral hamstrings and gastroc (2/4 on Modified Ashworth Scale)
Range of motion – Full range in all joints; with exception of moderate tightness of bilateral hamstrings (approximately 60° straight leg raise)
Muscle strength – Strength not formally assessed using manual muscle testing, but no specific muscle weaknesses noted during task performance that appeared to be a limiting factor
Movement patterns – Chorea: frequent choreic movements during walking with either leg occasionally flexing upward (hip and knee flexion) during swing phase; dystonia: during walking hands forming fists intermittently, posturing of shoulder into external rotation with elbow flexion (noted bilaterally); bradykinesia: observed during all tasks, especially ambulation, sit to stand and reaching tasks; rigidity: none noted; resting tremor: absent
Gait assessment (base of support, tonal changes, deviations, etc.) – Slow walking speed (1.67 ft/second); frequent choreic movements during walking with either leg occasionally flexing upward (hip and knee flexion) during swing phase
Mobility – Primary means of mobility: able to walk independently at home, despite his frequent falls and episodes of loss of balance
Endurance – Not assessed formally.

Impairments in body structure and function

B1 Global and specific mental functions

Notable cognitive deficits, including delayed processing speed and short-term memory; able to communicate concerns and feelings, and could converse with the therapist and carer; had experienced some depression and anxiety, both effectively managed through medication.

B7 Neuromusculoskeletal and movement functions

Slow gait with impaired balance. Significant difficulties with turning to look behind, one legged stance, tandem stance and alternating foot on step.

Bradykinesia observed during all tasks, especially ambulation, sit to stand and reaching tasks; frequent choreic movements during walking with either leg occasionally flexing upward (hip and knee flexion) during swing phase.

Functional abilities

Activities and participation

D4 Mobility. Able to walk independently at home, despite frequent falls and episodes of loss of balance; four falls in the 3 months prior to this assessment.

D5 Self care. Independent with washing and dressing. Requires assistance for cleaning, household tasks and cooking. Some swallowing difficulties, but able to handle different food consistencies and thin liquids. Tends to eat softer foods that are easier to swallow. Uses a covered cup with a straw for drinking most liquids.

D6 Domestic life. Limited ability to manage finances, needing assistance for monthly finance management.

D7 Interpersonal interactions. Enjoys spending time with family and friends, and travels by plane twice a year to visit relatives in different parts of the country.

D8/9 Major life areas and community life. General health was worse than it was a year ago, and patient is concerned about his frequent falls. Most notable difficulties in role limitations related to his physical health (significantly limited in his daily activities because of problems with his balance and walking ability).

Environmental factors

Assistive and adaptive devices

Bath transfer bench, grab bars in bathroom, a walking stick for outdoor mobility.

Environmental, home, and work (job/school) barriers

Home environment appropriately clutter-free.

Additional considerations

Behaviour – No problems noted
Cooperation – Patient cooperative and well motivated; has appropriate support at home
Safety concerns and problem solving – No specific concerns noted.

Treatment planning

A 49-year-old, mid-stage HD patient very concerned about recent falls and his declining functional abilities; limited ambulation ability; history of falls secondary to impaired balance, dystonia and gait disturbances attributable to HD; good candidate for a home-based programme as very motivated and has daily carer support.

Proposed

Home-bas ry
videotape D.
The video ists

demonstrating a full exercise routine to music. Instructions to use the video 5 days/week (Monday–Friday) with carer support at a mutually agreed time. Instructions of required equipment (chair, a theraband, 1 kg weights, and a towel for floor exercises) and safety precautions. In addition to the exercise video, patient was given three additional exercises to perform daily: (1) standing on one foot for up to 2 minutes on each leg, standing near kitchen counter, using hands for support only if he started to lose his balance; (2) tandem walking – walking with one foot in front of other, down length of hallway (10 m), five times; and (3) throwing and catching a tennis ball (standing approximately 3 m away from the wall, then throwing the ball at the wall, letting it bounce once and catching it).

Outcome measures and goal setting

Outcome measures utilized:

Initial assessment:

1. Falls: four in the 3 months prior to assessment
2. Gait speed: 1.67 ft/second
3. Modified Falls Efficacy Scale: 82%
4. Berg Balance Scale total score: 39/65
5. Motor section of the UHDRS total score: 69/124

Mutually agreed goals:

1. No falls within 14-week period
2. Walk on level pavement with gait speed of > 0.62/s
3. Berg Balance Scale score will be >42/56
4. Independent in performing home exercise programme with assistance of carer.

Summary of progress

Patient participated in a home exercise programme over a 14-week period. Patient was contacted every 2 weeks to answer any questions about his exercise programme, and to encourage continued compliance. Asked at each phone call if he had missed any sessions, and also if he had any falls. Visited in his home twice by the physiotherapist during the 14-week period (questions were asked regarding proper execution of exercises and patient observed performing components of the exercise programme).

Outcomes

Improvements were noted at the level of both activity limitations and impairments (walking speed, number of falls – 0, falls efficacy – 87%, Berg Balance Scale, UHDRS motor score). Specifically, the Berg Balance Score improved by 9 points, and improvements in dystonia, chorea and bradykinesia were seen as measured by the UHDRS. The patient and his carer reported that they noted significant improvements in his walking ability and balance over the past 3 months. Specifically, the patient reported that he 'doesn't fall', and 'people don't worry about me as much'. He had one reported fall during the intervention period (in contrast to four in the 3 months prior to the initial evaluation), which occurred whilst on holiday and he fell while walking on the beach. He was not injured during this fall. He enjoyed participating in the exercise programme and planned to continue with the entire exercise programme on a daily basis.

CASE HISTORY 3: Late-stage Huntington's disease

Subjective assessment

Patient information and demographics

Mr V. aged 58 years in late stage Huntington's disease. He has had a series of illnesses and hospitalizations over the past year due to urinary tract infections (UTI) or chest infections, and has numerous setbacks in terms of his ability to ambulate, speak and eat, and through weight loss. Mr V. was evaluated with his wife present. His wife contacted the physiotherapist for this evaluation, regarding difficulties he is having due to HD. The consultation took place in their home. Past medical history included right knee surgery secondary to a patellar fracture following a fall 1 year ago.

Social history and participation restrictions

Mr V. lives with his wife in a two-story home. His bedroom and a toilet are on the first floor. He is not working and has not worked for over 8 years. He stays at home most days and enjoys watching television and spending time with his wife. He goes outside once or twice per week, for which he uses a wheelchair. He also has a commode next to his bed. Mr V.'s primary caregiver is his wife, who is very dedicated to him and his needs. He also is seen by home health aides who provide assistance 4 hours/day.

Objective assessment

Posture and range of motion – Mr V. is able to sit up in a supported cushion chair, but tends to slide down in the chair after about 2–3 minutes and leans over to one side. In supine, he often positions himself diagonally in the bed, and seeks out support for his feet. He much prefers to have the head of the bed elevated about 45°. Full range of motion noted in both upper extremities and lower extremities
Respiratory function – Not assessed
Skin integrity – A hard, slightly protruding area was noted just lateral to the patella, which is likely to be scar tissue. Mr V. also has redness around his buttocks medial to the ischial tuberosities bilaterally, in a fairly large area. Up until 1 week ago he had open wounds, which are now

healing. Mrs V. reports that she has been applying cortisone cream as prescribed
Pain – Mr V. reports pain in his right knee (unable to use a pain scale but states his knee hurts 'a lot'
Sensation – Not assessed due to communication difficulties, however appears intact to light touch and pain
Muscle strength – Able to move all four limbs against gravity in supine and sitting. Unable to perform bridging in supine, suggesting gluteal weakness. Muscle wasting noted in bilateral gluteals and quadriceps muscles, and decreased strength evidenced by difficulties in standing from sitting position
Movement patterns – Chorea, dystonia, bradykinesia, tremor and rigidity. Mr V. demonstrates choreic movements in his hands bilaterally and his legs at rest, although there can be very little movement at times. If he becomes upset or anticipates a change, his choreic movements are exaggerated. He has moderate bradykinesia and dystonic posturing in his trunk and arms, particularly noticeable in standing
Endurance – Mrs V. reports that Mr V. has limited endurance for both upright sitting (20 minutes maximum) and walking (10 minutes).

Impairments in body structure and function

B1 Global and specific mental functions

Mr V. is able to speak, but with great difficulty. He was able to answer questions with one or two word responses, which were intelligible 50% of time. Mr V. demonstrated good receptive language skills and could follow simple instructions.

Functional abilities

Activities and participation

D4 Mobility. Mr V. spends most of his day in bed, which is a hospital bed with bed rails. He requires minimal-moderate assistance to roll bilaterally, and moderate-maximal assistance to achieve sitting on edge of the bed. He can sit on the edge of the bed with minimal assistance for up to 5 minutes prior to fatiguing. He requires moderate assistance to transfer to a wheelchair from the bed. His wheelchair has a pressure-relieving cushion, padded foot box and supportive back. Mrs V. reports that he is comfortable in the chair and it seems to fit him well, but he only uses it for transportation. He is able to walk for short distances with physical assistance from his wife and a caregiver (moderate assistance – two-hand hold typically). He can not walk unassisted. Mr V. used to enjoy walking outside, but this has become more difficult and requires two-person assistance for balance and stability.

D5 Self care. Mr V. requires maximum assistance for dressing and bathing, which are all done by his wife or by the nursing aide. He is on PEG feeding, and is currently only drinking occasional thickened milkshakes two to three times per week. He has a commode, however Mrs V. reports he becomes anxious and she feels it may not be comfortable for him. He instead uses inconsistence pads which may have contributed to his skin breakdown. Mrs V. showed the physiotherapist a padded supportive toilet cushion which she recently purchased but has not yet tried for him. Barthel Index: 3/20

Environmental factors

Mr V.'s home environment is well designed for his current needs. His bed is on the ground floor, as is the living room. He has a TV in his room and spends most of his day in bed.

Additional considerations

Mr V. appears underweight and his wife reports that he seems to continue to lose weight. Over the past 1 month she thinks he has lost at least 5–7 kg, although she has not weighed him.

Treatment planning

Mr V. would benefit from physiotherapy two to three times per week for 8 weeks. Treatment to include:

1. Walking in household and shorts distances outdoors for up to 10 minutes. Training caregivers in proper guarding techniques
2. Transfers to a chair or to the wheelchair for upright sitting, for as long as tolerated (maximum 20–30 minutes in any one position to prevent skin breakdown). Assess for pressure-relieving cushion to be used in recliner chairs, assuring that his buttocks are all the way back in the chair and his feet have support
3. Active range of motion and strengthening exercises, particularly to strengthen gluteals and quadriceps
4. Trial of a customized seating systems to provide comfortable upright sitting position.

Instructions for caregivers:

1. Use the cushioned toilet seat and/or commode chair as tolerated
2. Apply heat two times per day to right knee, and use elastic support as tolerated for comfort

3. Mr V.'s weight loss needs to be addressed, as has been mentioned by other professionals. The physiotherapist forwarded Mrs V. a research article which discusses calorie requirements in people with HD and discussed specific recommendations with her. Mr V. would benefit from a speech/language consultation to determine his swallowing ability, and to advise Mrs V. on potential food and drink recommendations.

Outcome measures and goal setting

Goals (8 weeks)

Mr V. will:

1. walk with minimal assistance of caregiver indoors
2. walk for 10 minutes on sidewalk outside his home daily
3. transfer from bed to wheelchair with minimal assistance of one caregiver
4. demonstrate ability to perform bridging in supine position with minimal assistance, for pressure relief
5. be able to sit upright for 20–30 minutes in a supportive chair.

Summary of progress

Mr V. was seen by physiotherapy two times per week for a total of 8 weeks. A trial of a specialized seating system was performed over 2 weeks, and Mr V. and his wife both felt that it improved his sitting posture and his overall mood as he appeared more comfortable. A letter of medical justification was written and approval was granted for purchase of a system (to be delivered in 4 weeks time). Mr V. enjoyed the therapy sessions and became increasingly verbal and engaging. Speech therapy consultation occurred during week 4, at which time an increase in PEG feeding was recommended and initiated. Mr V. is now using the toilet with the toilet seat for all toileting, eliminating need for pads. Skin integrity on buttocks has improved with minor redness noted. Mr V. continues to have difficulty with ambulation, and requires two persons to assist in order to assure his safety when walking outside.

REFERENCES

American Thoracic Society, 2002. ATS/ERS Statement on Respiratory Muscle Testing. Am. J. Respir. Crit. Care Med. 166, 518–624.

The American College of Medical Genetics/American Society of Human Genetics Huntington Disease Genetic Testing Working Group Statement (ASHG/AMCG), 1998. Laboratory guidelines for Huntington disease genetic testing. The American College of Medical Genetics/American Society of Human Genetics Huntington Disease Genetic Testing Working Group 1998. Am. J. Hum. Genet. 62 (5), 1243–1247.

Albin, R.L., Young, A.B., Penny, J.B., 1989. The functional anatomy of disorders of the basal ganglia. Trends Neurosci. 12 (10), 366–374.

Aubeeluck, A., Wilson, E., 2008. Huntington's disease. Part 1: essential background and management. Br. J. Nurs. 17 (3), 146–151.

Bates, G., Harper, P., Jones, L., 2002. Huntington's Disease, third ed. Oxford University Press, Oxford.

Bassile, C., Bock, C., 1995. Gait training. In: Craik, R., Oatis, C. (Eds.), Gait Analysis: Theory and Application. Mosby, St. Louis.

Berg, K.O., Wood-Dauphinee, S., Williams, J.L., et al., 1992. Measuring balance in the elderly: validation of an instrument. Can. J. Public Health 83 (Suppl. 2), S7–S11.

Bilney, B.M., Morris, M., Denisenko, S., 2003a. Physiotherapy for people with movement disorders arising from basal ganglia dysfunction. NZ. J. Physiother. 31 (2), 94–100.

Bilney, B.M., Morris, M., Perry, A., 2003b. Effectiveness of physiotherapy, occupational therapy, and speech pathology for people with Huntington's disease: a systematic review. Neurorehabil. Neural. Repair. 17 (1), 12–24.

Busse, M.E., Hughes, G., Wiles, C.M., et al., 2008a. Use of hand-held dynamometry in the evaluation of lower limb muscle strength in people with Huntington's disease. J. Neurol. 255 (10), 1534–1540.

Busse, M.E., Khalil, H., Quinn, L., et al., 2008b. Physical Therapy Intervention for Patients with Huntington's disease. Phys. Ther. 88 (7), 820–831.

Busse, M.E., Rosser, A.E., 2007. Can directed activity improve mobility in Huntington's disease? Brain Res. Bull. 72 (2–3), 172–174.

Busse, M.E., Wiles, C.M., Rosser, A.E., 2009. Mobility and Falls in Huntington's Disease. J. Neurol. Neurosurg. Psychiatry 80 (1), 88–90.

Cervo, F.A., Bryan, L., Farber, S., 2006. To PEG or not to PEG. A review of evidence for placing feeding tubes in advanced dementia and the decision-making process. Geriatrics 61 (6), 30–35.

Chartered Society of Physiotherapy (CSP), 2002. Curriculum Framework for Qualifying Programmes in Physiotherapy. Chartered Society of Physiotherapy, London.

Churchyard, A.J., Morris, M., Georgiou, N., et al., 2001. Gait dysfunction in Huntington's disease: parkinsonism and a disorder of timing. Implications for movement rehabilitation. Adv. Neurol. 87, 375–385.

Conneally, P.M., 1984. Huntington disease: genetics and epidemiology. Am. J. Hum. Genet. 36, 506–526.

Davies, S.W., Turmaine, M., Cozens, B.A., et al., 1997. Formation of neuronal intranuclear inclusions underlies the neuronal dysfunction in mice transgenic for the HD mutation. Cell 90 (3), 537–548.

Delval, A., Krystkowiak, P., Blatt, J.L., et al., 2006. Role of hypokinesia and bradykinesia in gait disturbances in Huntington's disease: a biomechanical study. J. Neurol. 253 (1), 73–80.

Delval, A., Krystkowiak, P., Blatt, J.L., et al., 2007. A biomechanical study of gait initiation in Huntington's disease. Gait Posture 25 (2), 279–288.

Delval, A., Krystkowiak, P., Delliaux, M., et al., 2008a. Effect of external cueing on gait in Huntington's disease. Mov. Disord. 23 (10), 1446–1452.

Delval, A., Krystkowiak, P., Delliaux, M., et al., 2008b. Role of attentional resources on gait performance in Huntington's disease. Mov. Disord. 23 (5), 684–689.

DiFiglia, M., Sapp, E., Chase, K.O., et al., 1997. Aggregation of huntingtin in neuronal inclusion and dystrophic neurites in brain. Science 277, 1990–1993.

Dite, W., Temple, V.A., 2002. A clinical test of stepping and change of direction to identify multiple falling older adults. Arch. Phys. Med. Rehabil. 83 (11), 1566–1571.

Dobrossy, M.D., Dunnett, S.B., 2005. Optimising plasticity: environmental and training associated factors in transplant-mediated brain repair. Rev. Neurosci. 16 (1), 1–21.

Foroud, T., Gray J Ivashina, J., et al., 1999. Differences in duration of Huntington's disease based on age at onset. J. Neurol. Neurosurg. Psychiatry 66, 52–56.

Goodwin, V.A., Richards, S.H., Taylor, R.S., et al., 2008. The effectiveness of exercise interventions for people with Parkinson's disease: a systematic review and meta-analysis. Mov. Disord. 23, 631–640.

Grimbergen, Y., Knol, M., Bloem, B.R., et al., 2008. Falls and gait disturbances in Huntington's disease. Mov. Disord. 23 (7), 970–976.

Grimbergen, Y., Munneke, M., Bloem, B.R., 2004. Falls in Parkinson's disease. Curr. Opin. Neurol. 17 (4), 405–415.

International Huntington's Association/ World Federation of Neurology Research Group on Huntington's chorea, 1994. Guidelines for the molecular genetics predictive test in Huntington's disease. J. Med. Genet. 31, 555–559.

Harper, P.S., 2002. The epidemiology of Huntington's disease. In: Bates, G., Harper, P., Jones, L. (Eds.), Huntington's disease 2ed. third ed. Oxford University Press, Oxford, pp. 159–197.

Harper, P.S., Quarrell, O.W.J., Youngman, S., 1988. Huntington's disease: prediction and prevention. Philosophical Transactions of the Royal Society 319, 285–298.

Hausdorff, J.M., Cudkowicz, M., Firtion, R., et al., 1998. Gait variability and basal ganglia disorders: stride-to-stride variations of gait cycle timing in Parkinson's disease and Huntington's disease. Mov. Disord. 13 (3), 428–437.

Henley, S.D., Bates, G.P., Tabrizi, S.J., 2005. Biomarkers for neurodegenerative disease. Curr. Opin. Neurol. 18, 698–705.

Hockly, E., Cordery, P.M., Woodman, B., et al., 2002. Environmental enrichment slows disease progression in R6/2 Huntington's disease mice. Ann. Neurol. 51 (2), 235–242.

Huntington's Disease Society of America (HDSA), 2000. A Physicians Guide to The Management Of Huntington's Disease. Huntington's Disease Society of America, New York.

Huntington's Disease Collaborative Research Group, 1993. A novel gene containing a trinucleotide repeat that is expanded and unstable on Huntington's disease chromosomes. Cell 26;72(6), 971–983.

Huntington Study Group, 1996. Unified Huntington's Disease Rating Scale: reliability and consistency. Mov. Disord. 11 (2), 136–142.

Koller, W.C., Trimble, J., 1985. The gait abnormality of Huntington's disease. Neurology 35 (10), 1450–1454.

Lanska, D.J., Lavine, L., Lanska, M.J., et al., 1988. Huntington's disease mortality in the United States. Neurology 38 (5), 769–772.

Lin, F., Parthasarathy, S., Taylor, S., et al., 2006. Effect of Different Sitting

Postures on Lung Capacity, Expiratory Flow, and Lumbar Lordosis. Arch. Phys. Med. Rehabil. 87 (4), 504–509.

Louis, E.D., Lee, P., Quinn, L., et al., 1999. Dystonia in Huntington's disease: prevalence and clinical characteristics. Mov. Disord. 14 (1), 95–101.

Mangarini, L., Shasivam, K., Seller, M., et al., 1996. Exon 1 of the HD gene with an expanded CAG repeat is sufficient to cause a progressive neurological phenotype in transgenic mice. Cell 87, 493–506.

Marder, K., Zhao, H., Myers, R.H., et al., 2000. Rate of functional decline in Huntington's disease. Huntington Study Group. Neurology 54 (2), 452–458.

Miller, M., Hankinson, J., Brusasco, V., et al., 2005. Standardisation of Spirometry. Eur. Respir. J. 26 (2), 319–338.

Moskowitz, C.B., Marder, K., 2001. Palliative care for people with late-stage Huntington's Disease. Neurol. Clin. 19 (4), 849–865.

Myers, A.M., Powell, L.E., Maki, B.E., et al., 1996. Psychological indicators of balance confidence: relationship to actual and perceived abilities. J. Gerontol. A Biol. Sci. Med. Sci. 51 (1), M37–M43.

Nieuwboer, A., Kwakkel, G., Rochester, L., et al., 2007. Cueing training in the Home improves gait-related mobility in Parkinson's disease: the RESCUE trial. J. Neurol. Neurosurg. Psychiatry 78 (2), 134–140.

Podsiadlo, D., Richardson, S., 1991. The timed "Up & Go: a test of basic functional mobility for frail elderly persons". J. Am. Geriatr. Soc. 39 (2), 142–148.

Powell, L.E., Myers, A.M., 1995. The Activities-specific Balance Confidence (ABC) Scale. J. Gerontol. A Biol. Sci. Med. Sci. 50 (A1), M28–M34.

Quarrell, O., 2009. Huntington's disease - the facts 2ed. Oxford University Press, Oxford.

Quarrell, O., Brewer, H.M., Squitieri, F., et al., 2009. Juvenile Huntington's Disease and other trinucleotide repeat disorders. Oxford University Press, Oxford.

Quinn, L., Gordon, A., Reilmann, R., et al., 2001. Altered Movement Trajectories and Force control during object transport in Huntington's disease. Mov. Disord. 16 (3), 469–480.

Quinn, L., Rao, A.K., 2002. Physical therapy for people with Huntington disease: current perspectives and case report. Neurology Report 3, 145–153.

Rao, A.K., Quinn, L., Marder, K.S., 2005. Reliability of spatiotemporal gait outcome measures in Huntington's disease. Mov. Disord. 20 (8), 1033–1037.

Rao, A.K., Muratori, L., Louis, E.D., et al., 2008. Spectrum of Gait impairments in Presymptomatic and Symptomatic Huntington's disease. Mov. Disord. 23 (8), 1100–1107.

Rao, A.K., Muratori, L., Louis, E.D., et al., 2009. Clinical measurement of Mobility and Balance impairments in Huntington's disease: validity and responsiveness. Gait Posture 29 (3), 433–436.

Reuben, D., Siu, A., 1990. An Objective measure of Physical function of Elderly outpatients. The Physical Performance Test. J. Am. Geriatr. Soc. 38 (10), 1105–1112.

Ribchester, R.R., Thomson, D., Wood, N.I., et al., 2004. Progressive abnormalities in skeletal muscle and neuromuscular junctions of transgenic mice expressing the Huntington's disease mutation. Eur. J. Neurosci. 20 (11), 3092–3114.

Roos, R.A.C., Hermans, J., Vegter-van der Vlis, M., et al., 1993. Duration of illness of Huntington's disease is not related to Age at onset. J. Neurol. Neurosurg. Psychiatry 56, 98–100.

Royal College of Physicians and British Society of Gastroenterology, 2010. Oral feeding difficulties and dilemmas: A guide to practical care, particularly towards the end of life. Royal College of Physicians, London.

Royal Dutch Society for Physical Therapy (KGNF), 2004. Guidelines for Physical Therapy in Patients with Parkinson's Disease. Dutch Journal of Physiotherapy 114, S3.

Shoulson, I., Fahn, S., 1979. Huntington disease: Clinical care and Evaluation. Neurology 29 (1), 1–3.

Shumway-Cook, A., Woollacott, M., 2001. Clinical Management of the Patient With a Postural Control Disorder. In: M. Biblis (Ed.), Motor control: theory and application. Lippincott Williams and Wilkins, Baltimore, pp. 397–445.

Simpson, S.A., 2007. Late stage care in Huntington's disease. Brain Res. Bull. 72 (2–3), 179–181.

Smith, M., Danoff, J., Jain, M., & Long, T., 2007. Genetic Disorders: Implications for Allied Health Professionals: Two Case Studies. Internet Journal of Allied Health Sciences and Practice. http://ijahsp.nova.edu. Vol 5, No 4 ISSN 1540-580X'.

Snowden, J.S., Craufurd, D., Griffiths, H.L., Neary, D., 1998. Awareness involuntary movements in Huntington's disease. Arch. Neurol. 55 (6), 801–805.

Sorensen, S., Fenger, K., 1992. Causes of death in patients with Huntington's disease and in unaffected first degree relatives. J. Med. Genet. 29 (12), 911–914.

Tassicker, R.J., Teltscher, B., Trembath, M.K., et al., 2009. Problems assessing uptake of Huntington disease predictive testing and a proposed solution. Eur. J. Hum. Genet. 17, 66–70.

Thaut, M.H., Miltner, R., Lange, H.W., et al., 1999. Velocity modulation and rhythmic synchronization of gait in Huntington's disease. Mov. Disord. 14 (5), 808–819.

Tinetti, M.E., 1986. Performance-oriented assessment of mobility problems in elderly patients. J. Am. Geriatr. Soc. 34 (2), 119–126.

Travers, E., Jones, K., Nichol, J., 2007. Palliative care provision in Huntington's disease. Int. J. Palliat. Nurs. 13 (3), 125–130.

van Dellen, A., Cordery, P., Spires, T.L., et al., 2008. Wheel running from a juvenile age delays onset of specific motor deficits but does not alter protein aggregate density in a mouse model of Huntington's disease. BMC Neurosci. 9, 34.

Walker, F.O., 2007. Huntington's disease. Lancet 369 (9557), 218–228.

Ware, J.J., Sherbourne, C., 1992. The MOS 36-item Short-form Health survey (SF-36). I. Conceptual Framework and Item Selection. Med. Care. 30 (6), 473–483.

Watson, M., 2002. Refining the Ten-metre walking test for use with neurologically impaired People. Physiotherapy 88 (7), 386–397.

World Health Organization, 2001. International Classification of Functioning, Disability and Health. World Health Organization, Geneva.

Zinzi, P., Salmaso, D., De Grandis, R., et al., 2007. Effects of an Intensive Rehabilitation Programme on Patients with Huntington's disease: a pilot study. Clin. Rehabil. 21 (7), 603–613.

Chapter | 8 |

Motor neurone disease

Samantha Orridge, Emma Stebbings

CONTENTS

DEFINITION

Motor neurone disease (MND) is a degenerative neurological condition characterized by damage at three main sites through the nervous system. Degeneration of anterior horn cells of the spinal cord causes lower motor neurone symptoms. Progressive damage to the corticospinal

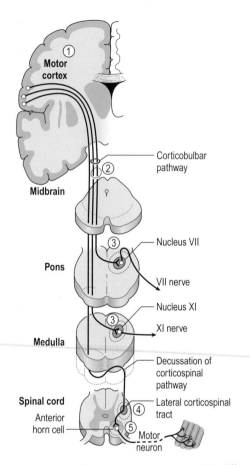

Figure 8.1 Functional neuroanatomy in MND and the different variants; 1, Cortical changes in Motor area or frontal/temporal lobes as evident in those with cognitive changes. 2, Pseudobulbar palsy. 3, Progressive Bulbar Palsy. 4, Primary Lateral Sclerosis. 5, Progressive Muscular Atrophy. (Illustration from Lindsay K, Bone I Neurology and neurosurgery Illustrated, 4th Edition. Edinburgh; Elsevier, 2004, p. 551. Reprinted with permission.)

tracts causes upper motor neurone signs and some motor nuclei in the brainstem are affected causing bulbar palsy (see Figure 8.1).

AETIOLOGY AND EPIDEMIOLOGY

The aetiology of sporadic MND is unknown. A mutation of the superoxide dismutase (SOD1) gene has been identified in approximately 20% of families with a familial manifestation of MND. Although familial forms account for only 5% of cases and SOD1 mutation cases for only 1%, genetic mutation is the only well-described cause. Some lifestyle and environmental factors have been linked with the condition, such as exposure to toxins in the workplace or extreme physical exercise, but there is no conclusive evidence.

Although there is no official register of MND patients in the UK, the incidence is thought to be 2 per 100 000 and the prevalence, 7 per 100 000 (Borasio & Miller, 2001). This equates to approximately 5000 people affected in the UK at any one time. Occurrence is slightly higher in men and onset is most common between the ages of 50 and 70 years. Survival and prognosis are discussed later in the chapter (see section on 'Progression and Prognosis').

ANATOMY AND PATHOPHYSIOLOGY

Motor neurone disease is characterized by progressive and irreversible deterioration of upper and lower motor neurons, resulting in both upper and lower motor signs. Degeneration within the corticospinal and corticobulbar tracts gives rise to upper motor weakness and hypertonia. The hardening of the tracts as the degenerated neurons are replaced by gliosis explains the term 'lateral sclerosis'.

Involvement of the anterior horn cells and cranial nuclei typically leads to lower motor weakness, wasting and involuntary flickering of muscle fibres, which is known as fasciculations. This atrophy of denervated muscle fibres leads to the use of the term 'Amyotrophy'(Charcot & Joffroy, 1869).

The exact triggers and pathological processes causing neuronal degeneration remain unknown but current theories suggest it is due to an interaction of multiple factors including genetic predisposition, autoimmune responses, glutamate excitotoxicity and abnormal muscle protein arrangements (Rocha et al., 2005).

CLINICAL PRESENTATION

MND describes a group of disorders where clinical presentation varies and each syndrome or variant is classified depending on the area of the central nervous system involved and the resulting signs with symptoms affecting speech, swallowing, limbs and respiratory muscles (see Figure 8.1):

- Classical amyotrophic lateral sclerosis
- Bulbar onset amyotrophic lateral sclerosis (ALS)
- Progressive muscular atrophy (PMA)/flail limb variant
- Primary lateral sclerosis (PLS).

More recently MND has been found to affect more than just motor neurons and individuals may demonstrate cognitive changes ranging from impaired higher level executive processing in up to one-third to fronto-temporal dementia in approximately 5% (Strong, 2001).

Classical amyotrophic lateral sclerosis

ALS makes up approximately two-thirds of the MND population and is more common in men, with a male:female ratio of 3:2 (Kato et al., 2003). There is involvement of both upper and lower motor neurons in ALS resulting in a mixed picture of upper and lower motor signs in limbs, trunk, respiratory muscles and affecting bulbar functions. Typically there is sparing of certain areas until the later stages of the disease (i.e. Cranial nerves III, IV, VIand spinal nerve S1-S3). This explains the preservation of ocular movement and bladder and bowel function (David, 2002).

Presentation at diagnosis varies but early signs often include progressive limb weakness, reduced dexterity and wasting of the hands (see Figure 8.2) and approximately two-thirds of those with ALS initially present with symptoms within the limbs. People may also complain of cramps or general fatigue and observe muscle fasciculations. Those with additional bulbar involvement present with wasting of the tongue, muscles of articulation and swallowing, leading to dysarthria and dysphagia. The presence of hyperreflexia in wasted limbs or brisk jaw jerk would indicate the upper motor neuron damage (see Figure 8.2).

Bulbar onset amyotrophic lateral sclerosis

One-third of patients with ALS present with progressive bulbar palsy (Ferguson & Elman, 2007), which affects the action of cranial nerves IX to XII causing dysarthria and dysphagia. When the cranial nerves are affected, the tongue has reduced mobility, is atrophied and fasciculates. Swallowing is often impaired. If the corticobulbar tract is affected, pseudobulbar weakness occurs and the tongue can become spastic leading to dysarthria. Emotional lability may also occur. Bulbar onset ALS is more common in older females with a male: female ratio 2:3 (Mandrioli et al., 2006).

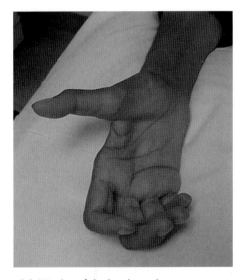

Figure 8.2 Wasting of the hand muscles

Although initial symptoms are bulbar, the disease usually progresses to include arm, leg and respiratory muscles. The majority of those with ALS have limb or bulbar onset but a small percentage (approximately 5%) may present primarily with respiratory weakness and minimal limb or bulbar involvement (Chen et al., 1996). These patients present with type 2 respiratory failure or signs of nighttime hypoventilation (respiratory issues are discussed in detail later in the chapter).

Overall the above two subsets comprise approximately 90% of the total MND population (Rocha et al., 2005). Typically life expectancy is between 3 and 5 years from symptom onset with an average of 36 months (Haverkamp et al., 1995).

Progressive muscular atrophy/flail limb variant

PMA accounts for 5–10% of those with MND who present with lower motor neurone changes only. This is usually in the limbs, but bulbar palsy may develop later in the disease. It mainly affects men (male:female ratio 2:1) and the rate of progression is slower than in the other variants with average survival 5–10 years (MND association).

Syndromes also exist where only one region is involved, e.g. anterior horn cell degeneration in the cervical region leading to flail arm syndrome, or lumbosacral region causing flail leg syndrome. If symptoms are limited to one region the prognosis is significantly better than it is for ALS or PMA where both upper and lower limbs are affected (Talman et al., 2008; Wijesekera et al., 2009).

Primary lateral sclerosis

PLS is a relatively rare condition (affecting 1–3% of those with MND) and presents with upper motor neurone involvement only. Diagnosis is often delayed to exclude potential other causes, but clinically those with PLS have only upper motor neurone signs and normal electromyography of limbs and bulbar muscles (Gordon et al., 2006). The condition can progress to ALS, but if no LMN signs are seen after 4 years prognosis is good with life expectancy comparable to normal, although this is rare.

Other presentations less commonly seen are hereditary conditions such as the spinal muscular atrophies, affecting both sexes, and bulbospinal muscular atrophy (Kennedy's disease), which affects males only.

DIAGNOSIS

At present there is no specific test for MND and therefore diagnosis relies on comprehensive history taking, clinical presentation and investigations including neuroimagery and blood tests to exclude other potential causes such as cervical cord compression or any other infective, inflammatory or autoimmune process that may cause similar symptoms.

Nerve conduction studies (NCS) and electromyography (EMG) help to confirm motor neurone degeneration (Schwartz & Swash, 1995). The motor nerve conduction speed is not affected until advanced stages but the motor action potentials may have reduced amplitude consistent with reduced number of motor axons. Sensory nerve action potentials are usually normal. EMG can identify LMN involvement or denervation prior to clinical signs of wasting and weakness. Multiple areas of denervation are consistent with ALS. If limited to just one nerve root or territory it is more likely to be radiculopathy or a mononeuropathy (Ferguson & Elman, 2007).

At present the diagnosis of ALS is aided by the revised El Escorial criteria where the combination of upper and lower motor neuron signs in the different body regions help guide certainty in diagnosis (Brooks, 2000), although this is not definitive.

PROGRESSION AND PROGNOSIS

For those with MND rates of progression vary dramatically and the life expectancies mentioned above are average values and do not reflect the range of individuals. As mentioned above, classification of the disease into different variants can help guide prognosis. Subsequently this may help target therapeutic intervention most effectively and help professionals, patients and families in utilizing resources at the most appropriate time to maximize function and quality of life, and to prevent crises.

To evaluate disease progression it is necessary to establish a baseline using objective measures. Suitable to clinic and research settings the Amyotrophic Lateral Sclerosis Functional Rating Scale (ALSFRS) is a subjective questionnaire regarding functional abilities including speech and swallowing, mobility, personal care and respiratory support (ALS CNTF, 1996). However, a revised version ALSFRS-R (Cederbaum et al., 1999) with an expanded section on respiration has proved more sensitive, better able to predict survival and is now more commonly used. Other outcome measures are discussed relevant to symptoms later in the chapter.

In general, there are several factors indicative of better prognosis: younger age at onset (<65 years), limb as opposed to bulbar onset of symptoms and a longer period between onset of symptoms to diagnosis of MND suggesting a less aggressive disease process (Mandrioli et al., 2006).

At time of writing Riluzole is the only disease-modifying drug available in the UK. A Cochrane review concluded that Riluzole provided modest benefits and increased survival by 2–3 months on average (Miller et al., 2007). Riluzole is a glutamate antagonist thought to inhibit the influx of calcium into the cells, which triggers a series of events that results in neuronal cell death (Lacomblez et al., 1996; Rowland & Shneider, 2001).

Although MND is a progressive, incurable disease it is important to note that quality of life does not directly correspond to level of impairment or disease progression and it does not necessarily decline over time (Simmons, 2005). This further enforces the key role of coordinated support and individualized therapy at all stages of the disease to optimize quality of life.

MULTIDISCIPLINARY APPROACH

Optimal management of patients with MND requires a team approach, with early referral for clinical assessment and prompt intervention. Multidisciplinary management has been associated with improved quality of life (Van den Berg, 2005) and potentially increased survival time (Traynor et al., 2003). Patients with MND are often seen by several different teams, i.e. community teams, hospice care teams, wheelchair services and social services. Good communication is essential to provide appropriate care for this client group. Clear, patient centred goals are the key to this communication process. The patient must always be included in goal setting and the needs of the carers must also be considered.

There are now seventeen specialist MND centres in the UK (see Appendix). The primary responsibility of the team at these MND care and research centres is to ensure that care is coordinated across the range of health, social care and voluntary agencies. The teams are also involved in research in partnership with people affected by MND.

ROLE OF THE PHYSIOTHERAPIST

As all patients manifest with some physical impairment, the physiotherapist is an essential member of the multidisciplinary team. The physiotherapist's overall aim is to maintain optimal function and quality of life for the patient throughout the course of the disease. This may include:

1. providing a baseline assessment and ensuring monitoring throughout the course of the disease
2. optimizing muscle strength, muscle length and joint range of motion, and managing muscle tone to maximize function
3. promoting mobility and independence by provision of treatment, aids and adaptations
4. providing advice about exercise
5. providing information, education and support to the patient and carer

6. providing or advising on pain management
7. providing or advising on fatigue management
8. treating and monitoring any respiratory dysfunction.

Any input must be guided by the patient's own goals and tailored to the patient's individual needs. This will sometimes necessitate an innovative and unconventional approach to patient management. The physiotherapist should have involvement in goal setting, treatment planning and other aspects of case management. They should also be prepared to advise, teach and to be an advocate for the patient, the carers and the other members of the multidisciplinary team.

SYMPTOMS AND THEIR MANAGEMENT

The symptom management described below is a multidisciplinary process and it is inappropriate to divide it into arbitrary professional areas but the emphasis in this instance is on the physical management. Drug treatments are mentioned briefly. All aspects of management should be directed towards addressing the patient's needs in a holistic way. This includes psychosocial and spiritual aspects as well as the physical.

The motor system

MND presents with a varied and sometime complex combination of motor problems. The various changes in muscle structure and function will impact upon each other and ultimately give rise to a high level of disability.

Weakness

Damage to the anterior horn cells leads to a typical lower motor neurone presentation of weakness, flaccidity and atrophy. Suspicion of MND as a potential diagnosis often arises where the classical atrophy of the thenar eminence and dorsal interossei are noticed. In addition to the weakness arising directly from the pathological process of the disease, the MND patient may also face disuse atrophy arising from inactivity and the loss of muscle power that accompanies aging in any individual. Physical inactivity is linked to a decrease in the number of available satellite cells within a muscle and, therefore, a decline in the muscle's ability to regenerate or recover from damage (Ambrosio et al., 2009).

The extent and distribution of the weakness will depend on the type of MND and the initial presentation.

The role of exercise

Exercise remains a debatable aspect of MND therapy despite an increasing raft of research to underpin its use (Dal Bello-Haas et al., 2008). The fear that it is ineffectual and may even cause further tissue damage still leads therapists to be cautious in its use. However, the benefits of exercise for people affected by MND are not dissimilar to those experienced by the rest of the population (see Ch. 18 for review) and it should feature in the treatment programme of most patients (Dal Bello-Haas et al., 2007). Exercise programmes have been shown to improve ALSFRS scores and to slow decline in physical function (Drory et al., 2001).

Damage to both the upper and lower motor neurones is seen in MND. A summary of the changes in motor neurone activation from each type of damage is presented in Table 8.1. When the motor neurones are damaged by the disease process, the muscle tissue that they innervate can no longer be activated and, therefore, atrophies. These motor units are permanently damaged and cannot be changed by exercise (Peruzzi & Potts, 1996). Other parts of the muscle, however, may have an intact motor neurone and still be functioning. As the patient becomes less mobile and less active due to, for example, fatigue, these otherwise healthy fibres may start to show signs of disuse atrophy. These disused fibres will respond to exercise and may allow the patient to develop a small reserve of healthy, usable muscle. Other factors may affect the muscles of a patient with MND, including increased likelihood of fatigue, impaired respiratory function (resulting in poor delivery of oxygen to the tissues), impaired nutritional intake and hypertonicity. These confounding factors, as well as poor recruitment and retention of subjects in studies amongst this patient group, make clinical research into the effects of exercise very difficult to conduct.

The primary effect of exercise training is to improve the neural control of the muscle, which will allow more effective recruitment and, therefore, stronger contractions (Sanjak et al., 1987). Since it is only the disused muscle tissue and not the diseased parts that can be strengthened in MND patients, the best results are seen in the least affected muscles.

Studies in other neuromuscular conditions and in mouse models of ALS show that exercise at a submaximal level can be safe and effective (see Ch. 18; Aitkens et al., 1993; Kilmer et al., 1994; Kirkinezos et al., 2003). High-resistance work is thought to be unnecessary and can be damaging to the muscles, particularly with eccentric (muscle-lengthening) contractions, which can cause delayed-onset muscle soreness (Lieber & Friden, 1999). Normal muscle recovers from such damage but repair in diseased muscle may not be possible (Ambrosio et al., 2009). Although eccentric contractions are difficult to avoid within an exercise programme, consideration should be given to how eccentric activity is used to avoid unnecessary strain.

Muscles in patients with MND will fatigue more rapidly than those in healthy individuals. It has not been established whether this is due to impaired central control (Kent-Braun & Miller, 2000) or to impaired activation at a muscular level (Sharma et al., 1995). For this reason, short but frequent exercise sessions may be preferable to prolonged activity.

Recommendations for exercise

- Allow patients to continue with sports or activities that they participated in prior to diagnosis, for as long as they are safely able to do so.
- Encourage low-stress, low-impact activities such as walking or swimming, in preference to high-impact or contact sports.
- Encourage an active lifestyle when sport and other exercise activities become impracticable.
- Avoid high-resistance exercises that increase the risk of muscle damage, without providing any additional benefits above a moderate-resistance programme.
- Advise patients to build up their programme slowly and to monitor the effects of their exercise on fatigue and pain. Teach patients to recognize delayed-onset muscle soreness as a sign of overuse.

Hypertonicity

Hypertonia, a feature of upper motor neurone syndrome, is defined as an increase in resistance to passive stretch and has both a neural (spasticity) and non-neural component (inherent viscoelastic properties of the muscle) which provides resistance to movement and contributes to muscle tone (see Ch. 14). The result of tonal changes can lead to inappropriate movement, discomfort, decreased mobility, reduced function and difficulty with positioning. Spasticity is managed in the same way as for other neurological patients (e.g. stroke, brain injury and multiple sclerosis) and there needs to be a multidisciplinary approach to treatment.

Medical management includes the use of oral medication to reduce tone, such as baclofen, diazepam, dantrolene and tizanadine (Ashworth et al., 2006). Careful monitoring of the effects of medication is needed, as excessive weakness caused by the medication can lead to flaccidity and a reduction in the patient's functional ability. Intramuscular botulinum toxin injection can be used to reduce focal spasticity (Richardson & Thompson, 1999). The drug weakens the muscle by inhibiting the release of acetylcholine at the neuromuscular junction, preventing muscle contraction. Some patients in the United States have received intrathecal baclofen pumps and achieved a decrease in tone and pain reduction as a result (McLelland et al., 2008). This can be considered but is rarely done in the UK.

Physical management of tone includes careful positioning and the interventions outlined below. The physiotherapist aims to maximize a patient's functional ability and comfort. A comprehensive assessment of the patient's main problems needs to be completed.

Tissue changes

Optimal tissue length is essential if muscle activation and the resultant function are to be maximized. Due to the weakness that results from MND, muscle imbalance causes changes in muscle length. Muscle shortening is especially likely where upper motor neurone involvement leads to increased muscle tone. Therefore, it is imperative that steps are taken early on to prevent changes in tissue length. These may include preventive splinting, stretching programmes and active exercise, positioning, appropriate seating and antispasmodic medication (see other sections of this chapter and Ch. 14).

Where muscle imbalance is seen, joints are at risk of being held in malalignment. This may be due to high muscle tone pulling them out of line or weakness and low muscle tone allowing the joints to be hypermobile. In either case, splinting may be necessary to prevent further malalignment and the risk of damage.

It is important to make a differential diagnosis to ascertain whether limb stiffness is due to joint stiffness, muscle inelasticity or, indeed, predisposing factors such as osteoarthritis, as the physical management and medication are different depending on the cause.

Physiotherapy management of hypertonicity and resultant tissue changes

- Stretching programme
    - A home exercise programme can be devised for the patient, incorporating stretches to maintain muscle length. As the patient becomes less active, passive stretches can be taught to the carer. Although there is little substantial evidence to support the use of this type of stretching in order to maintain tissue length or influence tone, it may be beneficial in terms of mobilizing joints, providing sensory input and relieving discomfort. Prolonged stretch is required in order to influence muscle length. Splinting may also be used as a means of imposing this sustained stretch (Edwards & Charlton, 2002). Guidelines have been prepared by the Association of Chartered Physiotherapists Interested in Neurology (ACPIN) and these provide information regarding the assessment, procedure, risk factors and protocols for casting. Guidelines for casting patients with complex neurological conditions have also been produced (Young & Nicklin, 2000). Adequate training in splinting techniques is essential.
- Standing
    - The theory behind weight-bearing activities is to maintain joint range and stimulate antigravity muscle activity (Brown, 1994). Standing exercises can be performed independently by the patient, with assistance, or with the use of specialized equipment such as a tilt table or Oswestry standing frame.

- Positioning/seating
  - Different postures and positions have an influence on tone and movement. If a patient is uncomfortable, then this may lead to an increase in muscle tone. Therefore, correct positioning over a 24-hour period is vital. Liaison with the local wheelchair team is important to provide the patient with a suitable wheelchair (see 'Positioning and seating' section).
- Activity modification
  - If a task is very effortful for a patient, then this may increase muscle tone and lead to difficulties completing the task. Therefore, activity modification is advised. Decreasing the effort of the task by either activity modification or the use of aids and adaptations may assist with reducing tone.
- Removing noxious stimuli
  - A noxious stimulus such as constipation, skin breakdown or an in-growing toenail may lead to an increase in tone. Poor positioning or an ill-fitting orthotic appliance may also increase tone unnecessarily. Therefore, it is important to identify any cause and make adjustments or withdraw the cause when managing patients with hypertonia.

Fatigue

Patients with MND frequently experience generalized fatigue, which can be one of the most disabling features of the condition. However, with good advice, they can learn how to minimize the effect of this problem. Activity should be encouraged but not so as to exhaust the patient (see 'The role of exercise", above).

Management strategies should include organizing the environment to minimize unnecessary energy expenditure, leading a healthy lifestyle, adopting good posture and positioning and employing relaxation techniques. Activity modification can be very effective. This encourages patients to eliminate unnecessary tasks from their day, plan ahead and divide the tasks into manageable sections, allowing rest periods in between. Adapted equipment and appropriate packages of care should also be considered.

Cramps

People with MND may experience painful cramps, often at night. These can be alleviated with stretching and massage. In severe cases, Quinine Sulphate can be given to prevent the cramping (Miller et al., 2005). Cramps will often be worse in patients who display hypertonicity and good management of the tone problems will help to minimize the other muscle-based problems.

Resultant disabilities

Any combination of the above impairments may lead to significant disability. These include:

- immobility
- loss of head control
- loss of upper limb function.

Immobility

Although maintaining ambulation is a priority for many patients, the physiotherapist has a responsibility to ensure that this does not become too energy-inefficient and fatiguing or unsafe. This may necessitate the use of walking aids such as sticks, crutches, zimmer or delta frames, or wheelchairs. It is important to gauge the patient's feelings on this subject before issuing an aid. It is not unusual for patients to refuse aids on grounds of cosmesis, and wheelchairs and crutches are often perceived as socially unacceptable symbols of disability. Mobility and independence are clearly linked with self-esteem and it is sometimes difficult for a patient to acknowledge that he or she has deteriorated enough to require a stick or a chair.

If a patient is unable to stand from sitting unaided, but can still walk, then a chair with an electric seat raise may overcome this problem.

It is necessary to consider arm function as well as lower-limb activity when selecting an aid, as poor grip, for example, will preclude the use of many walking aids. Patients who fatigue may prefer wheeled frames that have an integral seat, so that they can rest at stages in their journey.

Transfers may become difficult and advice from the physiotherapist on safe and effective technique may help to maintain independence in this activity. Many devices are commercially available to improve transfers, such as sliding boards, transfer belts and hoists. Transfer belts placed around the lower thorax/pelvis can be particularly useful where the patient has flail arms or painful shoulders, allowing the carer to have a firm hold on the patient without the risk of trauma to the limbs. However, this requires the patient to be able to maintain an upright posture and, therefore, may not be appropriate in the late stages of the disease. Consideration of comfort, type of transfer and environment should be made when selecting a hoist. Manual handling legislation must be part of the reasoning process when selecting transfer techniques (RCN, 1999).

Orthoses may also be necessary to maximize mobility. Lively or rigid splints and light weight orthoses can be of use, but careful assessment of their value must be made frequently. An ankle-foot orthosis is often provided for loss of active dorsiflexion (Figures 8.3A & B) and a 'foot–up' orthosis (Figure 8.4) is often beneficial in the early stages where mild or fatiguing footdrop presents.

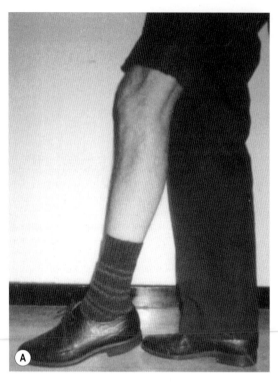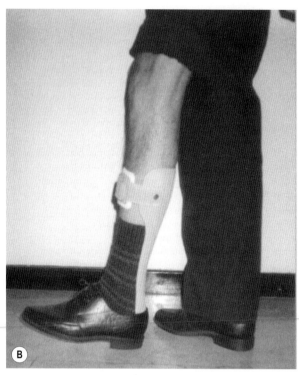

Figure 8.3 (A) Left foot drop due to weakness of the ankle dorsiflexors. (B) Use of ankle–foot orthosis to correct foot drop.

Insoles, calipers and knee braces can all improve the efficiency of gait and protect the soft tissues from the trauma of repeated malalignment.

Due to the progressive nature of MND, early referral for wheelchair provision is essential. Patients' local wheelchair service should be able to provide a chair that meets their mobility and postural needs, but if the patient desires something beyond this remit, there is a large selection of wheelchairs available commercially which have other features. If a wheelchair is being bought privately, it is worthwhile seeking advice from the wheelchair service to ensure it fully meets the patient's requirements and to investigate voucher scheme funding. The wheelchair may be manually propelled by the patient or attendant, or powered for indoor and/or outdoor use. Scooters are not currently provided by the National Health Service, but may provide another mobility option. Consideration must be given to postural requirements, function and pressure care when providing a wheelchair and seating system (Trail et al., 2001).

Loss of head control

Neck weakness causes many problems for the patient with MND. It causes stress on the muscles and ligaments of the neck, resulting in pain, impaired breathing and swallowing, increased drooling and decreased interaction with the environment, and it is cosmetically unpleasant.

There are several specially designed collars available that may offer a solution to these problems (Figure 8.5). These include two specifically designed rigid head supports, the Headmaster and the MNDA (Mary Marlborough Lodge) collar. Both provide a flexible platform for the chin that allows a small amount of anteroposterior movement for speaking and chewing, but prevents the head falling forwards, and they are open at the front to avoid throat compression.

Patients who side-flex as well as fall forwards often prefer a soft foam collar, such as the Adams collar (Johnson & Johnson), that feels supportive in all directions. These need to be replaced frequently to maintain good support and patients who drool can be given lengths of stockingette to cover the collar; these may be removed and washed. Sometimes a collar cut from block foam to act as a wedge on which the chin can rest may help.

Wheelchairs can be adapted to minimize the effects of neck weakness. A chair with a tilt-in-space arrangement will allow the neck to be relieved of load, whilst a good seated position is maintained. Head supports can be made integral to the chair and there is a wide range of available head rests. The patient's local wheelchair service should be able to provide advice on this subject. Positioning the upper limbs on a tray or pillows may allow the patient better control of the neck and decrease pull on the muscles.

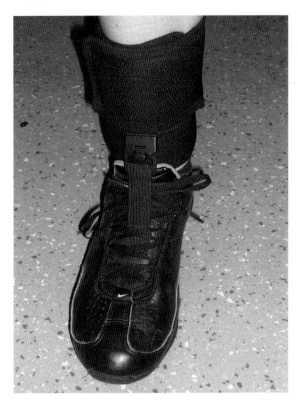

Figure 8.4 'Foot up' orthosis

Loss of upper limb function

The seating position has a significant effect on ability to use the upper limbs functionally. It is, therefore, advisable to position the patient well, prior to attempting any upper limb activities. Patients with decreased activity may find that leaning their elbows on a table or wheelchair tray allows them more hand function or that mobile arm supports help them with activities such as feeding. Splints, such as thumb spicas (Figure 8.6), may improve alignment and give better ability to grip.

There are a multitude of adapted devices that will allow patients to participate in or be independent in activities of daily living, such as feeding, washing, writing and domestic tasks. For patients with marked bulbar signs, hot plates and heated food dishes make slow eating more palatable. Anti-slip tablemats and thickened handles on cutlery, pens and toothbrushes aid independence. Anti-slip floor mats and the Rotastand aid transfers, and the use of Velcro and zip fasteners will help dressing.

In order to maximize both function and quality of life it is necessary to provide patients with knowledge of the various types of aids and equipment available to them. Again, such aids may be seen as a sign of deterioration and not readily accepted by the patient. Careful

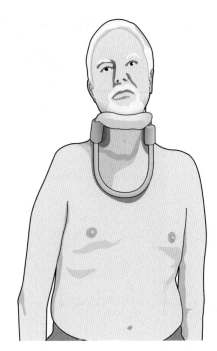

Figure 8.5 Headmaster collar

consideration when introducing these devices is important to assist acceptance, as they serve a number of purposes.

Referral to the occupational therapist early after diagnosis will mean that the patient has access to these devices and the necessary advice as the need arises.

Positioning and seating

Positioning is an essential part of the management of the patient with MND. Good positioning will help to maintain joint range and soft-tissue length, prevent deformity, improve comfort, prevent pressure areas and maximize function (Pope, 2002). Positioning is a 24-hour approach that includes lying and standing positions, as well as static and mobile seating. The combined resources of nurses, physiotherapists, occupational therapists and family are needed to achieve this.

When the antigravity muscles, which maintain an erect head, neck and trunk, become weakened, it becomes increasingly difficult to maintain the upright position. This applies whether the patient is standing, sitting in a wheelchair or sitting in bed. It is not sufficient to place more and more pillows behind and around the patient. In order to minimize the effect of gravity on the body, the patient should be reclined back from the vertical at the hips, so that the line of gravity passes in front of the head and neck through the thorax. This position also

171

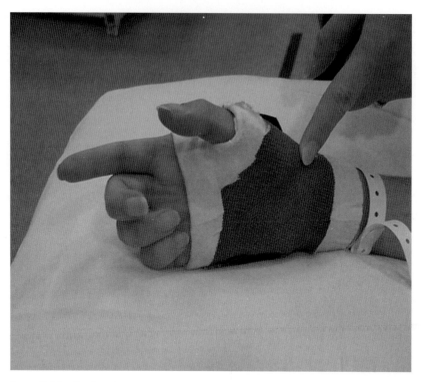

Figure 8.6 Opposition splint for the thumb

enables the diaphragm to work more efficiently and so aid breathing.

Equipment used for positioning can range from the simple use of pillows and wedges to complex seating systems. Electric adjustable beds, pressure-relieving mattresses and cushions plus one-way glide sheets will all assist comfort as well as facilitating easy adjustment of the patient's position. Small neck or support pillows could also be used. The patient's positioning in the environment must also be considered to allow the greatest degree of function, social interaction and stimulation.

Pain

Pain is a commonly reported problem in MND with between 23 and 73% of patients affected (Simmons, 2005). There are a variety of sources of pain experienced by this patient group.

Muscle weakness or hypertonus may lead to muscle imbalance and altered mechanics at joints. These abnormal stresses can cause damage and discomfort. Immobility and reduced ability to relieve pressure will lead to further mechanical stresses and pressure on the skin and soft tissues. Shoulder joints are particularly vulnerable to

malalignment problems (Figure 8.7), due to their large and multidirectional range of movement, and mishandling during functional tasks and transfers. Lower back pain is another commonly reported problem.

Prevention should be the main aim of treatment. Positioning and handling advice should be provided for the patient and carers, and provision of appropriate aids and appliances should be ensured. This includes seating and sleep systems, where appropriate, that have good postural support and sufficient pressure relief systems.

Standard symptomatic medical management may be appropriate with both opiate and non-steroidal anti-inflammatory drugs providing some relief. Regular use may be required to manage ongoing pain. Intra-articular steroid and anaesthetic injections may be used where a single joint is particularly affected. Pain secondary to spasticity can be managed with antispasmodic drugs such as baclofen or tizanidine and that related to cramping can be alleviated with quinine sulphate. Antidepressant medication and medications such as gabapentin and pregabalin can alleviate chronic pain.

The physiotherapy role in prevention and treatment of pain should not be forgotten (see Ch. 16). Good positioning and handling is the key to this problem. Well established physiotherapeutic treatments such as

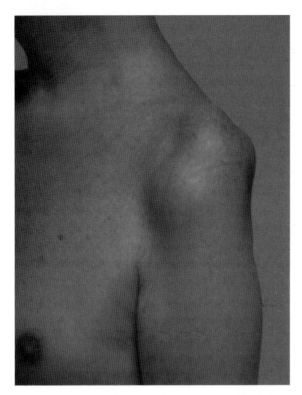

Figure 8.7 Subluxed shoulder – showing that the head of the humerus has dropped.

mobilizations, exercises and stretches may alleviate pain. Acupuncture may also be considered (Pan et al., 2000).

The respiratory system

Respiration requires the normal functioning of the muscles of inspiration, the muscles of expiration and the muscles that control the upper airway or bulbar muscles. Bulbar weakness is discussed in more detail in 'Bulbar symptoms' below.

Respiratory failure remains the most common cause of death in MND (Francis et al., 1999; Lyall et al., 2001; Vender et al., 2007). Respiratory symptoms (see Table 8.1) can be distressing for both the patient and carers, and assessment, early intervention and education are essential in preventing crisis and maximizing quality of life. Dyspnoea and secretion management is a primary area in palliative care and respiratory intervention has a major impact on both quality of life and survival (Tripodoro & De Vito, 2008).

Ventilatory failure occurs when the load placed on the respiratory muscle pump exceeds the capacity of the respiratory muscles (Lyall et al., 2001), and due to neuronal

degeneration within the cortex, brainstem and anterior horn cells those with MND are especially vulnerable to respiratory weakness. Reduced activity, poor mobility and postural changes that occur with disease progression can lead to secondary respiratory problems such as increased areas of lung atelectasis and secretion retention. The cough mechanism can be affected by both respiratory weakness and bulbar dysfunction so that whilst the demand to cough increases the effectiveness decreases (Hadjikoutis, 1999).

Signs of increasing respiratory weakness may not always be noticed due to reduced physical mobility associated with disease progression and therefore pulmonary function tests have an important role in assessing respiratory muscle strength, guiding management options and determining prognosis. A number of objective tests and subjective questionnaires such as the Epworth sleepiness score (Johns, 1994) are used to provide an overall picture of respiratory function (see Ch. 15).

Vital capacity (VC) is the most commonly used measure and hand-held spirometers enable this to be taken in clinic or ward setting, although they may be inaccurate in those with orofacial weakness who cannot form an adequate seal. VC is the volume of gas exhaled after a full inspiration and indicates inspiratory muscle strength (mainly diaphragmatic function). Normal values vary between 3 and 6 L depending on age, sex, height and weight.

Miller at al. 1999 suggests A VC of >1.5 L is required for an effective cough and that a VC <1 L (or < 25% of predicted) indicates significant risk of respiratory failure and that ventilatory support is required.

Another measure of inspiration is the sniff inspiratory nasal pressure (SNIP) a natural maneuver where a full breath out precedes a maximal inspiration. This technique may be easier to perform than VC using a mouthpiece for those with bulbar weakness and is more sensitive to inspiratory muscle weakness. Normal values are 70 cm H_2O for men and 60 cm H_2O for women and age predicted values are available to aid identification of respiratory weakness (Uldry & Fitting, 1995).

Other investigations include arterial blood-gas analysis to detect hypercapnia or venous blood gas analysis where a raised serum bicarbonate level indicates compensation of chronic hypoventilation (Lyall et al., 2001). Nocturnal oximetry can detect hypoventilation, as reflected by reduced oxygen saturations, which often occurs prior to daytime symptoms.

Additionally auscultation, checking the effectiveness of a patient's cough and clinical observations of respiratory muscle use are important aspects of the respiratory assessment. Any changes noted should be shared with the multidisciplinary team (MDT) and respiratory tests requested to optimize management as the rate of decline in respiratory function is an indicator of rate of disease progression and survival (Czaplinski et al., 2006).

Table 8.1 Respiratory problems

RESPIRATORY SIGNS AND SYMPTOMS	CAUSE
Dyspnoea at rest	Inspiratory (diaphragm and accessory muscles) weakness
Orthopnoea and/or paradoxical abdominal movement	Diaphragm weakness
Disturbed sleep, daytime sleepiness	Inspiratory muscle weakness→ Hypoventilation Reduced restful sleep as unable to rely solely on diaphragm
Morning headaches and/or altered cognition/ confusion	Hypoventilation → carbon dioxide retention
Reduced cough	Expiratory (abdominal and accessory muscle) weakness
Reduced vocal volume and/or few words per breath	Expiratory muscle weakness
Reduced chest wall movement and excessive use of accessory muscles	Inspiratory muscle weakness
Paradoxical breathing: Supine-upper abdominals move inwards on inspiration Sitting-intercostals move inwards on inspiration	Negative intrathoracic pressure pulls weak muscles inwards: Diaphragm weakness noted in supine Intercostal weakness noted in sitting
Retained secretions	Reduced lung volumes due to inspiratory muscle weakness Reduced cough effort due to expiratory muscle weakness Reduced bulbar function (poor cough trigger and/or poor airway protection- see Bulbar symptoms)

The role of the physiotherapist in management of respiratory symptoms

In the early stage the aim is to help educate the patient and carer and provide prophylactic advice. As the disease progresses, the physiotherapist has a key role in intervention to maximize ventilation and gas exchange and aid secretion clearance. Respiratory symptoms are best addressed by the MDT where there are clear communication links and any changes can be relayed immediately to the other members.

Prophylactic management

In the early stages, active exercise to maintain trunk mobility, as well as deep-breathing exercises can increase chest expansion and prevent atelectasis (lung collapse; Peruzzi & Potts, 1996). Maintaining activity such as standing or walking even if not the main mode of mobility can aid respiratory function as the patient becomes less mobile. Postural management and seating is also of importance in maintaining spinal mobility, chest compliance and maximizing lung volumes.

Education on how to prevent choking or aspiration (inhalation of fluid or food) is important in those with bulbar involvement. Full assessment by a speech and language therapist is essential to establish guidance for safe eating and drinking if oral intake is still appropriate. Recommendations to modify the consistency of the diet or to use a 'chin tuck' position to swallow may be given. The patient and carer should also be advised how to recognize signs of a chest infection so that prompt action can be taken (Tripodoro& De Vito, 2008).

Management of dyspnoea

Breathlessness is a common symptom as the disease progresses and most patients with MND will experience dyspnoea at some stage. One important aspect to recognize and educate patient and carers about is the fact that anxiety can exacerbate dyspnoea.

If dyspnoea occurs on exertion then modifying activity to reduce the effort, e.g. provision of mobility aids, can help alleviate symptoms. If orthopnoea (difficulty breathing in lying) is reported, positioning in bed to avoid supine is essential. The inclusion of an occupational therapist within the MDT can maximize positioning options and can provide energy-saving equipment and activity modification advice.

Seating and positioning can significantly affect respiratory function (Landers et al., 2003). Therefore, addressing these factors may relieve dyspnoea in those with MND. If there is neck weakness collars can support the head and seating to help stabilize the body and shoulder-girdle can ease the work of breathing. Options may include provision of a tilt-in-space wheelchair to reduce neck and postural muscle activity so reducing the demands on the respiratory system. Tailored positioning advice to the patient and carer to optimize ventilation-perfusion matching whilst not increasing the physiological demands can also aid dyspnoea.

The use of non-invasive positive pressure ventilation (NIPPV) can reduce symptoms of chronic hypoventilation by providing positive pressure to reduce the work of the respiratory muscles. This can help alleviate symptoms such as morning headache and daytime sleepiness, in addition to reducing the feelings of dyspnoea (Lyall et al., 2000). Objectively a VC of less than 50% of predicted is associated with poor prognosis and respiratory symptoms in those with MND, and therefore NIPPV may be introduced at this stage, although deterioration in other respiratory markers or subjective symptoms may indicate earlier use (Simmons, 2005).

NIPPV has been shown to improve various aspects of quality of life in MND patients and increase length of survival (Bourke et al., 2006). However, deterioration in function continues and some elements of carer burden and stress may be adversely affected; therefore, support systems should be facilitated and close monitoring is required (Mustfa et al., 2006). NIPPV can increase the risk of aspiration in those with significant bulbar involvement where there is difficulty protecting their own airway.

Secretion management

Retained secretions or thick secretions at the back of the throat can also cause dyspnoea and may be a result of several factors: immobility, bulbar dysfunction and reduced effectiveness of cough.

Physiotherapy interventions (see Ch. 15) include:

- breathing exercises
- positioning
- augmented cough
- suction.

Active cycle of breathing techniques

Breathing exercises can be used to aid lung expansion, prevent atelectasis and help secretion clearance (Prasad & Pryor, 2002), especially in those less mobile. The forced expiratory technique (FET) may also be used in early stages of the disease as a less effortful option to coughing, although this is less effective with disease progression where an assisted cough is required. Manual techniques may be used in addition to ACBT to further aid mobilization of secretions (Prasad & Pryor, 2002) during an acute chest infection.

Maximal insufflation or inspiration techniques such as breath stacking (taking several small breaths without breathing out in between) can help maintain vital capacity and aid lung and chest wall compliance. Glossopharyngeal or 'frog breathing', where air is gulped into the lungs, is an alternative method to increase maximum inspiration and aid cough effectiveness (Bott et al., 2009).

Positioning

Optmimizing ventilation–perfusion matching through positioning can help prevent development of atelectasis and retention of secretions. Gravity-assisted positions may be used, if appropriate, to aid drainage of secretions, although traditional positions may need to be modified to increase tolerance, especially in the presence of orthopnoea (Prasad & Pryor, 2002).

All the above interventions can aid secretion clearance however, if the cough is impaired the secretions will not be fully evacuated, therefore, techniques have been developed to augment cough effort.

The assisted cough technique is a useful physiotherapy intervention and can be taught to the patient and/or carer where appropriate (Polkey et al., 1999). The aim of the assisted cough is to imitate the function of the weak abdominal and internal intercostal muscles and to help clear secretions. It has been shown to increase cough flow by 11–13% in those with MND (Mustfa et al., 2003).

Contraindications include a paralytic ileus, internal abdominal damage or bleeding and rib fractures (Prasad & Pryor, 2002). The physiotherapist should liaise with nursing/medical staff regarding contraindications prior to teaching or performing the techniques. It is important to inform and explain the procedure to the patient and carer, to obtain informed consent and help sychronize the manoeuver with the patients own cough effort.

Self-assisted cough

- The patient should start with a good upright position, placing their forearms under the ribcage.
- As the patient coughs, he or she leans forward and uses the forearms to apply pressure in and upwards (bucket-handle action).
- The patient's cough should sound stronger and louder.

Assisted cough in sitting (Figure 8.8)

- Start with a good upright position.
- The assistant brings one arm in front and one arm behind to support the trunk.

175

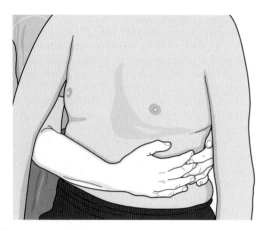

Figure 8.8 Assisted cough in sitting.

- The front arm is placed just below the ribcage with hand curved around the opposite side of the chest.
- Pressure is applied in an inwards and upwards direction (bucket handle) as the patient coughs.
- Coordination between the patient and assistant is important.
- The patient's cough should sound stronger and louder.

The assisted cough technique can be maximized by insufflation techniques, as discussed above, or use of NIPPV, or manual hyperventilation with bag and mask to aid deeper breaths prior to cough (Bott et al., 2009).

Where the patient has difficulty clearing thick secretions or has a large thorax two people may assist the cough (Figures 8.9A & B).

Mechanical insufflation/exsufflation

A mechanical insufflator/exsufflator (MIE) machine or cough-assist® (Figure 15.2) uses positive pressure to aid lung expansion on inspiration and then a rapid change to negative pressure on expiration. This process attempts to imitate the flow changes that occur during a cough and so help secretion clearance in those with neuromuscular disease. Use of MIE produces 26–28% greater peak cough flow than coughing without assistance in those with MND (Chatwin et al., 2003; Mustfa et al., 2003).

Contraindications are similar to use of any positive pressure intervention, e.g. undrained pneomothorax (air in the pleural cavity), large bullae (cystic-like lesions), proximal airway obstruction, recent barotrauma (Prasad & Pryor, 2002). In those with advanced bulbar dysfunction MIE can cause dynamic collapse of the upper airways and is therefore not effective in clearing secretions (Sancho et al., 2004).

Cough can be further enhanced by several positive pressure inspiratory breaths prior to cough and manual assisted cough on exsufflation.

Suction

If the patient is unable to clear secretions with assisted cough or bulbar dysfunction is so advanced that the individual cannot close the glottis to generate enough pressure to cough, suction to the back of the throat may be

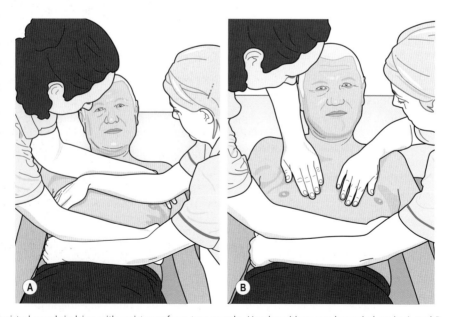

Figure 8.9 Assisted cough in lying with assistance from two people. Hand positions can be varied, as in A and B.

used. Patients may be provided with a suction machine to use at home.

Adequate hydration should be ensured (oral, systemic, use of nebulizers) to aid secretion clearance. Humidified air or NIPPV with humidifier and can also help clear thick secretions (Leigh et al., 2003).

Medical management

Antibiotics should be considered where there is evidence of pulmonary infectionand mucolytics can help loosen tenacious secretions making them easier to clear (Heffernan et al., 2006).

Medication such as hyoscine or glycopyrronium bromide can be used to dry secretions.

Anxiety that enhances the feelings of breathlessness can be treated with short-acting anxiolytics or in the palliative stages dyspnoea may be managed with benzodiazepines and opioids (see 'Palliative management' below).

The MND Association provides a 'Breathing Space Kit' containing advice and information for patient, carers and GP. This can include medications for use in respiratory emergency.

As the disease progresses it is important to initiate discussions and enable advanced planning prior to an emergency situation. Options such as non-invasive, invasive ventilation and end of life plans should be broached when respiratory deterioration is first noted. Invasive ventilation may be considered if non-invasive ventilation is not tolerated or is no longer effective. It has been shown to improve quality of life and survival, but both patient and carers should be fully aware of all implications (Heffernan et al., 2006). This aims to prevent potentially regrettable ventilation in emergency where it then becomes impossible to wean off the ventilation and the person risks becoming 'locked in' (Hayashi, 2000).

A coordinated team who can provide advice and education, physical therapy and adjuncts, respiratory investigations and support, such as non-invasive ventilation and instigatation of appropriate drug therapy, best manages respiratory symptoms. Management will vary depending on stage of disease and whether the individual is experiencing an acute episode of reversible deterioration, i.e. a chest infection, or disease progression.

Bulbar symptoms

Speech and swallowing difficulties are a common symptom in MND due to involvement of brainstem nuclei in the medulla with over 80% experiencing bulbar problems at some stage (Rocha et al., 2005). Damage can occur in the corticobulbar tract or within the cranial nerve nuclei leading to a mixed presentation of weakness, wasting and hypertonicity affecting the muscles of the tongue, lips and soft palate.

Dysarthria

Speech difficulties such as slowed rate of speech, poor formation of consonants, reduced volume and altered tone are experienced by over 80% of those with MND (Leigh et al., 2003). Assessment and intervention from a speech therapist is essential to ensure communication methods are available to enable the individual's autonomy to direct their own care.

Initial strategies may emphasize the use of breathing to aid articulation and volume, avoiding distracting background sounds, use of closed questions, facing the listener and education of carers to allow the person time to express themselves (Leigh et al., 2003).

As the disease progresses supplementary communication aids will be required. These can range from the use of pen and paper to sophisticated mechanical or computerized technology as discussed below.

Augmented communication

- Simple communication charts including pictures devised for the individual by the speech and language therapist or alphabet boards can provide simple and portable solutions to communication difficulties.
- The 'Lightwriter'® (Figure 8.10) available from Toby Churchill Ltd. is widely used and enables the user to produce speech by typing.
- With deterioration of dexterity and hand function, it is possible to link such machines to single switches for easier use.

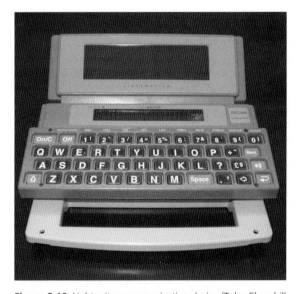

Figure 8.10 Lightwriter communication device (Toby Churchill Ltd) for people with impaired intelligibility. (Courtesy of G Derwent, Compass, Electronic Assistive Technology Service, Royal Hospital for Neuro-disability, London).

- Switches can be modified to enable use by various movements depending on the individual's strengths. For example a large sensitive hand switch may be used where there is loss of fine hand movement but gross movement is retained, alternatively switches may be placed close to the head for activation by head rotation.
- Sophisticated eye gaze and blink switches can also be linked to light writers or more complex computer systems.
- Advancing technology and the common use of email and mobile phone texts also provide further options.

Several of the above switch options may be linked to other systems to enable the individual to control their environment (e.g. lights, radio, door activation, etc.). For safety a personal alert button can be worn that once activated will contact either a carer or relative or central help centre.

For those with respiratory weakness, speech can be affected without bulbar impairment resulting in reduced volume and phonation time, and they may also benefit from assistive technologies such as voice amplifiers.

Ongoing review by the speech and language therapist, assistive technology and environmental controls teams are essential to ensure communication options are maximized. Further advice is available from expert charities such as Ability net (www.abilitynet.org) and the MND Association.

Dysphagia

Referral to the speech and language therapist for a full assessment should be completed at the first signs of swallowing difficulties, such as patient or carer reports of coughing or choking when eating, wet sounding voice after swallowing, reduced appetite and increased meal times. Reported weight loss should trigger additional referral to a dietician. Monitoring of body weight should be routinely included in assessment.

Clinical assessment may include observation of mastication and palpation of swallowing phases using varying food consistencies. Observations of voice quality before and after oral intake are also made. More detailed information can be gained by completing a videofluoroscopy, which visualizes the pharyngeal stage of swallowing and objectively detects aspiration of food or fluid, or by the use of auscultation during swallowing, where a change in breathing or vocalization having a wet quality may indicate secretions in the airway (Palovcaka et al., 2007).

Initial interventions may include postural strategies, such as chin tuck whilst swallowing to help protect the airway, and modified food consistencies. Soft moist food and thickened liquids require less control by the oral muscles and are therefore easier and safer to eat (Palovcaka et al., 2007). The patient and carer should also be advised on safe feeding strategies.

Eventually these strategies become ineffective and supplementary feeding needs to be explored. Ideally the options of alternative feeding via a tube such as a percutaneous endoscopic gastrostomy (PEG) or nasogastric tube (NG) are mentioned to the patient early in the process to enable advanced planning and awareness of the advantages and disadvantages (Galaszewski, 2007).

PEG is usually indicated when patients have significant bulbar impairment with episodes of aspiration or weight loss of >10% of baseline. It is suggested that PEG be inserted prior to marked respiratory decline and that those with VC <50% should have the gastrostomy inserted radiologically where no sedation is required and an upright position can be maintained. Post gastrostomy weight and nutritional status can be stabilized and survival time increased (Radunovic et al., 2007; Rocha et al., 2005). A nasogastric feeding tube can provide a short-term option (Leigh et al., 2003).

Those with an impaired swallow not only have an increased risk of aspiration and further respiratory complications, but also can have the mechanism of cough trigger affected (Hadjikoutis, 1999). It is worth noting that, although alternative feeding routes will reduce aspiration of food and drink, the patient may still not be able to protect their airway from oral secretions.

Excessive saliva or sialorrhea is mainly due to reduced reflex swallowing rather than increased production of saliva; however, this can be a distressing symptom as it not only causes drooling, but also can be a risk of aspiration. Treatment may include the use of hyoscine or glycopyrronium medication in liquid or patch form to dry secretions or botulinum toxin injections into the salivary glands may be considered (Verma & Steele, 2006). The patient may also be provided with suction equipment for use at home.

Understandably, coughing and choking are major concerns to those with MND and those with upper motor bulbar involvement tend to have more episodes of coughing or choking than those without, but they do not have significantly more chest infections. It is therefore unlikely that they are aspirating during a coughing episode and merely have difficulty suppressing the cough reflex (Hadjikoutis, 2000). The MDT has a key role in education and advice on positioning and diet modification for safe feeding and prevention of complications.

Other systems

Nutrition

For most people with MND the most common cause of weight loss and malnutrition is swallowing difficulty, but this is not the only cause. Anxiety and depression can lead to loss of appetite, as can immobility and constipation. Reduced arm function and dependence on others for food preparation and feeding often leads to prolonged meal times and reduced oral intake (Radunovic et al., 2007). Respiratory muscle weakness can lead to dyspnoea during and after eating with the effort of eating exacerbating their breathlessness and leading to fatigue after eating a small amount (Golaszewski, 2007).

A dietician is a key member of the MND MDT and in addition to their input for those with swallowing difficulties as mentioned above, assessment and advice as to nutritional supplements and small, frequent, calorie-dense meals for those with weight loss due to other factors is also important. The multiple contributing factors to poor nutrition in MND and the fact that nutritional status is linked to survival supports the need for weight to be monitored regularly.

Skin

As sensation is not impaired in MND, pressure sores are rarely a problem. However, decreased mobility and poor nutrition can compromise the skin. Pressure-relieving cushions and mattresses may minimize the risk. Patients should be taught how to relieve pressure in the wheelchair and the bed, and turning regimes should be initiated if they are unable to reposition themselves.

Bowels

Constipation resulting from inactivity, dietary changes or weakened abdominal muscles may be managed with a standard aperient. More severe cases may require enemas or manual evacuation. Members of the nursing team will be able to provide advice on a suitable bowel regime. Constipation may cause secondary problems such as exacerbation of spasticity, discomfort and impaired diaphragmatic movement. The root cause of the problem must be addressed as well as the symptom.

Urinary tract

Urinary incontinence does not result directly from MND. Problems with toileting arise from immobility and impaired function. Catheterization is sometimes considered for practical convenience, to facilitate social inclusion and to avoid skin damage.

Eyes

Muscle weakness may result in decreased blinking. Sore and infected eyes can be treated with artificial tears and antibiotic eye drops.

Sleep

Chronic insomnia is reported in approximately 66% of patients with neurological disease (Taylor et al., 2007). It is a significant problem for the MND population and has consequences for physical, psychological and social health.

Insomnia may arise from breathlessness, sleep apnoea, discomfort, fear or distress. Sleeplessness due to respiratory dysfunction may be alleviated by good positioning or nocturnal NIPPV NIV. Discomfort can be minimized with regular repositioning and pain medication if indicated. Fear and distress can be addressed in a number of ways. The following may help:

- A regular and familiar nighttime routine
- Use of relaxation techniques
- A means of calling help such as a switch, buzzer or bell being available to the patient
- Reassurance and recognition of realistic worries and counselling about unrealistic ones
- Sedatives, antidepressants and analgesics may all be considered.

PSYCHOSOCIAL FACTORS

Cognition

It is now well established that cognitive problems can arise from MND. Frontotemporal involvement has been confirmed with imaging studies (Ellis et al., 2001; Neary et al., 2000). Damage in this area may result in executive dysfunction and impaired social interaction (Strong, 2008). These problems must be considered when making all choices and decisions in the patient's care (see Ch. 17). Impulsiveness and impaired judgement, for example, may lead to safety concerns which could impact on home set up or care provision requirements. Clearly, this patient group will need a great deal of support for end-of-life decision-making. Assessment and advice for these problems can be provided by a neuropsychologist or an occupational therapist.

Emotion

A diagnosis of MND brings with it a plethora of fears and concerns. Issues of disability, changing roles, dependence and dying face the patient and their family. How the patient deals with these worries depends on many factors. It has been shown that perceived quality of life is higher in people with strong social and family bonds and those who have an established faith (Walsh et al., 2003).

Delivery of bad news in a sympathetic and accurate manner will make it easier for the patient to accept the diagnosis, deal with subsequent issues and seek help from the team. All team members should be skilled in communicating bad news, informal counselling and providing accurate information about the disease.

Expression of emotion may be difficult due to dysarthria, emotional lability, cognitive problems or facial weakness. Inappropriate or disproportionate expressions of emotion through laughing or crying, also known as pseudobulbar affect or emotional lability, can cause embarrassment and block communication. Although this is not a mood disorder in itself, it can sometimes be treated with either tricyclic or SSRI antidepressants. The patient and carers will need reassurance that this frustrating problem is physiological and not due to lack of comprehension or denial. Aids and strategies to facilitate appropriate communication will allow the patients to share their thoughts and fears with others.

Where anxiety or depression exceed that which would be expected in the circumstances and are causing the patient significant concern, drug therapies should be considered. Sedatives can be used for acute anxiety, low doses of SSRI antidepressants for longer-term anxiety and a whole range of antidepressant medication is available for depressive conditions. Treatment with medication should usually be paired with counselling or other psychological support.

Family care

The psychological, social and emotional impact of MND extends beyond the patient. Families will have to address the same issues of disability, dying and changing roles. Ideally, a family will be able to openly discuss concerns and share the burden of their worries, but where this is not possible, external help may be required. Families and carers should have access to counselling and support as needed.

Families may have concerns such as financial problems, housing issues and child care. Children may need to be supported through the disease process and death of a family member. The primary care giver to the child may previously have been the patient or be now involved in caring for the patient as well as the child. Specialist social work teams will be able to support the family and children.

Where packages of care are required, the family must be involved in the planning. Their burden as carers must be part of the considerations and many people are uncomfortable with accepting help or having strangers come into their home.

Sexual issues may also face the patient and their partner. Sexual drive is not normally affected but the disease will impact upon physical performance. Frontal lobe involvement may also lead to changes in sexual behaviours. Support and advice on all aspects of sexuality should be available and include information on alternative positions and means of expressing sexuality.

Every family needs to be provided with accurate information, therapeutic contact with the MDT and a realistic and supported vision of the future.

Spiritual aspects

Many people with a life-limiting disease turn to their religious beliefs for comfort, support and explanation, even if they are not normally practicing members of their faith. Religious belief has been linked to higher quality of life in this patient group (Walsh et al., 2003). The patient and/or their carers and family may need help accessing religious support. Local religious leaders will usually be happy to help and hospital chaplains will give spiritual help to anyone regardless of faith.

Counselling

As physiotherapists frequently have close physical contact with their patients during treatments and the patient often senses a familiarity which allows them to broach difficult topics. The patient may look for further information or advice about any aspect of the disease. The physiotherapist must be able to provide accurate information in a sensitive and open way when appropriate to do so and know when and where to seek help otherwise. It is important that the MDT works cohesively and that all information received by the patient is fed back to the team. Whilst repetition of some facts may aid absorption, contradicting information or advice misguides the patient and erodes their faith in the MDT. Where important information is being passed, it may be appropriate to have a family meeting with several members of the team to ensure good communication.

Information given should be responsive to the patient's immediate concerns, sensitively delivered and broken down into manageable amounts to avoid overwhelming or confusing the patient. The physiotherapist must recognize that they are dealing with a person whose life has been changed dramatically and may be grieving for their losses and that communication is a two-way process requiring good listening skills as well as skillful expression.

TERMINAL MANAGEMENT

Although the care of the MND patient is largely palliative throughout the course of the disease, symptomatic management becomes increasingly important towards the time of death. Death usually occurs as a result of respiratory failure, most commonly following infection (Neudert et al., 2001). The final decline is usually rapid and death frequently occurs in the night. Throughout this time, it is essential to ensure that the patient's comfort is maintained, and the psychological welfare of the whole family is attended to.

It is vital that all members of the team are aware of the change in the patient's status and that the approach to treatment is consistent between all professionals involved. It is important to anticipate all eventualities and to adhere to the patient's wishes as laid down in management plans or advance directives as far as possible. It is also important that invasive ventilation and some other radical, lifesaving measures are avoided should the patient be admitted via the emergency department. Otherwise, this can result in the terminal stages of the disease being prolonged and provide some difficult choices for the family or medical team to make.

The management should be responsive to the patient's symptoms using the methods described previously (Houseman, 2008). Opioid analgesics and anxiolytic agents are often employed at this stage to minimize pain and distress. Ready availability of team members and necessary treatments avoid crisis situations and unnecessary distress.

The Motor Neurone Disease Association has developed the Breathing Space Programme to help patients at this time. The patient and family can discuss the use of the Breathing Space Kit (see 'Medication', above) with their own doctor, who can then prescribe the medication so that it is immediately available at home if there is an episode of pain, breathlessness or choking.

Specialized palliative care units should be involved with the patient and family from early after diagnosis. Many can offer a range of services such as day centres, hospice care and hospice at home schemes. The patient's wishes with regard to location during their final days should be respected.

The patient and family may require heightened psychological or spiritual support during this phase and systems should be put in place to ensure that the family has access to support and counselling after the death (Hebert et al., 2005).

The Motor Neurone Disease Association

The MND Association acts as a support and information service as well as funding research. It publishes a number of leaflets for the patient and the family, as well as for professionals involved in care. Regional support groups for patients and carers are available throughout the UK. There is also a 24-hour help line and the association is able to loan equipment (see Appendix).

CASE HISTORY

Imagine you are assessing this patient in an outpatient or clinic setting.

At each stage of disease consider:

- What therapy interventions might you use?
- Which other members of the MDT might you refer to and why?
- What psychosocial issues are there to consider? How might these impact on therapy intervention?

Early stage

Mr L. is a 34-year-old man with a history of progressive left arm weakness of approximately 1 year and more recent distal weakness in his right arm. He was diagnosed with flail arm variant MND 1 month ago and has not had any therapy input.

He lives with his wife and young 3-year-old child in a 2nd floor council owned flat.

Prior to his illness he worked full time as a security officer for a high street store and played football two times per week. He is independent with all personal activities of daily living, but is unable to work and has been on sick leave for the past 6 months.

Problem list

Impairments

Left arm weakness and wasting (power 0–1/5 throughout)
Left shoulder pain with 2 cm subluxation when dependent
Right arm weakness and wasting thenar eminence (power 2–3/5)
Cramps throughout body
Fatigue.

Activity limitations

Independent indoor, outdoor and stair mobility, but distance limited by fatigue
Assistance required in performing bilateral dexterity tasks, e.g. buttons or zips
Poor sleeping pattern due to pain and cramps.

Participation restrictions

Home

Unable to fulfill physical care role for children.

Work

Unable to carryout previous employment.

Leisure

Unable to play football.

Potential interventions

- Education on role of therapy and positive effects of exercise
- Positioning advice for shoulder pain and range.

DO NOT overload with information. There is a fine balance between education and overload.

Other referrals

- Community physiotherapy. To help access gym-based activity to maintain activity levels and fitness. Possible use of hydrotherapy pool to aid maintenance of upper limb range.
- Social services. To review housing and equipment needs now and future. Plus provide advice on benefits, etc.
- Occupational therapist assessment for assistive aids, activity planning/fatigue management to maximize quality of life.

Psychosocial considerations

- Provide information about MNDA or 'patients like me' website so the patient is able to access peer support and further information when ready.
- Encourage attendance of wife/family at appointments for emotional support and re-enforce idea of him as important family member.
- Inclusion of family in activity, e.g. hydrotherapy to enable him to play with his son.

Disease progression (18 months after diagnosis)

Mr L.'s symptoms have now progressed in the right arm and to the legs. He has also noticed weight loss (115 kg to 105 kg in the past 6 months). He has started taking Riluzole 50 mg daily.

He recently retired from work on medical grounds and is awaiting rehousing.

Problem list

Impairments

Left arm weakness and wasting (power 0–1/5 throughout)
Left shoulder pain with 2 cm subluxation when dependent
Right arm weakness and wasting (power 0–1/5)
Fatigue and cramps throughout body
Lower limb weakness and fatigue grade 3–4/5 proximally
Respiratory muscle weakness FVC=65% of predicted.

Activity limitations

Independent indoor, outdoor and stair mobility but distance limited by fatigue
Assistance required to wash, dress and feed self
Difficulty in adjusting clothing after toileting
Poor sleeping pattern due to pain and cramps and inability to turn independently
Sit to stand from raised seat independently
Dependent on wife for all domestic and community tasks
Unable to get down/up from floor to play with child.

Participation restrictions

Home

Unable to fulfill physical care role for children.

Work

Unable to carryout previous employment.

Leisure

Unable to play football
Difficulty using telephone or accessing community, therefore dependent on others for social activities and query as to whether he is able to raise alarm if alone with child.

Potential interventions

- Teach self-assisted cough in sitting with good cough effort, to enable him to clear secretions adequately
- Advise about oral hydration to aid secretion clearance
- Advice to patient and career regarding safe feeding to prevent aspiration and maximize oral intake.

Other referrals

- Community physiotherapy. Positioning options for interaction with children
- Social work assessment of Mr L. and child – for assistance with personal care, childcare tasks, domestic chores ·
- Occupational therapy (OT) involvement regarding aids and equipment to facilitate drinking and oral hydration, a 'closomat' toilet. Electric Riser recliner chair ensuring Mr L. can operate controls. OT involvement to ensure that new property is appropriately adapted to meet long-term needs, i.e. wheelchair accessible. Fabrication of splint to aid grip with right hand and independence in some personal care, e.g. adjusting clothing after toilet use
- Assistive technology and environmental controls assessment with a view to the provision of equipment that facilitates feeding, using the telephone, using light switches, accessing the television and computer without arm use
- Dietetics review and prescription of nutritional supplements.

Psychosocial considerations

- Referral to palliative care services especially for family support – young children and wife especially as disease progressed faster than expected
- Potential involvement of MNDA volunteer to visit
- Use of assistive technology to ensure able to communicate and maintain organization of social activities to reduce isolation.

Multi-system involvement (3 years after diagnosis)

37-year-old male diagnosed with MND 3 years ago initially thought to have flail arm syndrome, but now progressed to ALS with all limbs and respiratory involvement.

He reports further weight loss.

He had a recent trial of NIPPV and is now using 8 hours overnight.

Mr L., his wife and child have been rehoused to a wheelchair accessible ground floor flat. He is spending a lot of time alone in the flat and is generally withdrawn.

Problem list

Impairments

Bilateral upper limb weakness with associated shoulder and neck pain
Bilateral lower limb weakness (3/5 distally)
Fatigue
Respiratory muscle weakness (FVC= 54%) and retained secretions
Weak neck extensors.

Activity limitations

Mobilizes <10 m indoors without aid. Occasional trips
Transfers with minimal assistance in sit-to-stand
Full assistance required to wash, dress, toileting and feeding
Mobilizes outdoors in electric wheelchair
Dependent on wife for all domestic and community tasks.

Participation restrictions

Home

Unable to fulfill physical care role for child.

Work

Retired on ill health grounds as unable to carry out previous employment.

Leisure

Unable to play football, requires accompanying in community as unable to raise alarm
Avoids social situations as unable to maintain head position and eye contact for conversation.

Potential interventions

- Teach assisted cough to patient and wife in sitting
- Plus cough with NIPPV breaths before to maximize secretion clearance. Advice re: oral hydration. Advice re: positioning to maintain passive range of movement (PROM) shoulders to reduce pain and aid washing and dressing. Humidifer for NIV.
- Trial and fitting of headmaster collar – ensuring wife or carer available to help donn/doff
- Trial of ankle-foot orthosis (AFO) to reduced tripping.

Other referrals/liaison with other services

- Social work. Request care needs assessment for help with personal care. Ideally via direct payment scheme to enable flexibility and personal autonomy
- Children and family social work team – for support with childcare, transport to school, etc.
- Social services occupational therapy team to assess for equipment, and to facilitate independent drinking and oral hydration

- Wheelchair service. Possible alternative control, e.g. head/voice to maintain independence, chair that can recline with head support and option to place ventilator on
- Referral to assistive technology and environmental control team for assessment for equipment that facilitates feeding, door access, using the telephone, using light switches, accessing the television and computer
- Orthotics: shoulder support to aid pain, AFOs
- Dietetics. Discussion regarding PEG/RIG before respiratory system deteriorates further. Likely RIG due to respiratory status
- Ensure links with palliative care services for general emotional support and specific counselling. Additional symptom management, e.g. saliva management, respite options and advanced planning.

Psychosocial considerations

- Ensuring seating and head position to enable social interaction
- MNDA emotional support for patient and family. Financial support funding. Accessible holiday accommodation or assistive technology/computer related
- Sensitivity about end-of-life discussions and planning and impact of how emotional responses to this may affect participation in all multiple agency involvement.

The above case history demonstrates the importance of the physiotherapist within the team, the need for understanding of disease variants and progress, i.e. initially factors such as age and limb-onset symptoms suggested increased survival and, therefore, early management focused on maximization of function and use of exercise to maintain activity. However, the respiratory decline and development of symptoms in various body regions suggested more aggressive disease progression, and the approach became much more supportive in symptom management and proactive in crisis prevention.

Appropriate and timely intervention by the physiotherapist as part of the MDT in addition to an appreciation of the individual's choices and autonomy is essential in providing therapeutic input and maximizing quality of life for those with MND.

ACKNOWLEDGMENTS

The Authors would like to thank Dr Cathy Ellis, Consultant Neurologist, Academic Neurosciences Centre, Kings College Hospital, London, for her help and comments on the chapter.

REFERENCES

Aitkens, S., McCrory, M., Kilmer, D., Bernauer, E., 1993. Moderate resistance exercise program: its effect in slowly progressive neuromuscular disease. Arch. Phys. Med. Rehabil. 74, 711–715.

ALS CNTF Treatment Study Phase I–II Group, Brooks, B.R., Sanjak, M., Ringel, S., England, J., Brinkmann, J., Pestronk, A., et al., 1996. The ALS functional rating scale: assessment of activities of daily living in patients with amyotrophic lateral sclerosis. Arch. Neurol. 53, 141–147.

Ambrosio, F., Kadi, F., Lexell, J., Fitzgerald, G.K., Boninger, M.L., Huard, J., 2009. The effect of muscle loading on skeletal muscle regenerative potential: an update of current research findings relating to aging and neuromuscular pathology. Am. J. Phys. Med. Rehabil. 88 (2), 145–155.

Ashworth, N.L., Satkunam, L.E., Deforge, D., 2006. Treatment for spasticity in amyotrophic lateral sclerosis/motor neuron disease. Cochrane Database Syst. Rev. (Issue. 1).

Borasio, G.D., Miller, R.G., 2001. Clinical characteristics and management of ALS. Semin. Neurol. 21, 155–166.

Bott, J., Blumenthal, S., Buxton, M., et al., 2009. Guidelines for the physiotherapy management of the adult, medical, spontaneously breathing patient. Thorax 64 (Suppl. 1), i1–i51.

Bourke, S.C., Tomlinson, M., Williams, T.L., Bullock, R.E., Shaw, P.J., Gibson, G.J., 2006. Effects of non-invasive ventilation on survival and quality of life in patients with amyotrophic lateral sclerosis: a randomised controlled trial. Lancet Neurol. 5, 140–147.

Brooks, B.R., Miller, R.G., Swash, M., Munsat, T.L., 2000. El Escorial revisited: revised criteria for the diagnosis of amyotrophic lateral sclerosis. Amyotroph. Lateral Scler. Other Motor Neuron. Disord. 1, 293–299.

Brown, P., 1994. Pathophysiology of spasticity. J. Neurol. Neurosurg. Psychiatry 57, 773–777.

Charcot, J.M., Joffroy, A., 1869. Deaux cas d.atrophie musculaire progressive avec lesions de la grise et des faisceaux antrerolateraux de la moelle epiniere. Arch. Physiol. 2, 629–760.

Chatwin, M., Ross, E., Hart, N., Nickol, A.H., Polkey, M.I., Simonds, A.K., 2003. Cough augmentation with mechanical insufflation/exsufflation in patients with neuromuscular weakness. Eur. Respir. J. 21 (3), 385–386.

Chen, R., Grand'Maison, F., Strong, M.J., Ramsay, D.A., Bolton, C.F., 1996. Motor neuron disease presenting as acute respiratory failure: a clinical and pathological study. J. Neurol. Neurosurg. Psychiatry 60, 455–458.

Czaplinski, A., Yen, A., Appel, S., 2006. Forced vital capacity (FVC) as an indicator of survival and disease progression in an ALS clinic population. J. Neurol. Neurosurg. Psychiatry 77, 390–392.

Dal Bello-Haas, V., Florence, J.M., Kloos, A.D., Scheirbecker, J., Lopate, G., Hayes, S.M., et al., 2007. A randomized controlled trial of resistance exercise in individuals with ALS. Neurology 68, 2003–2007.

Dal Bello-Haas, V., Florence, J.M., Krivickas, L.S., 2008. Therapeutic exercise for people with amyotrophic lateral sclerosis or motor neuron disease. Cochrane Database Syst. Rev. (Issue 2).

David, C., 2002. Electrodiagnostic approach to the patient with suspected motor neuron disease. Neurol. Clin. N. Am. 20, 527–555.

Drory, V.E., Goltsman, E., Reznik, J.G., Mosek, A., Korczyn, A.D., 2001. The Value of Muscle Exercise in Patients with Amyotrophic Lateral Sclerosis. J. Neurolog. Sci. 191, 133–137.

Edwards, S., Charlton, P., 2002. Splinting and the use of orthoses in the management of patients with neurological disorder. In: Edwards, S. (Ed.), Neurological Physiotherapy: A Problem-solving Approach. second ed. Churchill Livingstone, London, pp. 219–253.

Ellis, C.M., Suckling, J., Amaro, E., 2001. Volumetric analysis reveals corticospinal tract degeneration and extramotor involvement in ALS. Neurology 57, 1571–1578.

Ferguson, T.A., Elman, L.B., 2007. Clinical presentation and diagnosis of Amyotrophic Lateral Sclerosis. Neurorehabilitation 22, 409–416.

Francis, K., Bach, J.R., DeLisa, J.A., 1999. Evaluation and rehabilitation of patients with adult motor neurone disease. Arch. Phys. Med. Rehabil. 80, 951–963.

Galaszewski, A., 2007. Nutrition throughout the course of ALS. Neurorehabilitation 22, 431–434.

Gordon, P.H., Cheng, B., Katz, I.B., Pinto, M., Hays, A.P., Mitsumoto, H., 2006. The natural history of primary lateral sclerosis. Neurology 66, 647–653.

Hadjikoutis, S., Eccles, R., Wiles, C.M., 2000. Coughing and choking in motor neuron disease. J. Neurol. Neurosurg. Psychiatry 68, 601–604.

Hadjikoutis, S., Wiles, C.M., Eccles, R., 1999. Cough in motor neuron disease: a review of mechanics. Q. J. Med. 92, 487–494.

Haverkamp, L.J., Appel, V., Appel, S.H., 1995. Natural history of amyotrophic lateral sclerosis in a database population. Validation of a scoring system and a model for survival prediction. Brain 118, 707–719.

Hayashi, H., 2000. ALS care in Japan. In: Oliver, D., Borasio, G.D., Walsh, D. (Eds.), Palliative Care in Amyotrophic Lateral Sclerosis. Oxford University Press, Oxford, pp. 152–154.

Hebert, R.S., Lacomis, D., Easter, C., Frick, V., Shear, M.K., 2005. Grief support for informal caregivers of patients with ALS: A national survey. Neurology 64, 137–138.

Heffernan, C., Jenkinson, C., Holmes, T., Macleod, H., Kinnear, W., Oliver, D., et al., 2006. Management of respiration in MND/ALS patients: An evidence based review Amyotrophic Lateral Sclerosis 7, 5–15.

Houseman, G., 2008. Symptom Management of the Patient with Amyotrophic Lateral Sclerosis: A Guide for Hospice Nurses. Journal of Hospice and Palliative Nursing 10 (4), 214–215.

Johns, M., 1994. Sleepiness in different situations as measured by the Epworth sleepiness scale. Sleep 17, 703–710.

Kato, S., Shaw, P., Wood-Allum, C., 2003. Amyotrophic lateral sclerosis. Neurodegeneration. In: Dickson, D.W. (Ed.), The molecular pathology of dementia andmovement disorders. ISN Neuropath Press, Basel, pp. 350–368.

Kent-Braun, J.A., Miller, R.G., 2000. Central fatigue during isometric exercise in amyotrophic lateral sclerosis. Muscle Nerve 23, 909–914.

Kilmer, D., McCrory, M., Wright, N., 1994. The effect of a high resistance exercise program in slowly progressive neuromuscular disease. Arch. Phys. Med. Rehabil. 75, 560–563.

Kirkinezos, I.G., Hernandez, D., Bradley, W.G., Moraes, C.T., 2003. Regular exercise is beneficial to a mouse model of amyotrophic lateral sclerosis. Ann. Neurol. 53, 804–807.

Lacomblez, L., Bensimon, G., Leigh, P.N., Guillet, P., Meininger, V., 1996. Dose-ranging study of riluzole in amyotrophic lateral sclerosis. Amyotrophic Lateral Sclerosis/Riluzole Study Group II. Lancet 347, 1425–1431.

Landers, M., Barker, G., Wallentine, S., McWhorter, J., Peel, C., 2003. A comparison of tidal volume, breathing frequency, and minute ventilation between two sitting postures in healthy adults. Physiother. Theory Pract. 19, 109–119.

Leigh, P.N., Abrahams, S., Al-Chalabi, A., Ampong, M.-A., Goldstein, L.H., Johnson, J., et al., 2003. The Management of Motor Neurone disease. J. Neurol. Neurosurg. Psychiatry 74 (Suppl. 4), iv32–iv47.

Lieber, R.L., Friden, J., 1999. Mechanisms of muscle injury after eccentric contraction. J. Sci. Med. Sport. 2, 253–265.

Lyall, R.A., Donaldson, N., Polkey, M.I., 2001. Respiratory muscle strength and ventilatory failure in amyotrophic lateral sclerosis. Brain 124, 2000–2013.

Lyall, R., Moxham, J., Leigh, N., 2000. Dyspnoea. In: Oliver, D., Borasio, G.D., Walsh, D. (Eds.), Palliative Care in Amyotrophic Lateral Sclerosis. Oxford University Press, Oxford, pp. 43–56.

Mandrioli, J., Faglioni, P., Nichelli, P., Sola, P., 2006. Amyotrophic lateral sclerosis: Prognostic indicators of survival. Amyotroph. Lateral Scler. 7, 217–226.

McClelland 3rd S., Bethoux, F.A., Boulis, N.M., Sutliff, M.H., Stough, D.K., Schwetz, K.M., et al., 2008. Intrathecal Baclofen for spasticity-related pain in amyotrophic lateral sclerosis:efficcy and factors associated with pain relief. Muscle Nerve 37 (3), 396–398.

Miller, T.M., Layzer, R.B., 2005. Muscle Cramps. Muscle Nerve 32 (4), 431–442.

Miller, R.G., Mitchell, J.D., Lyon, M., Moore, D.H., 2007. Riluzole for amyotrophic lateral sclerosis (ALS)/ motor neuron disease (MND). Cochrane Database Syst. Rev. (1) Jan 24, 2007.

Miller, R.G., Rosenberg, J.A., Gelinas, D.F., 1999. Practice parameter: The care of the patient with amyotrophic lateral sclerosis (an evidence-based review). Neurology 52, 1311–1323.

Mustfa, N., Aiello, M., Lyall, R.A., et al., 2003. Cough augmentation in amyotrophic lateral sclerosis. Neurology 61, 1285–1287.

Mustfa, N., Walsh, E., Bryant, V., et al., 2006. The effect of Non invasive ventilation on ALS patients and their caregivers. Neurology 66, 1211–1217.

Neary, D., Snowden, J.S., Mann, D.M.A., 2000. Cognitive changes in motor neurone disease/amyotrophic lateral sclerosis. J. Neurolog. Sci. 180, 15–20.

Neudert, C., Oliver, D., Wasner, M., 2001. The course of the terminal phase in patients with amyotrophic lateral sclerosis. J. Neurol. 248, 612–616.

O'Gorman, B., Oliver, D., Nottle, C., Prisley, S., 2004. Disorders of nerve I: motor neurone disease. In: Stokes, M. (Ed.), Physical Management in Neurological Rehabilitation. second ed. Elsevier, London, pp. 233–251.

Palovcaka, M., Mancinellib, J.M., Elmana, L.B., McCluskey, L., 2007. Diagnostic and therapeutic methods in the management of dysphagia in the ALS population: Issues in efficacy for the out-patient setting. Neurorehabilitation 22, 417–423.

Pan, C.X., Morrison, R.S., Ness, J., Fugh-Berman, A., Leipzig, R.M., 2000. Complementary and alternative medicine in the management of pain, dyspnea, and nausea and vomiting near the end of life. A systematic review. J. Pain Symptom Manage. 20 (5), 374–387.

Peruzzi, A.C., Potts, A.F., 1996. Physical therapy intervention for persons with amyotrophic lateral sclerosis. Physiother. Can. 48, 119–126.

Pope, P.M., 2002. Postural management and special seating. In: Edwards, S. (Ed.), Neurological Physiotherapy: A Problem Solving Approach. second ed. Churchill Livingstone, London, pp. 189–217.

Polkey, M.I., Lyall, R.A., Davidson, A.C., 1999. Ethical and clinical issues in the use of home non-invasive mechanical ventilation for the palliation of breathlessness in motor neurone disease. Thorax 54, 367–371.

Prasad, S., Pryor, J., 2002. Physiotherapy for Respiratory and Cardiac Problems, third ed. Churchill Livingstone, London.

Radunović, A., Mitsumoto, H., Leigh, P.N., 2007. Clinical care of patients with amyotrophic lateral sclerosis. Lancet Neurol. 6 (10), 913–925.

Richardson, D., Thompson, A.J., 1999. Botulinum toxin: its use in the treatment of acquired spasticity in adults. Physiotherapy 85, 541–551.

Rocha, J.A., Reich, C., Similes, F., Fonsie, J., Menes Ribbentrop, J., 2005. Diagnostic investigation and multidisciplinary management in motor neuron disease. J. Neurol. 252, 1435–1447.

Rowland, L.P., Schneider, N.A., 2001. Amyotrophic lateral sclerosis. N. Engel. J. Red. 344, 1688–1700.

RCN code of practice for patient handling. Royal College of Nursing (London).

Sancho, J., Servers, E., Daze, J., Marín, J., 2004. Efficacy of Mechanical Insufflation-Exsufflation in Medically Stable Patietns With ALS. Chest 125, 1400–1405.

Sanjak, M., Reddan, W., Rix Brooks, B., 1987. Role of muscular exercise in amyotrophic lateral sclerosis. Neurol. Clin. 5, 251–267.

Schwartz, M.S., Swash, M., 1995. Neurophysiological changes in motor neurone disease. In: Leigh, P.N., Swash, M. (Eds.), Motor Neurone Disease: Biology and Management. Springer Verlag, London, pp. 31–344.

Sharma, K.R., Kent-Braun, J.A., Majumdar, S., 1995. Physiology of fatigue in amyotrophic lateral sclerosis. Neurology 45, 733–740.

Simmons, Z., 2005. Management strategies for patients with ALS from diagnosis to death. Neurologist 11 (5), 257–270.

Strong, M.J., 2001. Progress in clinical neurosciences: the evidence for ALS as a multisystems disorder of limited phenotypic expression. Can. J. Neurol. Sci. 28, 283–298.

Strong, M.J., 2008. The syndromes of frontotemporal dysfunction in amyotrophic lateral sclerosis. Amyotroph. Lateral Scler. 9, 323–338.

Talman, P., Forbes, A., Mathers, S., 2008. Clinical Phenotypes and Natural Progression for MND: analysis from an Australian Database. Amyotroph. Lateral Scler. 9, 1–6.

Taylor, D.J., Mallory, L.J., Lichstein, K.L., 2007. Comorbidity of chronic insomnia with medical problems. Sleep 30 (2), 213–218.

Trail, M., Nelson, N., Van, J.N., Appel, S.H., Lai, E.C., 2001. Wheelchair use by patients with Amyotrophic Lateral sclerosis: a survey of user characteristics and selection preferences. Arch Phys. Med. Rehabil. 82 (1), 98–102.

Traynor, B.J., Alexander, M., Corr, B., Frost, E., Hardiman, O., 2003. Effect of a multidisciplinary amyotrophic lateral sclerosis (ALS) clinic on ALS survival: a population based study, 1996-2000. J. Neurol. Neurosurg. Psychiatry 74, 1258–1261.

Tripodoro, V., De Vito, E., 2008. Management of dyspnoea in advanced Motor Neurone disease. Current Opinion in Supportive and Palliative Care 2, 173–179.

Uldry, C., Fitting, J.W., 1995. Maximal values of Sniff inspiratory pressure in healthy subjects. Thorax 50, 371–375.

Van den Berg, J., Kalmijn, S., Lindeman, E., et al., 2005. Multidisciplinary ALS care improves quality of life in patients with ALS. Neurology 65 (8), 1264–1267.

Vender, R., Maugher, D., Walsh, S., Alam, S., Simmons, Z., 2007. Respiratory Systems Abnormalities and clinical milestones for patients with ALS with emphasis upon survival. Amyotroph. Lateral Scler. 8, 36–41.

Verma, A., Steele, J., 2006. Botulinum toxin improves sialorrhea and quality of living in bulbar amyotrophic lateral sclerosis. Muscle Nerve 34 (2), 235–237.

Walsh, S.M., Bremer, B.A., Felgoise, S.H., 2003. Religiousness is related to quality of life in patients with ALS. Neurology 60, 1527–1529.

Wijesekera, L., Mathers, S., Talman, P., et al., 2009. Natural History and clinical Features of the flail arm and flail leg ALS variants. Neurology 72, 1087–1094.

Young, T., Nicklin, C., 2000. Lower Limb Casting in Neurology: Practical Guidelines, first ed. Royal Hospital for Neuro-disability, London.

RESOURCES

MND CARE CENTRES IN THE UK
www.mndassociation.org/
for_professionals/local_support/
care_centres

Please see the MND website for up-to-date contacts and their telephone numbers and e-mail addresses:

Barts & London
Barts & The London Queen Mary's School of Medicine & Dentistry
4 Newark Street
London E1 2AT

Belfast – Royal Hospital
Room 114, Bostock House
Royal Hospital
Grosvenor Road
Belfast BT12 6BA

Cambridge – Addenbrooke's Hospital
Addenbrooke's NHS Foundation Trust
Cambridge University Hospitals
Box 165
Hills Road
Cambridge CB2 2QQ

Birmingham – Queen Elizabeth Hospital
Dept of Neurosciences
Queen Elizabeth Hospital
University Hospitals
Birmingham NHS Foundation Trust
Edgbaston
Birmingham B15 2TH

Cardiff – University Hospital of Wales
MND Care Centre
Rookwood Hospital
Llandaff
Cardiff CF5 2YN

London – King's College Hospital
PO Box 41
Academic Neurosciences Building
Institute of Psychiatry
De Crespigny Park
London SE5 8AF

Leeds
The Leeds Teaching Hospitals
Dept of Neurology
E Floor Martin Wing
Leeds General Infirmary
Great George Street
Leeds LS1 3EX

Liverpool – The Walton Centre
Research Office
Neurological Rehabilitation Unit
The Walton Centre
Lower Lane
Fazakerley

Liverpool L9 7LJ

Manchester – Hope Hospital
Manchester MND Care Centre
Greater Manchester Centre for
Clinical Neurosciences
Department of Neurology
Hope Hospital
Stott Lane
Salford
Greater Manchester M6 8HD

London – National Hospital
Box 125
National Hospital
Queen Square
London
WC1N 3BG

**Newcastle – Newcastle General
Hospital**
MND Care & Research Centre
Lanercost
Newcastle General Hospital
Westgate Road
Newcastle Upon Tyne

NE4 6BE

**Nottingham – Queen's Medical
Centre**
MND Care and Research Centre,
Palliative Care Unit,
E Floor, East Block
Queen's Medical Centre
University Hospital
Nottingham NG7 2UH

Oxford – Radcliffe Infirmary
Oxford Centre for Enablement
Windmill Road
Oxford
OX3 7LD

Preston – Royal Preston Hospital
Preston MND Care Centre
Ward 17
Royal Preston Hospital
Sharoe Green Lane
Fulwood
Preston
PR2 9HT

**Sheffield – Royal Hallamshire
Hospital**
N Floor
Room N127
Royal Hallamshire Hospital
Glossop Road
Sheffield
S10 2JF

Southampton
Wessex Neurological Centre
B Level
Southampton General Hospital
Mailpoint 101
Tremona Road
Southampton
SO16 6YD

Peninsula MND Network
Building 2
Brest Road
Derriford Business Park
Plymouth
PL6 5QZ

Chapter | 9 |

Polyneuropathies

Gita Ramdharry

CONTENTS

KEY POINTS

Research in people with neuropathies indicates that the determinants of functional ability are not directly linked to physical fitness.

INTRODUCTION

Polyneuropathies are generalized disorders of the peripheral nerves and are a common neurological problem. The cause, pathology and presentation of this group of diseases are wide ranging and variable (England & Asbury, 2004). Some neuropathies have an acute onset and progression, whereas others have a more chronic, slower progressing picture. This chapter outlines the most common acute and chronic polyneuropathies, with examples given of disorders according to the structures involved in the pathological process. Evidence and best practice for rehabilitation interventions will be illustrated with a case history.

Polyneuropathies are most commonly mixed, affecting both motor and sensory neurones, but some can have a predilection for one modality. The key pathology is an impairment of transmission of nerve action potentials due to disruption of either the axon or the myelin sheath (Figure 9.1). Myelin and axonal damage can occur for a variety of reasons, such as infection, drug or environmental toxicity, metabolic and auto-immune disorders, malignancy and genetic factors (Hughes, 2008).

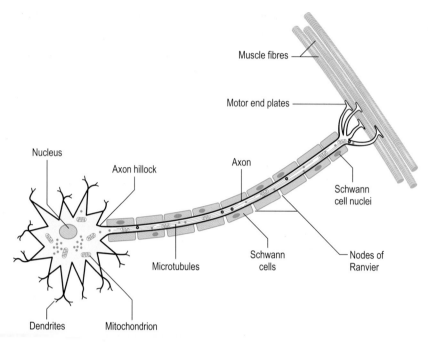

Muscle fibres

Motor end plates

Nucleus

Axon hillock

Axon

Schwann
cell nuclei

Schwann
cells

Nodes of
Ranvier

Microtubules

Dendrites   Mitochondrion

Figure 9.1 Schematic of a motor neuron showing the cell body and axon myelinated by the Schwann cells. The microtubules in the axon are important tracts to transport vital proteins, vesicles and mitochondrion to the periphery of the nerve.

BACKGROUND PHYSIOLOGY

To understand the pathology of nerve disease, a basic understanding of nerve physiology helps to explain the deficits and symptoms experienced by people with neuropathy (Figure 9.1) (England & Asbury, 2004). The health of the neuron from the proximal to the distal end is maintained by axonal transport. Transport of mitochondrion is important to meet the energy requirements of nerve conduction at the periphery. In fast conducting myelinated neurons, propagation of the action potential relies on the interaction between the nerve axon and myelin. In motor neurons, a clustering of voltage-gated sodium channels occurs at the axon hillock where the initial depolarization occurs. In sensory neurons depolarization occurs through stimulation of the sensory end organ. Clusters of channels also exist at the nodes of Ranvier in myelinated fibres. Action potentials are generated at the nodes by opening of the voltage-gated sodium (Na) channels leading to an influx of Na+ ions which depolarizes the membrane. Closure of the Na+ channels terminates the action potential by restoring the resting membrane potential (Vucic et al., 2009). This process is called saltatory conduction and allows the current to spread further and quicker between nodes so speeding up the action potential.

A commonly used diagnostic tool for investigating polyneuropathy is electrophysiological testing (England

& Asbury, 2004). A current is externally applied to a nerve and the speed of conduction, or conduction velocity, can be calculated. This indicates the presence of demyelination as slowing of conduction is seen where saltatory conduction is impaired by myelin degeneration (<38 m/s). Electrical studies also allow the measurement of the amplitude of the motor response, the compound muscle action potential (CMAP), or the sensory nerve action potential (SNAP). A reduction in the amplitude of the CMAP or SNAP indicates a loss of axons. These studies help to distinguish between different types of neuropathy but also help to understand how the structures involved in the pathology contribute to the presentation.

DEMYELINATING POLYNEUROPATHIES

Demyelinating neuropathies occur due to degeneration or destruction of myelin. Myelinated nerves tend to be larger and faster conducting, e.g. motor neurons and 1a sensory afferents, and a predilection for large fibre dysfunction is seen in demyelinating neuropathies (England & Asbury, 2004). It is worth noting, however, that prolonged periods of demyelination can lead to axonal degeneration, though the mechanism is not fully understood. Demyelination could cause an alteration of axonal ion channels and/or increased energy requirements that lead to disturbances in axonal transport and subsequent axonal degeneration. There are also reports of down regulation of neurotrophic factors in Schwann cells where structural changes in myelin are observed (Nicholson, 2006).

This section outlines the most common acute and chronic demyelinating polyneuropathies.

Acute demyelinating polyneuropathy

An acute polyneuropathy is described as one that reaches its highest point of severity, or nadir, in less than 4 weeks (Hughes, 2008). The most common type is Guillain Barré syndrome (GBS) or acute inflammatory polyradiculoneuropathy where there is a rapidly progressive paralysis, sensory impairment and areflexia (England & Asbury, 2004). The European incidence is 1.9 cases per 100 000, so it is a relatively rare condition (Vucic et al., 2009). GBS can affect any age group but is more prevalent in men and in older people, where the outcome after the acute period can be much worse (Vucic et ., 2009).

The cause is not clear but an infection precedes the onset of GBS in about two-thirds of cases (Hughes, 2008; Vucic et al., 2009). GBS is an autoimmune disorder where an immune response is directed towards unknown antigens triggered by the earlier infection. This immune response leads to an inflammatory process and destruction of the myelin sheath in the larger diameter motor and sensory neurons.

Presentation of Guillain Barré syndrome

The primary pathology in GBS is one of acute inflammatory demyelination which results in disruption of saltatory conduction leading to a slowing or block of nerve conduction (Figure 9.2). There is also a suggestion that the voltage-gated sodium channels are blocked by antibodies, also impacting on neuron function (Vucic et al., 2009).

GBS presents with proximal or distal weakness and sensory loss that either ascends or descends from onset. Symptoms can impact on functional abilities such as walking, standing or even sitting in severe cases. Facial and bulbar musculature is commonly involved in about 50% of cases (Vucic et al., 2009). In severe cases where there is extensive trunk weakness and bulbar dysfunction, respiratory function and vital capacity (below 20 mL/kg) can be compromised with up to one-third of cases needing respiratory support to maintain lung volumes and manage any secondary respiratory infections (England & Asbury, 2004; Vucic et al., 2009). Tracheostomy is commonly performed and associated with more severe symptoms and extended critical care admission (Ali et al., 2006). Autonomic involvement is commonplace causing fluctuations in blood pressure and cardiac arrhythmias. This can impact on the rehabilitation process, particularly in the early stages.

Urgent diagnosis is required because of the severity of complications. Blood tests demonstrate elevated immunoglobulin anti-bodies in 25% of cases, elevated protein in the cerebrospinal fluid (CSF) is observed in 80% of people with GBS, though this may not be apparent in the first week (Hughes, 2008). Nerve conduction studies show decreased conduction velocity and a partial conduction block due to the demyelination (Figure 9.2), though this may not be apparent in the very early stages. In addition, a decreased CMAP is observed where there is axonal loss (Vucic et al., 2009).

In the early phase the nadir is usually reached in up to 4 weeks with a progressive recovery thereafter (Figure 9.3), though relapses can occur in approximately 16% of cases. Ten to 20% of cases are left with disabling symptoms (Vucic et al., 2009).

Although weakness and sensory loss are the major impairments, persistent fatigue is a common feature in the more chronic stage with 60% reporting severe fatigue after a year. The severity of fatigue, however, does not correlate with disease severity at the nadir, peripheral nerve function or prior infections. It is, however, more prevalent in females and people over 50 years or age (Garssen et al., 2006b; Garssen et al., 2006c). A relationship was found between fatigue and central activation with repeated muscle contraction that may be due to changes in motor unit size and myelination pattern on recovery from GBS (Garssen et al., 2007). A study of Amantadine therapy, a NMDA receptor agonist, was unsuccessful in reducing fatigue symptoms in people with GBS despite some evidence of its efficacy in other neurological disorders (Garssen et al., 2006a).

Pain is frequently reported in 89% of people with GBS that is often severe and may require medical intervention with analgaesics, opioids or anti-depressants such as Gabapentine or Carbomazepine (Hughes, 2008). Pain often originates from the joints and muscles, but there can also be hyperaesthesia (Atkinson et al., 2006).

Management of Guillain Barré syndrome

The initial management of GBS is to address any serious complications, e.g. reduced vital capacity and airway protection through critical care support (see Ch. 15). Drug treatment involves the administration of intravenous immunoglobulins (IVIg) as a first-line intervention with proven efficacy in intervention trials (Hughes, 2008). IVIg can be repeatedly administered, but only if there is a response to the initial intervention (Hughes, 2008). Plasma exchange, or plasmapheresis, is another therapy where the benefits have been established in multiple intervention trials (Vucic et al., 2009). The effect of plasma exchange is to improve disability, with an increased proportion of people making a full recovery and reduction in people requiring mechanical ventilation.

There are no studies of the efficacy of rehabilitation approaches in GBS. At present intervention is based on

191

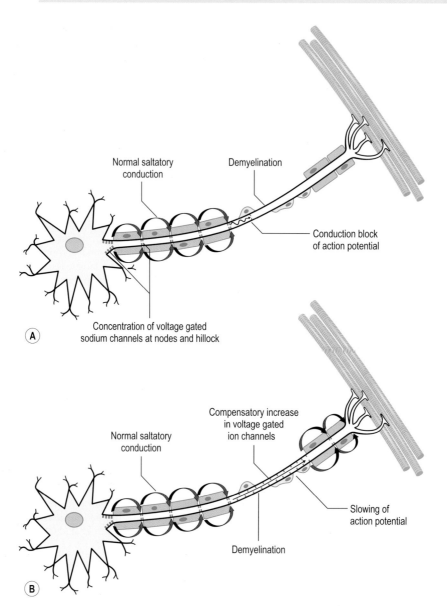

Figure 9.2 (A) Acute demyelination and conduction block. Saltatory conduction is effective where the myelin is intact, with fast propagation of the action potential. Where the axon has become demyelinated, the current is unable depolarize the membrane due to current leakage and fewer voltage-gated sodium channels. This results in a failure of conduction. (B) Chronic demyelination and conduction slowing. A compensatory increase in voltage-gated sodium channels along the demyelinated portion of the axon allows propagation of the action potential but this will be slower than saltatory conduction.

experience with other neurological conditions though the need for therapy input is recognized (Vucic et al., 2009). Physiotherapy management in the acute stage focuses on respiratory interventions and prevention of secondary complications (Khan, 2004). Respiratory treatments include sputum clearance techniques, maintenance of lung volumes and breathing exercises when the person is able to participate (see Ch. 15). Other interventions advocated are early mobilization, splinting, positioning, stretches to maintain joint range of motion and exercises to increase strength and endurance (Hughes, 2008; Khan, 2004; Meythaler, 1997). Fear, anxiety and sleep deprivation are common problems experienced by people with GBS in the early stages. Good two-way communication between the multidisciplinary team (MDT) and patient and carers is vital to ensure they are informed at every

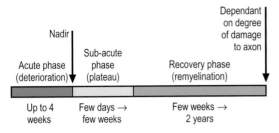

Figure 9.3 Phases and progression of Guillain Barré syndrome.

stage; though this may be challenging if a person is intubated, it can be supported by speech and language therapy intervention.

Approximately 40% of all people with GBS will need a period of multidisciplinary inpatient rehabilitation with the aim of maximizing functional recovery and participation (Khan, 2004; Meythaler, 1997). Two studies have found that the more severely affected people tend to access rehabilitation or physiotherapy services (Carroll et al., 2003; Davidson et al., 2009). The impact of therapy input may be important as a recent survey ($n>800$) of people with GBS found that 90% of people were treated by a physiotherapist, but this fell to 75% of people after discharge from hospital. The survey found that people who did not receive physiotherapy treatment as an outpatient or in the community had greater levels of disability than those who did (Davidson et al., 2009).

Chronic demyelinating polyneuropathy

Chronic demyelinating polyneuropathies can be acquired or inherited and are defined as taking more than 8 weeks to develop (Hughes, 2008). Two of the most common causes are inflammatory and genetic pathologies, and these are described in this section. The efficacy of rehabilitation of the chronic polyneuropathies will be discussed with a case study at the end of the chapter.

Chronic inflammatory demyelinating polyradiculoneuropathy

Chronic inflammatory demyelinating polyradiculoneuropathy (CIDP) is the most common acquired chronic demyelinating neuropathy affecting approximately 3 in 100 000 people (England & Asbury, 2004; Hughes, 2008). It occurs more frequently in adults aged 40 to 60 years with a slightly higher prevalence in men (Westblad et al., 2009).

CIDP has similarities to GBS in that it is an immunologically mediated neuropathy. It presents with multifocal demyelination that predominantly affects spinal nerve roots, proximal nerve trunks and plexuses leading to patchy regions of demyelination with some inflammatory infiltrates (Said, 2006). There is no genetic predisposition

to CIDP but a number of studies have suggested an infective episode or vaccination in the weeks prior to onset of the neuropathy. Approximately half of patients have antibodies against myelin-associated glycoprotein and protein levels in the CSF are raised (Said, 2006).

Presentation of chronic inflammatory demyelinating polyradiculoneuropathy

The course and presentation of CIDP is very variable and can be chronic progressive or relapse remitting. Electrophysiological testing reveals slowing and conduction block as indicative of an acquired demyelinating neuropathy (England & Asbury, 2004; Said, 2006). Reports of activity-dependant conduction block in CIDP could be functionally important as paresis can increase with repeated use (Pollard, 2002). Relapsing forms of CIDP tend to have a better prognosis than the more progressive types, but the degree of secondary axonal loss is most predictive of outcome.

Unlike some other polyneuropathies, CIDP is not length dependant, i.e. the longer nerves more affected. It is primarily a motor neuropathy that can affect distal and proximal muscles, though the distal ankle muscles are often the weakest (Westblad et al., 2009). Sensory impairment can also be present with some variants presenting with sensory ataxia. Symmetrical weakness and sensory changes develop in the limbs over more than 8 weeks, so differentiating from a diagnosis of GBS (Hughes, 2008). The majority of people have absent tendon reflexes and 4–15% can present with facial palsy (Said, 2006).

People with CIDP report problems with mobility and balance, but studies exploring the impact of the physical impairments are limited. In a study describing physical functioning, nearly 50% of subjects ($n=21$) reported that balance and walking difficulties were the worst consequences of having CIDP (Westblad et al., 2009). The same study found deficits in balance scores, timed up and go test, manual dexterity and the physical functioning domains of the SF-36 health status questionnaire.

Fatigue is reported as severe in people with CIDP and is one of the three most disabling symptoms in the majority (Merkies et al., 1999). The level of fatigue does not correlate with impairment measures of muscle strength and sensation or disease severity, so the cause of fatigue is not yet clear. The consequence of fatigue in this population, however, is the potential for a reduction in daily activity and secondary deconditioning.

Management of chronic inflammatory demyelinating polyradiculoneuropathy

Beneficial effects on the presentation of CIDP have been shown with corticosteroids, intravenous immunoglobulins and plasma exchange (Brannagan, 2009), but this is necessary over a prolonged period, which can be problematic. Long-term steroid use has difficult side-effects, IVIg is expensive and plasma exchange is inconvenient for the patient

(Hughes, 2008). The response to treatment will be determined by factors such as the degree of axonal loss. Evaluating the degree of improvement can also be hampered by a poor correlation between electrophysiological data and a lack of good, objective outcome measures (Said, 2006).

Charcot-Marie-Tooth disease type 1 (CMT1)

The most common hereditary neurological condition is a polyneuropathy called Charcot-Marie-Tooth disease (CMT) causing degeneration of the peripheral nerves and affecting about 36 in a 100 000 people (Krajewski et al., 2000; Pareyson et al., 2006). The name originates from the three neurologists who described it in 1886. The first gene causing the CMT phenotype was mapped in 1989. Since then many more have been identified and the common CMT phenotype can be caused by as many as a 100 gene mutations (Nicholson, 2006). The most common types of CMT show a slow decline in distal muscle strength and sensation that predominantly affects the longer peripheral nerves. Most genes causing CMT have autosomal dominant inheritance, though there are rarer autosomal recessive types. Family history is an important step in deciding if and how a neuropathy is inherited.

Type 1 CMT (CMT1) presents with demyelination of the more thickly myelinated, fast-conducting axons, for example the alpha motor neurons and 1a afferent sensory neurons. As with other demyelinating polyneuropathies, axonal loss occurs with prolonged demyelination. In CMT 1 there is an increase in the motor unit size, that is, an increase in the number of muscle fibres supplied by one motor axon. This occurs during the chronic, slow denervation process when unaffected motor axons are able to produce collateral sprouts that re-innervate previously denervated muscle fibres (Ericson et al., 2000).

CMT 1a refers to a type of CMT1 that is caused by the most common gene mutation. It accounts for up to 80% of people with CMT and is caused by the mutation of the PMP22 gene on the short arm of chromosome 17. Duplication of this gene affects the stability of the myelin sheath causing progressive demyelination (Pareyson et al., 2006).

The genetic test for type 1a CMT became available in the 1990s allowing diagnosis of a whole family with a simple blood test from one affected member. On electrophysiological examination, people with CMT1 have symmetrical, distal slowing of peripheral nerve conduction velocities due a reduction in saltatory conduction. They may also present with a reduction in the amplitude of compound motor action potentials (CMAP) and sensory nerve action potentials (SNAP), which will reflect the degree of secondary axonal degeneration.

Presentation of Charcot-Marie-Tooth disease type 1

Muscle wasting is one of the key signs described for people with CMT with the classic 'inverted wine bottle' appearance of the distal lower limb and 'claw hand' of the upper limb (Figure 9.4). Magnetic resonance imaging (MRI) reveals that atrophy of the distal lower limb muscles can occur even when an individual appears unaffected on clinical examination (Gallardo et al., 2006). The distal lower and upper limb muscles tend to weaken first showing a slow decline in strength over decades. The degree and extent of weakness have been correlated with axonal loss rather than demyelination in studies of the hand (Videler et al., 2008). The proximal limb muscles are less affected but some studies have found they are still weak compared to normative data (Carter et al., 1995).

In addition to weakness and wasting, a length-dependant gradual loss of sensation occurs. People with CMT1 show a principal impairment of the thickly myelinated large diameter sensory nerves that mediate the sensations of light touch and vibration (Nardone et al., 2000). However, sensations conveyed by smaller diameter fibres, e.g. pain, temperature or pin prick, may also be reduced (Carter et al., 1995).

Little has been written about hand deformity in people with CMT, but there has been interest in the presentation and evolution of foot deformity. Pes cavus is a common foot posture observed in people with CMT1 where the condition starts early in life and is described as a foot type with an excessively high longitudinal arch and foot supination (Figure 9.5). Pes cavus is often associated with hind foot varus, toe clawing and dorsiflexion of the metatarsophalangeal joints (MTPJs). These deformities are thought to evolve through muscle imbalances over time (Guyton & Mann, 2000; Holmes & Hansen, 1993; Mann & Missirian, 1988). In support of this theory, a significant correlation was found between a pes cavus foot structure and ankle dorsiflexion range in children with CMT (Burns et al., 2009).

Exploration of upper limb function has revealed that people with CMT can have impaired manual dexterity and upper limb functional tasks (Burns et al., 2008; Videler et al., 2007; Videler et al., 2008) that are related to muscle weakness (Selles et al., 2006). In the lower limb, distal weakness has been related to foot drop and failure of the plantarflexors (Vinci & Perelli, 2002), which influences the pattern of gait as people with CMT walk. Gait analysis has revealed primary distal gait impairments with problems with foot clearance during swing, and reduced contribution of the plantarflexor muscles to progression of the trunk and swing leg (Newman et al., 2007). Further exploration revealed that people with CMT utilize additional movements of the proximal joints during walking to compensate for the primary impairments of distal weakness and sensory loss (Don et al., 2007; Ramdharry et al., 2009).

Fatigue is well documented in people with CMT and 67% report severe fatigue (Kalkman et al., 2005). Self-reported fatigue has been shown to have an impact on specific functions, such as walking (Ramdharry et al., 2009), so there has been a lot of recent interest in the

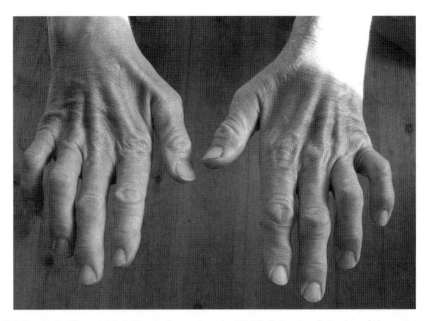

Figure 9.4 Hand deformity in Charcot-Marie-Tooth disease type 1a (CMT1a) showing flattening of the metacarpophalangeal (MCP) joints, clawing of fingers and wasting of the intrinsic hand muscles. (Reproduced with Permission from Charcot-Marie-Tooth UK.)

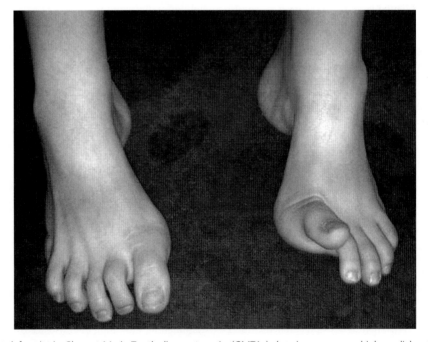

Figure 9.5 Foot deformity in Charcot-Marie-Tooth disease type 1a (CMT1a) showing pes cavus: high medial arch, midfoot supination, 1st metatarsophalangeal (MTP) dorsiflexion and toe clawing. (Reproduced with Permission from Charcot-Marie-Tooth UK.)

causes. Investigations of fatigue mechanisms have found that central fatigue exists, though no greater than healthy subjects, and there is a significant element of central activation failure that could be due to a long-standing reduction in sensory feedback (Kalkman et al., 2008; Schillings et al., 2007). As a group, people with CMT have been found to be less active than the general population (Kalkman et al., 2007) and are deconditioned, as measured by oxygen uptake during exercise (Carter et al., 1995). Aerobic deconditioning and disuse muscle atrophy are a likely consequence of reduced activity levels, which may also impact on fatigue and prolonged performance of daily tasks.

People with CMT complain of more pain than the general population (Padua et al., 2008a) though it is unclear whether the pain is directly due to the neuropathy or secondary musculoskeletal deformities. Burns et al. (2005a) found increased reports of pain in people with CMT who had a pes cavus foot deformity suggesting that musculoskeletal alignment may be a cause of foot pain.

Problems with balance are reported in the clinic by people with CMT. There have been limited investigations into balance impairments but reduced balance scores have been seen in children with CMT (Burns et al., 2009).

Investigations of quality of life for people with CMT have found lower scores than the general population and similar to those reported for people with stroke and other disabilities (Pfeiffer et al., 2001; Vinci et al., 2005). The reason for this is multi-factorial and measures of ambulation and axonal loss correlate with quality of life measures (Padua et al., 2008b). An interesting link has also been observed between quality of life and occupation in a study of 121 people. Using the short-form 36 measure, investigators found lower scores for physical functioning, physical role, emotional role and mental health for people who did not work (Vinci et al., 2005). It is unclear whether working improves these domains or whether the most physically, emotionally and mentally well people are able to continue to work for longer.

Management of Charcot-Marie-Tooth disease type 1

To date there is no drug therapy for people with CMT1, though there are currently a series of international trials investigating the efficacy of high doses of vitamin C in remyelination of axons in people with CMT1a. These trials were set up on the basis of work in a CMT mice model where high doses of vitamin C resulted in increased remyelination and improved physical function (Passage et al., 2004). There is also potential for future trials of progesterone and cucurium based on animal studies which are not yet at a stage for trials on humans (Khajavi et al., 2007; Sereda et al., 2003).

AXONAL POLYNEUROPATHIES

Chronic axonal neuropathies are the most common type of polyneuropathy. The causes vary from metabolic disorders, such as chronic renal failure and malignancy, to toxicity from chemical agents (England & Asbury, 2004). They are characterized by abnormality and degeneration of the nerve axons, so can affect nerves of any diameter and modality. Degeneration of the axon results in prevention of propagation of the nerve action potentials manifesting as reductions in amplitude of compound potentials on electrophysiological testing (Figure 9.6).

Two of the more common types of axonal neuropathy are highlighted: diabetic neuropathy and Charcot-Marie-Tooth disease type 2 (CMT2).

Diabetic neuropathy

In people over 40 years of age, the incidence of peripheral neuropathy is approximately 14%. Of these cases, half have neuropathy due to diabetes mellitus and half are idiopathic. Of the idiopathic group, it is now being suggested that pre-diabetes or impaired glucose tolerance (IGT) is a possible cause of neuropathy (Smith & Singleton, 2008).

Diabetic neuropathy is often just sensory or sensorimotor in presentation. Common complaints are burning and numbness in the feet due to the involvement of the smaller diameter, unmyelinated fibres from the cutaneous pain receptors (England & Asbury, 2004). Skin biopsies reveal reduced density of unmyelinated fibres in the epidermis indicating degeneration (England & Asbury, 2004).

The pathological process is initiated through hyperglycaemia which has a toxic effect on the nerves via oxidative stress, impaired axonal transport and accumulation of end products from glycation (Smith & Singleton, 2008). There is also an effect on the microvascular structures supporting the nerves with defects in the capillary endothelia (Smith & Singleton, 2008).

Recent work has also implicated dyslipidaemia as a possible trigger for diabetic neuropathy through oxidative stress mechanisms causing neurovascular injury. In mouse models, high fat feeding results in glucose intolerance and the development of neuropathy (Feldman, 2009). High levels of serum triglycerides in humans correlate with the progression of diabetic neuropathy (Feldman, 2009).

Presentation of diabetic neuropathy

Diagnosis of diabetic neuropathy is from neurological examination, indicating the existence of a peripheral neuropathy, and glucose tolerance testing (Hughes, 2008). The progression is slow and prognosis often depends on diabetic management.

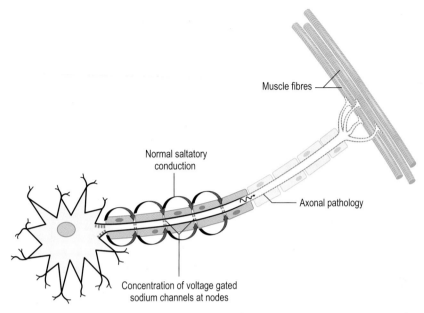

Muscle fibres

Normal saltatory
conduction

Axonal pathology

Concentration of voltage gated
sodium channels at nodes

Figure 9.6 Axonal pathology and conduction failure. Degeneration of the axon will prevent propagation of action potentials to the neuromuscular junction.

Where there is a loss of protective sensation, particularly in the foot, plantar ulceration is an unwelcome complication which can lead to partial foot or major lower extremity amputation (Kanade et al., 2006; van Deursen, 2008). Increases in pressure over the plantar surface can occur due to changes in the gait pattern and increased double support. Elevated plantar pressures can increase the risk of injury to the skin and plantar ulceration. Some concerns have been raised that if walking is encouraged as part of exercise/lifestyle advice there could be an increase in plantar pressures, so protective footwear is recommended in conjunction with this (Kanade et al., 2006). A decline on physical fitness and activity levels have been observed with increased foot complications so prevention is also important for general management of diabetes through an active lifestyle (Kanade et al., 2006).

Another consequence of sensory loss is postural instability and falls due to reduced proprioception and cutaneous sensation. Posturography studies have highlighted an increase in postural sway in people with diabetic neuropathy during static standing. One study found a modest correlation between sway and measures of sensation over the plantar surface (Ducic et al., 2004). A comparison with people with diabetes but no neuropathy demonstrated a deterioration in balance performance with static standing but no different with dynamic balance tests (Emam et al., 2009). This may be due to the various roles of the different-sized sensory afferents. The prevalence of falls in older people with neuropathy has been associated with severity of the neuropathy and body mass index.

Deficits in temporal and spatial gait parameters are also reported due to sensorimotor impairment (Paul et al., 2008). A study of muscle activation patterns in people with diabetic neuropathy revealed a delay in the first activation peaks of tibialis anterior, the peronei and soleus with treadmill walking, leading to a longer support phase (Sacco & Amadia, 2003). The investigators hypothesized that reduced sensation would lead to a delay in the loading response following initial contact. Cognitive and motor load during walking caused deterioration in temporal spatial gait parameters in people with diabetes and a group with diabetic neuropathy (Paul et al., 2008). This implies that gait impairment and falls risk may increase under dual task situations.

Management of diabetic neuropathy

The standard therapy for IGT and diabetes is diet and lifestyle advice (Smith & Singleton., 2008). In a study of 32 people with IGT neuropathy improvements in body mass index and intra-epidermal nerve fibre density (demonstrated using biopsies from proximal skin samples) were seen following a one-year diet and exercise counselling intervention. This study was not controlled but indicates that there could be changes at a fibre level with these interventions. Randomized controlled trials of exercise as an intervention to reduce neuropathy in people with diabetes are currently ongoing and preliminary results are encouraging with improvements in pain, proprioception and intra-epidermal nerve fibre density (Kluding et al., 2009; Singleton et al 2009).

Neuropathic pain and dysaesthesia can be difficult to treat, but is an important focus of medical management for people with diabetic neuropathy. Anti-epileptic drugs and anti-depressants, e.g. as Gabapentine and Amitriptyline, as well as opioids, such as Tramadol, may reduce symptoms. Topical Lidocaine can be useful where there are discreet areas of dysaesthesia (Hughes, 2008).

Charcot-Marie-Tooth disease type 2

Type 2 CMT (CMT2) presents with degeneration of the nerve axon. The axonal forms of CMT are less common than type 1; the most common mutation is of the mitofusin 2 gene, which accounts for about 20% of cases (Cartoni & Martinou, 2009). Mitofusin 2 is a mitochondrial protein that plays an important role in the process of mitochondrial fusion within a cell. In nerves, the long axon has high energy requirements far away from the nerve cell body which is provided by the mitochondria. Deficiency of mitofusin 2 seems to affect the transport of mitochondria down the axon (Cartoni & Martinou, 2009; Shy, 2004) (Figure 9.1). This can result in degeneration of the distal axon that is initially seen in longer nerves such as those supplying the foot and ankle muscles. The response to denervation seems to differ to CMT1, as people CMT2 show a compensatory increase in contractile tissue as reflected by muscle fibre hypertrophy. The reasons for the differences are not clear but it is suggested that in CMT2 there may be a reduced ability to form collateral sprouts (Ericson et al., 2000).

As with CMT1, family history is an important step to determine the inheritance but there are fewer opportunities for diagnostic genetic testing as genes for only 20% of CMT2 have been identified. Electrophysiology aids differentiation between CMT types, as people with CMT 2 have normal conduction velocities but show a symmetrical reduction in the amplitude of distal CMAPs and SNAPs due to primary axonal degeneration.

Presentation of Charcot-Marie-Tooth type 2

People with CMT2 have a very similar phenotype as people with CMT1 with slow progression of distal weakness, wasting and sensory loss. The onset of symptoms, however, may be later in life so the pes cavus foot type is not always present.

Another difference between the two types of CMT is balance. A posturography study of people with different types of CMT found that those with a more axonal presentation had increased postural sway during quiet standing. In dynamic balance situations people with both types of CMT demonstrated delays in segment co-ordination (Nardone et al., 2006).

Management of Charcot-Marie-Tooth type 2

To date, there are no specific medical interventions available or under investigation for people with CMT2. It is hoped that with a greater understanding of the biology and mechanisms of pathology, medical therapies will be developed. This is the current focus of research for this condition.

PHYSIOTHERAPY INTERVENTIONS FOR POLYNEUROPATHY

To date, much of the literature falls into two main areas: exercise and orthotics. The following section asks how efficacious exercise training and orthotic provision are in addressing the problems faced by people with polyneuropathy.

Exercise in polyneuropathy

Ascertaining the evidence for the efficacy of exercise training in people with polyneuropathy is challenging for a number of reasons. Some neuropathies are relatively rare conditions and research into exercise in neuropathy is fairly recent exploration. Two Cochrane reviews have included exercise training over the last 4 years. The first was a review of exercise for people with peripheral neuropathy (White et al., 2004) and the second was a review of treatment for people with Charcot-Marie-Tooth disease (Young et al., 2008). Both reviews found only a small body of literature on exercise in neuropathies and they both identified the same, single, randomized control trial as being the only study of sufficient quality for consideration.

The trial in question was an investigation into strength training in two patient groups, people with CMT and people with myotonic dystrophy (Lindeman et al., 1995). The 29 subjects in the CMT group were analysed separately to the dystrophy group. Subjects were randomized into training and control arms within each diagnostic group and training consisted of 60% of a maximal load for proximal lower limb muscles over a 24-week period. A moderate increase in knee extensor torques was observed in subjects with CMT which carried over into improvement in a 6 m walk.

A later study of exercise training in people with CMT was considered by the 2008 Cochrane review (Young et al., 2008), but was rejected as it did not have a control group. The study's 12 weeks of moderate strength training ($n=12$) demonstrated improvements in isometric strength in the elbow flexors and knee extensors with some carryover into functional measures (Chetlin et al., 2004).

A common feature of these two studies is that the training protocol focused on the proximal limb muscles. The primary impairment of weakness tends to be a more distal presentation in CMT and the proximal muscles are relatively spared. It is possible that the improvements seen in the strengthening studies are due to improvements in disuse atrophy, in this underactive population. The question of whether more profoundly weakened muscles will respond to training has not been fully answered. An early study suggested that muscles less than 10% of normal strength did not respond to strength training, though this was based on an investigation of a small sample of twelve people with mixed neuromuscular pathology (Milner-Brown & Miller, 1988).

Exercise training to improve aerobic fitness is deemed important in addressing the problem of de-conditioning that is prevalent in people with neuropathy. Improvements in cardiopulmonary function have been observed in other slowly progressive neuromuscular diseases (Fowler, 2002), but this has not been explored with good-quality randomized control trials. A recent study of a 24-week programme of bicycle-based interval training found improvements in oxygen uptake ($VO_{2\ peak}$) and functional measures in eight men with CMT (El Mhandi et al., 2008). There was no control group and a small sample size so the intervention requires further study, though the results are promising. This study also found decreases in reported fatigue measured by a visual analogue scale.

Two studies have investigated the effect of exercise in inflammatory neuropathy. A 12-week bicycle training programme was prescribed to sixteen people with GBS, who had made a good functional recovery, and four people with CIDP. They trained three times a week with a peak intensity of 70–90% of maximum heart rate. Participants reported significant improvements in reported fatigue, fitness levels, functional outcomes and quality of life. This was a small study with no control group, but the positive results warrant further study with randomized controlled trials (Garssen et al., 2004). Interestingly, this research team looked at the relationships between the different measurement domains and found that there was no correlation between physical fitness and functional outcomes. They found a relationship between reported fatigue and perceived physical function (Bussmann et al., 2007). This indicates that the determinants of functional ability do not necessarily correlate with fitness.

A community-based exercise study also had a mixed sample of people with stable CIDP and people 1 year post GBS nadir (Graham et al., 2007). A 12-week, unsupervised training programme was instigated that included aerobic exercise, strength training and task-specific training. Participants demonstrated significant improvements in knee extensor strength and total workload with exercise testing. There were also significant reductions in fatigue, anxiety and depression post exercise. A sub-group of five subjects showed increased activity levels, as measured by accelerometer activity monitors. This study demonstrated the feasibility and safety of such a programme, as there were no adverse events; however, again randomized controlled trials are required to determine the efficacy.

These studies highlight the need for further investigation but are beginning to demonstrate the positive benefits of exercise for people with polyneuropathy. We have seen, however, that this group comprises less active, deconditioned individuals and the reasons for this need to be explored. One of the traditional barriers to exercise for people with some neuropathies is a concern that exercise will worsen their condition. In the past, people were actively discouraged from exercising. In CIDP, people were advised not to exercise during the inflammatory phase of the condition, though evidence for increased deterioration has not been presented. In CMT, a specific pathological mechanism has not been suggested. In other conditions with enlarged motor units, e.g. post-polio syndrome, there are concerns that oxidative stress during exercise can damage already overburdened motor units (Tews, 2005). A small randomized control study of people with post polio syndrome ($n=10$) demonstrated improvements in thenar muscle MVC with strength training (Chan et al., 2003). Motor unit number estimation techniques were used to monitor any potential loss of motor units with exercise with no changes found with training. As mentioned, this has not been tested in such detail for people with CMT and other neuropathies, but other papers have explored the issue. A study assessing hand strength in 106 people with CMT claimed that increased weakness of the dominant hand was evidence of overwork weakness (Vinci et al., 2003). In this study, the MRC scale was used to assess muscle strength. Quantitative measures have been recommended in studies of people with CMT, as the MRC scale has been criticized for being unreliable and lacking in sensitivity (Burns et al., 2005b). This theory was tested in a later paper comparing hand strength using quantitative strength measurement in 28 people with CMT (Van Pomeren et al., 2009). No significant difference was found between the dominant and non-dominant hands. None of the exercise trials of people with CMT, GBS or CIDP have demonstrated any deterioration in muscle strength with training. For the time being, there is no convincing evidence of over work weakness and the problem of disuse atrophy in these deconditioned populations will probably have more functional impact. Chapter 18 outlines the growing use of exercise for managing neurological disorders and the increasing body of research.

Balance training

Balance training has been explored in people with CMT in one small randomized control trial ($n=16$) of a 12-day programme using a mechanical balance trainer/dynamic standing frame (Matjai & Zupan, 2006). The exercise group demonstrated significant improvements in the Berg balance score, the timed up and go test and the 10 m timed walk. The control group also improved their Berg balance score, but to a lesser degree. This is a small study of a very specific balance intervention, but it shows promise for future larger studies. Such studies may also be enhanced by the addition of posturography measures to help understand the mechanisms altered by training plus follow-up measures to explore longer-term effects.

Orthotic management

The provision of orthotic devices is common for people with neuropathy, although problems with non-use of splints are often reported (Vinci & Gargiulo, 2007). This section explores the evidence for the efficacy of orthotic devices and the problem of poor uptake of this intervention is also considered.

Foot orthoses have been recommended for people with foot deformity to either distribute pressure under the plantar surface or correct flexible pes cavus using lateral posting (Alexander & Johnson, 1989; Younger & Hansen, 2005). One good-quality randomized control trial investigated the effects of foot orthoses in painful pes cavus (Burns et al., 2006). As such, the main outcome measures were foot pain and function using the Foot Health Status questionnaire. The sample size was powered and the group interventions included a prescribed, custom-made foot orthosis and a flat sham insole. Groups were randomized and participants were blinded. The results demonstrated a significant improvement in foot pain and function. Analysis of plantar pressure distribution demonstrated that the customized orthoses reduced plantar pressure, particularly at the fore and hind foot, and it was concluded that this was the mechanism of the successful intervention. This study looked at a number of different conditions presenting with pes cavus, and only 16 of the subjects had CMT. In addition, there was no functional gait measure and it would have been interesting to investigate if the reduction in pain had a positive effect on parameters such as gait speed or maximal distance.

A key area of management for people with diabetic neuropathy is foot care. To reduce plantar pressures foot orthoses, custom-made shoes or casts are used to redistribute pressure, and to provide soft padding and shock absorbance through total plantar contact (van Deursen, 2008). Some of the materials used in these devices, however, could potentially threaten postural stability due to the thickness and compliance. A study using posturographic measures found that there were no differences in postural sway with foot orthoses or shoes. Total contact casts, however, did reduce postural stability, probably due to immobilization of the ankle (van Deursen, 2008). The risk of falls versus the risk of foot ulceration should be ascertained prior to the prescription of these devices.

Very few studies have investigated the use of ankle foot orthoses (AFO) in people with neuropathy. A single case study examined perceived exertion, oxygen consumption and cardiac stress for an individual with CMT when wearing a basic posterior leaf AFO and a custom-made device (Bean et al., 2001). The study found improvements in all three variables when the subject wore the custom-made AFO. Although this was a good A-B-A single case study design, it was investigating a very specific situation and individualized intervention parameters making generalization to other people difficult. A small proof of principle study used 3D motion analysis to investigate the effect of three commonly used pre-fabricated AFOs in 14 people with CMT (Ramdharry et al., 2007). Significant improvements in foot drop were seen with all of the splints immediately the devices were worn. There were no follow-up measures, the numbers were small and there was no control group so the application of these findings is limited. The study does, however, provide initial positive findings that warrant further investigation with longitudinal, controlled studies.

Another study of AFO intervention in people with CMT was an investigation of standing, although the subject group also included people with other lower motor neurone disorders (Hachisuka et al., 1997). The intention of this study was to investigate people who were able to walk but not stand still on the spot. They found that people who showed this feature had severe bilateral weakness of the posterior tibial muscles. When ankle foot orthoses were worn, 14 out of 16 subjects demonstrated a significant reduction in the path length of the centre of pressure over 30 seconds. The study did not report a group effect so it is unclear if this was significant and there was no functional measure to see if this extra support assisted the subjects in activities of daily living.

The only other study of external support was actually an investigation of the effect of night splinting to stretch the Achilles tendon (Refshauge et al., 2006). Stretching programmes have been recommended in people with flexible deformity, but it is not known if they are effective in assisting gait (Alexander & Johnson, 1989). The night splinting study recruited 14 adults and children with CMT to a randomized, cross over trial. The intervention phase involved wearing a night splint set into maximum dorsiflexion on one leg for a period of 6 weeks. The cross over process involved the splint being worn on the other leg so the non-splinted side acted as the control. The main outcome measure was passive dorsiflexion and eversion range of motion and was powered to show a change of 5° dorsiflexion. The study found no significant effects on range of motion. The authors attributed the lack of effect to problems with positioning the foot within the splint that could have affected the efficacy of the stretch applied. They acknowledge that positive subjective reports from subjects were received. This could be because of a change in stiffness of the muscles rather than passive range, but this was not measured in this study. In addition there were no functional measures to see if these subjectively reported benefits carried over into activities of daily living.

One of the challenges in rehabilitation research for people with polyneuropathy is that some of them are relatively rare conditions, so recruitment to studies can be difficult. Because there is a lot of variation in presentation, some orthotic devices will be more effective for certain presenting impairments depending on the construction and material properties of the device. In order to investigate this fully, large numbers of subjects would be required to be stratified according to their disease severity and presentation to see which devices give the best outcome. In view of the limited evidence for the efficacy of orthotic provision, clinicians should review any devices prescribed with appropriate outcome measures, depending on the aim of the device. People with polyneuropathy may be reluctant to accept orthoses, so consideration of the person's opinion and inclusion in decision-making will help to ensure that a device is prescribed that is acceptable to that individual. Measures of comfort should also be recorded over time, as ill-fitting splints can be another reason for non-use.

CASE HISTORY

A case history is outlined to explore intervention strategies for a person with CMT. Relevant evidence and clinical reasoning is presented to support the rehabilitation approaches.

Mr V. is a 32-year-old man who presented to a neuro-outpatient clinic via referral from a neurologist. He was diagnosed with type 1a CMT from family history, clinical examination, electrophysiological tests and genetic testing. Neurophysiological testing revealed slowed nerve conduction velocity in the bilateral median, ulnar and common peroneal nerves with reductions in the amplitude of the compound muscle action potential (CMAP) and sensory nerve action potentials (SNAP). Genetic testing of Mr V. and his family revealed that he had a duplication of the peripheral myelin protein 22 gene (PMP22) on chromosome 17.

Presenting impairments

a. *Musculoskeletal integrity and alignment:* Mr V. had marked distal upper limb muscle wasting in the forearm musculature, thenar eminences and intrinsic hand muscles. The hand adopted a 'claw'- like posture with flexion of the proximal and distal interphalangeal joints (PIPs and DIPs) and hyperextension of the metacarpophalangeal joints (MCPJs). In the lower limb there was marked wasting of the calf, peroneal and intrinsic foot muscles, as well as extensor digitorum brevis on the dorsum of the foot. The feet adopted a pes cavus position with calcaneal varus, dorsiflexed metatarsophalangeal joints (MTPJs) and clawed toes. Thick callous had formed on the plantar aspect under the metatarsal heads and under the lateral border of the foot. He had tight Achilles tendons and calf muscles bilaterally with restricted passive dorsiflexion of the right ankle to 2° plantar flexion (knee flexed), 5° plantar flexion (knee extended); and the left ankle to 0° (knee flexed), 2° plantar flexion (knee extended).

b. *Muscle strength and sensation:* MRC muscle testing revealed symmetrical, distal weakness of the hands and feet (see Table 9.1). Mr V. was unable to stand on his heels but could raise them from the floor when standing by 3 cm. Sensory testing revealed reduced light touch cutaneous sensation in a glove and stocking distribution. He had reduced joint position sense to the PIPs and 1st MCP of the hand and to the ankle. Pin prick and temperature sensation were intact. In standing the Romberg's test revealed increased body sway with the eyes closed.

Table 9.1 Summary of manual muscle strength testing using the Medical Research Council (MRC) scale

UPPER LIMB	MRC GRADING	LOWER LIMB	MRC GRADING
Thumb opposition, flexion, abduction	Grade 1	Toe extensors	Grade 1
Long finger flexors	Grade 3	Dorsiflexion	Grade 1
Long finger extensors	Grade 3	Plantarflexion	Grade 3+
Wrist flexors	Grade 4	Quadriceps	Grade 5
Wrist extensors	Grade 4	Hamstrings	Grade 4
Biceps	Grade 5	Hip flexors	Grade 5
Triceps	Grade 5	Hip extensors	Grade 4+

Observation of activities

a. *Upper limb function*: Mr V. demonstrated difficulties with pinch grip and power grip with the palmer aspect remaining flattened during many dexterity tasks. He demonstrated difficulty managing small fastenings and tied shoe laces by using his thumbs as a hook.

b. *Gait*: Mr V. walked with reduced step length, velocity and cadence. His gait pattern was high stepping with bilateral foot drop and delayed heel rise at pre-swing. Initial contact was with the lateral border of the mid foot. His knees hyperextended during mid stance and there was increased lateral trunk sway. Objective tests demonstrated that Mr V. walked at comfortable speed of 1.19 m per second, over 10 m, and he cover 356 m during 6 minutes of walking. During the 6-minute walk he reported his level of effort as 11 out of 20 on the Borg perceived exertion scale (Borg, 1970).

Mr V.'s reported problems and impact on participation

a. *Fatigue*: Mr V. worked full time for a recruitment company. He reported general fatigue where he would wake tired and not be refreshed by rest. He felt exhausted after a day's work and did little in the evening as a result. Mr V. also reported increased fatigue related to activity, e.g. prolonged walking or standing and needed to take breaks on shopping trips. He scored 37 out of 63 of the Fatigue Severity Scale indicating moderate levels of self-reported fatigue (Krupp, 2003).

b. *Balance*: Mr V. complained of difficulty standing for long periods on the spot, e.g. at work-related functions and when queuing for a bus. He reported falling approximately four to five times per month. These problems were long standing with Mr V. admitting clumsiness, falling and poor performance in school sports as a child. On assessment, Mr V. achieved 50 out of 56 on the Berg Balance Scale (Berg et al. 1989).

c. *Pain*: Mr V. reported diffuse pain anterior to the right lateral malleolus and metatarsal heads with prolonged walking that reached 4/10 on a visual analogue scale.

Physiotherapy options for Mr V.

In order to ascertain the best interventions for the problems Mr V. presented with, we must turn to the literature exploring rehabilitation for people with polyneuropathy (see above).

Management of gait and balance impairments

Orthotic prescription

Foot orthoses have been seen to be effective for reducing pain for people with pes cavus (Burns et al., 2006). Mr V. was prescribed full foot orthoses with medial, lateral and transverse arch pads to support the plantar surface and spread weight bearing. The insoles also had a small, 5° lateral wedge under the calcaneus and midfoot to de-weight the lateral border of the foot.

Mr V. was also prescribed bilateral Push ankle braces (Nea International, Maastricht, Netherlands) which are braces originally designed for ankle instability. Push braces are made of neoprene with calcaneal and lateral support. Preliminary studies have found that Push braces reduce foot drop without compromising the action of the plantar flexor muscles (Ramdharry et al., 2007). Mr V. had grade 3+ strength of his plantar flexor muscles that could contribute to gait (Neptune et al., 2001), so this benefit was a consideration. It was also felt that the lateral support would be helpful when walking for longer distances in view of the right foot and ankle pain. Mr V. preferred the appearance of the Push braces as they looked more 'sporty' than plastic AFOs he'd tried previously. He reported they were more comfortable and caused less rubbing due to the softer materials, an important consideration for people with sensory impairment.

Range of movement

It was theorized that the knee hyperextension and early heel raise Mr V. experienced while walking was mainly due to tightness of the Achilles tendon and calf muscles rather than weakness. It was deemed safe to stretch the calf as he had reasonable strength of the calf muscles. There are some concerns about over stretching muscles in people with severe weakness, as the soft tissue tightness may have a role in supporting the ankle during mid to late stance phase (Salsich & Mueller, 2000). He was given weight-bearing calf stretches with the knee in flexion and extension with 1 minute holds. Mr V. was instructed to do the calf stretches only with the foot orthoses on as the wedging would bring the sub-talar joint into a more neutral position so avoiding overstretching of adjacent structures due to poor alignment. In view of Mr V.'s busy work schedule, he was advised to stand and do the stretches every time he made himself a cup of tea, while he was waiting for the kettle to boil. This amounted to approximately four times per day.

Muscle strength

Strengthening exercises were prescribed for his proximal lower limb muscles as the evidence demonstrates improvements in strength and gait function (Chetlin et al., 2004;

Lindeman et al., 1995). Mr V. joined a gym near work and went 1–2 times per week. He was prescribed a programme of resistance training for the proximal lower limb muscles starting at 8 repetitions at 12 RM, progressing to 12 repetitions then gradually increasing the load to 10 RM. This prescription was based on recommendations for improving muscle strength and endurance (ACSM, 2006). He was also cautiously given a heel-raise exercise at 5–8 repetitions, but was instructed to stop if he experienced excessive muscle soreness, muscle tightness or increased weakness. Since the evidence is not yet clear about strengthening muscles with primary weakness, this was closely monitored. In addition, combining this exercise with his stretching regime would ensure that the repeated heel raise exercise did not further tighten the plantar flexor muscles.

Balance

Mr V. was given a tandem standing exercise to challenge his balance when standing near a support. He added this to his calf-stretching programme. In addition, he had identified difficulty with prolonged standing in queues, etc. On discussion with Mr V., it was felt a collapsible walking stick would be helpful to carry in his work bag so he could use it for support and stabilize him in standing as required.

Outcomes

Mr V. gradually increased the length of time that he wore the orthotic devices over 1 week culminating in them being worn for most of his active day. He reported a marked reduction in pain to 1 out of 10 on a visual analogue scale with prolonged walking.

After 12 weeks of his exercise programme and new orthoses, improvements in gait quality were observed with better heel strike on initial contact and improved knee alignment on mid stance (wearing orthoses). His gait speed improved slightly to 1.22 m per second, but most improvement was seen in the 6-minute test where he walked 402 m. He reported a Borg level 9 out of 20 for exertion during the test.

His Berg balance score stayed the same at 50 out of 56, but he reported tripping less when wearing the ankle braces, resulting in fewer falls. The strategy of using the collapsible walking stick proved helpful for periods of prolonged standing, but Mr V. admitted he would also find other external supports if available. e.g. walls or rails.

Management of upper limb function

The evidence base for management of upper limb problems is very deficient. The following interventions were based on clinical judgment and best practice.

Orthotics and equipment

Mr V. was referred to the Occupational Therapy (OT) service and his upper limb function was managed in joint OT/Physiotherapy sessions. Mr V. trialled a neoprene thumb spica splint, applied in order to bring the thumb into abduction and flexion. This aided opposition with the other fingers and allowed a pinch grip with medium-sized objects. The OT obtained a button hook and elastic laces to help with his dressing issues.

Stretches

He was taught stretches on a table top to extend the DIP and PIP joints, while maintaining MCP joint flexion, and encouraged to perform this through the day while at work.

Outcome

Mr V. found the equipment useful to aid dressing. He decided to stop using the thumb spica as he felt it interfered with how he had learned to do particular tasks. CMT is a slowly progressing condition and people problem-solve tasks, developing compensatory strategies over time. In this case, the change imposed by the splint altered his movement strategies and impaired function.

Management of fatigue

Fatigue management

The referral to OT also included fatigue management, to address issues such as pacing and strategies to manage activities with limited energy resources. No studies to date have explored the efficacy of fatigue management strategies for people with CMT, but a focus group study found that participants recommended organization, taking breaks and prioritizing tasks as ways of managing their fatigue (Ramdharry et al., 2010).

Cardiovascular exercise

On joining the gym, Mr V. found he enjoyed using the static bicycle, starting at 10 minutes low resistance and increasing to 30 minutes by 1 minute per week. Preliminary studies of bicycle training have been found to be safe for people with CMT and may help with fatigue and deconditioning (El Mhandi et al., 2008).

Outcome

Mr V. said he found the fatigue management advice helpful and had trialled some of the strategies. He reported finding the exercise sessions at the gym 'refreshing' and felt he had more energy. He started walking from his train stop to work each morning rather than getting the bus, but felt too tired to do this in the evening. On reassessment, he scored 30 out of 63 using the Fatigue Severity Score.

Follow-up

Mr V. was followed-up to monitor progress with his programme of intervention. He was then discharged with open access to the service. This would enable him to self-refer in the future. People with progressive conditions often benefit from open access and self-referral systems so they can re-enter services quickly as new issues occur. When educated about their condition and therapy interventions that could help them in the future, they have more control over when and what assistance to seek.

CONCLUSION

The current level of research into exercise and orthotic management is only emerging, but exercise, splints and braces have been part of established practice for many years. In the absence of supporting literature, physiotherapists should try to be specific in regimes they prescribe to match with the goal of intervention. If there is a problem with peak strength or muscle endurance then the protocol of load and repetition should reflect this. If the aim is to improve function then an element of task-related training should also be incorporated into rehabilitation programmes. Where there is a gap in scientific support then rigorous assessment, measurement and review are important to ascertain responsiveness to an intervention, so building knowledge that can be used to inform larger, good-quality rehabilitation trials.

REFERENCES

Alexander, I.J., Johnson, K.A., 1989. Assessment and management of pes cavus in Charcot-Marie-Tooth disease. Clin. Orthop. Relat. Res. 246, 273–280.

Ali, M.I., Fernandez-Perez, E.R., Pendem, S., Brown, D.R., Widjdicks, E.F.M., Gajic, O., 2006. Mechanical ventilation in patients with Guillain-Barré syndrome. Respir. Care 51, 1403–1407.

American College of Sports Medicine, 2006. ACSM's Guidelines for Exercise Testing and Prescription. Lippincot, Williams & Wilkins, Philadelphia.

Atkinson, S.B., Carr, R.L., Maybee, P., Haynes, D., 2006. The challenges of managing and treating Guillain-Barré syndrome during the acute phase. Dimens. Crit. Care Nurs. 25, 256–263.

Bean, J., Walsh, A., Frontera, W., 2001. Brace modification improves aerobic performance in Charcot-Marie-Tooth disease. Am. J. Phys. Med. Rehabil. 80, 578–582.

Berg, K., Wood-Dauphinee, S., Williams, J.I., Gayton, D., 1989. Measuring balance in the elderly: preliminary development of an instrument. Physiother. Can. 41, 304–311.

Brannagan, T.H., 2009. Current treatments of chronic immune-mediated demyelinating polyneuropathies. Muscle Nerve 39, 563–578.

Borg, G.V., 1970. Psychosocial basis of perceived exertion. Med. Sci. Sports Exerc. 14, 377–381.

Burns, J., Bray, P., Cross, L.A., North, K. N., Ryan, M.M., Ouvrier, R.A., 2008. Hand involvement in children with Charcot-Marie-Tooth disease type 1A. Neuromuscul. Disord. 18, 970–973.

Burns, J., Crosbie, J., Hunt, A., Ouvrier, R., 2005a. The effect of pes cavus on foot pain and plantar pressure. Clin. Biomech. (Bristol, Avon) 20, 877–882.

Burns, J., Redmond, A., Ouvrier, R., Crosbie, J., 2005b. Quantification of muscle strength and imbalance in neurogenic pes cavus, compared to healthy controls, using hand held dynamometry. Foot Ankle Int. 26, 540–544.

Burns, J., Crosbie, J., Ouvrier, R., Hunt, A., 2006. Effective orthotic therapy for painful cavus foot. A randomised controlled trial. J. Am. Podiatr. Med. Assoc. 3, 205–211.

Burns, J., Ryan, M.M., Ouvrier, R.A., 2009. Evolution of foot and ankle manifestations in children with CMT1a. Muscle Nerve 39, 158–166.

Bussmann, J.B., Garssen, M.P.J., Van Doorn, P.A., Stam, H.J., 2007. Analysing the favourable effects of physical exercise: relationships between physical fitness, fatigue and functioning in Guillain-Barré syndrome and chronic demyelinating inflammatory demyelinating polyneuropathy. Neuromuscular Diseases 39, 121–125.

Carroll, A., McDonnell, G., Barnes, M., 2003. A review of the management of Guillain-Barré syndrome in a regional neurological rehabilitation unit. Int. J. Rehabil. Res. 26, 297–302.

Carter, G.T., Abresch, R.T., Fowler, W.M., Johnson, E.R., Kilmer, D.D., McDonald, C.M., 1995. Profiles of Neuromuscular Disease: Hereditary Motor and Sensory Neuropathy, Types I and II. Am. J. Phys. Med. Rehabil. 74 (Suppl.), S140–S149.

Cartoni, R., Martinou, J., 2009. Role of mitofusin 2 mutations in the physiopathology of Charcot-Marie-Tooth disease type 2A. Exp. Neurol. 218, 268–273.

Chan, K.M., Amirjani, N., Sumrain, M., Clarke, A., Strohschein, F.J., 2003. Randomised controlled trial of strength training in post-polio patients. Muscle Nerve 27, 332–338.

Chetlin, R.D., Gutmann, L., Tarnopolsky, M., Ullrich, I.H., Yeater, R.A., 2004. Resistance training effectiveness in patients with Charcot-Marie-Tooth disease:

recommendations for exercise prescription. Arch. Phys. Med. Rehabil. 85, 1217–1223.

Davidson, I., Wilson, C., Walton, T., Brissenden, S., 2009. Physiotherapy and Guillain-Barré syndrome: the results of a national survey. Physiotherapy 95, 157–163.

Don, R., Serrao, M., Vinci, P., Ranavolo, A., Cacchio, A., Ioppolo, F., et al., 2007. Foot drop and plantar flexion failure determine different gait strategies in Charcot-Marie-Tooth patients. Clinical Biomechanics 22, 905–916.

Ducic, I., Short, K.W., Dellon, A.L., 2004. Relationship between loss of pedal sensibility, balance and falls in patients with peripheral neuropathy. Ann. Plast. Surg. 52, 535–540.

El Mhandi, L., Millet, G.Y., Calmels, P., Ricahrd, A., Oullion, R., Gautheron, V., et al., 2008. Benefits of interval training on fatigue and functional capacities in Charcot-Marie-Tooth disease. Muscle Nerve 37, 601–610.

Emam, A.A., Gad, A.M., Ahmed, M.M., Assal, H.S., Mousa, S.G., 2009. Quantitative assessment of posture stability using computerised dynamic posturography in type 2 diabetic patients with neuropathy and its relation to glycaemic control. Singapore Med. J. 50, 614–618.

England, J.D., Asbury, A.K., 2004. Peripheral neuropathy. The Lancet 363, 2151–2161.

Ericson, U., Borg, J., Borg, K., 2000. Macro EMG and muscle biopsy of paretic foot dorsiflexors in Charcot-Marie-Tooth disease. Muscle Nerve 23, 217–222.

Feldman, E.L., 2009. Diabetic neuropathy: mechanisms to management. J. Peripher. Nerv. Syst. 14 (Suppl.), 2.

Fowler, W.M., 2002. Consensus conference summary. Role of physical activity and exercise training in neuromuscular diseases. Am. J. Phys. Med. Rehabil. 81 (Suppl.), S187–S195.

Gallardo, E., Garcia, A., Combarros, O., Berciano, J., 2006. Charcot-Marie-Tooth disease type 1A duplication spectrum of clinical and magnetic resonance imaging features in leg and foot muscles. Brain 129, 429–437.

Garssen, M.P.J., Bussman, J.B.J., Schmitz, P.I.M., Zandbergen, A., Welter, T.G., Merkies, I.S.J., et al., 2004. Physical training and fatigue, fitness, and quality of life in Guillain-Barré syndrome and CIDP. Neurology 63, 2393–2395.

Garssen, M.P.J., Schmitz, P.I.M., Merkies, I.S.J., Jacobs, B.C., van der Meché, F.G.A., van Doorn, P.A., 2006a. Amantadine for treatment of fatigue in Guillain- Barré Syndrome: a randomised, double blind, placebo controlled, crossover trial. J. Neurol. Neurosurg. Psychiatry 77, 61–65.

Garssen, M.P.J., Van Doorn, P.A., Visser, G.H., 2006b. Nerve conduction studies in relation to residual fatigue in Guillain-Barré Syndrome. J. Neurol. 253, 851–856.

Garssen, M.P.J., Van Koningsveld, R., Van Doorn, P.A., 2006c. Residual fatigue is independent of antecedent events and disease severity in Guillain-Barré Syndrome. J. Neurol. 253, 1143–1146.

Garssen, M.P.J., Schillings, M.L., van Doorn, P.A., van Engelen, B.G.M., Zwarts, M.J., 2007. Contribution of central and peripheral factors to residual fatigue in Guillain-Barré syndrome. Muscle Nerve 36, 93–99.

Graham, R.C., Hughes, R.A.C., White, C.M., 2007. A prospective study of physiotherapist prescribed community based exercise in inflammatory peripheral neuropathy. J. Neurol. 254, 228–235.

Guyton, G.P., Mann, R.A., 2000. The pathogenesis and surgical management of foot deformity in Charcot-Marie-Tooth disease. Foot Ankle Clin. 5, 317–326.

Hachisuka, K., Ohnishi, A., Yamaga, M., Dozono, K., Ueta, M., Ogata, H., 1997. The role of triceps weakness surae muscles in astasia without abasia. J. Neurol. Neurosurg. Psychiatry , vol. 62. pp. 496–500.

Holmes, J., Hansen, S.T., 1993. Foot and ankle manifestations of Charcot-Marie-Tooth disease. Foot and Ankle 14, 476–485.

Hughes, R., 2008. Peripheral nerve diseases. Practical Neurology 8, 396–405.

Kalkman, J.S., Schillings, M.L., van der Werf, S.P., Padberg, G.W., Zwarts, M.J., van Engelen, B.G.M., et al., 2005. Experienced fatigue in fascioscapulohumeral dystrophy, myotonic dystrophy, and HMSN-1. J. Neurol. Neurosurg. Psychiatry 76, 1406–1409.

Kalkman, J.S., Schillings, M.L., Zwarts, M.J., van Engelen, B.G.M., Bleijenberg, G., 2007. The development of a model of fatigue in neuromuscular disorders: a longitudinal study. J. Psychosom. Res. 62, 571–579.

Kalkman, J.S., Zwarts, M.J., Schillings, M.L., van Engelen, B.G.M., Bleijenberg, G., 2008. Different types of fatigue in patients with fascioscapulohumeral dystrophy, myotonic dystrophy and HMSN-1. Experienced fatigue and physiological fatigue. Neurol. Sci. 29, S238–S240.

Kanade, R.V., van Deursen, R., Harding, K., Price, P., 2006. Walking performance in people with diabetic neuropathy: benefits and threats. Diabetologia 49, 1747–1754.

Khajavi, M., Shiga, K., Wiszniewski, W., He, F., Shaw, C.A., Yan, J., et al., 2007. Oral curcumin mitigates the clinical and neuropathologic phenotype of the Trembler-J mouse: a potential therapy for inherited neuropathy. Am. J. Hum. Genet. 81, 438–453.

Khan, F., 2004. Rehabilitation in Guillain Barré syndrome. Aust. Fam. Physician 33, 1013–1017.

Kluding, P., Pasnoor, M., Rupali, R., Tseng, B., Moses, R., Herbelin, L., et al., 2009. Beneficial effects of exercise on diabetic neuropathy. J. Peripher. Nerv. Syst. 14 (Suppl.), 76.

Krajewski, K.M., Lewis, R.A., Fuerst, D.R., Turansky, C., Hinderer, S.R., Garbern, J., et al., 2000. Neurological dysfunction and axonal degeneration in Charcot-Marie-Tooth disease 1a. Brain 123, 1516–1527.

Krupp, L.B., 2003. Measurement of fatigue. Fatigue. Butterworth Heinemann, Philadelphia.

Lindeman, E., Leffers, P., Spaans, F., Drukker, J., Reulen, J., Kerckhoffs, M., et al., 1995. Strength training in patients with myotonic dystrophy and hereditary motor and sensory neuropathy: a randomized clinical trial. Arch. Phys. Med. Rehabil. 76, 612–620.

Mann, R.A., Missirian, J., 1988. Pathophysiology of Charcot-Marie-Tooth disease. Clin. Orthop. Relat. Res. 234, 221–228.

Matjai, Z., Zupan, A., 2006. Effects of balance training during standing and stepping in patients with hereditary sensory motor neuropathy. Disabil. Rehabil. 28, 1455–1459.

Merkies, I.S.J., Schmitz, P.I.M., Samijn, J.P.A., van der Meche, F.G.A., Van Doorn, P.A., 1999. Fatigue in immune mediated polyneuropathies. Neurology 53, 1648–1654.

Meythaler, J.M., 1997. Rehabilitation of Guillain-Barré syndrome. Arch. Phys. Med. Rehabil. 78, 872–879.

Milner-Brown, H.S., Miller, R.G., 1988. Muscle strengthening through high-resistance weight training in patients with neuromuscular disorders. Arch. Phys. Med. Rehabil. 69, 14–19.

Nardone, A., Grasso, M., Schieppati, M., 2006. Balance control in peripheral neuropathy: are patients equally stable under static and dynamic conditions. Gait Posture 23, 364–373.

Nardone, A., Tarantola, J., Miscio, G., Pisano, F., Schenone, A., Schieppati, M., 2000. Loss of large diameter spindle afferent fibres is not detrimental to the control of body sway during upright stance: evidence from neuropathy. Exp. Brain Res. 135, 155–162.

Neptune, R.R., Kautz, S.A., Zajac, F.E., 2001. Contributions of the individual ankle plantar flexors to support, forward progression and swing initiation during walking. J. Biomech. 34, 1387–1398.

Newman, C.J., Walsh, M., O'Sullivan, R., Jenkinson, A., Bennett, D., Lynch, B., et al., 2007. The characteristics of gait in Charcot-Marie-Tooth disease types I and II. Gait Posture 26, 120–127.

Nicholson, G.A., 2006. The dominantly inherited motor and sensory neuropathies: clinical and molecular advances. Muscle Nerve 33, 589–597.

Padua, L., Cavallaro, T., Pareyson, D., Quattrone, A., Vita, G., Schenone, A., 2008a. Charcot-Marie-Tooth and pain: correlations with neurophysiological, clinical and disability findings. Neurol. Sci. 29, 193–194.

Padua, L., Shy, M.E., Aprile, I., Cavallaro, T., Pareyson, D., Quattrone, A., et al., 2008b.

Correlation between clinical/neurophysiological findings and quality of life in Charcot-Marie-Tooth type 1a. J. Peripher. Nerv. Syst. 13, 64–70.

Pareyson, D., Scaioli, V., Laurà, M., 2006. Clinical and electrophysiological aspects of Charcot-Marie-Tooth disease. Neuromolecular Med. 8, 3–22.

Passage, E., Norreel, J.C., Noack-Fraissignes, P., Sanguedolce, V., Pizant, J., Thirion, X., et al., 2004. Ascorbic acid treatment corrects the phenotype of a mouse model of Charcot-Marie-Tooth disease. Nat. Med. 10, 396–401.

Paul, L., Ellis, B.M., Leeset, G.P., McFadyen, A.K., McMurray, B., 2008. The effect of a cognitive or motor task on gait parameters of diabetic patients, with and without neuropathy. Diabet. Med. 26, 234–239.

Pfeiffer, G., Wicklein, E.M., Ratusinski, T., Schmitt, L., Kunze, K., 2001. Disability and quality of life in Charcot-Marie-Tooth disease type 1. J. Neurol. Neurosurg. Psychiatry 70, 548–550.

Pollard, J.D., 2002. Chronic inflammatory demyelinating polyradiculoneuropathy. Curr. Opin. Neurol. 15, 279–283.

Ramdharry, G., Day, B., Reilly, M., Marsden, J., 2007. Walking in Charcot-Marie-Tooth disease: the role of proximal compensatory strategies and the impact of ankle foot orthoses. In: Charcot Marie Tooth disease Second International Charcot-Marie-Tooth Consortium Meeting. Snowbird, Utah, USA 18–20 July 2007.

Ramdharry, G., Day, B., Reilly, M., Marsden, J., 2009. Hip Flexor Fatigue limits walking in Charcot-Marie-Tooth disease. Muscle Nerve 40, 103–111.

Ramdharry, G.M., Reilly, M.M., Marsden, J.F., 2010. Exploring the experience of living with fatigue in people with Charcot-Marie-Tooth disease: a qualitative study. Neuromuscular Disorders 20S1, S18–19.

Refshauge, K.M., Raymond, J., Nicholson, G.A., van den Dolder, P.A., 2006. Night splinting does not increase ankle range of motion in people with Charcot-Marie-Tooth disease: a randomised, cross-over trial. Aust. J. Physiother. 52, 193–199.

Sacco, I.C., Amadia, A.C., 2003. Influence of the diabetic neuropathy on the behaviour of electromyographic and sensorial responses in treadmill gait. Clin. Biomech. (Bristol, Avon) 18, 426–434.

Said, G., 2006. Chronic inflammatory demyelinating polyneuropathy. Neuromuscul. Disord. 16, 293–303.

Salsich, G.B., Mueller, M.J., 2000. Effect of plantar flexor muscle stiffness on selected gait characteristics. Gait Posture 11, 207–216.

Schillings, M.L., Kalkman, J.S., Janssen, H.M.H.A., van Engelen, B.G.M., Bleijenberg, G., Zwarts, M.J., 2007. Experienced and physiological fatigue in neuromuscular disorders. Clin. Neurophysiol. 118, 292–300.

Selles, R.W., van Ginneken, B.T.J., Schreuders, T.A.R., Janssen, W.G.M., Stam, H.J., 2006. Dynamometry of intrinsic hand muscles inpatients with Charcot-Marie-Tooth disease. Neurology 67, 2022–2027.

Sereda, M.W., Meyer, Z.U., Hörste, G., Suter, U., Uzma, N., Nave, K.A., 2003. Therapeutic administration of progesterone antagonist in a model of Charcot-Marie-Tooth disease (CMT-1A). Nat. Med. 9, 1533–1537.

Shy, M.E., 2004. Charcot-Marie-Tooth disease: an update. Curr. Opin. Neurol. 17, 579–585.

Singleton, J.R., Marcus, R.L., Smith, S.B., Arsenault, C., Burch, A., Smith, A.G., 2009. Supervised exercise improves small fibre function in diabetic subjects without neuropathy. J. Peripher. Nerv. Syst. 14 (Suppl.), 136.

Smith, A.G., Singleton, J.R., 2008. Impaired glucose tolerance and neuropathy. Neurologist 1, 23–29.

Tews, D.S., 2005. Muscle-fibre apoptosis in neuromuscular diseases. Muscle Nerve 32, 443–458.

van Deursen, R., 2008. Footwear for the neuropathic patient: offloading and stability. Diabetes Metab. Res. Rev. 24 (Suppl. 1), S96–S100.

Van Pomeren, M., Selles, R.W., Van Ginneken, B.T.J., Schreuders, T.A.R., Janssen, W.G.M., Stam, H.J., 2009. The hypothesis of overwork weakness in Charcot-Marie-Tooth: a critical evaluation. J. Rehabil. Med. 41, 32–34.

Videler, A.J., Beelen, A., Nollet, F., 2007. Manual dexterity and related functional limitations in hereditary motor and sensory neuropathy. An explorative study. Disabil. Rehabil. 30, 634–638.

Videler, A.J., van Dijk, J.P., Beelen, A., de Visser, M., Nollet, F., van Schaik, I.N., 2008. Motor axon loss is associated with hand dysfunction in Charcot-Marie-Tooth disease 1a. Neurology 71, 1254–1260.

Vinci, P., Esposito, C., Perelli, S.L., Antenor, J.A.V., Thomas, F.P., 2003. Overwork weakness in Charcot-Marie-Tooth disease. Arch. Phys. Med. Rehabil. 84, 825–827.

Vinci, P., Gargiulo, P., 2007. Poor compliance with ankle-foot-orthoses in Charcot-Marie-Tooth disease. Eura. Medicophys. 43, 1–5.

Vinci, P., Perelli, S.L., 2002. Foot drop, foot rotation, and plantarflexor failure in Charcot-Marie-Tooth disease. Arch. Phys. Med. Rehabil. 83, 513–516.

Vinci, P., Serrao, M., Didda, A., De Santis, F., Capici, S., Martini, D., et al., 2005. Quality of life in patients with Charcot-Marie-Tooth disease. Neurology 65, 922–924.

Vucic, S., Kiernan, M.C., Cornblath, D.R., 2009. Guillain-Barré syndrome: an update. J. Clin. Neurosci. 16, 733–741.

Westblad, M.E., Forsberg, A., Press, R., 2009. Disability and health status in patients with chronic inflammatory demyelinating polyneuropathy. Disabil. Rehabil. 31, 720–725.

White, C.M., Pritchard, J., Turner-Stokes, L., 2004. Exercise for people with peripheral neuropathy (review). Cochrane Database Syst. Rev. [Online] Issue 4.

Young, P., De Jonghe, P., Stogbauer, F., Butterfass-Bahloul, T., 2008. Treatment for Charcot-Marie-Tooth disease. Cochrane Database Syst. Rev. [Online] Issue 1.

Younger, A.S.E., Hansen, S.T., 2005. Adult cavovarus foot. J. Am. Acad. Orthop. Surg. 13, 302–315.

USEFUL WEBSITE

Charcot-Marie-Tooth UK, www.cmt.org.uk.

Chapter | **10** |

Muscle disorders

Nicola Thompson, Ros Quinlivan

CONTENTS

INTRODUCTION

Muscle diseases include a number of rare, often progressive conditions leading to physical disability and, frequently, reduced life expectancy. Although each condition is rare, the overall prevalence of muscle disease is 1:1000 and individual disorders tend to present at around the same age, although there may be a wide range. Significant improvements in management means that affected children are surviving to middle age where previously they would have died and they are now presenting for care in adulthood (Wagner et al., 2007). Knowledge of these conditions tends to be poor outside the specialist area of paediatric physiotherapy. This chapter gives an overview of the most frequently seen disorders so the physiotherapist is aware of the different diagnoses which can influence overall management. For many conditions, management strategies are transferable and knowledge of the most frequently seen conditions will be relevant even to the most rare disorder. For a comprehensive text on muscle disorders the reader is referred to Dubowitz (1995).

CLASSIFICATION AND DIAGNOSTIC INVESTIGATIONS

Since the 1980s tremendous advances in genetics and molecular biology have enhanced our understanding of the pathogenesis of muscle disorders. This has led to the availability of genetic testing for many conditions which has broadened our concept of classical phenotypes to include milder, even subclinical presentations. Becker muscular dystrophy (BMD) is a good example, whereby the disorder can result in loss of mobility as early as 16 years of age or as late as the sixth decade (Bradley et al., 1978), yet some patients present only with exertional cramps and myoglobinuria (Gospe et al., 1989). The limb girdle muscular dystrophies (LGMD) are another example. They are a heterogeneous group of disorders classified according to age of onset, inheritance pattern, and molecular and genetic defect, as shown in Table 10.1. The classification of congenital muscular dystrophies (CMD), based on clinical and/or pathological features, is also expanding and several forms are alleic with LGMD as shown in Table 10.2.

Other conditions included within the diagnostic category of muscle disease are the congenital myopathies, myotonic disorders, spinal muscular atrophies (SMA),

Table 10.1 Classification of the limb girdle and sex-linked muscular dystrophies in relation to the genetic defect

TYPE	GENE LOCUS	GENE PRODUCT
Autosomal dominant		
LGMD1A	5q22-q34	Myotilin
LGMD1B	1q11-21	Lamin A/C
ADEDMD	1q11-21	Lamin A/C
LGMD1C	3p25	Caveolin 3
Autosomal recessive		
LGMD2A	15q15.1-q21.1	Calpain 3
LGMD2B	2p13	Dysferlin
LGMD2C	13q12	γ Sarcoglycan
LGMD2D	17q21	α Sarcoglycan
LGMD2E	4q12	β Sarcoglycan
LGMD2F	5q33-q34	δ Sarcoglycan
LGMD2G	17q11-12	Telethonin
LGMD2H	9q31-34.1	Not yet known
LGMD2I	19q13.3	FKRP
LGMD2J	2q31	Titin
LGMD2K	9q34.1	POMT1
LGMD2L	11p13-p12	
LGMD2M	9q31	POMT2
Sex-linked		
Dystrophinopathy	Xp21	Dystrophin
(DMD, BMD)		
EDMD	Xq28	Emerin

LGMD, limb girdle muscular dystrophy; ADEDMD, autosomal dominant Emery Dreifuss muscular dystrophy; DMD, Duchenne muscular dystrophy; BMD, Becker muscular dystrophy; EDMD, Emery Dreifuss muscular dystrophy.

Table 10.2 Classification of congenital muscular dystrophies

TYPE	GENE	PROTEIN	DISEASE
MDC1A (LAMA2)	6q2	Laminin α 1 chain of merosin	Merosin deficient CMD
FCMD	9q31-33	Fukutin	Fukuyama CMD
ITGA7	12q	Inegrin α deficiency	
MEB	1q3	POMGnT1	Muscle eye brain disease
WWS	9q34 14q24.3	POMT1 POMT2	Walker Warburg syndrome
RSMD1	1q36	SEPN1	Rigid spine syndrome
MDC1B	1q42	Secondary merosin deficiency	CMD with secondary merosin deficiency 1
MDC1C	19q1	FKRP	CMD with secondary merosin deficiency 2
UCMD	21q22.3 21q32 2q37	COL6A1 COL6A2 COL6A3	Ulrich CMD

and mitochondrial and metabolic myopathies, as well as disorders affecting the neuromuscular junction, which can be inherited or acquired. Despite many advances in the field, a definitive diagnosis will still be lacking for some individuals other than the finding of clinical and pathological features of a myopathy.

Acquired neuromuscular disorders are more common in adults than children. Polymyositis and dermatomyositis are inflammatory conditions presenting with weakness and pain. The onset is either acute or subacute and may be precipitated by infections in children or malignancy in adults. Myasthenia gravis is an autoimmune disorder presenting in adults or older children, frequently associated with a thymoma (a benign enlargement of the thymus); there may be a history of diplopia (double vision), ptosis (droopy eyelids), bulbar symptoms and weakness precipitated by repetitive tasks. In adults, endocrine disorders, especially hypothyroidism, can present as a myopathy.

The history will most often elicit functional difficulites such as frequent tripping or legs giving way and difficulty climbing stairs. Examination may reveal muscle hypertrophy or wasting or a combination of both and nearly always muscle weakness involving facial, axial, proximal, distal or global muscles, depending on the disorder. Some disorders, such as Emery Dreifuss muscular dystrophy (EDMD), present with disproportionately severe joint contractures. Exercise-induced myalgia (muscle pain) is more likely to be the presenting complaint of a metabolic or mitochondrial myopathy, although it can be a feature of BMD. The development of a systemic complication, such as early-onset cataracts or cardiac rhythm disorder, can be the presenting feature of a muscle disorder such as myotonic dystrophy.

The severity of respiratory muscle involvement does not always correlate with the severity of skeletal weakness and it is, therefore, essential that all patients with neuromuscular disorders are monitored regularly for forced vial capacity (FVC) (Griggs et al., 1981; Hough, 1991; also see Ch. 15). Symptoms of incipient respiratory failure include recurrent chest infections, weight loss, early-morning headaches, sweating, disturbed nights and daytime somnolence. A sleep study will confirm nocturnal hypoventilation, and non-invasive respiratory support improves symptoms and can be life saving.

Diagnostic investigations include the serum concentration of creatine kinase (CK), which is raised in many muscle diseases, although a normal result does not exclude a muscle disorder. Where appropriate, biochemical analysis for metabolic disorders will include lactate, carnitine and acyl carnitine levels together with functional exercise testing. Electromyography (EMG) and nerve conduction studies may be useful in some cases, but this is by no means universal. Muscle biopsy is the definitive diagnostic test for most of the muscular dystrophies and myopathies. However, in some instances, such as spinal muscular atrophy and facioscapulohumeral muscular dystrophy, a blood test for DNA analysis is sufficient to confirm a diagnosis.

PRINCIPLES OF MANAGEMENT

Current therapeutic research is targeted towards finding ways of replacing the abnormal protein. Those individuals with fewer secondary complications of their disorder (e.g. contractures and spinal deformity) will almost certainly derive the greatest benefit if new effective treatments are discovered. Management is based upon the recognition of the patient's specific needs, together with monitoring for complications of the disorder, e.g. 24-hour cardiac monitoring in EDMD and respiratory monitoring in rigid spine syndrome (RSS1). Corticosteroids have been shown to improve muscle strength in Duchenne muscular dystrophy (DMD), thus prolonging independent walking and are now routinely prescribed from the age of 5 years (Manzur et al., 2008a). But side effects are significant, especially osteoporosis, and must be actively managed.

Generally, an approach to managing the family rather than the individual is an important factor that influences an integrated multidisciplinary and multispecialty approach (medical rehabilitation, neurology, clinical genetics, physiotherapy, paediatrics, orthopaedics, dietetics and orthotics). Close liaison with community therapists to provide care, support and adaptations to the home and school is an essential element in enabling independence and quality of life for the affected individual.

THE MUSCULAR DYSTROPHIES

The muscular dystrophies are a heterogeneous group of genetically determined disorders associated with progressive degeneration of skeletal muscle. They can be subdivided into a number of different conditions based upon the mode of inheritance, protein, enzyme and/or genetic defect (Tables 10.1). The Xp21 dystrophies or dystrophinopathies are allelic disorders with a wide spectrum of severity with DMD at the most severe end, a group of intermediate patients and BMD at the milder end of the spectrum. X-linked cardiomyopathy (XLDC) is caused by a deletion in the same gene and results in a severe life-limiting cardiomyopathy, but little, if any, muscle weakness. All of these disorders are caused by a defect of the protein dystrophin and are characterized by X-linked inheritance, in which males are affected and females are carriers, although up to 10% of carriers can manifest muscle weakness. Apart from muscle hypertrophy particularly affecting the calf muscles, there is a normal appearance in infancy, although the serum, CK is very high. With advancing age there is progressive muscle weakness and wasting leading to severe physical disability.

Duchenne muscular dystrophy

DMD was first described by Meryon in 1852 and later by Duchenne. It is rapidly progressive and is the most severe of all the muscular dystrophies. The incidence is 1:3500 live male births and there is a prevalence in the population of 1.9–4.8 per 100 000 (Emery, 1991).

Clinical and diagnostic features

Children with DMD almost always have delayed motor milestones and about one-third of patients will also have learning difficulties leading to global developmental delay. The child often walks after 18 months of age, and when he does begin to walk he may be clumsy, and rarely acquires the ability to run or jump. If there is no family history the diagnosis may not be suspected until muscle weakness is obvious, usually by 5 years of age.

Progressive hip and knee extensor weakness causes difficulty in getting up from the floor resulting in a typical Gowers' manoeuvre, whereby the child must give some assistance to hip and knee extension by pushing off from the thigh with the hand or forearm. With increasing weakness, the child climbs up his legs using both arms. An abnormal 'waddling' gait occurs because of early weakness of the hip abductors resulting in an inability to maintain a level pelvis when lifting one leg off the ground. The child inclines the trunk towards the stance leg to bring the centre of gravity of the body over that leg, and as he moves forward this action is continually repeated and accounts for the Trendelenburg sign. This is accompanied by widening of the base of support for increased stability, which contributes to the evolution of hip abduction contractures (iliotibial band tightness).

By 7–8 years of age, contractures of heel cords and iliotibial bands lead to toe walking. Without corticosteroid treatment ambulation is always lost by the 13th birthday and the mean age for loss of ambulation is 9.5 years (Emery & Muntoni, 2003). Prolonged sitting caused by wheelchair dependence leads to the rapid development of flexion contractures of the elbows, hips and knees.

In the early ambulatory phase of DMD, an equinus foot posture is precipitated by relative weakness of the ankle dorsiflexors compared with the better preserved plantarflexors. Gait analysis has shown that a dynamic equinus is a necessary biomechanical adaptation to maintain knee stability in the presence of gross quadriceps muscle weakness. Forceful action of the ankle plantarflexors provides a torque which opposes knee flexion (Khodadadeh et al., 1986). Thus, contracture of the Achilles tendon, which eventually accompanies disease progression, is secondary to dynamic equinus.

Muscle involvement is bilateral and symmetrical and the proximal muscles are more affected than the distal groups. As the condition progresses the tendon reflexes become depressed and are eventually lost. In the ambulatory stage, the pelvic girdle is slightly more affected than the shoulder girdle. There is more severe weakness in the extensor groups than in the flexors, although this differential muscle involvement becomes less clear as the disease progresses, so that ultimately such patterns of weakness are no longer obvious. Finally, contractures become fixed and a progressive scoliosis develops. Scoliosis exacerbates existing respiratory muscle weakness, and in severe cases may render the child bed-bound if it is not managed with spinal fusion.

Muscle imbalance (caused by the specific pattern of developing weakness) and postural malalignment (resulting from compensatory adjustments to maintain standing equilibrium) are factors precipitating the eventual development of contractures about weight-bearing joints. These are relatively mild while the child remains ambulant but progress rapidly once there is dependence on a wheelchair. These postures combine lumbar lordosis, hip flexion and abduction, and ankle equinus. The first alteration of body alignment in DMD is a lumbar lordosis due to early weakness of the hip extensors, so that active stabilization of the hip joint is compromised. In order to maintain the line of force behind the hip joint and prevent collapse into hip flexion, there is an initial posterior alignment of the upper trunk resulting in a compensatory lumbar lordosis. As weakness progresses this is accompanied by an exaggerated anterior tilt of the pelvis which predisposes to contractures of the hip flexors. By 18 years of age cardiomyopathy and respiratory insufficiency are the norm.

Thus, DMD is a severe life-limiting disease characterized by muscle weakness, contracture, deformity and progressive disability. However, 'incurable' is not synonymous with 'untreatable'. A variety of therapeutic and surgical measures are available that can help to minimize deformity, prolong independent ambulation and maximize functional capabilities. There is evidence that improved management strategies are resulting in increased survival rates (Eagle et al., 2002; Eagle et al., 2007). Corticosteroid treatment results in an increase in muscle strength followed by a slowing down of the dystrophic process (Manzur et al., 2008a). Most boys will die from respiratory or cardiac failure, but the introduction of nocturnal nasal ventilation has improved survival figures, such that the average life expectancy is now 25 years or more with non-invasive ventilation, compared with 19 years without this treatment (Eagle et al., 2002). The principles of successful management are based on an understanding of the natural evolution of patterns of weakness, contracture and deformity, so that intervention can be staged appropriately.

Pathology

Weakness in DMD results from the gradual loss of functional muscle fibres which are replaced by fat and connective tissue due to a lack of dystrophin, a protein encoded by the Xp21 gene, is the primary biochemical defect (Muntoni et al., 2003). Dystrophin is integral within a complex of proteins which stabilizes the integrity of the sarcolemmal membrane, particularly during the stress associated with repeated cycles of contraction and relaxation. Absence of dystrophin in the skeletal and cardiac muscle results in a reduction in permeability of the muscle cell membrane, so allowing excessive quantities of calcium to accumulate within the muscle fibre leading to myofibrillar over-contracture, breakdown of myofibrils and various metabolic disturbances that culminate in muscle fibre degeneration. Dystrophin isoforms are also expressed in Schwann and Purkinge cells found in the brain which is the reason for the high incidence of learning difficulty.

Diagnosis

Diagnosis is suspected by finding a raised serum creatine kinase usually in the region of 50–100 times the normal level. A muscle biopsy is necessary to confirm the diagnosis together with DNA analysis. Muscle biopsy can be undertaken as a percutaneous technique using a biopsy needle or as an open procedure, depending on the practice of the investigating unit. Muscle histology demonstrates dystrophic features which include: an increased variation of fibre size, evidence of necrosis with phagocytosis, an increase in central nuclei, hypercontracted eosinophillic hyaline fibres, and an increase in fat and connective tissue (Figure 10.1). Histochemical staining using antibodies to N, C and rod domain epitopes of dystrophin usually show complete absence of the protein, except for occasional revertent fibres (these are fibres which label normally with antibodies to dystrophin; their origin is not understood).

Weak or uneven labeling of dystrophin may be seen in BMD and intermediate phenotypes and thus can guide on prognosis. In manifesting carriers, dystrophin immunolabelling demonstrates a mosaic appearance with positive and negative fibres. Immunolabelling with other antibodies in both DMD and BMD shows a reduction of membrane proteins associated with dystrophin, and over expression of utrophin, a protein similar in structure to dystrophin.

DNA testing from a blood sample will demonstrate a frame-shift deletion within the dystrophin gene in approximately 60% of DMD patients, the rest will result from duplications and nonsense mutations (Mastaglia & Laing, 1996). Confirmation of the diagnosis by DNA testing allows carrier detection and prenatal diagnosis in the affected boy's mother and female relatives. In some cases DNA analysis is the only test required to confirm the diagnosis of DMD. In BMD the reading frame of the gene is preserved (in-frame). Exceptions to the frame-shift rule occur with some deletions and thus a muscle biopsy is recommended to confirm the diagnosis.

General management

Informing parents that their child has DMD causes extreme distress and should only be undertaken by the most senior member of the team, in an appropriate

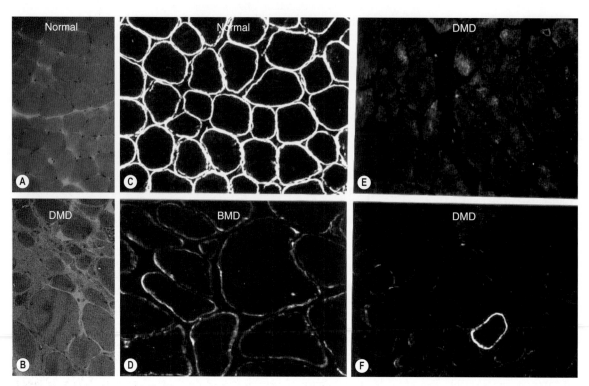

Figure 10.1 Biopsies of normal (A, C) and dystrophic muscle (B, D–F). Note the abnormal histology of the dystrophic muscle (B) with a wide variation in fibre size, fibrous tissue surrounding the fibres and nuclei within the fibres. An antibody to dystrophin has been used to label the muscle in panels (C–F). Note the normal intense sarcolemmal localization on all fibres in (C), the reduced patchy labelling of dystrophin in a case of Becker muscular dystrophy (BMD) in panel (D), and the absence of dystrophin in a case of Duchenne muscular dystrophy (DMD) in (E). One revertent fibre with apparently normal dystrophin is shown in (F). (Courtesy of Professor Caroline Sewry.)

environment, with a support worker present who can maintain contact with the family once they have left the hospital. The information given to the parents must be factual and honest, but delivered with sensitivity and empathy.

The long-term care of the child will require a specialist multidisciplinary team (MDT) liaising closely with community medical, educational and social agencies. As soon as the diagnosis is confirmed the child should have a MDT developmental assessment to screen for learning difficulty so that plans can be made for appropriate educational support. Social services will be required to become involved to ensure the family receives the correct State financial entitlements and will be paramount in arranging home adaptations, which are usually necessary by the time the child is 7 or 8 years of age, when the child has difficulty climbing stairs.

From an early age, tightness and subsequently contractures of the tendo-achilles (TA) develop. Daily passive stretching of the TA and provision of night splints are recommended as soon as any tightening is demonstrated. Later on, when significant pelvic girdle weakness is manifest by a waddling gait, the ilio-tibial bands and hip flexors may start to tighten. Care must be taken to ensure assessment at each outpatient visit with advice to undertake stretching exercises. The priority of physical management is to prolong ambulation for as long as possible, since once ambulation is lost scoliosis and joint contractures develop rapidly. At the point of loss of ambulation, light weight knee-ankle-foot orthoses (KAFOs) can be used to prolong walking (Figure 10.2). This usually involves a minor surgical procedure to percutaneously release any lower limb contractures, usually the TAs, together with an intensive rehabilitation programme. Where there are only moderate contractures of the TAs, serial casting may be an alternative to surgery to allow fitting of the KAFOs (Main et al., 2007). The parents and child must be both strongly motivated and well supported for this form of rehabilitation to be successful.

In recent years, there is growing evidence that treatment with corticosteroids (prednisolone or deflazacort) will stabilize muscle function for some time, therefore delaying the loss of ambulation by up to 2 years (Manzur et al., 2008a). Careful monitoring for side-effects is essential,

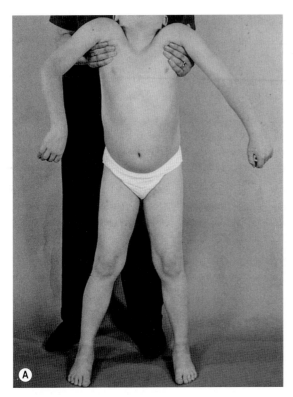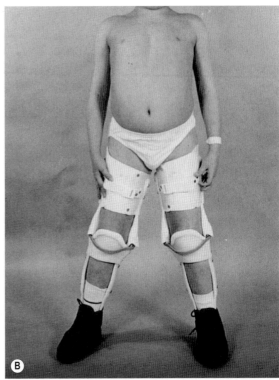

Figure 10.2 Boy with Duchenne muscular dystrophy. (A) At the point of loss of independent walking. (B) Following percutaneous Achilles tenotomies and rehabilitation in light-weight ischial weight-bearing knee–ankle–foot orthoses (KAFOs).

especially weight gain, which may potentially have a negative effect on function. The potential benefit of longer-term steroid treatment has yet to be evaluated, but some open studies suggest preserved respiratory and cardiac function (Manzur et al., 2008a). Premature loss of ambulation can follow lower limb fractures or ligament strains unless active management, such as internal fixation, is instigated to promote early mobility. Immobilizing any joint beyond the initial painful phase should be actively discouraged.

Once independent ambulation is lost, regular use of a standing frame is recommended to maintain good posture and reduce contracture development. Rigid ankle foot orthoses (AFOs) are recommended for daytime use to maintain a good foot position. Likewise it is essential to ensure that the wheelchair provides good back and neck support (Pope, 2002) and, ideally, the controls of an electric wheel chair should be centrally placed. Swimming and hydrotherapy are particularly useful and enjoyed by the boys who find they can move more easily in the water.

A rapidly progressive scoliosis requiring surgical stabilization will develop in up to 95% of boys. There is, however, a reduced incidence and severity of scoliosis in glucocorticosteroid-treated boys (Biggar et al., 2006) which is likely to be due to prolongation of walking and increase in trunk muscle strength. Posterior spinal fusion is highly successful in correcting the deformity, and in improving posture and the quality of life for both patient and carer (Mehdian et al., 1989). The timing of operation is crucial since a decline in vital capacity occurs at the same time as the development of scoliosis. To avoid undue anaesthetic risks the procedure must be undertaken when the vital capacity is greater than 30% of predicted height (Manzur et al., 2008b). Thus surgical correction is usually recommended when the degree of spinal curvature is still relatively mild.

Management of restricted participation

Restricted participation has replaced the term 'handicap' in the revised International Classification of Functioning, Disability and Health by the World Health Organization (WHO ICF, 2001; see Ch. 11) and its management must take into account psychosocial issues, mobility and education. Providing an electric wheelchair is essential to providing a degree of independence, but this requires appropriate home adaptations including: widened doors and indoor/outdoor wheelchair access. A hoist is required for lifting in and out of the wheelchair, and the child will require a ground floor bedroom and bathroom with shower and adapted toilet. An electric bed enables the child to alter his position and saves the parents many sleepless nights. An adapted motor vehicle is required for transport to enable the child to drive his own wheelchair in and out of the vehicle.

The revolution in computer technology and its application to assistive devices has transformed the lives of many disabled people, e.g. the POSSUM system (Patient Operator Selector Mechanisms) enables the child to open and close doors, windows, curtains and turn on and off lights, etc. Access to the internet allows friendships to develop and provides a source of information and various services. Electronic games enable the boys to play competitively alongside their able-bodied companions and probably have a major effect on building self-esteem and reducing boredom.

Respiratory problems

With advancing age, respiratory impairment becomes inevitable and, if not recognized early, is an important cause of unpleasant symptoms or death. Characteristically there is a restrictive defect, with a reduction in total lung capacity caused by a combination of diaphragmatic and intercostal muscle weakness. Chest wall stiffness, recurrent aspiration and an inability to cough effectively compound the respiratory insufficiency leading to an increased frequency of chest infections (Smith et al., 1991). The forced vital capacity is a reliable measure of respiratory function, provided the boy is able to undertake a good technique (in some boys with learning difficulty this may be a problem) (Griggs et al., 1981). The forced vital capacity, when corrected for height, plateaus and then falls progressively on average between 12 and 14 years of age. Once the vital capacity falls below 1 L, in a boy who has reached skeletal maturity, the average life expectancy without treatment is 3 years (Phillips et al., 2001).

Sleep-related respiratory abnormalities play a major role in ventilatory failure, resulting in symptoms of hypercapnia which include: early-morning headache, nausea and sweating, daytime somnolence and a loss of respiratory drive (resulting in rapid deterioration into coma if a high concentration of oxygen is administered). Chronic nocturnal hypoxaemia leads to cor pulmonale (right heart failure), the ECG may show evidence of pulmonary hypertension and right heart strain (Carroll et al., 1991). Once the vital capacity falls below 40% sleep studies should be undertaken at regular intervals to monitor for nocturnal hypoventilation. Treatment by non-invasive nasal ventilation is effective in alleviating symptoms and prolongs survival (Eagle et al., 2002; Jeppesen et al., 2003; Simonds, 2000). There is recent evidence that the cumulative effect of both spinal surgery and nocturnal ventilation further improves survival (Eagle et al., 2007).

Cardiac problems

Post-mortem studies show that all boys with DMD have evidence of cardiomyopathy by 18 years of age. In practice, however, symptomatic cardiomyopathy is less common than might be expected. It has been assumed the sedentary lifestyle of these boys contributes to the lack of symptoms (Hunsaker et al., 1982). Abnormalities of the electrocardiogram are evident from an early age and will be present in all boys by 18 years of age (Nigro et al., 1990); the most common abnormality is a resting tachycardia, which is almost universal. Cardiac arrhythmias occur and may be a cause of early sudden death. When congestive cardiac failure does occur the progression is rapid and relentless. Monitoring with cardiac echo is recommended once ambulation is lost. Early treatment with ACE (angiotensin-converting enzyme) inhibitors has been shown to be beneficial, although the results need to be confirmed (Duboc et al., 2007).

The final illness

Close monitoring and liaison with the general practitioner and palliative care services are paramount. Children's Respite Hospices play a vital role in supporting families and boys during this difficult time. Patient support groups, such as The Muscular Dystrophy Campaign, frequently fund care workers to support families (see Appendix 'Associations and Support Groups').

Becker muscular dystrophy

Becker muscular dystrophy (BMD) is allelic to DMD, but has a milder phenotype (see Table 10.1) and has a prevalence of 1 in 30 000. It is caused by a partial deficiency of the protein dystrophin (Karpati et al., 2001).

Clinical and diagnostic features

BMD has a wide spectrum of severity; at the severest end ambulation may be lost by 16 years of age compared with the mildest form which presents with non-progressive cramps and myoglobinuria (Gospe et al., 1989). Distribution of weakness is similar to DMD, but progression of the disease is much slower and contractures are often less severe than in DMD. As with DMD, muscle hypertrophy, especially of the calves, occurs. Up to 40% of patients will lose ambulation, and prolonging ambulation with long-leg calipers is more difficult than in DMD because of adult height.

In some patients, as with DMD, an unexpected malignant hyperthermia reaction following general anaesthesia may be the first manifestation of the disease. Cardiomyopathy is common and more likely to be symptomatic than in DMD. ECG and echocardiogram abnormalities may be evident in up to 50% of cases (Steare et al., 1992) and many patients have successfully undergone cardiac transplantation (Quinlivan & Dubowitz, 1992).

Because the life expectancy is much better than for DMD, genetic implications are more important for the patient who will not father affected sons, but will pass the faulty gene to all daughters who will be carriers for the disorder. The diagnosis is confirmed by finding a deletion, duplication or missense mutation in the dystrophin gene and/or abnormal dystrophin staining on a muscle biopsy.

General management

The management of BMD involves prevention of contractures and prolonging ambulation as with DMD. An active approach to management using low-intensity aerobic exercise has been shown to safely improve fitness and strength in individuals with mild BMD (Sveen et al., 2008). Home adaptations are essential in promoting independence and the patient may require support to continue working in an adapted environment. For those patients who are wheelchair dependent, regular standing, and preventing excessive weight gain and constipation are important. Prevention of respiratory infections by vaccination against influenza and pneumococcus, together with prompt antibiotic treatment of infection are important. Monitoring of respiratory function and overnight oximetry for sleep hypoxaemia are necessary. Symptoms of chronic ventilatory failure should be managed with non-invasive ventilation as for the DMD group. Regular cardiac monitoring with yearly ECGs and cardiac ECHOs every 2 or 3 years is necessary. Early intervention with ACE inhibitors for ventricular dysfunction may be helpful, but as yet has to be fully evaluated. If cardiac symptoms fail to respond to medical treatment, assessment for cardiac transplantation is warranted (Quinlivan & Dubowitz, 1992).

Emery–Dreifuss muscular dystrophy

This is a rare but clinically distinct form of MD. Two modes of inheritance exist. Firstly, a sex-linked form (EDMD) in which mutations in the Emerin gene located at Xq28 lead to a complete absence of the nuclear envelope protein Emerin (Mastaglia & Laing, 1996). Secondly, there is an autosomal dominant form (ADEDMD) in which the defective gene is at 1q11-q23 encoding for another nuclear envelope protein; Lamin A/C (LMNA) (Bonne et al., 1999).

Clinical and diagnostic features

The main feature of the nuclear envelope muscular dystrophies is the predominance of joint contractures and muscle weakness occurring in a scapulo-peroneal distribution. Contractures predominantly affect the neck and spine, elbows and tendo-achilles. Disturbances of cardiac conduction are universal by the second or third decades, and may result in sudden death unless detected and cardiac pacing instituted (Bialer et al., 1991). Thus, regular ECG and 24-hour ECG monitoring are essential. Muscle weakness is slowly progressive, however many patients retain some ambulation throughout adult life.

General management

Management of contractures involves passive stretching exercises and night splints, as discussed below. Provided the diagnosis is made sufficiently early, the insertion of a cardiac pacemaker may be life-saving. In the case of ADEDMD a defibrillator pace-maker is recommended.

The associated weakness is usually mild. However, due to rigidity of the spine throughout its length, the patient is unable to compensate for any hip extensor weakness with a lumbar lordosis, as is commonly seen in many of the other neuromuscular diseases. Instead, the patient maintains the centre of mass with increasing equinus at the ankles, leading to secondary contracture of the Achilles tendon. If these contractures become severe, they may in themselves jeopardize mobility and require percutaneous surgical correction. Management should be aimed at controlling the progression of deformity by appropriate strengthening, passive stretching and splinting techniques (see Ch. 12 & 14).

Limb girdle muscular dystrophy

The limb girdle muscular dystrophies (LGMDs) are a clinically and genetically diverse group of disorders, characterized by the predominance of limb girdle weakness, with or without contractures (Table 10.1). Inheritance can be either dominant or recessive, depending upon the specific disorder. Clinical heterogeneity also occurs within some of these disorders, for example LGMD2B is caused by mutations in the dysferlin gene on chromosome 2p13 and is allelic to Miyoshi distal myopathy (Illarioshkin et al., 1997).

The onset of LGMD can occur at any time between childhood and old age, although the average age of onset is in the second and third decades. The disorders are progressive, with weakness usually affecting the shoulder girdle and pelvic girdle. Many patients will lose independent ambulation within 10–20 years of onset. The CK is frequently greatly increased and a combination of muscle biopsy and DNA analysis will often lead to a precise diagnosis.

Dilated cardiomyopathy is a relatively frequent complication of the LGMDs: routine ECG and, where appropriate, echocardiogram (ECHO) are recommended. In autosomal dominant Emery Dreifuss muscular dystrophy (ADEDMD, allelic to LGMD1B), cardiac conduction block requiring a defibrillator pacemaker is almost universal by the third decade and can be life-saving. Respiratory failure from diaphragmatic weakness, leading to sleep hypoventilation syndrome, occurs in most of the muscular dystrophies and must be screened for regularly. Generally, if the FVC is less than 50% of that expected for height, or if there is a greater than 20% drop in FVC when the patient lies flat, sleep hypoventilation should be suspected and a sleep study should be arranged. Treatment with non-invasive mask ventilation is highly effective in alleviating symptoms. Scoliosis may occur in adolescents, necessitating spinal fusion. While skeletal contractures can occur in all patients once they become wheelchair-dependent, they are a particular problem in ambulant ADEDMD and calpain-deficient muscular dystrophy (LGMD2A). Severe lower-limb contractures may compromise mobility.

General management

As with other disabling neuromuscular diseases, patients with LGMD need help and support to adapt their environment to suit their needs. A self-raising chair or pneumatic cushion can be invaluable in assisting rising to standing. Adaptations to the patient's home may be required to ensure appropriate bathroom facilities, hoists or stair lifts. Adaptations to the patient's vehicle may also be required to maintain independence. Weight gain can be a major problem for some individuals, especially when they are confined to a wheelchair, and may compromise respiration. Encouraging exercise is important for general health and well being; swimming is an excellent example which also helps maintain strength. Low-intensity aerobic training has been show to improve exercise performance in patients with LGMD type 21 (Sveen et al., 2007). Many patients appreciate the benefit of regular passive stretching exercises and the opportunity to stand using either a tilt table or standing frame. Prevention of chest infections with pneumococcal vaccination and yearly flu vaccines is important for any patient with evidence of respiratory muscle weakness.

Congenital muscular dystrophies

There are several recognized forms of congenital muscular dystrophy depending upon the protein/gene defect and/or the association of central abnormalities (see Table 10.2). They are usually caused by autosomal recessive genes and present at birth or in infancy with hypotonia and joint contractures, often involving the spine. The serum CK may be normal in some groups, and elevated in others. Intellect may be normal or impaired depending upon the presence of neuronal migration defects. White matter changes may be seen on magnetic resonance imaging (MRI) in cases with merosin deficiency, although there is normal intellect. Muscle biopsy shows dystrophic features and in some types specific protein abnormalities.

Clinical and diagnostic features

Reduced fetal movements during pregnancy suggest that signs are already present before birth, such infants are frequently born with arthrogryposis. Features in early infancy consist of muscle weakness and generalized hypotonia, 'floppiness', poor suck and respiratory difficulty (Kobayashi et al., 1996). In childhood, motor milestones are delayed, with severe and early contractures and often joint deformities. Weakness is greater in the pelvic girdle and upper leg muscles than in the shoulder girdle and upper arm muscles. On the whole, with the exception of Fukuyama congenital muscular dystrophy (FCMD), these conditions are relatively slowly progressive and functional ability can initially improve over time. Contractures at birth are common, and may restrict function to a greater degree than weakness if not controlled. It is particularly important to be vigilant for the insidious development of contractures and to treat them promptly.

Other features of the disease are hip dislocation, pes cavus and kyphoscoliosis. The motor development is slow, leading to late sitting, standing and walking, which is achieved in some but not all. Intelligence is normal in merosin deficient CMD and Ullrich CMD, but will be reduced in the muscle eye brain forms of CMD, where there are structural brain abnormalities, such as polymicrogyria and cerebellar cysts. Serum CK activity is usually very high in the early stages. In this group of patients vision should be assessed to exclude myopia and cataracts. In the Ullrich form of CMD intelligence and vision are normal, but there may be skin changes such as keloid scars or follicular hyperplasia.

General management

Attention to feeding and breathing is important in the neonatal period. Some patients will require percutaneous endoscopic gastrostomy (PEG) feeding due to bulbar involvement. Later on, useful mobility should be maintained for as long as possible. Regular exercise should be encouraged and obesity avoided. Regular gentle stretching is required to avoid or control contractures (see below). Nocturnal hypoventilation may develop at any time but is most common in the second decade and responds well to nocturnal non-invasive ventilation.

Fascioscapulohumeral muscular dystrophy

This condition follows an autosomal dominant pattern of inheritance with a high degree of penetrance but variable expression. The clinical features are always present by 30 years of age. As many as 30% of cases present sporadically and are due to germ line mosaicism. The overall prevalence is estimated to be 1:20 000 (Kissell, 1999). In 95% of affected individuals, a short fragment on the telomeric portion of chromosome 4 (4q35) is identified (Wijmenga et al., 1991), which has been associated with a reduced number of 3.3-kb tandem repeat segments called D4Z4 in a non-protein-encoding region of the gene (Orrell et al., 1999). The size of the D4Z4 segment correlates inversely with clinical severity. The mechanism by which the reduced number of D4Z4 tandem repeats produce disease is unknown.

The age at onset, degree of severity and course of the disease are more variable than in many other neuromuscular diseases. Within a family it may range from someone who has minimal facial weakness with slow progression, to a condition which has a more marked progression of lower limb weakness that can cause severe disability early in life. Examination reveals facial weakness and a characteristic horizontal smile and inability to whistle. Shoulder-girdle weakness is often asymmetrical and more pronounced than lower limb weakness. Scapular winging with characteristic shoulder 'terracing' on abduction of the arms reflects weakness of serratus anterior, trapezius and rhomboids (Figure 10.3). The biceps and triceps muscles tend to be affected later.

The deltoid muscles are preserved in 50% of cases (Bunch & Siegel, 1993), but even if the deltoids are not involved the muscles lose their mechanical advantage due to lack of shoulder-girdle stability, causing limitation of active abduction and flexion. The patient may compensate surprisingly well, using trick movements to raise the hand above shoulder level, but can be more obviously compromised if the activity involves lifting objects of any weight. Foot drop may occur early in the disease due to peroneal and anterior tibial muscle weakness. Leg muscle weakness may progress to loss of ambulation, which occurs in approximately 20% of cases. Joint contractures are rare and mild.

Cardiac involvement is uncommon and reported to occur in about 5% of cases; atrial arrhythmias are the most usual manifestation (Laforet et al., 1998). Sometimes the severe facial weakness may be mistaken for Moebius syndrome (Miura et al., 1998). The serum CK may be normal or three to five times the normal value. Confirmation of diagnosis can now be made with DNA analysis so that muscle biopsy is rarely necessary. Congenital onset is rare and can be associated with deafness, learning difficulties and severe muscle weakness.

General management

Studies of specific treatment for FSH are limited. Patients often develop a marked lumbar lordosis and low back pain due to pelvic girdle weakness, so that strengthening the pelvic musculature plus passive stretching exercises to minimize hip flexion contractures may be helpful. A recent study of mildy affected patients with FSH showed that low-intensity aerobic training over a 12-week period improved exercise performance (Olsen et al., 2005). Ankle–foot orthoses (AFOs) can be provided to control

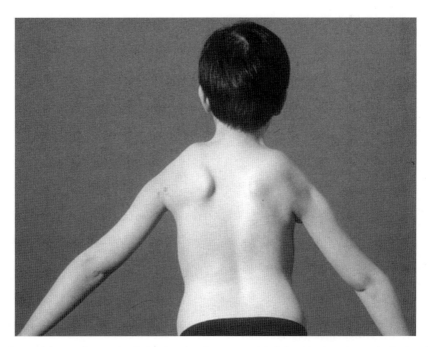

Figure 10.3 Fascioscapulohumeral muscular dystrophy, showing asymmetrical shoulder terracing and winging of the scapulae on abduction of the arms.

for foot drop, but may not be tolerated unless the ankle achieves plantigrade and quadriceps strength is at least antigravity (Eagle et al., 2001).

Thoracoscapular fusion can be effective in the long term for patients with scapular winging, provided the deltoid muscle remains functional (Rhee & Ha, 2006). More recently scapulothoracic fixation (scapulopexy) using wires to reposition the scapula over the ribs, without arthrodesis, has been shown to be successful (Gianinni et al., 2007). Both techniques result in improved range of movement and appearance of the shoulder and this is most beneficial for patients whose occupation specifically requires the ability to sustain flexion and abduction.

Myotonic dystrophy

Classical myotonic dystrophy (dystrophia myotonica; DM1) is a dominantly inherited multisystem disease that is relatively common, with a prevalence of 4 per 100 000 (Harper, 1989). DM1 is caused by an expansion of CTG repeats in the DMPK gene on chromosome 19q13 (Friedrich et al., 1987). The size of the expansion determines the severity of the phenotype and contributes to the phenomenon of anticipation, whereby the severity of the condition worsens in successive generations. This is especially obvious with the congenital form of the disease, where a severe and life-threatening phenotype occurs in the newborn infant, in contrast to the often presymptomatic mother.

The condition is classified according to the age of onset. The most severe congenital form presents at birth with contractures, respiratory and bulbar insufficiency and learning difficulty. The juvenile and classic forms of the disease present insidiously in the second and third decades with ptosis, frontal balding, myotonia (muscle stiffness) and muscle weakness (especially involving the facial, sternocleidomastoid and distal lower-limb muscles). Other features include: hypersomnolence, dysarthria, dysphagia, immune suppression, testicular atrophy, cataracts, digestive problems and diabetes. The most serious systemic complication is a cardiac conduction disorder, which can be a cause of sudden death.

At the mildest end of the spectrum cataracts or diabetes may be the only feature of the condition. Anaesthetic risks are significant in all cases, depolarizing muscle relaxants can lead to severe laryngospasm, and when given in combination with potent inhalational anaesthetics, a malignant hyperthermia reaction can occur (Moore & Moore, 1987). Myotonia is demonstrable by asking the patient to clench his or her fist and then let go quickly, the patient has to release their grip using the other hand. The EMG shows widespread myotonic discharges, which produce a classical dive-bomber sound caused by gradual fluctuations in frequency and amplitude (Fawcett & Barwick, 1994). The diagnosis is confirmed by DNA analysis.

General management

Education, monitoring and avoidance of complications remain the cornerstone in the management of patients with myotonic dystrophy. Cardiac arrhythmias are the most serious complication and permanent cardiac pacing may sometimes be required. A 12-lead electrocardiogram (ECG) should be undertaken annually and 24-hour ECG monitoring is necessary once there is evidence of conduction abnormalities, such as prolongation of the PR interval.

Speech and language therapy input may help with the bulbar symptoms. Foot drop can be improved by the use of AFOs. Sleep studies should be contemplated if there is a change in the pattern of daytime somnolence. Anaesthesia and surgery require special attention because of the general anaesthesia risk. In addition to the risks already mentioned, patients may slip into respiratory failure in the postoperative period and are at risk of aspiration pneumonia as a consequence of their abnormal bulbar function. All patients should be advised to carry an alert card outlining the anaesthetic risks. Several drugs, such as phenytoin, can be used to relieve the myotonia, although in practice the side-effects often outweigh any benefit.

SPINAL MUSCULAR ATROPHIES

The spinal muscular atrophies (SMAs) are a group of disorders in which there is degeneration of the anterior horn cells of the spinal cord, resulting in muscle weakness. They are the most common neuromuscular disease in childhood after DMD and affect both sexes. The mode of inheritance is mainly autosomal recessive but can vary, with dominant or X-linked traits (Emery, 1971). The genetic defect for the recessive form is a deletion in exon 7 and or exon 8 of the SMN1 gene on chromosome 5q (Ogino et al., 2004). Weakness is symmetrical, is greater proximally than distally, and the pelvic girdle is weaker than the shoulder girdle. Weakness is generally non-progressive, although as a result of increasing height and weight there may be some loss of functional activities over time. There is no facial weakness and intellectual development is often above normal. Classification of 5q SMA is most usefully based on clinical severity (Dubowitz, 1995):

- Severe (type 1) – Unable to sit unsupported
- Intermediate (type 2) – Able to sit unsupported; unable to stand or walk unaided
- Mild (type 3) – Able to stand and walk.

Severe spinal muscular atrophy (type 1 or Werdnig–Hoffman disease)

Infants with severe type 1 SMA present within the first 6 months of life and usually by 3 months with hypotonia and feeding difficulties. The condition progresses rapidly and leads to severe muscle weakness with marked respiratory and bulbar involvement. As a result affected infants rarely survive beyond 2 years of age. Treatment is directed towards palliative care to control symptoms and support feeding. The infant is unable to move out of a lying position and the upper limbs adopt an internally rotated 'jug-handle' position and the lower limbs are flexed and abducted 'frog position'. Limb contractures may develop related to these positions and, if untreated, activities such as dressing and lifting can become uncomfortable. Regular passive stretching techniques can become part of the daily routine at bath times and nappy changes. Moulding of the ribs can occur if the infant is always positioned on one particular side. This will further compromise respiratory capacity, and so alternation of sleeping positions is recommended.

The intercostal muscles are severely affected and breathing is almost entirely diaphragmatic, giving a characteristic bell-shaped chest. Cough is weak and bulbar weakness may give rise to sucking and swallowing difficulties. The child will be prone to recurrent respiratory infections. Parents should be taught secretion management techniques and they should be provided with suction. There is no place for spinal bracing or orthopaedic management in this group. Severe type 1 SMA is a devastating diagnosis and families need to be supported as much as possible. These very sick infants do not travel well and care should be delivered as close to home as possible.

Intermediate spinal muscular atrophy (type 2)

These children appear to develop normally until about 12 months when the child presents with inability to stand or walk. Long-term prognosis is dependent on respiratory function, and rapidly progressive scoliosis is a common complication associated with this group. Early spinal bracing will help to control the rate of progression, but spinal fusion may be necessary. Limb joints are often hyperextendable, particularly at the elbow and hands, but are prone to contractures related to positioning.

A major aim of management is to promote standing and the ability to achieve this will be dependent on residual muscle strength, particularly in the trunk and pelvic girdle, which should be carefully assessed. Some children show functional improvement and, with appropriate training, progression from standing in a frame to walking with orthoses is possible. Since muscle strength is relatively stable, the ability to walk using knee–ankle–foot orthoses (KAFOs) can be maintained over many years, helping to control both joint contractures and scoliosis. It should be noted that spinal bracing and spinal fusion

are not normally compatible with continued mobility in calipers, since they limit compensatory trunk side flexion which aids weight transference when the hip abductors are weak.

Mild spinal muscular atrophy (type 3 or Kugelburg–Welander disease)

In Type 3 SMA the ability to walk is achieved at the normal age or slightly late, and the child often presents with a deterioration of motor skills often around the time of the pubertal growth spurt. Proximal weakness is more marked in the lower, rather than the upper limbs, and particularly in the hip abductors. Individuals are therefore dependent on compensatory pelvic and trunk motion for forward propulsion. Strengthening programmes focusing on the pelvic girdle would be functionally beneficial for type 2 and type 3 SMA (Armand et al., 2009). Joint contractures and progressive scoliosis are rare in this group (Carter et al., 1995). Weakness is generally relatively static, but rapid periods of growth may result in loss of ambulation, and rehabilitation can be achieved in some using lightweight KAFOs.

MUSCLE SODIUM CHANNEL AND MUSCLE CHLORIDE CHANNEL DISEASES

The muscle channelopathies comprise two groups of disorders – those where the muscle is hyperexcitable, leading to stiffness (myotonia), and those conditions where there is reduced muscle excitability leading to weakness (the periodic paralyses). Both symptoms are caused by a temporary depolarization of the skeletal muscle membrane (Karpati et al., 2001).

The muscle channelopathies include:

* myotonia congenita
* paramyotonia congenita
* myotonia fluctuans
* hyperkalaemic periodic paralysis
* normokalaemic periodic paralysis.

Depending upon the specific condition, patients will present with either episodic weakness or stiffness, or both, made worse by cold weather and exercise. Paradoxically, there is a warm-up phenomenon with exercise but people with paramyotonia congenita will subsequently worsen. Patients with hyperkalaemic periodic paralysis and paramyotonia congenita benefit from treatment with acetazolamide or a thiazide diuretic to manage the serum potassium levels. Those with myotonia congenita respond to membrane-stabilizing drugs, such as Mexiletine which can have a pronounced beneficial effect.

GLYCOGEN STORAGE DISEASES

The glycogen storage diseases (GSDs) are characterized by abnormal glycogen metabolism.

Pompe disease

Pompe disease (acid maltase deficiency, GSD11) is a lysosomal storage disorder affecting muscle glycogen metabolism. The condition can present in infancy with a severe phenotype, resulting in progressive muscle weakness and cardiomyopathy. Death usually occurs by 2 years of age from cardiac and respiratory failure. Early diagnosis is essential for a good outcome with enzyme replacement with myozyme (Nicolino et al., 2009). Less severe forms of GSD11 present during childhood (juvenile-onset) and adulthood. The condition is milder with a slower progression, causing limb girdle weakness, which closely resembles LGMD or mild SMA. Respiratory failure due to both diaphragmatic involvement and cardiomyopathy occurs and can be disproportionate to the skeletal weakness. Regular cardiorespiratory monitoring is therefore recommended. Enzyme replacement therapy is available for all forms of Pompe disease, although the evidence for benefit is currently based upon the treatment of the severe infantile form.

McArdle disease

McArdle disease (glycogen storage disorder type V; GSDV) is caused by a deficiency of the enzyme muscle phosphorylase, resulting in impaired utilization of muscle glycogen during anaerobic exercise. Muscle pain and fatigue occurring early during exercise are the cardinal symptoms. Often the patient will describe a second wind, whereby muscle pain occurs within the first few minutes of exercise, but when the patient slows down or stops, pain-free exercise can be resumed. This phenomenon is probably due to a switch from glycolytic metabolism to aerobic oxidative phosphorylation.

If exercise is continued despite pain, an electrically silent contracture occurs where the muscle seizes and later becomes swollen. This is followed by myoglobinuria, a dark red/brown or black discoloration of the urine caused by rhabdomyolysis (muscle damage), which, if severe, can cause acute renal failure. The serum CK is invariably raised at rest and there is a lack of rise in venous lactate during a forearm exercise test. Muscle biopsy demonstrates a subsarcolemmal accumulation of glycogen and absent muscle phosphorylase activity. The condition is caused by mutations in the muscle phosphorylase gene on chromosome 11q13 (Beynon et al., 2002). Strenuous anaerobic exercise should be avoided to prevent muscle damage; however, regular gentle aerobic exercise is recommended, to upregulate fatty acid oxidation, thus conditioning the muscles and improving performance.

INFLAMMATORY MYOPATHIES

Inflammatory myopathies can be divided into three distinct groups:

- Dermatomyositis (DM)
- Polymyositis (PM)
- Inclusion body myositis (IBM).

DM and PM have an autoimmune aetiology and respond well to immuno-suppressive agents; IBM occurs in older people, it is usually sporadic and does not always respond to immunesuppression. There are two rare subtypes of inherited IBM in younger patients, caused by homozgous mutations in the GNE gene, while in older patients a rare genetic form with mutations in VCP is associated with Pagets disease and dementia (Phadke et al., 2009; Vesa et al., 2009).

DM is an inflammatory muscle condition associated with a characteristic facial rash occurring around the eyes (heliotrope rash). The condition affects children between the ages of 5 and 15 years. A second peak in incidence occurs in middle and old age, and is frequently associated with an underlying malignancy (Callen, 1988). The disease is characterized by muscle pain and proximal weakness, joint contractures can develop rapidly. The serum CK and erythrocyte sedimentation rate may be elevated, and a muscle biopsy confirms the inflammatory process. Treatment includes immune suppression and physiotherapy to minimize contractures.

PM presents with subacute proximal weakness, without myalgia and rash. The condition may occur as part of a more generalized autoimmune connective tissue disease and can also be precipitated by some drugs, including penicillamine and zidovudine (AZT). Muscle biopsy confirms an inflammatory myopathy and patients respond to corticosteroids and immune suppression.

IBM occurs more commonly in males most often over the age of 50. IBM should be suspected when a patient with an inflammatory myopathy fails to respond to corticosteroids. Unlike DM and PM, there may be facial weakness and there is frequently distal weakness, especially of the finger flexors and foot extensors, in addition to proximal weakness. About 20% of cases will be associated with an underlying autoimmune connective tissue disorder.

PHYSICAL MANAGEMENT OF NEUROMUSCULAR DISORDERS

This section highlights the areas of management which are specific to muscle disorders, both in adulthood and childhood. Details of treatment concepts and techniques are found in Chapters 11 & 12, respectively. A problem-solving approach is preferable and treatment planning should involve the multidisciplinary team (MDT), the patient, parents and carers.

Assessment

Thorough, standardized and regular assessment of neuro-muscular patients is essential because of the progressive nature of many conditions and the superimposed effect of growth on children. Assessment will guide clinical management and evaluate therapeutic outcome for research purposes. The key aspects of assessment are mea-surement of muscle strength and performance and lung function; the principles of assessment are discussed in Chapter 1 (also see Ryerson, 2009; Stokes, 2009).

Measurement of muscle strength

Strength assessment provides information for the planning and monitoring of intervention as well as diag-nostic information.

Manual muscle testing

Manual muscle testing is the most widely used means of assessing muscle strength and has been recommended as an outcome measure for therapeutic trials in neuromuscu-lar disease (Brooke et al., 1981). The Medical Research Council scale of grading muscle strength is the most widely known grading system and is based on an ordinal scale of 0 to 5. No special equipment is required and manual muscle testing is a rapid method of determining the distribution and severity of weakness over a large number of muscle groups. However, the major criticism of this method is its subjectivity. There are no standardized joint positions at which testing should be performed and the point at which counterforce is administered is also self-selected. The proportion of maximum strength required to overcome gravity is markedly different between muscle groups (Wiles et al., 1990), and a loss of strength in excess of 50% may develop before weakness can be detected by manual muscle testing (Fisher et al., 1990).

Dynamometry

Force can be measured directly with dynamometers; these quantitative measurements of muscle force are supe-rior to manual muscle testing and provide the most direct method of assessing a particular muscle group. A hand-held dynamometer can measure maximal isometric strength and the results are highly reproducible provided standardized techniques are used and the same observer performs the measurement on each occasion (Bohannon, 1986; Lennon & Ashburn, 1993). Serial measurements of a single patient will be the most useful means of evaluating the distribution and rate of change of muscle weakness, whilst the degree of weakness can be estab-lished by comparison with published normal values of muscle strength (Beenacker et al., 2001). Hand-held dynamometers are useful only when muscles are weak, since their use is restricted by the strength of the operator to oppose the patient's efforts. Strain gauges attached to rigs, and also commercially available isometric and isoki-netic machines, are available.

Measurement of joint range

The development of joint contractures should be moni-tored carefully and joint ROM can be measured using a goniometer. However, caution must be taken with this method as it shows variable inter-rater reliability and measurements should be made by the same assessor where possible (Pandya et al., 1985).

Measurement of functional performance

The quantification of muscle strength has proved to be of value in the assessment and management of many muscle diseases, but it can be seen that this is a measure of impairment and is incomplete without concomitant mea-sures of disability and ultimately the handicap to the patient. Measures of functional performance range from simple tests such as the ability to rise from the floor to more detailed measures of motor ability including gait analysis (D'Angelo et al., 2005; Khodadadeh et al., 1986; Sutherland et al., 1981). These measurements are suscep-tible to the effects of impairments other than strength, but it is important in terms of patient management to determine whether a change in disability can properly be attributed to a change in the strength of the muscles measured.

There may be disparities between strength and disabil-ity in muscle for a variety of reasons. These include: a fail-ure to assess the relevant muscle groups that cause disability; a failure to note progressing severe weakness in an important group, perhaps because of the averaging of many groups; or the intrusion of other factors, such as the development of compensatory biomechanical man-oeuvres or a gain in weight or height. It is of paramount importance that the measure of physical performance is both valid and reliable, and these factors need to be recognized.

Motor ability tests

Classically the most commonly used measures of motor ability have been those developed for DMD by Vignos et al. (1963), Brooke et al. (1981) and the Hammersmith Motor Ability Scale (HMAS) (Scott et al., 1982). The Vig-nos scale was originally designed as a functional classifica-tion and its sensitivity as an objective measure of function is doubtful. The HMAS has been widely used in clinical practice, although there is little published information about its reliability and validity. This scale has recently been modified, is now known as the 'North Star Ambulatory Assessment' and been shown to have excellent inter-observer reliability (Mazzone et al., 2009). Its 17 motor activities are biased towards activities involving the lower limbs, making it suitable for assessment of ambulant patients (Table 10.3). The patient sequentially performs a succession of movements that are scored on a 3-point scale which can be completed in 15 minutes. A functional test, the EK scale, for non-ambulant patients with DMD has been shown to be reliable by Steffensen et al. (2002).

Table 10.3 North Star Amulatory Assessment	
TEST ITEM	**SCORE**
1. Stand	
2. Walk (10 m)	
3. Sit to stand from chair	
4. Stand on one leg – R	
5. Stand on one leg – L	
6. Climb step – R	
7. Climb step – L	
8. Descend step – R	
9. Descend step – L	
10. Gets to sitting	
11. Rise from floor	
12. Lifts head	
13. Stand on heels	
14. Jump	
15. Hop – R	
16. Hop – L	
17. Run	
TOTAL SCORE	

Scores: 2 – 'Normal': achieves goal without assistance; 1 – Modified method but achieves goal independent of physical assistance from another; 0 – Unable to achieve independently. R, right leg; L, left leg
(Reprinted from Mazzone ES, Messina S, Vasco G et al. Reliability of the North Star Ambulatory Assessment in a multicentric setting. Neuromuscular Disorders, 2009; 19:458-461, with permission from Elsevier.)

Timed tests

Timed performance tests are commonly used as supplementary measures of physical performance as a means of reflecting progressive weakness (Brooke et al., 1981). A timed walk over a fixed distance or time, such as the 10 m test or the 6 minute walk test, can reliably detect changes over time (Mazzone et al., 2009). The 10 m walk test can predict loss of ambulation (McDonald et al., 1995). Timing the Gowers' manoeuvre is a useful measure of changing function and supine lying is a more reproducible starting position than is sitting.

Lung function

Spirometry forms part of the regular assessment to monitor changes in lung function. Inspiratory and expiratory mouth pressures can also be measured to assess the strength of the respiratory muscles. Details of lung function tests can be found elsewhere; see Chapter 15 and also Griggs et al. (1981) and Hough (1991).

Treatment principles

The benefits of an active approach to the physical management of neuromuscular disease are increasingly recognized. These include not only minimizing complications in order to maximize abilities, but also maintaining the patient in the best possible physical condition so that he or she could benefit from new treatments; developments in translational research make this a realistic possibility.

The main principles of treatment are:

- to maintain muscle strength and retard contracture progression to maximize function
- to promote or prolong ambulation with appropriate orthoses
- to delay or control the development of scoliosis
- to treat promptly any respiratory and cardiac complications.

Treatment concepts (see Ch. 11) and details of techniques (see Ch. 12) are not discussed here, but the principles relevant to patients with muscle disorders are outlined.

Maintenance of muscle strength

There are very few controlled studies on the effect of exercise in neuromuscular disease and many are not disease specific. The results of mild to moderate resistance exercise programmes in muscular dystrophies have shown limited increases in strength, with no negative effect on muscle function (Ansved, 2003). Greatest effects occur in patients with mild to moderate weakness and in the more slowly progressive conditions, whilst patients with severely weak muscles do not generally benefit from strengthening programmes. It appears in normal subjects that a prerequisite for successful strength training is a high content of type II fibres (Jones et al., 1989). The relative deficiency of type II fibres in DMD (Dubowitz, 1985) may contribute to the poor force-generating capacity of dystrophic muscle and could also be a limiting factor in the eventual benefit of a strengthening programme.

Consistent reductions in maximal or peak oxygen uptake, pulmonary ventilation, work capacity and endurance have been reported in both rapidly and slowly progressive neuromuscular disorders (Kilmer, 2002). Short-term studies in disease-specific patients (Olsen et al., 2005; Sveen et al., 2007; Sveen et al., 2008) indicate low to moderate intensity aerobic exercise is well tolerated with functional improvements in aerobic capacity.

Eccentric muscle training is increasingly being used in the training of athletes to facilitate the development of muscle power, i.e. the rate of force generation. However, eccentric exercise can cause appreciable morphological damage to muscle fibres (Newham et al., 1986) and damage of this nature is commonly seen in the muscles of patients with myopathic diseases. Whilst normal muscle recovers from this damage, eccentric exercise would seem best avoided in muscle disease in favour of more traditional concentric protocols.

Edwards et al. (1987) documented important differences in the rate of progression of various muscle groups and highlighted a particularly rapid loss of force in the hip and knee extensors. Insufficiency of these muscle groups has been shown to be the key deficit in functional decline and gait deterioration in DMD (Sutherland et al., 1981). Whilst maximizing muscle strength to achieve optimal or improved functional ability is a primary objective of treatment, the effect of specific muscle strengthening programmes on function in neuromuscular disorders awaits objective evaluation. To devise a strengthening programme, the required functional gain should be considered and appropriate muscle groups targetted.

It is well accepted that in normal individuals physical exercise increases muscle strength, whilst inactivity causes de-conditioning, and there is also widespread observation amongst clinicians that severe restriction of activity causes rapid weakening of muscle in dystrophic conditions and should be avoided. It is therefore important that the duration of enforced immobilization during any acute illness, and after surgery, should be kept to a minimum so that the patient's return to mobility is not compromised by muscle atrophy. Exercise and strength training in patients with neuromuscular disorders is discussed in Chapter 18.

Weakness occurs when a muscle is held in a shortened position due to joint deformity, and also when it is contracting over a reduced range (Gossman et al., 1982). The establishment of compensatory postures, long before the development of fixed contracture, means that the muscle is biomechanically disadvantaged earlier than is obvious, since it is continually contracting over a shortened range. This could be a major factor in further progression of the disease as optimal function of the muscle is prevented. Joint positioning during strengthening may therefore be important but research in these patients is still required.

Electrical stimulation of normal muscle can improve strength and fatiguability but evidence that the technique is safe, as well as beneficial, in muscle disorders has yet to be produced (see Chapter 12).

Retarding contracture progression

The management of contractures is one of the major contributions of physiotherapy in neuromuscular disease. The aim is not only to retard the progression of contracture, but also and more importantly to promote or prolong independent ambulation and functional ability. Impairment of mobility caused by contractures compromises the strength of the muscles working across the involved joint or joints. The force-generating ability of a muscle is influenced by the length at which it contracts (Jones & Round, 1990) and thus the strength of a muscle held in a shortened position is reduced. In the presence of profound weakness, the maintenance of full joint range of motion is essential for optimal muscle function.

A sustained programme of night splinting and passive stretching in the early stages of DMD can retard the development of lower limb contractures. Two studies have specifically evaluated the effect of passive stretching and the use of orthoses on the development of contractures. Both concluded that the combination of passive stretching and night splints are more effective than passive stretching alone at delaying contractures and prolonging independent ambulation (Hyde et al., 2000; Scott et al., 1981).

Whilst independently ambulant, the provision of AFOs for control of Achilles tendon contracture should be confined to night use only. Gait analysis has shown that an equinus position of the foot is used as a compensatory manoeuvre to increase knee stability during walking. Khodadadeh et al. (1986) observed that boys with DMD necessarily adopt a dynamic equinus during gait in order to maintain a knee-extending moment in the presence of gross quadriceps weakness. AFOs intended to correct the foot position by reducing the equinus during walking will have biomechanical effects which will de-stabilize the knee. If there is significant quadriceps weakness the knee will buckle. Thus AFOs used in this way reduce the available compensatory manoeuvres and result in premature loss of ambulation.

Promoting or prolonging ambulation

Following the cessation of independent walking, the duration of useful ambulation in children can be prolonged with an immediate programme of percutaneous Achilles tenotomy and rehabilitation in lightweight KAFOs and intensive physiotherapy (Figure 10.2). The gains in additional walking time have varied in different centres but on average an extra 2 years of walking can be achieved and sometimes up to 4 years (Bakker et al., 2000). This approach is now generally accepted as a means of maintaining mobility after independent walking ceases and has been shown to impede the development of both lower limb contractures (Vignos et al., 1996) and scoliosis (Rodillo et al., 1988).

The accurate timing of intervention and prompt provision of orthoses are crucial to the success of prolonging ambulation (Thompson et al., 2007). The optimal time for the provision of the orthoses is when the child has lost useful walking but is still able to stand or walk a few steps. There is no advantage in providing orthoses earlier than this. Two of the important factors used to predict successful outcome are the absence of severe hip and knee contractures, and the percentage of residual muscle strength (Hyde et al., 1982). Swivel walkers may be appropriate to allow movement over short distances at home or school. Once the child has been wheelchair-bound for even a short time, fixed lower limb deformities and muscle weakness rapidly progress, and therefore any delay in undertaking this programme may compromise a successful outcome.

Maintenance of activities

A positive management strategy is to introduce a variety of aids to sustain a broad range of normal activities for as long as possible, as outlined above. In children, KAFOs are used to minimize contractures and sustain upright standing posture and prolong walking. Later, a standing frame allows the patients to stand for several hours a day with a view to delaying spinal curvature and contractures of hips, knees and ankles. Lastly, a wheelchair can be introduced as a means to improve mobility and independence. Adults should be encouraged to perform exercise to reduce contractures and thus be able to enjoy physical leisure activities.

Management of scoliosis

Scoliosis is a serious complication of DMD and intermediate SMA. Whilst scoliosis is also associated with other neuromuscular disorders, it is rapidly progressive in these two conditions unless it is treated.

In DMD, a progressive scoliosis almost always develops once the child loses the ability to walk. The period of most rapid deterioration corresponds most closely with the adolescent growth spurt between the ages of 12 and 15 years (McDonald et al., 1995). Progressive scoliosis is also a threat in the adolescent years of patients with type 3 SMA, but due to the profound weakness that is present from early infancy in patients with type 2 SMA it may become a problem at a much earlier age.

The curve often develops in a paralytic long C pattern in the thoraco-lumbar areas and is associated with increasing pelvic obliquity. It further compromises respiratory capacity, which is already restricted by involvement of the respiratory muscles (Kurz et al., 1983). An increasing scoliosis also leads to difficulty in sitting and maintaining head control, and can cause discomfort and pressure areas. Patients will often need to use their elbows for support in maintaining an upright position, so preventing them from using the arms for other functions such as feeding. Untreated, the scoliosis may cause patients to become bedridden.

One of the major benefits of treatment aimed at maintaining an upright posture is that it will help to delay the progression of scoliosis. Once the patient is dependent on a wheelchair, the main means of managing scoliosis are conservative, using a spinal orthosis, or by spinal fusion. The spine should be monitored carefully where scoliosis is a likely complication of the disease, in conjunction with the respiratory capacity using simple spirometry. Once a curve is clinically apparent, any progression is most accurately measured from radiographs using Cobb's angle. Prompt provision of a spinal orthosis is advisable, to be worn during the day whilst the patient is upright and should be corrective rather than supportive. It is recognized that spinal bracing is not the definitive treatment in curves that are known to be rapidly progressive, but it is important in slowing the rate of progression of the curvature (Seeger et al., 1990) and can be used effectively for skeletally immature patients in whom spinal fusion is not yet indicated.

Posterior spinal fusion is used widely in the management of progressive scoliosis in neuromuscular disease and provides rigid fixation without the need for postoperative immobilization or orthoses. It is effective in achieving maximum curve correction and minimizing respiratory complications. Early surgery is the treatment of choice while respiratory and cardiac function is adequate to undergo the procedure safely. In DMD vital capacity increases with age and growth in the early years, reaches a plateau, and then declines in the early teens. There is therefore a window of opportunity when surgery can be performed safely and this is usually when the curve is 20–40° (Cobb angle) and forced vital capacity is above 30% (Manzur et al., 2008b). Spinal fusion is associated with slowing of the rate of respiratory decline postoperatively, as well as enhanced comfort and seating (Velasco et al., 2007). It has recently been reported that patients with low vital capacity can safely undergo spinal surgery provided it is undertaken in a specialist centre (Gill et al., 2006; Marsh et al., 2003).

In the immediate postoperative period, respiratory therapy to aid removal of secretions will be necessary in patients with a poor cough (see Ch. 15). It is possible for a lumbar lordosis and dorsal kyphosis to be moulded into the rods (Galasko et al., 1992), which helps prevent loss of head control in sitting when weakness of the neck and trunk musculature is likely to be advanced. However, seating requirements will need to be reassessed postoperatively, for example, due to significant upper limb weakness the child is likely to utilize upper trunk flexion to help get his or her mouth down to his or her hands for feeding purposes. Following surgery the height of wheelchair arm supports or table height will need to be adjusted to compensate for a fused spine.

Management of respiratory complications

Chest infections are a serious complication to vulnerable patients with respiratory muscle weakness and a poor cough. Longstanding weakness may lead to more serious secondary problems including widespread microatelectasis with reduced lung compliance, a ventilation perfusion imbalance, and nocturnal hypoxaemia (Smith et al., 1991).

Chest infections should be treated promptly with physiotherapy, postural drainage, antibiotics and, when appropriate, assisted ventilation (see Ch. 15). Spinal orthoses that control scoliosis may reduce respiratory capacity and should be temporarily removed if causing distress or interfering with treatment. The aim of treatment is to help clear the lungs of secretions effectively in the shortest possible time without causing fatigue. Thoracic expansion exercises will allow increased airflow through small airways and the loosening of secretions, while forced expiration techniques, the use of intermittent positive pressure breathing (IPPB) and assisted coughing will aid removal of secretions (Webber, 1988). Diaphragmatic weakness may limit the use of supine or tipped positions for postural drainage. Parents of children prone to recurrent chest infections can become competent at administering chest physiotherapy but will require support that is readily accessible if children become distressed.

Inspiratory muscle training has been reported by some to improve respiratory force and endurance (Martin et al., 1986; Wanke et al., 1994), an effect which may be dose dependent (Topin et al., 2002), whereas others report no significant effects (Rodillo et al., 1989; Stern et al., 1989). Overall training is best started in the early stages of DMD where there is only moderate impairment of lung function. This approach does not appear to be used regularly in clinical practice and has probably been superceded by the successful use of nocturnal ventilation at a later stage.

Respiratory failure may be precipitated by chest infection or it may occur as a result of increasing nocturnal hypoventilation and hypoxia. The onset is often insidious but symptoms include morning drowsiness, headache or confusion and nighttime restlessness, and can be confirmed by sleep study. Life expectancy is less than 1 year once diurnal hypercapnia develops. Symptoms, quality of life and survival can be improved by non-invasive nasal ventilation (Eagle et al., 2002; Simonds, 2000).

'SOCIAL' AND PSYCHOLOGICAL ISSUES IN NEUROMUSCULAR DISORDERS

A complexity of factors influences management at different stages of the patient's life. For lifelong disorders, these influences pose similar problems as in other disabling conditions, such as cerebral palsy or spina bifida (see Shepherd, 1995). The need for more training and support for professionals managing these patients was highlighted in a survey by Heap et al. (1996).

Preschool years

The time of diagnosis will be traumatic for the parents and sensitive support will be needed. If not already known to the family, the genetic implications will need to be discussed and family members offered genetic counseling. A realistic picture of the future should be given with appropriate information to prepare for each stage as it comes. Precise details of the end stages would not be appropriate, for obvious psychological reasons; also because medical advances may alter the prognosis with time.

The school years

Optimal management can be achieved only if there is good communication between the medical team, parents and carers at school. Facilities at school and integration with able-bodied children are important. Physical management programmes should involve realistic goals and take into account other aspects of life which may demand the child's time, particularly, for example, at exam times. The timing of surgery should also consider such issues and not just the medical considerations. Preparation for leaving school should include organization for continuation of support services as well as careers advice.

Transition from childhood to adulthood

There is a lack of provision of services for the young disabled adult. On leaving school, the support system often ceases and, apart from occasional visits to the hospital consultant, physiotherapy and other services are not always offered. Patients whose disorder begins in adulthood may never be offered any services or treatment, or even referred to a specialist, despite having a significant disability.

There is a need for specialist centres to provide advice and treatment from experienced therapists and offer an environment for social interaction and training for vocational and leisure activities. This would enable children to continue with their physical management programmes as adults, taking responsibility for their own treatment but receiving help for monitoring and modification of treatment. Those with disorders of adult onset could be educated in physical management strategies by therapists and other patients, and learn how to maximize their abilities and remain functional for as long as possible. Other areas, such as weight control and sexual counselling, could also be dealt with or referral made where appropriate.

Patients with neuromuscular disorders, particularly adults, often feel isolated in the community and some do not lead as full a life as they have the potential for because of a lack of support and education about their condition. Some give up employment or even going out of the house. Specialist centres could provide an important function and fill a major gap in care and support.

In the terminal stage of illness, support from the care team, particularly the general practitioner, is essential and bereavement counselling may be required. The Muscular Dystrophy Campaign Family Care Officers (see 'Association and Support Groups') play a very important role at all stages, particularly during the final illness, in guiding and supporting families.

ACKNOWLEDGEMENTS

Dr Quinlivan gratefully acknowledges the support of the Muscular Dystrophy Campaign and the AGSDUK.

REFERENCES

Ansved, T., 2003. Muscular dystrophies: influence of physical conditioning on the disease evolution. Curr. Opin. Clin. Nutr. Metab. Care 6, 435–439.

Armand, S., Mercier, M., Watelain, E., Patte, K., Pelissier, J., Rivier, F., 2009. Gait pattern in Duchenne muscular dystrophy. Gait Posture 29 (1), 36–41 Epub 2008 Jul 25.

Bakker, J.P.J., De Groot, I.J.M., Beckerman, H., de Jong, B.A., Lankhorst, G.J., 2000. The effects of knee-ankle-foot-orthoses in the treatment of Duchenne muscular dystrophy: review of the literature. Clin. Rehabil. 14, 343–359.

Bialer, M.G., McDaniel, N.L., Kelly, T.E., 1991. Progression of cardiac disease in Emery–Dreifuss muscular dystrophy. Clin. Cardiol. 14 (5), 411–416.

Beenakker, E.A., van der Hoeven, J.H., Fock, J.M., et al., 2001. Reference values of maximum isometric force obtained in 270 children aged 4-16 years by hand-held dynamometry. Neuromuscul. Disord. 11 (5), 441–446.

Beynon, R., Quinlivan, R.C.M., Sewry, C.A., 2002. Selected disorders of carbohydrate metabolism. In: Karpati, G. (Ed.), Structural and Molecular Basis of Skeletal Muscle Diseases. ISN Neuropath Press, Basel, pp. 182–188.

Bertorini, T.E., et al., 2002. Diagnostic Criteria for Duchenne's Muscular Dystrophy. In: Clinical Evaluation and Diagnostic tests for Neuromuscular Disorders. Butterworth-Heinemann Press, p. 784.

Biggar, W.D., Harris, V.A., Eliasoph, L., et al., 2006. Long term benefits of deflazacort treatment for boys with Duchenne muscular dystrophy in their second decade. Neuromuscul. Disord. 16, 249–255.

Bohannon, R.W., 1986. Test–retest reliability of hand-held dynamometry during a single session of strength assessment. Phys. Ther. 66, 206–209.

Bonne, G., Di Barletta, M.R., Varnous, S., et al., 1999. Mutations in the gene encoding lamin A/C cause Autosomal Dominant Emery-Dreifuss muscular dystrophy. Nat. Genet. 21, 285–288.

Bradley, W.G., Jones, M.Z., Fawcett, P.R.W., 1978. Becker Type muscular dystrophy. Muscle Nerve 1, 111–132.

Brooke, M.H., Griggs, M.D., Mendell, J.R., et al., 1981. Clinical trial in Duchenne dystrophy. 1. The design of the protocol. Muscle Nerve 4, 186–197.

Bunch, W.H., Siegel, I.M., 1993. Scapulothoracic arthrodesis in Fascioscapulohumeral Muscular Dystrophy. J. Bone Joint Surg. Am. 75A, 372–376.

Callen, J.P., 1988. Malignancy in polymyositis / dermatomyositis. Clinical Dermatology 2, 55–63.

Carroll, N., Bain, R.J.I., Smith, P.E.M., et al., 1991. Domiciliary investigation of sleep-related hypoxaemia in Duchenne muscular dystrophy. Eur. Respir. J. 4, 434–440.

Carter, G.T., Abresch, R.T., Fowler, W.M., et al., 1995. Profiles of neuromuscular disease: Spinal muscular atrophy. Am. J. Phys. Med. Rehabil. 74, 150–159.

D'Angelo, M.G., Berti, M., Piccinini, L., et al., 2005. A comparison of gait in spinal muscular atrophy, type II and Duchenne muscular dystrophy. Gait Posture 21 (4), 369–378.

Duboc, D., Meune, C., Pierre, B., Wahbi, K., Eymard, B., Totain, A., et al., 2007. Perindopril preventive treatment on mortality in Duchenne muscular dystrophy: 10 years follow-up. Am. Heart J. 154, 596–602.

Dubowitz, V., 1985. Muscle biopsy: A practical approach, second ed. Ballière Tindall, London.

Dubowitz, V., 1995. Muscle disorders in childhood, second ed. WB Saunders, London.

Eagle, M., Baudouin, S.V., Chandler, C., et al., 2002. Survival in Duchenne muscular dystrophy; improvements in life expectancy since 1967 and the impact of home nocturnal ventilation. Neuromuscul. Disord. 12, 926–930.

Eagle, M., Bourke, J., Bullock, R., et al., 2007. Managing Duchenne muscular dystrophy – the additive effect of spinal surgery and home ventilation in improving survival. Neuromuscul. Disord. 17, 470–475.

Eagle, M., Peacock, C.K., Bushby, K., Major, R., Clements, P., 2001.

Fascioscapuohumeral muscular dystrophy: gait analysis and effectiveness of ankle foot orthoses (AFOs) (abstract). Neuromuscul. Disord. 11 (6–7), 631.

Edwards, R.H.T., Chapman, S.J., Newham, D.J., et al., 1987. Practical analysis of variability of muscle function measurements in Duchenne Muscular Dystrophy. Muscle Nerve 10, 6–14.

Emery, A.E.H., 1971. The nosology of the spinal muscular atrophies. J. Med. Genet. 8, 481–495.

Emery, A.E.H., 1991. Population frequencies of inherited neuromuscular diseases– a world survey. Neuromuscul. Disord. 1, 19–29.

Emery, A.E., Muntoni, F., 2003. Duchenne Muscular Dystrophy. Oxford University Press, Oxford.

Fawcett, P.R.W., Barwick, D.D., 1994. The clinical neurophysiology of neuromuscular disease. In: Walton, J.N., Karpati, G., Hilton-Jones, D. (Eds.), Disorders of voluntary muscle. sixth ed. Edinburgh, Churchill Livingstone, pp. 1033–1104.

Fisher, N.M., Pendergast, D.R., Calkins, E.C., 1990. Maximal isometric torque of knee extension as a function of muscle length in subjects of advancing age. Arch. Phys. Med. Rehabil. 71, 729–734.

Friedrich, U., Brunner, H., Smeets, D., et al., 1987. Three points linkage analysis employing C3 and 19cen markers assign the myotonic dystrophy gene to 19q. Hum. Genet. 75, 291–293.

Galasko, C.S.B., Delaney, C., Morris, P., 1992. Spinal stabilisation in Duchenne Muscular Dystrophy. J. Bone Joint Surg. 74B, 210–214.

Gianinni, S., Faldini, C., Pagkrati, S., Grandi, G., Digennaro, V., Luciani, D., et al., 2007. Fixation of winged scapula in facioscapulohumeral muscular dystrophy. Clin. Med. Res. 5 (3), 155–162.

Gill, I., Eagle, M., Jwalant, S., et al., 2006. Correction of neuromuscular scoliosis in patients with pre-existing respiratory failure. Spine 21, 2478–2483.

Gospe, S.M., Lazaro, R.P., Lava, N.S., et al., 1989. Familial X linked myalgia and cramps: a non-progressive myopathy associated with a deletion in the dystrophin gene. Neurology 39, 1277–1280.

Gossman, M.R., Sahrmann, S.A., Rose, S.J., 1982. Review of length associated changes in muscle. Phys. Ther. 62, 1799–1808.

Griggs, R.C., Donohoe, K.M., Utell, M.J., et al., 1981. Evaluation of pulmonary function in neuromuscular disease. Arch. Neurol. 38, 9–12.

Harper, P.S., 1989. Myotonic dystrophy, second ed. WB Saunders, Philadelphia.

Heap, R.M., Mander, M., Bond, J., et al., 1996. Management of Duchenne muscular dystrophy in the community: views of physiotherapists, GP's and school teachers. Physiotherapy 82, 258–263.

Hough, A., 1991. Physiotherapy in respiratory care. Chapman & Hall, London.

Hunsaker, R.H., Fulkerson, P.K., Barry, F.J., et al., 1982. Cardiac function in Duchenne's muscular dystrophy. Results of 10–year follow up study and noninvasive tests. Am. J. Med. 73, 235–238.

Hyde, S.A., Fløytrup, I., Glent, S., et al., 2000. A randomised comparative study of two methods of controlling tendo achilles contracture in Duchenne muscular dystrophy. Neuromuscul. Disord. 10, 257–263.

Hyde, S.A., Scott, O.M., Goddard, C.M., et al., 1982. Prolongation of ambulation in Duchenne muscular dystrophy. Physiotherapy 68, 105–108.

Illarioshkin, S.N., Ivanova-Smolenskala, I.A., Tanaka, H., 1997. Refined genetic location of the chromosome 2p linked progressive muscular dystrophy gene. Genomics 42, 345–348.

Jeppesen, J., Green, A., Steffensen, B.F., Rahbek, J., 2003. The Duchenne muscular dystrophy population in Denmark, 1977–2001: prevalence, incidence and survival in relation to the introduction of ventilator use. Neuromuscul. Disord. 13 (10), 804–812.

Jones, D.A., Round, J.M., 1990. Skeletal muscle in health and disease, Manchester University Press, Manchester.

Jones, D.A., Rutherford, O.M., Parker, D.F., 1989. Physiological changes in skeletal muscle as a result of strength training. Q. J. Exp. Physiol. 74, 233–256.

Karpati, G., Hilton-Jones, D., Griggs, R.C., 2001. Disorders of Voluntary Muscle,

seventh ed. Cambridge University Press.

Khodadadeh, S., McClelland, M.R., Patrick, J.H., et al., 1986. Knee moments in Duchenne muscular dystrophy. Lancet 6 (September), 544–555.

Kilmer, D.D., 2002. Response to aerobic exercise training in humans with neuromuscular disease. Am. J. Phys. Med. Rehabil. 81 (Suppl. 11), S187–S195.

Kissell, J.T., 1999. Fascioscapulohumeral dystrophy. Semin. Neurol. 19, 35–43.

Kobayashi, O., Hayashi, Y., Arahata, K., et al., 1996. Congenital muscular dystrophy. Neurology 46, 815–818.

Kurz, L.T., Mubarek, S.J., Schultz, P., 1983. Correlation of scoliosis and pulmonary function in Duchenne muscular dystrophy. J. Pediatr. Orthop. 3, 347–353.

Laforet, P., De Toma, C., Eymard, B., et al., 1998. Cardiac involvement in genetically confirmed Fascioscapulohumeral muscular dystrophy. Neurology 51, 1454–1456.

Lennon, S.M., Ashburn, A., 1993. Use of myometry in the assessment of neuropathic weakness: testing for reliability in clinical practice. Clin. Rehabil. 7, 125–133.

Main, M., Mercuri, E., Haliloglu, G., et al., 2007. Serial casting of the ankles in Duchenne muscular dystrophy: can it be an alternative to surgery? Neuromuscul. Disord. 17, 227–230.

Manzur, A.Y., Kuntzer, T., Pike, M., Swan, A., 2008a. Glucocorticosteroids for Duchenne muscular dystrophy. The Cochrane Library (1), CD 003725.

Manzur, A.Y., Kinali, M., Muntoni, F., 2008b. Update on the management of Duchenne muscular dystrophy. Arch. Dis. Child. 93, 986–990.

Marsh, A., Edge, G., Lehovsky, J., 2003. Spinal fusion in patients with Duchenne's muscular dystrophy and a low forced vital capacity. Eur. Spine J. 12 (5), 507–512.

Martin, A.J., Stern, L., Yeates, J., et al., 1986. Respiratory muscle training in Duchenne Muscular Dystrophy. Dev. Med. Child. Neurol. 28, 314–318.

Mastaglia, F.L., Laing, N.G., 1996. Investigation of muscle disease. J. Neurol. Neurosurg. Psychiatry 60, 256–274.

Mazzone, E.S., Messina, S., Vasco, G., et al., 2009. Reliability of the North Star Ambulatory Assessment in a multicentric setting. Neuromuscul. Disord. 19, 458–461.

McDonald, C.M., Abresch, R.T., Carter, G.T., et al., 1995. Profiles of neuromuscular disease. Duchenne muscular dystrophy. Am. J. Phys. Med. Rehabil. 74, 70–92.

Mehdian, H., Shimizu, N., Draycott, V., et al., 1989. Spinal stabilisation for scoliosis in Duchenne muscular dystrophy. Experience with various sub-laminar instrumentation systems. Neuro-Orthopedics 7, 74–82.

Miura, K., Kumagai, T., Matsumoto, A., Iriyama, E., Watanabe, K., Goto, K., et al., 1998. Two cases of chromosome 4q35-linked early onset fascioscapulohumeral muscular dystrophy with mental retardation and epilepsy. Neuropaediatrics 29, 239–241.

Moore, J.K., Moore, A.P., 1987. Postoperative complications of dystrophia myotonica. Anaesthesia 42, 529–533.

Muntoni, F., Torelli, S., Ferlini, A., 2003. Dystrophin and mutations: one gene, several proteins, multiple phenotypes. Lancet Neurol. 2, 731–740.

Newham, D.J., Jones, D.A., Edwards, R.H.T., 1986. Plasma creatinine kinase changes after eccentric and concentric contractions. Muscle Nerve 9, 59–63.

Nicolino, M., Byrne, B., Wraithe, J.E., Leslie, N., Mendel, H., Freyer, D.R., et al., 2009. Clinical outcomes after long-term treatment with alglucosidase alfa in infants and children with advanced Pompe disease. Genet. Med. 11, 210–219.

Nigro, G., Comi, L.I., Politano, L., et al., 1990. The incidence and evaluation of cardiomyopathy in Duchenne muscular dystrophy. Int. J. Cardiol. 26, 271–277.

Ogino, S., Wilson, R.B., Gold, B., 2004. New insights on the evolution of the SMN1 and SMN2 region simulation and meta-analysis for allele and haplotype frequency calculations. Eur. J. Hum. Genet. 12, 1015–1023.

Olsen, D.B., Orngreen, M.C., Vissing, J., 2005. Aerobic training improves exercise performance in fascioscapulohumeral dystrophy. Neurology 64, 1064–1066.

Orrell, R.W., Forrester, J.D., Tawil, R., et al., 1999. Definitive molecular diagnosis of fascioscapulohumeral muscular dystrophy. Neurology 52, 1822–1826.

Pandya, S., Florence, J.M., King, W.M., et al., 1985. Reliability of goniometric measurements in patients with Duchenne muscular dystrophy. Phys. Ther. 65, 1339–1342.

Phadke, A.P., Jay, C., Chen, S.J., Haddock, C., Wang, Z., Yu, Y., et al., 2009. Safety and in vivo Expression of a GNE-Transgene: A Novel Treatment Approach for Hereditary Inclusion Body Myopathy-2. Gene Regulation and Systems Biology 3 (May), 89–101.

Phillips, M.F., Quinlivan, R.C.M., Edwards, R.H.T., et al., 2001. Changes in spirometry over time as a prognostic marker in patients with Duchenne Muscular Dystrophy. American Journal of Critical Care Medicine 164, 2191–2194.

Pope, P.M., 2002. Postural management and special seating. In: Edwards, S. (Ed.), Neurological physiotherapy: a problem solving approach, second ed. Churchill Livingstone, London, pp. 189–217.

Quinlivan, R.M., Dubowitz, V., 1992. Cardiac transplantation in Becker muscular dystrophy. Neuromuscul. Disord. 2 (3), 165–167.

Rhee, Y.G., Ha, J.H., 2006. Long-term results of scapulothoracic arthrodesis of fascioscapulohumeral muscular dystrophy. J. Shoulder Elbow Surg. 15 (4), 445–450.

Rodillo, E.B., Fernandez-Bermejo, E., Heckmatt, J.Z., et al., 1988. Prevention of rapidly progressive scoliosis in duchenne muscular dystrophy by prolonging walking with orthoses. J. Child. Neurol. 3, 269–274.

Rodillo, E., Noble-Jamieson, C.M., Aber, V., et al., 1989. Respiratory muscle training in Duchenne muscular dystrophy. Arch. Dis. Child. 64, 736–738.

Ryerson, S., 2009. Neurological assessment: the basis of clinical decision making. In: Lennon, S., Stokes, M. (Eds.), Pocketbook of Neurological Physiotherapy. Churchill Livingstone, pp. 113–126.

Scott, O.M., Hyde, S.A., Goddard, C., et al., 1981. Prevention of deformity in Duchenne muscular dystrophy. Physiotherapy 67, 177–180.

Scott, O.M., Hyde, S.A., Goddard, C., et al., 1982. Quantitation of muscle function in children: a prospective study in Duchenne Muscular Dystrophy. Muscle Nerve 5, 291–301.

Seeger, B.R., Sutherland, A., Clark, M.S., 1990. Management of scoliosis in Duchenne muscular dystrophy. Arch. Phys. Med. Rehabil. 65, 83–86.

Shepherd, R.B., 1995. Physiotherapy in Paediatrics, third ed. Butterworth Heinnemann, Oxford.

Simonds, A.K., 2000. Nasal ventilation in progressive neuromuscular disease: experience in adults and adolescents. Monaldi Archives of Chest Disease 55 (3), 237–241.

Smith, P.E.M., Edwards, R.H.T., Calverley, P.M.A., 1991. Mechanisms of sleep-disordered breathing in chronic neuromuscular disease: implications for management. Q. J. Med. 296, 961–973.

Steare, S.E., Benatar, A., Dubowitz, V., 1992. Subclinical cardiomyopathy in Becker muscular dystrophy. Br. Heart J. 68, 304–308.

Steffensen, B.F., Hyde, S.A., Attermann, J., et al., 2002. Reliability of the EK scale; a functional test for non-ambulatory individuals with Duchenne muscular dystrophy. Adv. Physiother. 4, 47.

Stern, L.M., Martin, A.J., Jones, N., et al., 1989. Training inspiratory resistance in Duchenne dystrophy using adapted computer games. Dev. Med. Child. Neurol. 31, 494–500.

Stokes, E.K., 2009. Outcome measurement. In: Lennon, S., Stokes, M. (Eds.), Pocketbook of Neurological Physiotherapy. Churchill Livingstone, pp. 192–201.

Sutherland, D.H., Olshen, R., Cooper, L., et al., 1981. The pathomechanics of gait in Duchenne muscular dystrophy. Dev. Med. Child. Neurol. 23, 3–22.

Sveen, M.L., Jeppesen, T.D., Hauersley, S., Krag, T.O., Vissing, J., 2007. Edurance training. An effective and safe treatment for patients with LGMD21. Neurology 68, 59–61.

Sveen, M.L., Jeppesen, T.D., Hauerslev, et al., 2008. Endurance training improves fitness and strength in patients with Becker muscular dystrophy. Brain 131, 2824–2831.

Thompson, N., Porter, S., Morris, C., 2007. Muscular Dystrophies, Spinal Muscular Atrophies and Peripheral Neuropathies. In: Morris, C., Dias, L. (Eds.), Paediatric Orthotics. Mac Keith Press, London.

Topin, N., Matecki, S., Le Bris, S., et al., 2002. Dose dependent effect of individualized respiratory muscle training in Duchenne muscular dystrophy. Neuromuscul. Disord. 12, 576–583.

Velasco, M.V., Cloin, A.A., Zurakowski, D., et al., 2007. Posterior spinal fusion for scoliosis in Duchenne muscular dystrophy diminishes the rate of respiratory decline. Spine 4, 459–465.

Vesa, J., Su, H., Watts, G.D., Krause, S., Walter, M.C., Martin, B., et al., 2009. Valosin containing protein associated inclusion body myopathy: abnormal vacuolization, autophagy and cell fusion in myoblasts. Neuromuscul.

Disord. 19 (11), 766–772 Epub 2009 Oct 13.

Vignos, P.J., Spencer, G.E., Archibald, K.C., 1963. Management of progressive muscular dystrophy in childhood. JAMA 13, 89–96.

Vignos, P.J., Wagner, M.B., Karlinchak, B., et al., 1996. Evaluation of a program for long-term treatment of Duchenne muscular dystrophy: experience at the University Hospitals of Cleveland. J. Bone Joint Surg. Am. 78 (12), 1844–1852.

Wagner, K.R., Lechtzin, N., Judge, D.P., 2007. Current treatment of adult Duchenne muscular dystrophy. Biochim. Biophys. Acta 1772 (2), 229–237. Epub 2006 Jul 8.

Wanke, T., Toifl, K., Merkle, M., et al., 1994. Inspiratory muscle training in patients with Duchenne Muscular Dystrophy. Chest 105, 475–482.

Wijmenga, C., Padberg, G.W., Moerer, P., et al., 1991. Mapping of fascioscapulohumeral gene to chromosome 4q35-qter by multipoint linkage analysis and *in situ* hybridization. Genomics 9, 570–575.

Webber, B.A., 1988. The Brompton Hospital guide to chest physiotherapy. Blackwell Scientific Publications, Oxford.

Wiles, C.M., Karni, Y., Nicklin, J., 1990. Laboratory testing of muscle function in the management of neuromuscular disease. J. Neurol. Neurosurg. Psychol. 53, 384–387.

World Health Organization (WHO), 2001. International classification of functioning, disability and health (ICF). World Health Organization, Geneva. Online. Available: http://www.who.int/classification/icf.

Section | 2 |

Treatment approaches in neurological rehabilitation

Chapter | **11** |

The theoretical basis for evidence-based neurological physiotherapy

Sheila Lennon

INTRODUCTION

This chapter aims to explain the theoretical framework underlying current practice in neurological physiotherapy for adults with damage to the nervous system. The text below will explain why theory and evidence-based practice are important, clarify the role of the neurological physiotherapist and discuss the key neurophysiological, motor learning and behavioural principles that guide practice. These guiding principles are derived from the theoretical framework proposed by Lennon and Bassile (2009).

Why are theory and evidence-based practice important?

Therapists need to subscribe to a theoretical framework for intervention, as theory provides the explanation not only for the behaviour of people following neurological damage, but also for the actions and decisions of therapists in clinical practice (Shephard, 1991). There are several neurological treatment approaches that influence the content, structure and aims of therapy. In the past therapists may have implemented care based on their preferred treatment approaches. However, to date there is no evidence to suggest that one therapy approach is superior to another (Kollen et al., 2009; Pollock et al., 2007). Therapy delivered in practice is always composed of multiple components tailored to suit each individual patient; therefore, research trials should aim to evaluate the active ingredients or components within physiotherapy, as similarities between approaches may actually outweigh their differences. In order to implement evidence-based practice, therapists are expected to incorporate a wide range of strategies that are supported by the current evidence base into their treatment programmes (Pollock et al., 2007).

There are many examples of specific training strategies such as strength training or task-specific practice, which are effective at improving movement and function (Van Peppen et al., 2007 see www.cochrane.org for relevant systematic reviews). There are also many clinical guidelines that provide a comprehensive review of all the available evidence to date for multidisciplinary management of people post-stroke (NCGS, 2008), with Parkinson's disease (Keus et al., 2006) and with multiple sclerosis (MS Society, 2008). These guidelines, developed by multidisciplinary panels and subjected to peer review, and are based on the best available evidence.

Components selected within therapy sessions should be evidence-based rather than based on therapist preference for a specific treatment approach. However, it is also important to realize that there are still many key areas of clinical practice with no evidence or conflicting evidence; therefore, therapists continue to rely on their clinical reasoning skills to select treatment techniques appropriate to the needs, wishes and goals of patients and their carers. This is why evidence-based practice is defined as the integration of best evidence with clinical expertise and patient values (Bernhardt & Legg, 2009).

Evidence-based guidelines rather than therapist preference for any named therapy approach should serve as a framework from which therapists should derive the most effective treatment (Kollen et al., 2009). However, there are many methodological shortcomings in the current evidence base and further high-quality trials need to be conducted (Kollen et al., 2009).

KEY POINTS

- Theory can explain therapist and patient behaviour in relation to intervention.
- No single treatment approach has been shown to be the best.
- Components selected within therapy sessions should be evidence-based rather than based on therapist preference for a specific treatment approach.
- Evidence-based practice involves three components: evidence available, clinical judgement and service user values.
- The components involved in physiotherapy interventions need to be defined and evaluated.
- There are many methodological flaws in the current evidence base; more research is essential.

Role of the physiotherapist

One of the key roles of the physiotherapist working in neurology is to help the patient experience and relearn optimal movement, and function in everyday life within the constraints imposed by the disease process and presenting impairments. Physiotherapists are not only interested in which functional activities patients can or cannot perform, but also in how the patient moves (the quality of movement) to execute these activities.

Physiotherapists help patients, their carers and the multidisciplinary team to identify potential for change following damage to the nervous system. Physiotherapists provide stimulus via movement to engage patient response; physiotherapists make movement and activity possible by using a variety of strategies such as therapeutic handling, or elimination of gravity and activity in mid range to elicit motor activity even when patients are

unable to demonstrate movement to command (Kilbride & Cassidy, 2009).

The aims of neurological physiotherapy can be summed up using the acronym RAMP for Recovery, Adaptation, Maintenance and Prevention (see Figure 11.1).

Physiotherapy ideally aims to restore movement and function in people with neurological pathology, but this may not always be possible. Adaptation (compensation) refers to the use of alternative movement strategies to complete a task (Shumway-Cook & Woollacott, 2007, pp. 152–153). Therapists focus on promoting compensatory strategies that are necessary for function and discouraging those that may be detrimental to the patient, e.g. promoting musculoskeletal damage, such as knee hyperextension (Edwards, 2002, p. 2). Interventions aimed at recovery of function need to be emphasized over compensation if the patient has the potential to change. Maintenance of function is just as important as recovery, and should be viewed as a positive achievement; several reviews have now confirmed that functional ability can be maintained despite deteriorating impairments in progressive neurological disease (Keus et al., 2006). Physiotherapy also aims to prevent the development of complications such as contracture, swelling and disuse atrophy. There are different stages in patient management, where these aims may have differential priorities. Understanding the nature of the pathology, and the prognosis for recovery in collaboration with patients and care givers to establish desired goals will help determine which of these aims should be emphasized in physiotherapy.

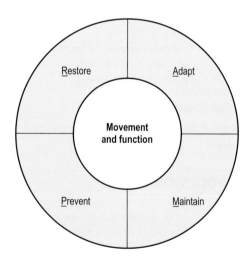

Figure 11.1 RAMP – aims of neurological physiotherapy. (Reproduced from Lennon S, Bassile C. Guiding Principles for neurological physiotherapy. In Lennon S, Stokes M (eds). Pocketbook of Neurological Physiotherapy. Elsevier Ltd, London, 2009, pp. 97-111, with permission from Elsevier Ltd.)

KEY POINTS

- Movement re-education and functional task practice are essential components of neurological physiotherapy.
- Physiotherapists provide stimulus via movement to engage patient response.
- The core aims of neurological physiotherapy are: Restoration, Adaptation, Maintenance, and Prevention (RAMP).

GUIDING PRINCIPLES

Lennon and Bassile (2009) have identified eight principles to guide physiotherapy practice (see Figure 11.2): (1) the World Health Organization (WHO) *International Classification of Functioning, Disability and Health* (ICF); (2) team work; (3) patient-centred care; (4) neural plasticity; (5) a systems model of motor control; (6) functional movement re-education; (7) skill acquisition; and (8) self-management (self-efficacy). Each of these principles will be discussed in this chapter.

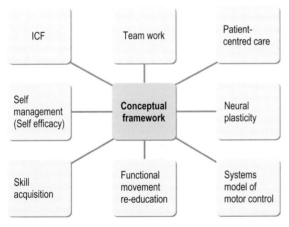

Figure 11.2 Guiding principles for neurological physiotherapy. (Reproduced from Lennon S, Bassile C. Guiding Principles for neurological physiotherapy. In: Lennon S, Stokes M, eds. Pocketbook of Neurological Physiotherapy. Elsevier Ltd, London, 2009, pp. 97-111, with permission from Elsevier Ltd.)

Principle 1: The ICF

The WHO has developed the ICF (2001; www.who.int/classifications/icf), which provides a systematic way of understanding the problems faced by patients, illustrating the multiple levels at which therapy may act. The activities dimension covers the range of activities performed by an individual. The participation dimension classifies the areas of life in which there are societal opportunities or barriers for each individual.

This framework provides a mechanism to document the impact of the environment on a person's functioning. Impairment is defined as a deficit in body structure or function. Following a CVA, an example of impairment would be weakness, with a restriction in the activity of walking thus requiring the use of a wheelchair for mobility. Being in a wheelchair may limit the individual's ability to resume his or her job, a restriction in participating in that individual's previous role in society.

Within the ICF framework, neurological physiotherapy may directly target both impairment (a loss or abnormality of body structure) and activity (performance in functional activities) with the overall aim of improving quality of life and enabling participation in desired life roles. Most large randomized controlled trials agree that patients need to have a minimum level of residual movement to demonstrate functional improvement (Van Peppen et al., 2004). This means that therapists will need to use both impairment and function focused strategies depending on the patient.

Principle 2: Team work

Neurological physiotherapists use their clinical reasoning skills combined with current evidence to assess, develop and evaluate an appropriate plan of care in collaboration with the patients and their carers, and the multidisciplinary team (Ryerson, 2009).

Team work is required to coordinate rehabilitation, as a variety of health-care professionals are involved to exchange information with the patients and their families. Team meetings are held to agree a common plan of care in order to reduce the risk of conflicting information, and to work towards common goals (Sivaraman Nair & Wade, 2003). Interdisciplinary rehabilitation refers to the activities of the health-care team, where there is a high level of communication, mutual goal planning and evaluation (Long et al., 2003). The Stroke Unit Trialists Collaboration (SUTC, 2006) has identified that patients who receive organized stroke unit care provided in hospital by nurses, doctors and therapists who specialize in looking after stroke patients and work as a coordinated team are more likely to survive their stroke, return home and become independent in looking after themselves. Thus it would appear that team working is an essential factor in improving patient outcomes.

Goal setting

Developing an appropriate plan of care revolves around collaborative goal setting within the team. Setting goals by the interdisciplinary team is recognized as a core component of neurorehabilitation (Wade, 2009). Setting goals aims to:

- motivate the team and the patient
- coordinate activities
- ensure that all important goals are identified.

Although there is limited evidence as to the best approach to use in goal setting, there is strong evidence that prescribed, specific and challenging goals lead to improved patient performance on simple cognitive and motor tasks (see Levack et al., 2006, for a review of goal planning in rehabilitation). Team goals need to be based on patient's wishes, expectations, priorities and values in line with the SMART acronym, which recommends that goals should be specific, measurable, achievable/ambitious, relevant and timed (Playford et al., 2009). Also see Bovend'Eerdt et al. (2009) for some practical guidance on how to set SMART goals.

Principle 3: Patient-centred care

Patient and carer involvement is a key component of neurological rehabilitation (Cott et al., 2007; Laverty et al., 2009). There is little consensus regarding a definition. Lewin et al. (2009) has suggested that patient-centred care is based on shared control and shared decisions about interventions or the management of health problems with the focus on the whole patient in their psychosocial context.

Although patient-centred care is not a new concept, it is increasingly evidence-based, with studies showing improvements in self-care, quality of life, satisfaction with care, increased engagement and reduced anxiety (Laverty et al., 2009; Whalley Hammell 2009). The physiotherapist, working in collaboration with the interdisciplinary rehabilitation team, discusses and explains treatment options; patients and their care givers (as appropriate) use this information to make decisions about their goals and select treatment solutions. Thus the emphasis should be placed on the patient as the problem solver and the decision maker. The process of goal setting provides a mechanism for patient-centred care by enabling autonomy, and appropriate pacing of information and responsibility (Playford et al., 2009).

Principle 4: Neural plasticity

Although there is always a degree of spontaneous recovery following brain damage, advances in neuroimaging have confirmed that plasticity (enduring changes in structure and function) can occur following damage to the nervous system, and also as a result of experience and therapy. The brain responds to injury by adaptation aimed at restoring function. Thus cortical maps can be modified by a variety of inputs such as sensory inputs, experience, learning and therapy, as well as in response to injury (Nudo, 2007). This ability for neuroplastic change implies that recovery

of movement and function should be the main aim of therapy rather than the promotion of independence using the unaffected side, e.g. compensation.

Therapists use different techniques to promote neuroplasticity. There is sound neurophysiological evidence to support the use of afferent information, in particular from the proximal regions, such as the trunk and the hip, as well as the foot, to trigger both postural adjustments and planned sequences of muscle activation during goal-directed movements (Allum et al., 1995; Bloem et al., 2002; Park et al., 1999). The evidence base for applying exercise therapy in functional activities within a meaningful environment and context is also strong (Kwakkel et al., 2004), for example a systematic review by French et al. (2007), has suggested that interventions based on task practice and repetition are more effective than conventional therapy in improving lower limb function after stroke.

Studies have shown that plasticity occurs in association with rehabilitation but further research is required to establish direct links between interventions, neuroplastic change and functional improvement in people following brain damage (see Kleim, 2009, for an overview of animal and human evidence in neurorehabilitation)

Principle 5: A systems model of motor control

Textbooks recommend that a systems model of motor control be adopted, integrating evidence from neurophysiology, biomechanics and motor learning (Carr & Shepherd, 2003). There are many different models of motor control. Shumway-Cook and Woollacott (2007, pp.16–17) recommend a systems model, which considers that solutions to the patient's motor problems change according to the interaction between the individual, the task and the environment. Although it is important to understand the role of major circuits and pathways of the nervous system (see Kandel et al., 2000, for an overview) and the effects of lesions on these structures and circuits, it is important to understand that there are many subsystems and multiple connections within the nervous system that work in hierarchy and in parallel to generate movement. The actions of a person with damage to the motor control are a consequence of the impairments caused by the damage, the compensatory strategies that enable function to be achieved in the presence of impairments and the effects of the environment the person has been experiencing since the lesion (Bate, 2009).

The key points to remember when designing therapy programmes are that therapists can change the environment, or the task, in such a way that enables the patient to elicit or practice both actions and the tasks required to achieve their goals. See Bate (2009) for an overview of how the motor control system generates movements based on a systems model.

Principle 6: Functional movement re-education

Physiotherapists use observed deviations from normal movement to plan treatment. Normal movement appears to be a logical model for therapy, provided that the patient has the potential to recover movement, for several reasons. Firstly, these movement patterns, used in everyday life, are already well engrained in each individual's motor system, as they have been practised throughout an individual's motor development at an early stage, and, secondly, they are more energy efficient.

Guidelines of critical features for training actions and functional tasks have been published in expert text books (Carr & Shepherd, 2003; Edwards, 2002). Normative data for everyday activities help therapists to understand motor performance and the impact of impairments on these everyday activities (Carr & Shepherd, 2006); therapists place an emphasis on training control of muscles, and promoting learning of relevant actions and tasks. Therapists aim to optimize movement and function. However, with the majority of neurological conditions, recovery of normal movement and function is not achievable for many patients; this depends to some extent on whether or not the patient has a progressive condition (Edwards, 2002, p. 256).

Physiotherapists use an array of techniques to make movement and function possible, and therapeutic handling is only one of many techniques (see Ch. 12). There is a role for hands-on practice or therapeutic handling, where the therapist manually guides the patient's movements and activities; as well as a role for hands-off practice where the therapist acts more in the role of a coach to correct movement and functional task performance. It is always preferable to prioritize the practice of functional activities selected in collaboration with the patient. However, if the patient has impairments that make it difficult to practice these tasks directly, therapists may also need to address impairments or practice specific movements, either before or during a modified version of functional task practice (Lennon & Bassile, 2009). For example, a patient may not have any signs of motor activity in the lower limb in order to practice the task of walking. In this case the patient may require either hands on assistance from therapists or support from assistive technologies, e.g. a partial body weight system in order to practice the task of walking. A comprehensive physiotherapy programme may include a wide range of components, such as postural control training, movement re-education (trunk/pelvis/limbs), aerobic training, strengthening exercises, flexibility exercises, and functional task practice, e.g. reach and grasp, bed mobility, transfer and ambulation activities (Lennon & Bassile, 2009). The choice and emphasis of the components will vary depending on the results of each patient's assessment.

> ### KEY POINTS
>
> - Physiotherapy targets both impairments and functional activities.
> - Therapists may need to use a combination of impairment- and function-focused strategies.
> - There is a role for both hands-on and hands-off practice.

Principle 7: Skill acquisition

There is mounting evidence that task-specific training is required in therapy in order to improve functional recovery (French et al., 2007; Hubbard et al., 2009). Evidence from motor learning and skill acquisition can provide some guiding principles about how to structure practice within therapy sessions (Marley et al., 2000). Motor learning literature differentiates between whole and part practice of a task; yet current evidence does not suggest that whole-task practice is more effective at regaining function than part practice activities (Majsak, 1996; Shumway-Cook & Woollacott, 2007, pp.538-539). Research has highlighted practice and feedback as two crucial issues for therapists. The type of practice used may depend on the task at hand; for example, part practice of fast, discrete tasks or tasks with interdependent parts is less effective than practising the whole task. It has also been suggested that patients need to rely on both intrinsic and extrinsic information to learn new skills (Schmidt et al., 2005).

Motor skill learning can be divided into three phases (Marley et al., 2000):

- An early cognitive phase
- An intermediate associative phase
- An autonomous phase.

Certain types of feedback should be used at different points in skill acquisition. For example, manual guidance should mainly be used at the early cognitive stage of motor learning, whereas physical and verbal guidance may actually interfere with motor learning in the later associative and autonomous stages of skill acquisition (Schmidt et al., 2005). Different techniques may work better with different patients; sometimes it will be necessary to practise the components of normal movement that comprise an activity such as pelvic tilting. Sometimes it will work best to break tasks down into the different parts before getting the patient to practise the whole sequence of activity in a functional task. On other occasions it will work best to practise the functional task.

A critical issue for physiotherapy is how much practice is required to improve functional skills (Kwakkel, 2006). Carryover from therapy sessions into everyday activities can be problematic; generalization of treatment effects should be sought by giving the patient activities to practise outside therapy (Lennon, 2003; Marley et al., 2000). The majority of motor learning research is based on normal populations; much more research is required in patients with neurological impairments to determine the most effective ways in which to structure practice and provide feedback.

Principle 8: Self management (self-efficacy)

Whilst it is acknowledged that physiotherapists aim to target both impairments and functional limitations, they also have a role to play in enabling people to return towards meaningful roles in the wider community, with a focus on health and wellness, as well as on ill health and disability (Cott et al., 2007; Dean 2009). Ultimately this means that neurological physiotherapy within rehabilitation involves changing behaviour.

Self-management (the maintenance of health and wellbeing; see Ch. 19) is important as it involves developing skills required to cope with disability and change behaviours necessary to resume desired lifestyles (DoH, 2006). Self-efficacy is a cornerstone of self-management; it is defined as people's beliefs about their capabilities to influence key events that affect their lives (Bandura, 2007). People with a strong sense of self-efficacy set themselves challenging goals and maintain strong commitment to them; they continue to sustain their efforts in the face of failure or setbacks (Bandura, 2007). A review specific to physiotherapy by Barron et al. (2007) has shown that self-efficacy can be related to better health, higher achievement, more social integration and higher motivation to act.

Growing evidence provides support for the importance of self-efficacy as a correlate of adherance to therapy (Rhodes & Fiala, 2009). However, evidence is scarce regarding the most effective ways of supporting and enabling individuals with neurological problems to manage ways of living with their chronic disability (Jones, 2006). Physiotherapists need to consider how they can promote self-efficacy and enhance their patients' self-management skills (see Jones, 2009, for an overview).

CONCLUSION

Physiotherapists have a key role to play in enabling patients to experience and relearn optimal movement, and function in everyday life within the constraints imposed by neurological disease and presenting impairments. Neurophysiological, motor learning and behavioural principles need to be taken into account in the theoretical framework underlying neurological physiotherapy. This chapter has discussed eight principles derived from Lennon and Bassile (2009) to guide current practice in neurological physiotherapy: the ICF, team work, patient-centred care, neural plasticity, a systems model of motor control, functional movement re-education, skill acquisition and self-management (self-efficacy).

Developing an appropriate plan of care revolves around collaborative goal setting with the patient and carers within the interdisciplinary team. This process of goal setting provides a key mechanism for patient-centred care. As well as focusing on the physical activities required to re-educate movement and promote skill acquisition, physiotherapists also need to understand how to facilitate behavioural change, by promoting self-efficacy and enhancing their patients' self-management skills. It is crucial to link clinical practice to quality research. Components selected within therapy sessions should be evidence-based rather than based on therapist preference for a specific treatment approach.

REFERENCES

Allum, A., Honegger, F., Acuna, H., 1995. Differential control of leg and trunk muscle activity by vestibulo-spinal and proprioceptive signals during human balance corrections. Acta Otolaryngol. (Stockholm) 115, 124–129.

Bandura, A., 2007. Self efficacy in health functioning. In: Ayers, S. et al., (Ed.), Cambridge handbook of Psychology, Health and Medicine, second ed. Cambridge University Press, New York, pp. 191–193.

Barron, C.J., Klaber Moffett, J.A., Potter, M., 2007. Patient expectations, of physiotherapy: definitions, concepts and theories. Physiother. Theory Pract. 23, 37–46.

Bate, P., 2009. Motor Control. In: Lennon, S., Stokes, M. (Eds.), Pocketbook of Neurological Physiotherapy. Elsevier Science, London, pp. 31–40.

Bernhardt, J., Legg, L., 2009. Chapter 1. Evidence-based practice. In: Lennon, S., Stokes, M. (Eds.), Pocketbook of Neurological Physiotherapy. Elsevier Science, London, pp. 3–15.

Bloem, B.R., Allum, J.H., Carpenter, M.G., et al., 2002. Triggering of balance corrections in a patient with total leg proprioceptive loss. Exp. Brain Res. 142, 91–107.

Bovend'Eerdt, T.J.H., Botell, R.E., Wade, D.T., 2009. Writing SMART rehabilitation goals and achieving goal attainment scaling: a practical guide. Clin. Rehabil. 23, 352–361.

Carr, J.H., Shepherd, R.B., 2003. Stroke rehabilitation: guidelines for exercise and training to optimise motor skills. Butterworth Heinemann, Oxford.

Carr, J.H., Shepherd, J.H., 2006. Neurological rehabilitation. Disabil. Rehabil. 28, 811–812.

Cott, C.A., Wiles, R., Devitt, R., 2007. Continuity, transition and participation: Preparing clients for life in the community post-stroke. Disabil. Rehabil. 29, 1566–1574.

Dean, E., 2009. Foreword from the Special Issue Editor of 'Physical Therapy Practice in the 21st Century: A New Evidence-informed Paradigm and Implications. Physiother. Theory Pract. 25, 328–329.

Department of Health (DoH), 2006. Supporting people with long term conditions to self-care: a guide to developing local strategies and good practice. March.

Edwards, S., 2002. Neurological Physiotherapy. Edinburgh, Churchill Livingstone.

French, B., Thomas, L.H., Leathley, M.J., Sutton, C.J., McAdam, J., Forster, A., et al., 2007. Repetitive task training for improving functional ability after stroke (Review). The Cochrane Library (4).

Hubbard, I.J., Parsons, M.W., Neilson, C., Carey, L.M., 2009. Task-specific training: evidence for and translation to clinical practice. Occup. Ther. Int. 16, 175–189.

Jones, F., 2006. Strategies to enhance chronic disease self-management: how can we apply this to stroke? Disabil. Rehabil. 28, 841–847.

Jones, F., 2009. Continuity of care. In: Lennon, S., Stokes, M. (Eds.), Pocketbook of Neurological Physiotherapy. Elsevier Science, London, pp. 203–210.

Kandel, E.R., Schwartz, J.A., Jessell, T.M., 2000. Principles of Neural Science, fourth ed. McGraw Hill, New York.

Keus, S., Bloem, B., Hendriks, E., et al., 2006. Evidence-based analysis of physical therapy in Parkinson's Disease with recommendations for practice and research. Mov. Disord. 22, 451–460.

Kilbride, C., Cassidy, E., 2009. The acute patient before and during stabilisation; stroke, traumatic brain injury, Guillain Barre Syndrome. In: Lennon, S., Stokes, M. (Eds.), Pocketbook of Neurological Physiotherapy. Elsevier Science, London, pp. 127–135.

Kleim, J.A., 2009. Neural plasticity in motor learning and motor recovery. In: Lennon, S., Stokes, M. (Eds.), Pocketbook of Neurological Physiotherapy. Elsevier Science, London, pp. 41–50.

Kollen, B.J., Lennon, S., Lyons, B., Wheatley-Smith, L., Scheper, M., Buurke, J., et al., 2009. The effectiveness of the Bobath Concept in stroke rehabilitation: what is the evidence. Stroke 40, e89–1e87.

Kwakkel, G., 2006. Impact of intensity of practice after stroke: issues for consideration. Disabil. Rehabil. 28, 823–830.

Kwakkel, G., Kollen, B., Lindeman, E., 2004. Understanding the pattern of functional recovery after stroke. Restor. Neurol. Neurosci. 22, 281–299.

Laverty, A.M., Jones, Z., Rodgers, H., 2009. Ensuring patient and carer-centred care. In: Lennon, S., Stokes, M. (Eds.), Pocketbook of Neurological Physiotherapy. Elsevier Science, London, pp. 17–24.

Lennon, S., 2003. Physiotherapy practice in stroke rehabilitation: a survey. Disabil. Rehabil. 25, 455–461.

Lennon, S., Bassile, C., 2009. Guiding Principles for neurological physiotherapy. In: Lennon, S., Stokes, M. (Eds.), Pocketbook of Neurological Physiotherapy. Elsevier Ltd, London, pp. 97–111.

Levack, W.M.M., Dean, S.G., Siegert, R.G., McPherson, K.M., 2006. Purposes and mechanisms of goal planning in rehabilitation: the need for a critical distinction. Disabil. Rehabil. 28, 741–749.

Lewin, S., Skea, Z., Entwistle, V.A., Zwarenstein, M., Dick, J., 2009. Interventions for providers to promote a patient-centred approach in clinical consultations (Review). The Cochrane Library (3).

Long, A.F., Kneafsey, R., Ryan, J., 2003. Rehabilitation practice: challenges to effective team working. Int. J. Nurs. Stud. 40, 663–673.

Majsak, M.J., 1996. Application of motor learning principles to the stroke population. Top. Stroke Rehabil. 3, 27–59.

Marley, T.L., Ezekiel, H.J., Lehto, N.K., Wishart, L.R., Lee, T.D., 2000. Application of motor learning principles: the physiotherapy client as a problem solver. II. Scheduling practice. Physiother. Canada 52, 315–320.

MS Society, 2008. Translating the NICE MS Guideline into practice: a physiotherapy guidance document, London, second ed. MS Society, Chartered Society of Physiotherapy and Association of Physiotherapists in Neurology, London.

NCGS, 2008. National Clinical Guidelines for Stroke. Royal College of Physicians, London. Available online at: http://www.rcplondon.ac.uk/pubs/books/stroke.

Nudo, R., 2007. Post-infarct cortical plasticity and behavioural recovery. Stroke 38, 840–845.

Park, S., Toole, T., Lee, S., 1999. Functional roles of the proprioceptive system in the control of goal-directed movement. Percept. Mot. Skills 88, 631–647.

Playford, E.D., Siegert, R., Levack, W., freeman, J., 2009. Areas of consensus and controversy about goal setting in rehabilitation: a conference report. Clin. Rehabil. 23, 334–344.

Pollock, A., Baer, G., Pomeroy, V., Langhorne, P., 2007. Physiotherapy treatment approaches for the recovery of postural control and lower limb function following stroke. The Cochrane Library (1).

Rhodes, R.E., Fiala, B., 2009. Building motivation and sustainability into the prescription and recommendations for physical activity and exercise therapy: the evidence. Physiother. Theory Pract. 25, 424–441.

Ryerson, S., 2009. Neurological assessment: the basis of clinical decision making. In: Lennon, S., Stokes, M. (Eds.), Pocketbook of Neurological Physiotherapy. Elsevier Science, London, pp. 113–126.

Schmidt, R.A., Lee, T., 2005. Motor Control and Learning: A Behavioural Emphasis, fourth ed. Human Kinetics, Illinois.

Shepard, K., 1991. Theory: criteria, importance and impact. In: Proceedings of the 2nd STEP Conference on Contemporary Management of Motor Control Problems. Foundation for Physical Therapy, Virginia, pp. 5–10.

Shumway Cook, A., Woollacott, M.H., 2007. Motor Control translating research into clinical practice. Williams & Wilkins, Baltimore.

Sivaraman Nair, K.P., Wade, D.T., 2003. Satisfaction of members of interdisciplinary rehabilitation teams with goal planning meetings. Arch. Phys. Med. Rehabil. 84, 1710–1713.

Stroke Unit Trialists Collaboration (SUTC), 2006. Organised inpatient (stroke unit) care for stroke(review). The Cochrane Library (3).

Van Peppen, R.P.S., Kwakkel, G., Wood-Dauphinee, S., et al., 2004. The impact of physical therapy on functional outcomes after stroke: what's the evidence? Clin. Rehabil. 18, 833–862.

Van Peppen, R.P.S., Hendriks, H.J., van Meeteren, N.L., Helders, P.J., Kwakkel, G., 2007. The development of a clinical practice stroke guideline for physiotherapists in The Netherlands: a systematic review of available evidence. Disabil. Rehabil. 29, 767–783.

Wade, D.T., 2009. Goal setting in rehabilitation: an overview of what, why and how. Clin. Rehabil. 23, 291–295.

Whalley Hammell, K., 2009. The wider context of neurorehabilitation. In: Lennon, S., Stokes, M. (Eds.), Pocketbook of Neurological Physiotherapy. Elsevier Science, London, pp. 25–30.

World Health Organization (WHO), 2001. International Classification of Functioning, Disability and Health (ICF). World Health Organization, Geneva. Available online at: http:/www.who.int/classification/icf.

Chapter | **12** |

Specific treatment techniques

Joanna Jackson

CONTENTS

INTRODUCTION

Physiotherapists working in neurological rehabilitation employ a large variety of techniques. When examining treatment approaches from different philosophical backgrounds, it is apparent that similar techniques may be being utilized (see Ch. 11). A technique can be defined as a 'method or skill used for a particular task' (Collins English Dictionary). With this definition in mind it is important to consider to what purpose different techniques are employed. It is also important that the technique is appropriate in order to help meet the treatment goals.

This chapter illustrates the diversity of the techniques used by physiotherapists. It is clear that there is a wealth of research supporting the use of some techniques and a lack of a clear evidence base to justify the use of others. Many techniques continue to rely on anecdotal evidence to support their use. In this chapter a variety of techniques are reviewed and the evidence available to support their use is considered. Physiotherapists are challenged to provide best practice based on evidence. However, such evidence may be unavailable or incomplete (Jones et al., 2006) and this is reflected in the field of specific treatment techniques used in neurological physiotherapy.

The chapter is divided into sections: some techniques have mixed effects such that they could be included in more than one section; they will be found in the section which reflects their main usage. This is not intended as a recipe-type guide to treatments but rather as a brief overview of the different treatments available, their proposed effects and their indications for use. Details of how to apply the techniques can be found in the relevant literature, some of which is cited here. Examples of where the techniques may be applied, and illustrations of their use, can be seen in the chapters on specific neurological conditions in this text.

FACILITATION

Many of the techniques used in neurological rehabilitation are applied to facilitate and enhance muscle activity, and thus help achieve improved control of movement. It is also proposed that these interventions are chosen to facilitate neuroplasticity (Umphred et al., 2007a). Many of the specific techniques used for facilitation have their origins in the work of Margaret Rood. For a comprehensive examination of the Rood approach and the most recent interpretation of its relevance, the reader is directed to Baily Metcalfe and Lawes (1998) and Schultz-Krohn et al. (2006). Some of those most commonly used techniques are outlined below.

Brushing

In the 1950s Rood proposed that fast brushing, using a battery-operated brush, of the skin overlying a muscle could be used to facilitate a muscle contraction. Brushing has been used widely by physiotherapists, applied either using an electrically operated brush or manually using a bottle brush, but there is little indication given about the required rate or duration of the brushing, or pressure to be applied. It would make sense that the skin being brushed and the muscle being facilitated should be supplied by the same spinal segment. Although Garland and Hayes (1987) observed an effect of brusing in hemiplegic subjects with foot drop, there is little evidence to support its effectiveness. In subjects who received a combination of brushing preceded by voluntary contraction of the tibialis anterior, a significant change in electromyographic (EMG) activity was seen both immediately and 30 minutes after stimulation.

Brushing may be a powerful method of facilitation but it is clearly not well researched in terms of its continued effects, particularly as much of the work has been carried out on subjects with no neurological impairments. It is worth noting that caution in its use has been advised (Farber, 1982) and that Schultz-Krohn et al. (2006) consider it beyond the scope of entry-level practice.

KEY POINTS

- Little evidence exists for effectiveness of brushing.
- Caution is advised.

Ice – brief

Ice can be used to facilitate a response from muscle. Ice uses a combination of coolness and pain sensations to produce the desired response.

In order to facilitate a motor response, an ice cube is quickly swept over the chosen muscle belly (Umphred et al., 2007a). Following each swipe the iced area is blotted with a towel. After three swipes the patient is asked to produce an active muscle contraction. If ice is being used to facilitate lip closure and encourage feeding and sucking, an ice lolly can be placed in the mouth with pressure on the tongue (Farber, 1982).

When using ice as a stimulating technique it is important to remember that it can be a potent stimulus and results can be unpredictable. Putting ice on the face above the level of the lips and to the midline of the trunk should be avoided, as it has been reported that undesirable behavioural and autonomic responses may be provoked (Umphred et al., 2007a; Schultz-Krohn et al., 2006).

Retraining of sensory function has received little attention in the physiotherapy literature. However, the use of repeated ice water immersions of the affected hand in chronic stroke patients was investigated by Bohls and McIntyre (2005) in a small scale study. Although wrist position sense was not improved by the intervention it was suggested that a positive effect may be found in relation to the sensation of light touch and temperature discrimination.

KEY POINTS

♦ Brief ice can be a potent stimulus with unpredictable effects.
♦ Avoid applying ice to the face above the level of the lips and to the midline of the trunk.

Tapping

Tapping is the use of a light force applied manually over a tendon or muscle belly to facilitate a voluntary contraction. Tapping over a tendon would usually be used to assess reflex activity. A normal response would be a brisk muscle contraction. It is not therefore recommended that tendon tapping be used in a treatment situation, as the response is a crude muscle contraction and will be of little use to help a patient produce a graded, functional movement (Umphred et al., 2007a).

Rood recommended three to five taps over the belly of the muscle being facilitated. In addition, tapping can be applied to a muscle that has been stretched by the effect of gravity. Once the muscle responds to the stretch produced by gravity the therapist taps the muscle, using the hand, facilitating further activity (O'Sullivan, 2007). For example, with a patient who is standing, weight-bearing through both legs, if one knee gives way gravity will stretch the quadriceps muscle group. The therapist can then tap the muscle, facilitating a return to full knee extension.

Sweep tapping is a light touch sweeping movement applied by the back of the therapist's fingers over the dermatomal area innervating the muscles the patient is required to contract (Umphred et al., 2007a). Davies (2000) described the use of sweep tapping to provide an excitatory stimulus to activate the finger extensors in hemiplegia. This is applied by providing support to the affected upper limb with one hand, while the other hand sweeps firmly and briskly over the extensors of the wrist and fingers; the sweep commences just below the elbow and continues over the dorsum of the hand and fingers. In common with other tapping techniques, an active response is requested from the patient following its application.

The use of tapping, like many of the other sensory facilitatory techniques, is mainly supported by anecdotal evidence.

KEY POINT

♦ Tapping, like many of the other sensory facilitatory techniques, is mainly supported by anecdotal evidence.

Passive stretching – fast

Stretching may be applied in different ways to patients with neurological dysfunction to achieve different effects. A quick stretch is applied to facilitate a muscle contraction, and a slow or sustained stretch is given to reduce spasticity or prevent or reduce contractures. It is not within the scope of this chapter to consider the anatomy and physiology of the structures involved, including muscle, tendons, joints and the stretch reflex, as there are comprehensive texts devoted entirely to such topics.

A quick stretch is facilitatory and achieves its effect via stimulation of the muscle spindle primary endings. Quick stretching of the agonist muscle will, therefore, result in reflex facilitation of that muscle via the monosynaptic reflex arc. This stretch is normally applied manually by the physiotherapist. Fast stretching is one of the core procedures employed during proprioceptive neuromuscular facilitation (PNF) techniques (see below).

Joint compression

Receptors in joints and muscles are involved with the awareness of joint position and movement. Compression of a joint stimulates these receptors and can produce both inhibitory and facilitatory effects. Joint compression (approximation) is achieved either by normal body weight (or less) being applied through the longitudinal axis of the bone (light compression) or as heavy joint compression, where the approximation is greater than that produced by body weight (Schultz-Krohn et al., 2006). Heavy joint compression is thought to facilitate cocontraction at the joint undergoing compression, whereas light joint compression is reported to produce an inhibitory (relaxing) effect on spastic muscles around joints (Schultz-Krohn et al., 2006).

KEY POINTS

♦ Heavy joint compression is thought to facilitate muscle cocontraction.
♦ Light joint compression is thought to inhibit (relax) muscle spasticity.
♦ Evidence for effectiveness of joint compression is anecdotal.

Bone pounding or jamming is used to inhibit plantar-flexion and facilitate cocontraction around the ankle. It can be applied with the patient sitting, by pounding the heel on the floor whilst supporting the knee. Alternatively, with the patient lying prone over a pillow with some degree of flexion at the hips and knees, force can be applied to the heel by the therapist using the ulnar side of a clenched fist (Umphred et al., 2007a).

Other techniques that use joint compression include weight-bearing through a hemiplegic arm to facilitate cocontraction and activation of the muscles around the shoulder joint (Davies, 2000). Weight belts and weighted wrist or ankle cuffs have also been used to increase joint compression. Joint compression can be applied to many joints using a variety of positions or patterns of movement. For example, using four-point kneeling as a starting position, joint compression can be applied to the shoulders and/or hips. Ideally, joint compression should be applied in a functional position, but if this is not possible treatment should quickly progress to using the joint in a functional manner. Joint compression is also a procedure used in PNF and is considered in this context below.

Several authors described joint compression, either in terms of normal weight approximation or by other means, but only anecdotal evidence is given to support its use (Davies, 2000; Farber, 1982; Schultz-Krohn et al., 2006; Umphred et al. 2007a).

Vibration

Muscle vibration

Therapeutic vibration is a directly applied stimulus of high frequency (100–300 Hz) and low amplitude, which stretches the muscle spindle and activates type 1a afferent fibres. Vibration is generally applied directly to the chosen muscle or its tendon. Bishop (1974) identified three motor effects achievable by vibrating a muscle: (1) a sustained contraction of the vibrated muscle (via the tonic vibration reflex); (2) the depression of the motoneurones innervating the antagonistic muscles (reciprocal inhibition or antagonist inhibition); and (3) suppression of the monosynaptic stretch reflexes of the vibrated muscle (during the period of vibration). There appears to be disagreement, however, as to whether vibration has a sustained effect on muscle contractility (Umphred et al., 2007a) and thus any long-term benefit.

It would appear that vibration has potential clinical applications via agonist facilitation or antagonist inhibition. Bishop (1974) identified four factors that influenced the strength of the tonic vibration reflex (TVR):

1. The location of the vibrator
2. The initial length of the muscle

3. The level of excitability of the central nervous system (CNS)
4. The parameters of the vibratory stimulus.

Application of the vibrator to the belly of a stretched muscle or over the tendon allows easy facilitation of the TVR. It appears that the tonic neck reflexes and body-righting reflexes (Rothwell, 1994; Shepherd, 1994) interact with the TVR; so, treatment in the supine position results in an improved extensor TVR, and that in the prone position results in increased flexor TVR. Finally, increasing the amplitude of the vibration increases the stretch on the muscle but, more significantly, the TVR is greater as the frequency of the vibratory stimulus increases.

Despite the apparent theoretical basis for its use, there are few reports of vibration being used in clinical practice to facilitate muscle contraction.

Another quite different investigation involving vibration was made by Lovgreen et al. (1993), who studied the effects of muscle vibration on the voluntary movements of patients with cerebellar dysmetria. Part of the study was to consider whether vibration could improve movement accuracy and reduce hypermetria. They found that antagonist vibration reduced the amplitude of patients' movements and suggested that vibration had potential for use in both hyper- and hypometria, although the feasibility of its application would require careful thought.

Vibration has the potential to be a potent treatment technique but there are various precautions that must be considered when using it. Key points to remember include: vibration will generate heat at its point of application and there is potential to cause damage to the skin, particularly at high amplitudes (Farber, 1982). Vibration to augment a muscle contraction should not be applied with cutaneous pressure, which is known to cause inhibition as the two oposing effects could negate each other (Umphred et al., 2007a).

KEY POINTS

Muscle vibration:
- generates heat at the point of application
- can potentially damage skin, particularly at high amplitude
- should not be applied with cutaneous pressure
- has little evidence of effectiveness, despite theoretical basis.

Umphred et al. (2007a) recommend that vibrators registering 100–125 Hz be used and noted that most battery-operated hand-held vibrators register only 50–90 Hz. There is a wide range of commercially available vibrators, so the available frequency range should always be checked prior to purchase.

The use of more generalized vibration has also been considered. Its current use as part of exercise training formed the basis of a study by Jackson et al. (2008) examining its effect on lower limb performance in patients with multiple sclerosis, although results were inconclusive.

Whole body vibration

Whole body vibration is a relatively new modality in neurological rehabilitation, which involves the patient standing on a vibrating platform (Wunderer et al., 2008). The effect of vibration compared to conventional physiotherapy to improve balance and gait in Parkinson's disease was explored by Ebersbach et al. (2008). However, improvements were demonstrated in both groups, so its superior efficacy in comparison to a standard approach to rehabilitation was not established. Another study exploring its use in Parkinson's disease (Arias et al., 2009) concluded that any effect from whole body vibration in Parkinson's disease was solely due to a placebo effect. A systematic review by Wunderer et al. (2008) concluded that whole body vibration appeared to produce similar gains to traditional exercise and resistance training but also limited fatigue, so its use could therefore be considered beneficial in neurological patients.

> ### KEY POINTS
>
> Whole body vibration:
> - is a relatively new modality in physiotherapy.
> - may produce similar gains as traditional exercise and resistance training.

Vestibular stimulation

Any static position or movement will have an effect on the vestibular system, so many interventions will result in vestibular stimulation in some way or other. However, specific vestibular stimulation has not been widely used in neurological physiotherapy and was, until recently, mainly described in relation to a multisensory approach to neurological rehabilitation in paediatrics. Advocates of its use are anxious to remind others that vestibular stimulation is a powerful form of stimulation that should be used with care. Umphred et al. (2007a, p. 231) stated that it is important to remember that 'the rate of vestibular stimulation determines the effects. A constant, slow, repetitive rocking pattern, irrespective of plan or direction, generally causes inhibition of total-body responses, whereas a fast spin or fast linear movement tends to heighten both alertness and the motor responses.'

The management of vestibular dysfunction has evolved from increasing research to become recognized as a specialist area within physiotherapy. Chapter 13 explains that patients with a primary problem of vestibular dysfunction require vestibular rehabilitation, which involves specific assessment and treatment techniques.

> ### KEY POINTS
>
> - Vestibular stimulation is a powerful form of stimulation and should be used with care.
> - The rate of vestibular stimulation determines its effects.

Facilitation of movement

Facilitated movements do not require the patient to activate the nervous system to produce the required movement. This lack of self-initiation of movement has been criticized for not providing a basis for the learning of movement. However, it could be argued that once movement can be initiated in patients the possibility of the production of an active response then exists with the potential for learning of functional movements (Baily Metcalfe & Lawes, 1998). However, it must be remembered that eventually the patient must become independent of the physiotherapist in order to produce the movements required for functional indpendence.

NORMALIZATION OF TONE AND THE MAINTENANCE OF SOFT-TISSUE LENGTH

The Bobath approach is widely used as a treatment approach in neurological physiotherapy (Lennon, 2003; Sackley & Lincoln, 1996) and the control and normalization of tone clearly contribute to the theoretical assumptions of the Bobath concept of stroke rehabilitation (Raine 2007; also see Ch. 11). An awareness of the potential for changes in the musculoskeletal system and the subsequent loss of range of movement associated with neurological dysfunction (Ch. 14) is essential for effective management of patients with neurological disorders.

Passive stretching – slow

Slow stretch is applied to a muscle or joint such that a stretch reflex is not elicited and the effect is, therefore, inhibitory in terms of the neural response. The effect of prolonged, slow stretching on muscle is not entirely clear, although it certainly varies depending upon the time for which the stretch is maintained. It appears to have an influence on both the neural components of muscle, via the Golgi tendon organs and muscle spindles (O'Sullivan, 2007), and the structural components in the long term, via the number and length of sarcomeres (Hale et al., 1995).

Changes in muscle length

The presence of increased tone, possibly combined with paresis and/or weakness, can ultimately lead to joint contracture and changes in muscle length (see Ch. 14). Slow, prolonged stretching is therefore applied to maintain or prevent loss of range of movement (ROM). It has been demonstrated in animal studies that if a muscle is immobilized in a shortened position, sarcomeres will be lost and, conversely, a muscle immobilized in a lengthened position will add on sarcomeres (Goldspink & Williams, 1990). A shortened immobilized muscle will also show an increase in stiffness related to an increase in connective tissue within the muscle (Williams et al., 1988). However, it has been demonstrated in mice that a stretch of 30 minutes daily will prevent the loss of sarcomeres and changes in the connective tissue of an immobilized muscle (Williams, 1990). The timescale relating to changes in the mouse may not be relevant to humans.

Manual stretching

A prolonged muscle stretch can be applied manually, using the effect of gravity and body weight, or mechanically (by machine or splint). When applied, the stretch should provide sufficient force to overcome the hypertonicity and passively lengthen the muscle. When contractures are already present, it is doubtful whether the use of manual stretching alone will be sufficient to provide a sustained improvement in the ROM, if any was achieved. A systematic review exploring the effects of stretching in spasticity by Bovend'Eerdt et al. (2008) found some positive evidence to support the immediate effects of one stretching session, but the long-term effects were unclear. Overall the heterogeneic nature of the studies made a meta-analysis unfeasible and they concluded that the available evidence related to the clinical benefits of stretching and spasticity was inconclusive.

Splinting

Low-force stretching of long duration can be provided by splinting. The clinical practice guidelines on splinting adults with neurological dysfunction (Association of Chartered Physiotherapists Interested in Neurology (ACPIN), 1998) identified a paucity of research in the area, making it almost impossible to adopt an evidence-based approach to the use of splints. Over a decade later, little has changed.

Dynamic Lycra splints have been used as part of the management of patients with hemiplegia (Gracies et al., 2000). Lycra splints are custom-made, individually designed garments – it is claimed that Lycra splinting is effective in managing posture, and motor and sensory changes following a stroke. The study by Gracies et al. (2000) investigated acceptability and effects

on swelling, resting posture, spasticity, active ROM and passive ROM of an upper-limb Lycra garment when worn for 3 hours by patients with a hemiplegia. The findings from this small-scale study, using a convenience sample, indicate some support for the use of these garments in reducing spasticity and swelling. Overall the use of lycra splits or orthoses in adult patients with neurological dysfunction is not widespread. In contrast there is increasing use of lycra splinting in children with cerebral palsy, although a review by Attard and Rithalia (2004) identified a lack of scientific research to support their use.

Different types of splinting and the rationale for use are discussed in Chapter 14, with further details being provided by Edwards and Charlton (2002). Examples of splints used for peripheral nerve injuries are illustrated in photographs in Chapter 9.

Weight-bearing

Several studies report the use of weight-bearing to reduce contractures in joints of the lower limb (Bohannon, 1993; Richardson, 1991). These reports illustrate the effectiveness of using a tilt table to achieve a sustainable position in which a prolonged stretch is applied. The angle of table tilt needs to be considered when standing patients with knee joint contractures, as the supporting straps bear more of the body weight than when the knees are extended (Morgan et al., 2003). Force exerted at the supporting straps is greater the higher the degree of flexion, and is more pronounced with greater body weight, but can be modified by reducing table incline, thus reducing the pressure on underlying tissues. However, a study by Ben et al. (2005) challenged some of the assumptions about the benefits of standing where small changes to ankle mobility and little or none to mineral density were found during a single blinded randomized trial examining the effects of a 12-week standing programme in patients with recent spinal cord injuries. Illustrated examples of equipment to assist standing can be seen in Chapters 4 and 14.

Serial casting

Serial plaster casting is another technique used to prevent or reduce contractures (O'Sullivan 2007), which may be most effective when the contractures result from spasticity. Serial casting methods were described and illustrated by Edwards and Charlton (2002) and a comprehensive overview of the practicalities of casting the lower limb in neurology was provided by Young and Nicklin (2000).

The use of a soft splint has been shown to be effective in the acute management of elbow hypertonicity (Wallen & Mackay, 1995). This splint has certain advantages over casting in that it is more dynamic in nature, less likely to cause unwanted pressure and provides neutral warmth (Wallen & O'Flaherty, 1991). However, it is also easily removed and thus a level of compliance is necessary!

Moseley (1997) also demonstrated the effectiveness of serial casting and stretching on regaining ROM in the ankle due to established shortening of the calf muscles. Jones (1999) undertook a series of single-system studies to examine the efficacy of lower-extremity serial casts on gait in four adults with hemiparetic gait patterns. There was an improvement in walking speed and a reduction in the level of assistance required during walking following the intervention. Singer et al. (2004) reported a descriptive study of the non-surgical management of ankle contracture in patients with acquired brain injury. Serial casting was used when the contracture appeared to be worsening, despite standard physiotherapy. In some cases of serial casting this also included an injection of botulinum toxin type A.

When spasticity is present, physiotherapists are often reluctant to use splints or other externally applied devices for stretching as, despite the lack of supporting evidence, it is thought that splinting can lead to an increase in muscle tone. However, it has been demonstrated that inhibitory splinting can reduce contractures without causing detrimental effects to muscle tone (Mills, 1986). Indeed, the ACPIN guidelines (1998) recommend that patients suitable for splinting are those who may have, or be at risk of, contractures as a result of significant increases in muscle tone or immobility.

Duration of stretch to reduce spasticity

Although it has been shown that prolonged stretching can reduce spasticity, the time needed is not clear. Hale et al. (1995) found that the most beneficial duration of stretch applied to reduce spasticity was 10 minutes. This study used a variety of methods to assess the level of spasticity, including both subjective and objective measures. The results illustrated the difficulties that arise when measuring spasticity (see Ch. 14), and that perhaps the concurrent problems of length-associated changes in muscle required greater consideration.

Duration of stretch to prevent contracture

Tardieu et al. (1988) investigated how long it was necessary to stretch the soleus muscle each day to prevent contracture in children with cerebral palsy and concluded that it must be stretched for 6 hours a day.

Some work has been done to evaluate the effect of stretching, mainly on normal subjects (Harvey et al., 2002). However, it is clear that further work is still required to establish the appropriate stretching techniques and the duration required to produce the desired effect in different situations.

KEY POINTS

Passive stretching – slow:
- has a variable effect which is not entirely clear
- if applied manually is unlikely to be effective if contractures are already present
- may be applied by standing patients using a tilt table
- if applied via a splint may reduce the risk of patients developing contractures
- requires additional research to establish the required duration and best method of application to produce an effect.

Positioning

Positioning is used widely by physiotherapists to prevent the development of contractures (Fraser, 2009) and to discourage unwanted reflex activity (Carr & Kenney, 1992; Pope, 2002). A survey of practice of positioning for stroke patients identified that one of the most common aims of physiotherapists advocating its use was to modulate muscle tone and prevent damage to affected limbs (Chatterton et al., 2001). A study by Ada et al. (2005a) of stretching in patients with a recent stroke, in which the affected shoulders were positioned in 90° of flexion with the maximum external rotation tolerable for two 30 minute sessions a day, 5 days a week, for 4 weeks, found significantly reduced incidence of contracture when compared with a control group. This contrasted with Dean et al. (2000) who failed to demonstrate a significant effect of prolonged positioning of the shoulder, applied daily for 6 weeks, in patients undergoing a multidisciplinary rehabilitation programme. Turton et al. (2005), although supporting the principle that early treatment to prevent the loss of range of movement in the affected limb post stroke is essential, also raised the issue of patient compliance, which must be considered in any intervention requiring patients to adopt a sustained position. However, a recent meta-analysis of positioning to prevent loss of range of movement in the shoulder post stroke did not support its use (Borisova & Bohannon, 2009).

Specific positions are often adopted to achieve a slow maintained stretch on a particular muscle and the thinking behind this has already been explored. Bromley (2006) gave detailed guidelines for the positioning of patients following spinal cord injury and described its importance for: correct alignment of fractures, prevention of contractures, prevention of pressure sores and inhibiting the onset of severe spasticity.

Indeed, historically many of the positions advocated by physiotherapists relate to the desire to avoid the development of spastic patterns of movement (Bobath, 1990). Positions are chosen to minimize the influence of the primitive reflexes. The three reflexes, which are normally under cortical control and whose release can be influenced by careful choice and use of positions, are: (1) the symmetrical tonic neck reflex; (2) the asymmetrical tonic neck reflex; and (3) the labyrinthine reflex (Carr & Kenney, 1992).

Davies (2000) gave fairly detailed descriptions of desirable positions that should be used following stroke, urging the avoidance of supine lying, as in this position the influences of the tonic neck and labyrinthine reflexes are great and this could result in an overall increase in extensor activity throughout the body. Fraser (2009) advocates the use of good seating and positioning to facilitate appropriate alignment and stability of the trunk and limbs, thus avoiding compensatory responses to prevent falling.

Careful positioning to limit musculoskeletal changes is essential, but it appears that there is a lack of consensus about the precise positions necessary to limit the onset of spasticity and unwanted patterns of movement, particularly after stroke (Carr & Kenney, 1992; Chatterton et al., 2001). Certainly, Bobath (1990) identified a need to be more dynamic and advocated the use of reflex-inhibiting patterns of movement, rather than static postures, to inhibit abnormal postural reactions and facilitate automatic and voluntary movements.

These concepts are discussed in Chapter 11. Positioning is also discussed in Chapters 4 and 14, where illustrations show various types of equipment used for posture and seating.

> ### KEY POINTS
>
> ◆ Although positioning is widely used, its effectiveness has not been established.
> ◆ There is a lack of consensus about which positions should be adopted and why.

Pressure

Pressure is used by physiotherapists both to facilitate and inhibit a response in muscle, more especially in muscle tone (O'Sullivan, 2007). This pressure can be applied in a variety of ways, including the use of air-filled splints (Johnstone, 1995), tone-inhibiting casts (Zachazewski et al., 1982) or manually (Umphred et al., 2007a). Pressure can be applied directly over a tendon (Leone & Kukulka, 1988) or over the muscle itself (Robichaud et al., 1992). The pressure can be sustained or intermittent, and variable in terms of the degree applied.

Most of the research investigating the effects of a variety of pressure conditions has measured motoneurone excitability, via change in the Hoffman reflex (H reflex). Studies have suggested that the characteristic appearance of the H reflex reflects spinal motor function and, therefore, it can be used to evaluate the

effects of therapeutic interventions that aim to reduce motoneurone excitability (Suzuki et al., 1995). It is important to remember, however, the problems of quantifying that part of muscle tone that occurs as a direct result of reflex activity.

Leone and Kukulka (1988) investigated the effects of Achilles tendon pressure on the H reflex in stroke patients. The assumption was made that any change in motoneurone excitability would be reflected in an associated alteration in tone as, again, no direct measurement of tone was made. Pressure was applied both continuously and intermittently, and under both conditions depression of the H reflex occurred. Intermittent pressure, however, was significantly more effective than continuous. Further investigation revealed that increasing the amount of pressure had no greater effect, and the effect of the pressure was sustained only during its actual application. No carryover effect was observed, but it is suggested that tendon pressure could be used therapeutically, e.g. when a short-term reduction in tone would allow achievement of an improved patient position in bed.

The strongest proponent of the use of pressure during treatment was Johnstone (1995), who advocated the use of constant pressure provided by orally inflated splints and intermittent pressure produced by a machine. The uses of the splint are to: reduce the therapist's need for extra hands; provide stability to the limb; divert associated reactions; allow early weight-bearing through the affected limb; and increase sensory input (Johnstone, 1995). It was claimed that when the antigravity muscles of the upper limb are held in a position of sustained stretch using the air splints, tonic and phasic wrist flexor EMG activity is reduced (Johnstone, 1995).

Robichaud et al. (1992) supported the use of air-splint pressure to reduce motoneurone excitability of the soleus muscle when circumferential pressure was applied around the lower leg. As in the tendon pressure study, the reduction was not sustained once the pressure had been released. Conversely, an increase in motoneurone excitability following the application of muscle pressure has been reported (Kukulka et al., 1987). This may reflect the different methods employed to apply pressure, which can include tapping and massage (Umphred et al., 2007a).

It is clear that the application of pressure has many potential effects, some of which are still not understood. Externally applied pressure over muscle or tendon must also cause a disturbance in the cutaneous mechanoreceptors. Because of the wealth of afferent activity caused by pressure, its application poses many questions yet to be answered. Pressure is postulated to be one of the mechanisms supporting the therapeutic use of lycra body suits (Attard & Rithalia, 2004). The efficacy of using pressure as a technique has largely been supported by observations of therapists, but outcome studies are now required (Umphred et al., 2007a).

Neutral warmth

When considering exteroceptive input techniques, Umphred et al. (2007a) identified an additional use for air splints – that of the provision of neutral warmth. Johnstone (1995) also advocated their use to provide sensory stimulation of soft tissues, causing inhibition of the area under which the neutral warmth is applied. Alternative techniques used for achieving neutral warmth are tepid baths, whole-body wrapping and wrapping of isolated body parts (O'Sullivan, 2007). The required range of temperatures that should be utilized for this technique is 35–37°C (Farber, 1982).

There appears to be little research to support the use of this concept of neutral warmth. Baily Metcalf and Lawes (1998) suggested that the inhibition seen is due to inhibition of tonic muscles via the stimulation of low-threshold mechanoreceptors through light touch. One study looked specifically at the effect of a wrapping technique on a passive ROM in a spastic upper extremity (Twist, 1985). Wrapping (elastic wrap bandages and gloves) was applied to spastic upper limbs for 3 hours, three times a week on alternate days over a period of 2–4 weeks. Results showed statistically significant increases in passive ROM, with subjective reports of reduced pain. Although this study contained several shortcomings (small subject numbers and lack of control), it did indicate an effect.

Ice – prolonged

Prolonged use of ice reduces afferent and efferent neurotransmission. To be effective in reducing spasticity, the muscle spindles must themselves be cooled. The ice must be applied until there is no longer an excessive reflex response to stretching (Lehmann & De Lateur, 1990). It is considered that a reduction of spasticity lasting 1–2 hours can be achieved, such that stretching or active exercises can be applied to greater effect.

The most common form of application of ice to reduce spasticity is local immersion; this is particularly effective for reducing flexor spasticity in the hand. A mixture of tap water and flaked ice is used, in the ratio of one-third water to two-thirds ice. Davies (2000) advocated that the hand is immersed three times for 3 seconds, with only a few seconds between immersions. The therapist should hold the patient's hand in the ice–water mixture. This procedure can result in a dramatic reduction in spasticity.

General immersion, where the patient sits in a bath of cold water, has been used to reduce spasticity. Patients can tolerate water temperatures of 20–22°C for 10–15 minutes (Lee et al., 1978). Neither local nor general cooling has been found to have any long-term effect on spasticity, so any short-term reduction achieved must be fully exploited.

When using ice it is important to remember that the patient must be receptive to its use. If ice causes the patient distress and anxiety, the inhibitory effect may be blocked (Farber, 1982). A sensory assessment of the patient should be carried out before using ice and the presence of sensory deficits is a contraindication to its use (Umphred et al., 2007a).

Vibration

Vibration can also be used to produce inhibitory effects. In an effort to support the efficacy of its use to treat patients with disorders of muscle tone, Ageranioti and Hayes (1990) investigated the effects of vibration on hypertonia and hyperreflexia in the wrist joints of patients with spastic hemiplegia. They found that immediately after vibration, hypertonia and hyperreflexia were significantly reduced and concluded that in patients with spastic hemiplegia vibration gave short-term symptomatic relief. However, they also acknowledged that, despite using a relatively homogeneous group of subjects, there were many different patterns of hyperreflexia and this could possibly explain previous anecdotal reports where vibration was of no benefit in apparently similar cases.

Vibration has also been used at low frequencies (60–90 Hz) to normalize or reduce sensitivity in the skin (Farber, 1982; Umphred et al., 2007a). Hochreiter et al. (1983) found that in the 'normal' hand, vibration increased the tactile threshold, with the effect lasting for at least 10 minutes. There appears to be a lack of clinically applied studies in this area.

Certain precautions need to be considered when applying vibration (Farber, 1982), and these are outlined above in the section on facilitation.

KEY POINTS

◆ There is little evidence to support the use of vibration for inhibition.
◆ Care should be taken when applying vibration.

Massage

Massage was a core element of physiotherapy in the UK and has been described as one of the 'roots of our profession' (Murphy, 1993). How widely massage is used or should be used is the subject of much debate that will not be explored here. For an extensive overview of massage, its application and effects, the reader is directed to Holey and Cook (2003) or Hollis and Jones (2009).

Massage has two main physical effects – mechanical and physiological. The inhibitory effects of massage are of particular interest to the physiotherapist working in neurology when the aim is to achieve a reduction in muscle tone or muscle spasm. Slow stroking applied to patients with multiple sclerosis has been found to achieve a significant reduction in the amplitude of the H reflex (a measure of motoneurone excitability). The stroking was of light pressure and applied over the posterior primary rami (Brouwer & Sousa de Andrade, 1995).

Studies on neurologically healthy subjects have found similar results. Goldberg et al. (1992) found that deep massage produced a greater inhibitory response than light massage when applied to the leg. Sullivan et al. (1991) indicated, by their results, a specificity of the effect of massage on the muscle group being massaged. This was contrary to their expectations that the inhibitory effects of massage would extend beyond the muscle being massaged.

It is not clear whether the results of these studies could be transferred to subjects with neurological dysfunction; further studies are essential and must include measures beyond that of H-reflex amplitude as an indication of the efficacy of massage.

KEY POINT

◆ Little research has been undertaken exploring the effects of massage in patients with neurological disorders.

EXERCISE AND MOVEMENT

This section includes well-established treatments and those that are emerging in neurological rehabilitation (also see Ch. 18). A major area that is not included is gait re-education, which is a vast field and the reader is referred to the chapters in this book on the different neurological conditions, as well as to Kisner and Colby (2007), Whittle (2007) and Kerrigan and Sheffler (1995).

Hydrotherapy

Immersion in water can enhance the treatment of the neurologically impaired patient and has therapeutic, psychological and social benefits. Hydrotherapy can give an individual with limited independence on dry land an ability to move freely and with confidence. It also allows a recreational activity that can be easily enjoyed by many.

It must be remembered, when hydrotherapy is incorporated into a rehabilitation programme, that the effects of gravity are altered when in water. Many of the problems associated with neurological dysfunction arise from an individual's inability to respond normally to the effect of gravity and, therefore, hydrotherapy is unlikely to be the sole method of treatment. However, water is an environment that permits a freedom of movement seldom achieved elsewhere. Water is also quite unique in being able to take over some of the physiotherapist's work (Gray, 1997), particularly in terms of supporting the patient.

Muscle stretching, reducing contractures, re-education of motor patterns, re-education of balance and equilibrium reactions, gait retraining and breathing exercises are all areas covered by Gray (1997) and Bennie (1997), along with details of examples of suitable procedures used in hydrotherapy for neurological rehabilitation. Bad Ragaz techniques, where the buoyancy of the water is used to provide support rather than resistance to the patient, are covered by Davis and Harrison (1988). This approach has been advocated to achieve improvement in stability and motor control in neurological rehabilitation (Cameron, 2009).

As with any technique, careful assessment of the patient before and after treatment will allow the physiotherapist to monitor the effect of hydrotherapy. There are anecdotal reports of increased tone following exercise in hot water, but there is little evidence to substantiate this claim. The anxiety experienced by a patient being treated in water should be minimized by the reassurance provided by careful teaching skills (Reid Campion, 1997).

Swimming can form an integral part of hydrotherapy. The Halliwick method of swimming for the disabled (Lambeck et al., 2004; Reid Campion, 1997) is suitable for nearly any degree of disability at any age. A demonstrable improvement in postural balance and knee flexor strength was found by Noh et al. (2008) in stroke survivors undertaking an Ai Chi and Halliwick based exercise programme in water. Water-based exercise for improving cardiovascular fitness in people with chronic stroke was investigated by Chu et al. (2004) who demonstrated significant improvements in fitness and mobility. Both of these small-scale randomized trials of relatively short duration identify effects that warrant further investigation. Despite the widespread use of hydrotherapy with children with neurological impairments, a lack of evidence-based research was identified by Getz et al. (2006).

For further details of the principles, applications and techniques of hydrotherapy, the reader is directed to Schrepfer (2007), Cole and Becker (2004), Hecox and Leinanger (2006) and Reid Campion (1997).

KEY POINTS

Hydrotherapy:
♦ may give an individual the ability to move freely and with confidence
♦ has therapeutic, psychological and social benefits
♦ although used extensively lacks a sound evidence base.

Gymnastic balls

Gymnastic balls were originally used in orthopaedics, but are now used widely by physiotherapists working in neurology. These balls are light-weight, being inflated with air to a high pressure. The ball is used to provide some support to the patient; this could range from a patient lying supine with feet resting on the ball to a patient sitting on the ball with the feet on the ground. When using the gymnastic ball, the principle of action–reaction is followed. The patient is asked to achieve a specific action of the ball that will result in the desired reaction of body movement. With the patient sitting on the ball, feet on the floor, the action required is to roll the ball gently forwards and backwards. The reaction is flexion and extension of the lumbar spine, with associated pelvic tilt.

When using a ball it is important to remember several key points (below) so that its potential is fully exploited.

KEY POINTS

♦ A ball provides an unstable surface; if it is fixed and unable to roll, its effects are significantly altered.
♦ The stability of a ball is influenced by the horizontal location of the centre of gravity relative to the base of support.
♦ The ball can be used with the patient lying, sitting or standing.

♦ Its uses are so extensive that it can be used with patients who have a limited ability to move independently or those who are completely independent. For example, when sitting a patient on a ball, the ball supports the weight of much of the body.
♦ Achieving and maintaining a correct sitting position will require continual coordinated activity in the muscles of the trunk and limbs to prevent the ball from rolling. This would be more demanding than having the patient sit on a stable surface, yet easier than standing.
♦ The patient functioning at a higher level can use the ball in a more dynamic manner in which controlled movement of the ball is required.

A comprehensive description of the use of the gymnastic ball can be found in Carriere (1998, 1999) and Davies (1990), and an example of use is illustrated in Chapter 4 (Figure 4.15). A wide range of exercises using the gymnastic ball can be found in Kisner and Colby (2007).

Gymnastic balls are available in a variety of different sizes and are now produced by various manufacturers. They should be made of a resilient plastic and inflated to sufficient pressure to withstand adult body weight such that little deformation of the ball occurs. The gymnastic ball is a highly portable, versatile piece of equipment and is available in many neurological physiotherapy departments, yet there is no evidence of its effectiveness and research is required to support its continued use.

Proprioceptive neuromuscular facilitation

Proprioceptive neuromuscular facilitation (PNF) was developed as a therapeutic approach over 40 years ago. It is a very labour-intensive method of treatment, in which the physiotherapist facilitates the achievement of specific movement patterns by the patient with particular use of the therapist's hands. Some of the basic procedures and techniques that are utilized will be considered here in relation to their use in neurological rehabilitation. For a complete overview of PNF the reader is referred to Voss et al. (1985), Kisner and Colby (2007) and Adler et al. (2008); combined, these texts give an extensive theoretical and practical review of the thoughts of some of the proponents of PNF.

Ten basic procedures for facilitation have been identified by Adler et al. (2008):

1. Resistance
2. Irradiation and reinforcement
3. Manual contact
4. Body position and body mechanics
5. Verbal commands
6. Vision
7. Traction or approximation

8. Stretch
9. Timing
10. Patterns of movement.

The application of manual resistance has been one of the core features of PNF. There has been a shift away from the use of maximal resistance to the use of resistance appropriate to the needs of the patient. How the resistance is applied will reflect the type of muscle contraction being resisted. Concentric and eccentric muscle work should be resisted so the movement is smooth and coordinated. Resistance to an isometric contraction should be varied, with a gradual increase and decrease such that no movement occurs. By the correct application of resistance, irradiation or reinforcement will result. An example of this could be the use of resisted hip flexion, adduction and external rotation to facilitate weak dorsiflexion.

These two procedures of resistance and the resulting irradiation and reinforcement are possibly two of the reasons why PNF is no longer used extensively for neurological rehabilitation in the UK. The use of resistance does not fit comfortably with the other neurophysiological approaches, such as the Bobath approach. This, combined with the diagonal and spiral patterns of movement in the three anatomical planes, makes its relevance to normal movement difficult to comprehend. It is interesting to note, however, that Adler et al. (2008) felt that the patterns are not essential for the application of PNF and it is possible to use only the philosophy and appropriate procedures.

The other basic procedures appear to involve the use of techniques widely employed by physiotherapists using other approaches. The use of accurate handling is stressed in PNF; the lumbrical grip is advocated to give the appropriate stimulus to the patient. The therapist's manual contact should give information to the patient, facilitating movement in a specific direction. The position of the therapist relative to the patient allows the therapist to stay in line with the desired motion or force and to use body weight to give resistance. The use of visual feedback is promoted, with the patient following the movement to facilitate a stronger contraction. Traction and approximation may be applied to the trunk or extremities, eliciting a response via stimulation of the joint receptors.

The remaining three procedures – timing, stretch and the use of verbal commands – are extensively used in physiotherapy. Combining these in a variety of ways gives rise to the specific techniques of PNF.

Adler et al. (2008) grouped the techniques so that those with similar functions or actions were together. They gave detailed descriptions and examples of the techniques and indications for their use.

Although the core PNF texts previously cited gave examples of its use with neurological dysfunction, PNF is certainly not in common use in neurology gymnasia in the UK. One study investigated its effect on the gait of patients with hemiplegia of long and short duration and found its cumulative effects were more beneficial than the immediate effects (Wang, 1994). However, as no control groups were used, the possible inferences from this study are limited. An earlier study by Dickstein et al. (1986) compared three exercise therapy approaches including PNF and found that no substantial advantages could be attributed to any of the three therapeutic approaches used.

It has been identified that some of the underlying assumptions of the procedures and techniques used in PNF are now out of date (Morris & Sharpe, 1993), but there still appears to be a vast potential for research involving its use, especially in modified forms. An attempt has been made to explore the rationale behind the PNF relaxation techniques by studying postcontraction depression of the H reflex (Moore & Kukulka, 1991). The techniques did produce a strong but brief neuromuscular inhibition; however the results of this study, performed on subjects with no neurological dysfunction, cannot be directly applied to patients.

More recent publications are available via the International PNF Association (http://www.ipnfa.org).

KEY POINTS

Proprioceptive neuromuscular facilitation:
♦ is rarely used in neurological rehabilitation in the UK
♦ may be more useful used in a modified form.

Cardiovascular exercise, strength training and exercise on prescription

The use of exercise to increase muscle strength in neurological rehabilitation is controversial and many physiotherapists have believed that muscle strength is not appropriate for treatment or measurement. However, there is increasing evidence that use of exercise and strength training, including the use of treadmills and static bikes, is beneficial in the management of patients with neurological dysfunction. Refshauge et al. (2005) provide evidence of the importance of exercise and training for individuals with chronic disability. Chapter 18 reviews the emerging literature, which reveals the benefits of exercise without the adverse effects traditionally feared by physiotherapists, such as increasing muscle tone in patients with spasticity.

There are currently no UK guidelines for exercise prescriptions for people with chronic neurological conditions (Glynn & Fiddler, 2009) so any recommendations are usually based on those for cardiovascular training. The guidelines produced by the American College of Sports Medicine are widely recognized as a resource for those planning to undertake training with special populations (ACSM, 2009).

Treadmill training

Treadmill training has been used across a range of different neurological patient groups to improve locomotion (see Ch. 18). Treadmill training is based upon the principle of task-specific repetitive training in that to learn to walk or improve walking practice is essential. Partial bodyweight-supported treadmill training can be used with non-ambulatory patients following a stroke to enable them to practice the complex requirements of the gait cycle (Hesse, 2008). Treadmill training has also been investigated in chronic stroke where it was found to be more effective in improving walking speed than resisted leg cycling alone (Sullivan et al., 2007). A recent review by Damiano and Dejong (2009) of the effectiveness of treadmill training in paediatric rehabilitation concluded that its efficacy had been demonstrated in children with Down's syndrome, but although positive effects had been noted with other patient groups, including cerebral palsy, further research was required to support its use. This conclusion is supported in another review specific to children with cerebral palsy (Mutlu et al., 2009).

It should be acknowledged that the benefits of treadmill may extend beyond the improvement of walking ability. For some patient groups, for example spinal cord injured patients, it has been argued that the physiological and psychological benefits may justify its use even where it has not been shown to be superior to conventional physiotherapy in improving locomotor ability (Hicks & Martin Ginis, 2008). The potential contribution of treadmill training in relation to cardiorespiratory fitness should also be considered (Kilbreath & Davis, 2005).

Pilates-based rehabilitation

Pilates exercise has evolved from its use with elite dancers into different areas of rehabilitation (Anderson & Spector, 2000). Pilates-based rehabilitation was introduced from the USA in the 1990s and interest amongst physiotherapists is growing. For a summary of the principles behind its use and possible clinical applications the reader is directed to Anderson and Butler (2007). Despite the proliferation of Pilates courses for physiotherapists there is almost no research into its efficacy as part of a rehabilitation programme for patients with neurolocial dysfunction. A recent article by King and Horak (2009) included Pilates as part of a sensorimotor programme for patients with Parkinson's disease. Although a rationale for such an approach was presented it has not yet been tested.

As acknowledged in the above reviews, research is needed to provide evidence of its effectiveness. However, it has been claimed that one of the defining characteristics of Pilates-inspired exercises is to enhance core, shoulder girdle and limb control (Lange et al., 2000) and this philosophy in many cases has a good fit with the aims of physiotherapy. Pilates classes in sports gyms are also very popular but people with neurological conditions would be advised to seek specialist supervision from a physiotherapist trained in Pilates, at least initially.

Tai chi

Tai chi is increasingly being incorporated into the range of interventions recommended or used by physiotherapists. It is used across the world as a form of exercise for health and fitness (Wang et al., 2004) despite little evidence of its benefits. A systematic review by Wang et al. (2004) explored the physical and psychological effects of tai chi on various chronic conditions, concluding that due to the lack of rigour in the majority of the studies considered it was difficult to make recommendations to support its use despite the apparent benefits. However, it appeared safe and was useful in relation to balance control, flexibility and cardiovascular fitness. A more recent review by Harling and Simpson (2008) concluded that there was strong evidence to support the use of tai chi in reducing the fear of falling in older adults, although the evidence to support its effectiveness in actually reducing the incidence of falling was weak. Given the anxiety in relation to falling experienced by many people with neurological conditions, it would seem reasonable therefore to consider its use within such populations. There is clearly a need for additional research and this view was supported by Lee et al. (2008) who reviewed its use in relation to Parkinson's disease and found insufficient evidence to support its use.

KEY POINT

◆ Tai chi requires additional research to support its use.

Constraint-induced (forced-use) therapy

The principle of forced use to overcome the effects of 'learned non-use' is the basis for the increasing use of constraint therapy (Morris & Taub, 2001). It is used particularly in relation to rehabilitation of the upper limb in adults following a stroke and children with cerebral palsy and is discussed in Chapter 18. A systematic review (Hakkennes & Keating, 2005) of constraint-induced (forced-use) therapy (CIMT) following stroke concluded that it may improve upper limb function for some patients when compared to alternative or no treatment. This is reflected in the *National Clinical Guidelines for Stroke* (Intercollegiate Working Party for Stroke, 2008), which highlight the great commitment required from the patient when using CIMT and the need to use specific selection criteria and full patient agreement. There is considerably more research exploring its use in adults with stroke than children with cerebral palsy. However, a review by Hoare et al. (2007) also found positive trends supporting its use with children.

For a historical perspective and overview of the use of CIMT the reader is directed to Wolf (2007) who explores its theoretical underpinnings, the rationale behind its use and the associated strengths, uncertainties and limitations.

KEY POINTS

Constraint induced therapy:
◆ may improve upper limb function for some patients post stroke
◆ raises issues in relation to the commitment and compliance of patients.

Robotics

The use of robotics within neurorehabilitation provides an alternative method of enhancing both upper and lower limb function in patients with movement disorders (Umphred et al., 2007a). It is another form of an augmented intervention along with bodyweight-supported treadmill training and CIMT, and has the most potential to exploit the increasing use of technology in rehabilitation (Umphred et al., 2007a). As the most recent of these interventions, it has the most limited evidence base for its use. The majority of support exists where the focus is on rehabilitation of the upper limb and it has been suggested that it could complement conventional therapy (Masiero et al., 2007). A review by Kwakkel et al. (2008) highlighted the challenges of making sense of the existing research due to the heterogeneity of the studies available. However, it appeared that a significant improvement in upper limb motor function after stroke could be identified with the use of upper limb robotics.

KEY POINTS

◆ The use of robotics within physiotherapy is an area of emerging practice.
◆ Robotics utilizes developments in technology.

Cueing

Cueing can be thought of as a way of prompting a response. This prompt can be given in many different ways, including a verbal command, a noise, touch or visual stimulus. Its use has been explored extensively in Parkinson's disease, where it is used to circumvent the dopamine deficits associated with the disease (Rubinstein et al., 2002; also see Ch. 6). External cueing has been defined as, 'applying temporal (rhythmical) or spatial stimuli associated with the initiation and ongoing facilitation of motor activity.' (Lim et al., 2005). However, the evidence base is limited and in a systematic review by Lim et al. (2005) only one high-quality randomized controlled trial was identified exploring the effects of auditory rhythmical cueing. This study suggested that the walking speed of patients with Parkinson's disease could be positively influenced by such cueing, but it is unclear whether the effects would be translated into the real world. Insufficient evidence was found to support the use of visual or somatosensory cueing. In another study exploring bilateral arm training in chronic stroke, rhythmic auditory cueing appeared to induce significant changes identified by functional magnetic resonance imaging, although no significant functional outcomes were found (Luft et al., 2004).

More recently the RESCUE project has published a CD-ROM which provides guidelines for therapists using cueing to improve mobility in Parkinson's disease (http://www.rescueproject.org/).

ELECTRICAL STIMULATION TECHNIQUES

The uses of electrical stimulation (ES) include pain relief, muscle strengthening and improving endurance, and producing functional movement. Different terms are used for the different applications (see below).

Transcutaneous electrical nerve stimulation

Transcutaneous electrical nerve stimulation (TENS) is a term used to describe nerve-stimulating pulses of low intensity, often used to control pain but also to reduce spasticity.

Pain relief

The management of pain in neurological rehabilitation would possibly not be identified as a key area for the physiotherapist working in neurology. However, the physiotherpist may have a significant role in the management of a patient's pain. Chapter 16 reviews the specific management of pain in neurological rehabilitation.

TENS has been used specifically in the management of hemiplegic shoulder pain (Leandri et al., 1990). However a systematic review by Price and Pandyan (2000) concluded that it was not possible to confirm or refute the use of electrical stimulation for shoulder pain post stroke.

Details about TENS and its application in pain relief can be found in Kitchen (2002) and Robertson et al. (2006), which also provide a comprehensive overview of electrotherapy and its principles and practice.

Management of spasticity using transcutaneous electrical nerve stimulation

An alternative use of TENS has been in the treatment of spasticity. Studies investigating its effects on spasticity have had mixed results. Goulet et al. (1994) postulated that TENS would have an inhibitory effect on the amplitude of the soleus H reflex. They failed to demonstrate any consistent effects and no significant treatment effects were found following stimulation (at 50 or 99 Hz) on a mixed or sensory nerve. These results could reflect the difficulties of obtaining consistent H-reflex amplitudes in normal subjects and in those with neurological dysfunction.

Seib et al. (1994) used the spasticity measurement scale, in which neurophysiological and biomechanical responses are evaluated, to investigate the effect of cutaneous ES (over the tibialis anterior muscle) on spasticity of the gastrocnemius–soleus–achilles tendon unit. Using two groups of subjects, one with traumatic brain injuries and the other with spinal cord injuries; a significant reduction in spasticity was found which lasted for 6 hours or more following the stimulation. Based on these results the authors proposed that TENS could be of use for decreasing spasticity prior to other physiotherapeutic interventions such as stretching. Sonde et al. (2000) evaluated whether high-frequency TENS on a specific acupuncture point would influence the level of spasticity in the paretic leg after stroke. They found a reduction in spasticity, which was sustained in some patients for 2 weeks after treatment. Information about acupuncture points used with TENS is available in Fox and Sharp (2007).

More recently the effects of TENS and exercises on the sensorimotor and functional recovery of the upper limb in acute stroke were investigated by Yozbatiran et al. (2006). It was concluded that additonal stimulation of the hand and fingers improved sensorimotor outcome immediately after the intervention, although it was acknowledged that the implications of this finding in relation to functional performance were not investigated.

Electrical stimulation of muscle

Surface ES to produce a muscle contraction via the motor nerves has been widely used in physiotherapy. Muscle ES has five major uses in physiotherapy in general:

1. Strengthening and/or maintaining muscle bulk
2. Facilitating voluntary muscle contraction
3. Gaining or maintaining ROM
4. Reducing spasticity
5. As an orthotic substitute to produce functional movement.

The latter three uses are those most commonly seen in neurological rehabilitation. All types of ES that produce contraction tend to be termed functional electrical stimulation (FES), but this is inaccurate (see below).

Maintaining ROM is often an important goal in neurological dysfunction. If patients are unable to maintain range by moving a joint themselves, or having it moved passively, neuromuscular ES may be used to provide assistance or as a substitute. It can provide a consistent controlled treatment that the patient can apply and use at home (Baker, 1991).

The effects of ES on shoulder subluxation, functional recovery of the upper limb and shoulder pain in stroke patients have been studied (Faghri et al., 1994). Using radiographs to assess the degree of subluxation, a significant reduction in the amount of displacement was achieved in the experimental group who received ES to supraspinatus and posterior deltoid muscles. A larger study by Chantraine et al. (1999) also supported the early use of ES in order to reduce the degree of shoulder subluxation poststroke.

A review by De Kroon et al. (2002) of therapeutic electrical stimulation on the functional abilities of the upper limb post stroke was unable to draw specific conclusions due to limitations within the studies reviewed. However the positive effect noted on motor control did support the need for further research in this area.

Functional electrical stimulation

Functional electrical stimulation (FES) is the term used when the aim of treatment is to enhance or produce a functional movement (McDonough & Kitchen, 2002).

When used as an orthotic substitute, FES can possibly be considered to be truly functional. However, opinions vary as to the efficacy of its use in this area. Petrofsky (1988) identified that FES can be used, often in conjunction with lightweight braces, to provide a method of independent ambulation, but that walking in this way is only part of a comprehensive physical training programme. Melis et al. (1995) concluded that the use of ambulatory assistive devices and FES could help patients with spinal cord injuries to regain independent locomotion and improve their quality of life. Much of the literature available about FES of the lower limbs focuses on its use in spinal cord injury. Whalley Hammell (1995) considered the financial implications of FES which, despite two decades of research, still cannot produce a functional level of walking. However, research has continued and Kim et al. (2004) concluded that a combination of a hinged ankle-foot orthosis and FES provided greater benefits in overall gait function that either device used alone in patients with incomplete spinal cord injury. Another use of FES in this patient group is in the upper limb to improve hand function, but it appears that the fine control required here is as difficult to reproduce as the combination of balance and movement required in walking (Baker, 1991).

The use of FES as part of a rehabilitation programme must be accompanied by an accurate explanation to the patient, including setting achievable goals so that the patient's expectations are realistic. It should be noted that the *National Clinical Guidelines for Stroke* (Intercollegiate Working Party for Stroke, 2008) do not recommend the routine use of FES after stroke. This recommendation is based on the work of Handy et al. (2003) and De Kroon et al. (2002). However, a review by Roche et al. (2009) concluded that FES could have a positive orthotic effect for gait speed and physiological cost index in chronic post stroke patients, although the therapeutic effect (presence of the effect with the FES device removed) was less evident so it appears to be an area with potential for more research.

Electrical stimulation for reducing spasticity

Establishing the effect of ES on spasticity has been hindered by the difficulties of quantifying spasticity. Vang et al. (1995) used a single-case-study design to investigate the effect of ES on a patient experiencing problems with upper limb function due to spasticity, secondary to cerebral palsy. Using a test of hand function to evaluate the level of spasticity, ES resulted in a measurable reduction in spasticity. However, a systematic review of the literature relating to the use of ES for preventing and treating poststroke shoulder pain concluded that there was no significant effect on upper limb spasticity (Price & Pandyan, 2000).

Considerations when using electrical stimulation

It is important to be aware of the safety aspects of using ES and the adverse effects it may have on abnormal neuromuscular systems, as much of the research has so far been conducted on normal muscle. Stokes and Cooper (1989) considered the problems of fatigue when stimulating muscles, the physiological effects of ES and the potential dangers when ES is used indiscriminately for therapeutic stimulation. Indeed, initial studies using stimulation to allow paraplegic and quadriplegic subjects to stand and walk short distances found that fatigue limited the distance walked and excessive stress was placed on the cardiorespiratory system and the legs (Petrofsky, 1988). These problems have been partly overcome by the combined use of bracing and FES, and preparation of the muscle for FES by low-frequency conditioning stimulation to improve endurance.

Increased resistance to fatigue in response to conditioning stimulation is achieved by biochemical and physiological adaptations in the muscle (Pette, 1986). Furthermore, the frequency patterns used during conditioning stimulation are important, as a single low frequency can cause muscle weakness, but intermittent bursts of high frequency can maintain strength and still improve endurance (Rutherford & Jones, 1988). When ES is used to strengthen muscle, a stimulation pattern similar to the normal motor unit firing pattern has been shown to be more effective than uniform frequency or random frequencies (Oldham et al., 1995). This finding was in patients with rheumatoid arthritis and hand muscle weakness. Stimulation patterns have also been studied in the quadriceps in patients with patellofemoral pain (Callaghan et al., 2001). Whilst this approach appears promising, these studies involved conditions in which muscles and nerves were not diseased, so further research is required in patients with muscular and neurological disorders.

It also appears that further studies are necessary to monitor the effects of ES in specific neuromuscular disorders. Studies such as those which examined the effects of ES on patients with progressive muscular dystrophy (Zupan & Gregoric, 1995) and other neurological disorders (Scott et al., 1986) may allow physiotherapists to make informed decisions about the usefulness of ES as part of a therapeutic programme. Research is also needed to establish appropriate stimulation parameters for the different applications of ES. The reader is directed to McDonough and Kitchen (2002) and Fox and Sharp (2007) for specific guidance to the use of ES.

KEY POINT

◆ The use of electrical stimulation in patients with neurological disorders requires more research to support its use.

OTHER TECHNIQUES

In this section, various unrelated techniques are discussed. Two treatments that were mainly used in orthopaedics before being applied to neurology are acupuncture and neurodynamics (see below). Another orthopaedic treatment not discussed here is the correction of muscle imbalance (Sharmann, 2002).

Biofeedback

Biofeedback has been used widely in physiotherapy; a detailed description of its use in neurology can be found in Umphred et al. (2007a) and Robertson et al. (2006). It has been defined as 'procedures whereby information about an aspect of bodily functioning is fed back by some visual or auditory signal' (Caudrey & Seeger, 1981). External or augmented feedback can be used to provide patients with knowledge of results or knowledge of performance with the goal of improving motor control (Dutton, 2007). Biofeedback therapy seeks to allow subjects to gain conscious control over a voluntary but latent activity (Glanz et al., 1995).

The most commonly used form of biofeedback in neurological rehabilitation using technology is EMG using surface electrodes. Most EMG feedback equipment will provide both auditory and visual feedback to the patient and therapist. For the purposes of providing feedback, changes in the EMG signal can be taken to indicate changes in muscle activity. This does not provide a measure of changes in force, since EMG and force are known to dissociate when muscle fatigues, as shown by the classic experiment of Edwards and Lippold in 1956. EMG biofeedback therefore reflects muscular effort and not force.

Force can be reflected more accurately by recording the mechanical activity of muscle, using the technique of mechanomyography or MMG (Orizio, 1993; Stokes & Blythe, 2001). A small recording device is placed on the skin to record the vibrations (often referred to as muscle sounds) produced when a muscle contracts. This technique is currently used in research to examine the contractile properties of muscle and has been used clinically, including for biofeedback. MMG can be used to record from muscles in which force cannot be measured directly, e.g. paraspinal muscles. The potential for MMG as a clinical tool is, therefore, very promising but some technical limitations need to be overcome before it can be used in routine clinical practice.

It should be noted that the most recent *National Clinical Guidelines for Stroke* (Intercollegiate Working Party for Stroke, 2008) no longer recommend the use of biofeedback based on Woodford and Price (2007) and Van et al. (2005).

Caudrey and Seeger (1981) provided a clear review of biofeedback devices other than EMG, which could be used as adjuncts to conventional physiotherapy. These include posture control equipment and the head position trainer, the limb load monitor and devices for improving orofacial control.

Another technique that is becoming a useful biofeedback tool in physiotherapy is real-time ultrasound imaging of muscle (see Whittaker et al., 2007, for a review). For example, re-education of the lumbar multifidus muscle, which can be difficult to teach, was shown to be enhanced using ultrasound imaging as visual feedback (Hides et al., 1998). It is stressed that adoption of the ultrasound technique by physiotherapists requires training and knowledge of its technical aspects, and adherence to safety guidelines (see www.bmus.org).

Most biofeedback equipment provides immediate, precise feedback to the patient about some aspect of activity. It is important to remember that most physiotherapists utilize verbal feedback when treating patients, whether to provide praise, correction or instruction.

KEY POINTS

◆ The use of biofeedback in stroke rehabilitation is no longer recommended.
◆ The inclusion of real-time ultrasound imaging may provide a useful development in biofeedback.
◆ Verbal feedback is the most commonly used form of biofeedback in neurological rehabilitation.

Neurodynamics

With any form of neurological dysfunction, the normal adaptive lengthening or shortening which occurs within the nervous system may be interrupted (Shacklock, 2005). Maintaining and restoring a mobile, extensible nervous system and a knowledge of normal neurodynamics could therefore be considered an essential part of the management of the neurological patient. However, it should be noted that a review by Ellis and Hing (2008) concluded that there was a lack of evidence in terms of quality and quantity to support its use.

Orthoses

An orthosis is a device that, when correctly applied to the appropriate external surface of the body, will achieve one or more of the following (Leonard et al., 1989):

- Relief of pain
- Immobilization of musculoskeletal segments
- Reduced axial loading
- Prevention or correction of deformity
- Improved function.

In neurological rehabilitation, orthoses are most frequently used to improve function and occasionally to prevent or correct deformity. Using anatomical and physiological knowledge, functional and biomechanical abnormalities are identified and, as far as is possible, corrected.

A variety of materials and designs can be used in the construction of an orthosis. The word 'splint' suggests an orthotic device designed for temporary use (Edelstein, 2007); examples of some splints were considered above in the section on inhibitory stretching. Ideally, most orthoses are designed, made and fitted by an orthotist.

Orthoses tend to be named in relation to the joints they surround. Foot orthoses (FOs) are applied to the foot, either inside or outside the shoe (arch supports, heel lifts). Ankle–foot orthoses (AFOs) encompass the foot and ankle, generally extending to just below the knee (see Ch. 8, Figure 8.3). Knee–ankle–foot orthoses (KAFOs) extend from foot to thigh; those extending above the hip are hip–knee–ankle–foot orthoses (HKAFOs; Edwards & Charlton, 2002).

Orthoses should help the patient meet identified functional objectives; in the case of those applied to the lower limbs, this frequently relates to walking. In order to use orthoses effectively to improve walking, it is essential to consider the normal biomechanics of walking. When using an orthosis, forces are applied to the lower limb as a series of three-point force systems (Leonard et al., 1989). It is essential that these forces are correctly applied so that the desired effect is achieved.

Of particular biomechanical interest is the ability to visualize the ground reaction forces during activities of the lower limb. In a laboratory situation it is possible, using a force plate and video vector generator, to evaluate the effects of an orthosis, using a real-time ground reaction vector. Abnormal moments or turning effects on joints can be noted; energy demand is reduced by minimizing the moments that must be resisted during walking, and this can be achieved by altering the forces applied by the orthosis. Butler and Nene (1991) illustrated this clearly in relation to the application of fixed AFOs used in the management of children with cerebral palsy.

Upper limb orthoses used in neurological dysfunction are often employed to provide a dynamic force on a joint to reduce contractures (Leonard et al., 1989), a use already outlined above. Orthoses to enhance upper limb function are illustrated in Chapter 9. Perhaps the most common orthotic device used by physiotherapists working in neurology is some form of shoulder support for patients with subluxation following stroke. Various types of shoulder support have been used; one of the most commonly used supports in the UK is based upon a method outlined by Bertha Bobath (Leddy, 1981). There is currently insufficient evidence to support the use of a supportive device in the prevention and treatment of subluxation of the shoulder after stroke (Ada et al., 2005b). In a randomized controlled trial strapping patients 'at risk' of developing hemiplegic shoulder pain, Griffin and Bernhardt (2006) found that therapeutic strapping limited development of hemiplegic shoulder pain, although placebo strapping also had an effect.

> ### KEY POINTS
>
> - Orthoses should be used in neurological rehabilitation to achieve pre-determined objectives.
> - They are commonly used to improve function and occasionally to prevent or correct deformity.

Acupuncture

Acupuncture was recognized in 1979 by the World Health Organization (WHO) as a clinical procedure of value that should be taken seriously. Although increasingly used in the musculoskeletal field, acupuncture has not been used extensively by physiotherapists working in neurology.

The use of acupuncture for stroke rehabilitation was reviewed by Wu et al. (2006) who concluded that the quality of the trials was poor, so no definite conclusions could be reached. A similar judgement was reached by He et al. (2006) when considering its use in relation to Bell's palsy. More information and an overview of acupuncture is available in Umphred et al. (2007b). Electroacupuncture was investigated by Mukherjee et al. (2007) to ascertain whether it could be used to influence spasticity of the impaired wrist joint in chronic stroke patients. A combination of the electro-acupuncture and resisted exercise for 6 weeks was found to significantly reduce spasticity using a variety of outcome measures.

String wrapping

Flowers (1988) advocated the use of string wrapping, also referred to as compressive centripetal wrapping, to help control oedema. This is an easily applied method for reducing oedema, particularly in the swollen paralysed hand. Each digit, the thumb and hand, are wrapped from distal to proximal using string of 1–2 mm diameter. A loop is made as the wrapping commences and the wrapping is applied firmly and continuously. Once applied, the wrapping is immediately removed by pulling on the free end of the loop (Davies, 2000). The reduction of swelling allows greater facilitation of active movement. This is a treatment that can easily be applied by carers prior to, and in between, episodes of physiotherapy. It has very specific, local effects and may prove very useful when swelling is restricting functional improvement in the hand.

CONCLUSION

A variety of techniques used by physiotherapists working in neurology has been discussed. It is not possible to give detailed descriptions of their exact application but brief outlines have been given and references provided for further information. Many of the techniques used require further research either to validate their use and/or to establish appropriate guidelines for their application.

CASE HISTORIES

Case 1 – Stroke

History and problem

Mrs S. is a 62-year-old woman attending for outpatient physiotherapy following a left cerebrovascular accident (CVA). At the moment she is wheelchair-dependent and has little active movement in her right upper and lower limbs. Passive ROM on the right is within normal limits and there is no resistance felt to passive movement.

Treatment

Techniques of facilitation can be combined with the use of functional positions to try and facilitate a motor response on the right. Possible techniques include approximation and tapping.

To apply approximation, Mrs S. must be placed in a position that results in joint approximation. Sitting Mrs S. on a low plinth, the right upper limb is placed with the shoulder laterally rotated and abducted, with the elbow extended and the hand resting on the plinth. The physiotherapist may need to give manual support to the elbow and shoulder to maintain the position while weight is taken through the hand, and joint approximation occurs.

Alternatively, Mrs S. could be weight-bearing through her upper limb using a plinth in front of her while she stands and also takes weight through the lower limbs.

Tapping over the right knee extensors can be used to facilitate their action during standing. Continuing in standing, a ball could be placed on the plinth so that Mrs S. can achieve some dynamic upper limb weight-bearing, combined with continued weight-bearing through the lower limbs.

Case 2 – Head injury

History and problem

Mr P. is a 70-year-old man who has been an inpatient for some time following a head injury. He is currently working to improve his walking ability, which is severely hindered by a loss of extensibility in his right calf muscles.

Treatment

Before he starts his physiotherapy session, Mr P. comes down to the gym to stand on a tilt table in order to give his calf muscles a prolonged stretch. To make this even more effective, his left leg is placed on a stool to ensure that the right limb is fully loaded. When he starts his walking practise he has EMG biofeedback applied to his right ankle dorsiflexors to help him activate these muscles during the swing phase of gait. His physiotherapist has also been using ice on his dorsiflexors to facilitate movement. This is applied by sweeping an ice cube over the muscle belly and then asking Mr P. to try and dorsiflex his ankle.

REFERENCES

Ada, L., Goddard, E., McCully, J., Stavrinos, T., Bampton, J., 2005a. Thirty minutes of positioning reduces the development of shoulder external rotation contracture after stroke: a randomized controlled trial. Arch. Phys. Med. Rehabil. 86, 230–234.

Ada, L., Foongchomcheay, A., Canning, C.G., 2005b. Supportive devices for preventing and treating subluxation of the shoulder after stroke. Cochrane Database Syst. Rev. 1, CD003863.

Adler, S.J., Beckers, D., Buck, M., 2008. PNF in Practice. Springer Medizin Verlag, Heidelberg.

Ageranioti, S., Hayes, K., 1990. Effects of vibration in hypertonia and hyperreflexia in the wrist joint of patients with spastic hemiparesis. Physiother. Can. 42, 24–33.

American College of Sports Medicine, 2009. ACSM guidelines for exercise testing and prescription. Williams and Wilkins, Philadelphia.

Anderson, B.D., Butler, M.N., 2007. The Pilates Method. In: Umphred, D. A. (Ed.), Neurological Rehabilitation. Mosby, St Louis, pp. 1145–1148.

Anderson, B.D., Spector, A., 2000. Introduction to Pilates-based rehabilitation. Orthopedic Physical Therapy North America 9, 395–410.

Arias, P., Chouza, M., Vivas, J., Cudeiro, J., 2009. Effect of whole body vibration in Parkinson's disease: a controlled study. Mov. Disord. 24, 891–898.

Association of Chartered Physiotherapists Interested in Neurology (ACPIN), 1998. Clinical Practice Guidelines on Splinting Adults with Neurological Dysfunction. Chartered Society of Physiotherapy, London.

Attard, J., Rithalia, S., 2004. A review of the use of lycra pressure orthoses for children with cerebral palsy. International Journal of Therapy and Rehabilitation 11, 120–126.

Baily Metcalf, A., Lawes, N., 1998. A modern approach of the Rood approach. Phys. Ther. Rev. 3, 195–212.

Baker, L., 1991. Clinical uses of neuromuscular electrical stimulation. In: Nelson, R., Currier, D. (Eds.), Clinical Electrotherapy. Connecticut, Appleton and Lange, pp. 143–170.

Ben, M., Harvey, L., Denis, S., Glinsky, J., Goehl, G., Chee, S., et al., 2005. Does 12 weeks of regular standing prevent loss of ankle mobility and bone mineral density in people with recent spinal cord injuries? Aust. J. Physiother. 51, 251–256.

Bennie, A., 1997. Spinal cord injuries. In: Reid Campion, M. (Ed.), Hydrotherapy: Principles and Practice. Butterworth-Heinemann, Oxford, pp. 242–251.

Bishop, B., 1974. Neurophysiology of motor responses evoked by vibratory stimulation. Phys. Ther. 54, 1273–1282.

Bobath, B., 1990. Adult Hemiplegia: Evaluation and Treatment. Heinemann, Oxford.

Bohannon, R.W., 1993. Tilt table standing for reducing spasticity after spinal cord injury. Arch. Phys. Med. Rehabil. 74, 1121–1122.

Bohls, C., McIntyre, A., 2005. The effect of ice stimulation on sensory loss in chronic stroke patients – a feasibility study. Physiother. 91, 237–241.

Bovend'Eerdt, T.J., Newman, M., Barker, K., Dawes, H., Minelli, C., Wade, D.T., 2008. The effects of stretching in spasticity: a systematic review. Arch. Phys. Med. Rehabil. 89, 1395–1406.

Bromley, I., 2006. Tetraplegia and Paraplegia. A Guide for Physiotherapists. Elsevier, Churchill Livingstone.

Brouwer, B., Sousa de Andrade, V., 1995. The effects of slow stroking on spasticity in patients with multiple sclerosis: a pilot study. Physiother. Theory. Pract. 11, 13–21.

Borisova, Y., Bohannon, R.W., 2009. Positioning to prevent or reduce shoulder range of motion impairments after stroke: a meta-analysis. Clin. Rehabil. 23, 681–686.

Butler, P., Nene, A., 1991. The biomechanics of fixed ankle foot orthoses and their potential in the management of cerebral palsied children. Physiotherapy 77, 81–88.

Callaghan, M.J., Oldham, J.A., Winstanley, J., 2001. A comparison of two types of electrical stimulation of the quadriceps in the treatment of patellofemoral pain syndrome. A pilot study. Clin. Rehabil. 5, 637–646.

Cameron, M.H., 2009. Physical agents in rehabilitation. Saunders, St Louis.

Carr, E.K., Kenney, F.D., 1992. Positioning of the stroke patient: a review of the literature. Int. J. Nurs. Stud. 29, 355–356.

Carriere, B., 1998. The Swiss Ball: Theory, Basic Exercises and Clinical Applications. Springer Verlag, Berlin.

Carriere, B., 1999. The 'Swiss ball. Physiotherapy 85, 552–561.

Caudrey, D., Seeger, B., 1981. Biofeedback devices as an adjunct to physiotherapy. Physiotherapy 67, 371–376.

Chantraine, A., Baribeault, A., Uebelhart, D., et al., 1999. Shoulder pain and dysfunction in hemiplegia. Arch. Phys. Med. Rehabil. 80, 328–331.

Chatterton, H.J., Pomeroy, V.M., Gratton, J., 2001. Positioning for stroke patients: a survey of physiotherapists' aims and practices. Disabil. Rehabil. 23, 413–421.

Chu, K.S., Eng, J.J., Dawson, A.S., Harris, J.E., Ozkaplan, A., Gylfadottir, S., et al., 2004. Water based exercise for cardiovasucular fitness in people with chronic stroke: a randomized controlled trial. Arch. Phys. Med. Rehabil. 85, 870–874.

Cole, A.J., Becker, B.E., 2004. Comprehensive aquatic therapy. Butterworth Heinemann, Philadelphia.

Damiano, D.L., DeJong, S.L., 2009. A systematic review of the effectiveness treadmill training and body weight support in pediatric rehabilitation. J. Neurol. Phys. Ther. 33, 27–44.

Davies, P.M., 1990. Right in the Middle. Selective Trunk Activity in the Treatment of Adult Hemiplegia. Springer-Verlag, Berlin.

Davies, P.M., 2000. Steps to Follow: The Comprehensive Treatment of Patients with Hemiplegia. Springer-Verlag, Berlin.

Davis, B.C., Harrison, R.A., 1988. Hydrotherapy in Practice. Churchill Livingstone, Edinburgh.

Dean, C.M., Mackey, F.H., Katrak, P., 2000. Examination of shoulder positioning after stroke: a randomized controlled pilot trial. Aust. J. Physiother. 46, 35–40.

De Kroon, J.R., van der Lee, J.H., IJzerman, M.J., Lankhorst, G.J., 2002. Therapeutic electrical stimulation to improve motor control and functional abilities of the upper extremity after stroke: a systematic review. Clin. Rehabil. 16, 350–360.

Dickstein, R., Hocherman, S., Pillar, T., et al., 1986. Stroke rehabilitation three exercise therapy approaches. Phys. Ther. 66, 1233–1237.

Dutton, L.L., 2007. Adult nonprogressive central nervous system disorders. In: Cameron, M.H., Monroe, L.G. (Eds.), Phys. Rehabil. pp. 405–435.

Ebersbach, G., Edler, D., Kaufhold, O., Wissel, J., 2008. Whole body vibration versus conventional physiotherapy to improve balance and gain in Parkinson's disease. Arch. Phys. Med. Rehabil. 89, 399–403.

Edelstein, J.E., 2007. Orthotics. In: Cameron, M.H., Monroe, L.G. (Eds.), Physical rehabilitation. Elsevier, St Louis, pp. 897–917.

Edwards, S., Charlton, P., 2002. Splinting and the use of orthoses in the management of patients with neurological disorders. In: Edwards, S. (Ed.), Neurological Physiotherapy: A Problem-solving Approach. Edinburgh, Churchill Livingstone, pp. 219–253.

Edwards, R.G., Lippold, O.C.J., 1956. The relation between force and integrated electrical activity in fatigued muscle. J. Physiol. 312, 677–681.

Ellis, R.F., Hing, W.A., 2008. Neural mobilization: a systematic review of randomized controlled trials with analysis of therapeutic efficacy. J. Man. Manip. Ther. 16, 8–22.

Faghri, P.D., Rodgers, M.M., Glaser, R.M., et al., 1994. The effects of functional electrical stimulation on shoulder subluxation, arm function recovery and shoulder pain in hemiplegic stroke patients. Arch. Phys. Med. Rehabil. 75, 73–79.

Farber, S., 1982. A multisensory approach to neurorehabilitation. In: Farber, S. (Ed.), Neurorehabilitation: A Multisensory Approach. WB Saunders, Philadelphia, pp. 115–177.

Flowers, K., 1988. String wrapping versus massage for reducing digital volume. Phys. Ther. 68, 57–59.

Fox, J., Sharp, T., 2007. Practical electotherapy: a guide to safe application. Edinburgh, Churchill Livingstone.

Fraser, C., 2009. Exploring partnerships in the rehabilitation setting: the 24-hour approach of the Bobath concept. In: Raine, S., Meadows, L., Lynch-Ellerington, M. (Eds.), Bobath concept Theory and clinical practice in neurological rehabilitation. Wiley Blackwell, Oxford, pp. 182–204.

Garland, S.J., Hayes, K.C., 1987. Effects of brushing on electromyographic activity and ankle dorsiflexion in hemiplegic subjects with foot drop. Physiother. Can. 39, 239–247.

Getz, M., Hutzler, Y., Vermeer, A., 2006. Effects of aquatic interventions in children with neuromotor impairments: a systematic review of the literature. Clin. Rehabil. 20, 927–936.

Glanz, M., Klawansky, S., Stason, W., et al., 1995. Biofeedback therapy in poststroke rehabilitation: a meta-analysis of the randomised controlled trials. Arch. Phys. Med. Rehabil. 76, 508–515.

Glynn, A., Fiddler, H., 2009. The physiotherapist's pocket guide to exercise assessment, prescription and training. Churchill Livingstone, Edinburgh.

Goldberg, J., Sullivan, S.J., Seaborne, D. E., 1992. The effect of two intensities of massage on H-reflex amplitude. Phys. Ther. 72, 449–457.

Goldspink, G., Williams, P.E., 1990. Muscle fibre and connective tissue changes associated with use and disuse. In: Ada, L., Canning, C. (Eds.), Key Issues in Neurological Physiotherapy. Butterworth-Heinemann, Oxford, pp. 197–218.

Goulet, C., Arsenault, A.B., Levin, M.F., et al., 1994. Absence of consistent effects of repetitive transcutaneous electrical stimulation on soleus H-reflex in normal subjects. Arch. Phys. Med. Rehabil. 75, 1132–1136.

Gracies, J.M., Marosszeky, E., Renton, R., et al., 2000. Short-term effects of dynamic lycra splints on upper limb in hemiplegic patients. Arch. Phys. Med. Rehabil. 81, 1547–1555.

Gray, S., 1997. Neurological rehabilitation. In: Reid Campion, M. (Ed.), Hydrotherapy: Principles and Practice. Butterworth-Heinemann, Oxford, pp. 204–224.

Griffin, A., Bernhardt, J., 2006. Strapping the hemiplegic shoulder prevents development of pain during rehabilitation: a randomized controlled trial. Clin. Rehabil. 20, 287–295.

Hakkennes, S., Keating, J.L., 2005. Constraint-induced movement therapy following stroke: a systematic review of randomised controlled trials. Aust. J. Physiother. 51, 221–231.

Hale, L.A., Fritz, V.U., Goodman, M., 1995. Prolonged static muscle stretch reduces spasticity – but for how long should it be held? S. Afr. J. Physiother. 51, 3–6.

Handy, J., Salinas, S., Blanchard, S.A., Aitken, M.J., 2003. Meta analysis examining the effectiveness of electrical stimulation in improving functional use of the upper limb in stroke patients. Phys. Occup. Ther. Geriatr. 21, 67–78.

Harling, A., Simpson, J.P., 2008. A systematic review to determine the effectiveness of Tai Chi in reducing falls and fear of falling in older adults. Phys. Ther. Rev. 13, 237–248.

Harvey, L., Herbert, R., Crosbie, J., 2002. Does stretching induce lasting changes in joint ROM? A systematic review. Physiother. Res. Int. 7, 1–13.

Hecox, B., Leinanger, P.M., 2006. Hydrotherapy. In: Hecox, B., Andemicael Mehreteab, T., Weisberg, J., Sanko, J. (Eds.), Integrating physical agents in rehabilitation. Pearson Education, New Jersey, pp. 397–426.

He, L., Zhou, M., Zhou, D., Wu, B., et al., 2006. Acupuncture for Bell's palsy. Cochrane Database Syst. Rev. 2, CD002914.

Hesse, S., 2008. Treadmill training with partial body weight support after stroke: a review. NeuroRehabilitation 23, 55–65.

Hicks, A.L., Martin Ginis, K.A., 2008. Treadmill training after spinal cord injury: it's not just about the walking. J. Rehabil. Res. Dev. 45, 241–248.

Hides, J.A., Richardson, C.A., Jull, G.A., 1998. Use of real-time ultrasound imaging for feedback in rehabilitation. Man. Ther. 3, 125–131.

Hoare, B.J., Wasiak, J., Imms, C., Carey, L., 2007. Constraint-induced movement therapy in the treatment of the upper limb in children with hemiplegic cerebral palsy. Cochrane Database Syst. Rev. 2, CD004149.

Hochreiter, N.W., Jewell, M., Barber, L., et al., 1983. Effect of vibration on tactile sensitivity. Phys. Ther. 6, 934–937.

Holey, E., Cook, E., 2003. Evidence based therapeutic Massage. Churchill Livingstone, Edinburgh.

Hollis, M., Jones, E., 2009. Massage for therapists: a guide to soft tissue therapy. Wiley-Blackwell, Chichester.

Intercollegiate Working Party for Stroke, 2008. National Clinical Guidelines for Stroke, third ed. Royal College of Physicians, London. Available online at: http://www.rcplondon.ac.uk/pubs/contents/6ad05aab-8400-494c-8cf4-9772d1d5301b.pdf.

Jackson, K.J., Merriman, H.L., Vanderburgh, P.M., Brahler, C.J., 2008. Acute effects of whole body vibration on lower extremity muscle performance in persons with multiple sclerosis. J. Neurol. Phys. Ther. 32, 171–176.

Johnstone, M., 1995. Restoration of Normal Movement after Stroke. Edinburgh, Churchill Livingstone.

Jones, C.A., 1999. Case in point. Effect of lower extremity serial casts on hemiparetic gait patterns in adults. Phys. Ther. Case Rep. 2, 221–231.

Jones, M., Grimmer, K., Edwards, I., Higgs, J., Trede, F., 2006. Challenges to applying best evidence to physiotherapy. Internet Journal of Allied Health Science Practice 4 (3) Accessed from http://ijahsp.nova. edu/articles/vol4num3/jones.htm.

Kerrigan, D.C., Sheffler, L.R., 1995. Spastic paretic gait: an approach to evaluation and treatment. Crit. Rev. Phy. Rehabil. Med. 7, 253–268.

Kilbreath, S.L., Davis, G.M., 2005. Cardiorespiratory fitness after stroke. In: Refshauge, K., Ada, L., Ellis, E. (Eds.), Science-based rehabilitation Butterworth Heinemann Edinburgh. pp. 131–158.

Kim, C.M., Eng, J.J., Whittaker, M.W., 2004. Effects of a simple functional electric system and/or a hinged ankle-foot orthosis on walking in persons with incomplete spinal cord injury. Arch. Phys. Med. Rehabil. 85, 1718–1723.

King, L.A., Horak, F.B., 2009. Delaying mobility disability in people with Parkinson disease using a sensorimotor agility exercise program. Phys. Ther. 89, 384–393.

Kisner, C., Colby, L.A., 2007. Therapeutic Exercise: Foundations and Techniques. FA Davis, Philadelphia.

Kitchen, S. (Ed.), 2002. Electrotherapy Evidence Based Practice. Edinburgh, Churchill Livingstone, 2002.

Kukulka, C., Haberichter, P.A., Mueksch, A.E., et al., 1987. Muscle pressure effects on motoneuron excitability: a special communication. Phys. Ther. 67, 1720–1722.

Kwakkel, G., Kollen, B.J., Krebs, H.I., 2008. Effects of robot-assisted therapy on upper limb recovery after stroke: a systematic review. Neurorehabil. Neural Repair 22, 111–121.

Lambeck, J., Coffey Stanat, F., Kinnaird, D. W., 2004. The Halliwick Concept. In: Cole, A.J., Becker, B.E. (Eds.), Comprehensive Aquatic Therapy. Butterworth Heinemann, Philadelphia.

Lange, C., Unnithan, V., Larkham, E., Latta, P., 2000. Maximizing the benefits of Pilates-inspired exercise for learning functional motor skills. J. Bodyw. Mov. Ther. 4, 899–1008.

Leandri, M., Parodi, C.I., Corrieri, N., et al., 1990. Comparison of TENS treatments in hemiplegic shoulder pain. Scand. J. Rehabil. Med. 22, 69–72.

Leddy, M., 1981. Sling for hemiplegic patients. Br. J. Occup. Ther. 44, 158–160.

Lee, S.M., Lam, P., Ernst, E., 2008. Effectiveness of tai chi for Parkinson's disease: a critical review. Parkinsonism Relat. Disord. 14, 589–594.

Lee, J.M., Warren, M.P., Mason, A.M., 1978. Effects of ice on nerve conduction velocity. Physiotherapy 64, 2–6.

Lehmann, J., De Lateur, B., 1990. Application of heat and cold in the clinical setting. In: Lehmann, J. (Ed.), Therapeutic Heat and Cold. Williams & Wilkins, Baltimore, pp. 633–644.

Lennon, S., 2003. Physiotherapyapy practice in stroke rehabilitation: a survey. Disabil. Rehabil. 25, 455–461.

Leonard, J.A., Hicks, J.E., Nelson, V.S., et al., 1989. Prosthetics, orthotics, and assistive devices. 1. General concepts. Arch. Phys. Med. Rehabil. 70, S195–S201.

Leone, J., Kukulka, C., 1988. Effects of tendon pressure on alpha motoneuron excitability in patients with stroke. Phys. Ther. 68, 475–480.

Lim, I., van Wegen, E., de Goede, C., Deutekom, M., et al., 2005. Effects of external rhythmical cueing on gait in patients with Parkinson's disease: a systematic review. Clin. Rehabil. 19, 695–713.

Lovgreen, B., Cody, F.W.J., Schady, W., 1993. Muscle vibration alters the trajectories of voluntary movements in cerebellar disorders – a method of counteracting impaired movement accuracy? Clin. Rehabil. 7, 327–336.

Luft, A.R., McCombe-Waller, S., Whitall, J., Forrester, L.W., et al., 2004. Repetitive bilateral arm training and motor cortex activation in chronic stroke: a randomized controlled trial. JAMA 292, 1853–1861.

Masiero, S., Celia, A., Rosati, G., Armani, M., 2007. Robotic-assisted rehabilitation of the upper limb after acute stroke. Arch. Phys. Med. Rehabil. 88, 142–149.

McDonough, S., Kitchen, S., 2002. Neuromuscular and muscular electrical stimulation. In: Kitchen, S., (Ed.), Electrotherapy Evidence Based Practice. Edinburgh, Churchill Livingstone, pp. 241–258.

Melis, E.H., Torres-Moreno, R., Chilco, L., et al., 1995. Application of ambulatory assistive devices and functional electrical stimulation to facilitate the locomotion of spinal cord injured subjects. In: Proceedings of 12th International Congress of World Confederation for Physical Therapy. Washington, DC, p. 772.

Mills, V., 1986. Electromyographic results of inhibitory splinting. Phys. Ther. 64, 190–193.

Moore, M., Kukulka, C., 1991. Depression of Hoffmann reflexes following voluntary contraction and implications for proprioceptive neuromuscular facilitation therapy. Phys. Ther. 71, 321–333.

Morgan, C.L., Cullen, G.P., Stokes, M., et al., 2003. Effects of knee joint angle and tilt table incline on force distribution at the feet and supporting straps. Clin. Rehabil. 17, 871–878.

Morris, S.L., Sharpe, M., 1993. PNF revisited. Physiother. Theory Pract. 9, 43–51.

Morris, D.M., Taub, E., 2001. Constraint-induced therapy approach to restoring function after neurological injury. Top. Stroke Rehabil. 8, 16–30.

Moseley, A.M., 1997. The effect of casting combined with stretching on passive ankle dorsiflexion in adults with traumatic head injury. Phys. Ther. 77, 240–247.

Mukherjee, M., McPeak, L., Redford, J.B., et al., 2007. The effect of electro-acupuncture on spasticity of the wrist joint in chronic stroke survivors. Arch. Phys. Med. 88, 159–166.

Murphy, C., 1993. Massage – the roots of the profession. Physiotherapy 79, 546.

Mutlu, A., Krosschell, K., Gaebler Spira, D., 2009. Treadmill training with partial body-weight support in children with cerebral palsy: a systematic review. Dev. Med. Child Neurol. 51, 1157–1164.

Noh, D.K., Lim, J., Shin, H., Paik, N., 2008. The effect of aquatic therapy on postural balance and muscle strength in stroke survivors a randomized controlled pilot trial. Clin. Rehabil. 22, 966–976.

Oldham, J.A., Howe, T.E., Peterson, T., et al., 1995. Electrotherapeutic rehabilitation of the quadriceps in elderly osteoarthritic patients: a double blind assessment of patterned neuromuscular stimulation. Clin. Rehabil. 9, 10–20.

Orizio, C., 1993. Muscle sound: bases for the introduction of a mechanomyographic signal in muscle studies. Crit. Rev. Biomed. Eng. 21, 201–243.

O'Sullivan, S.B., 2007. Strategies to improve motor function. In: O'Sullivan, S., Schmitz, T. (Eds.), Physical Rehabilitation. FA Davis, Philadelphia, pp. 471–522.

Petrofsky, J., 1988. Functional electrical stimulation and its application in the rehabilitation of neurologically injured adults. In: Finger, S., et al., (Ed.), Brain Injury and Recovery: Theoretical and Controversial Issues. Plenum Press, New York.

Pette, D., 1986. Skeletal muscle adaptation in response to chronic stimulation. In: Nix, W.A., Vrbová, G. (Eds.), Electrical Stimulation and Neuromuscular Disorders. Springer-Verlag, Berlin, pp. 12–20.

Pope, P.M., 2002. Postural management and special seating. In: Edwards, S. (Ed.), Neurological Physiotherapy: A Problem-solving Approach. Edinburgh, Churchill Livingstone, pp. 189–253.

Price, C.I.M., Pandyan, A.D., 2000. Electrical stimulation for preventing and treating post-stroke shoulder pain (Cochrane Review). In: The Cochrane Library. issue 2. Update Software, Oxford.

Raine, S., 2007. The current theoretical assumptions of the Bobath concept as determined by the members of the BBTA. Physiother. Theory Pract. 23, 137–152.

Reid Campion, M., 1997. Hydrotherapy Principles and Practice. Butterworth-Heinemann, Oxford.

Refshauge, K., Ada, L., Ellis, E., 2005. Science-based rehabilitation theories into practice. Butterworth Heinemann, Edinburgh.

Richardson, D.L.A., 1991. The use of the tilt table to effect passive tendo-Achilles stretch in a patient with head injury. Physiother. Theory Pract. 7, 45–50.

Robertson, V., Ward, A., Low, J., Reed, A., 2006. Electrotherapy explained: principles and practices. Elsevier, Oxford.

Robichaud, J., Agostinucci, J., Vander Linden, D., 1992. Affect of air-splint application on soleus muscle

motoneuron reflex excitabilty in nondisabled subjects and subjects with cerebrovascular accidents. Phys. Ther. 72, 176–185.

Roche, A.O., Laighin, G., Coote, S., 2009. Surface-applied functional electrical stimulation for orthotic and therapeutic treatment of drop-foot after stroke – a systematic review. Phys. Ther. Rev. 14, 63–80.

Rothwell, J., 1994. Control of Human Voluntary Movement. Chapman & Hall, London.

Rubinstein, T.C., Giladi, N., Hausdorff, J.M., 2002. The power of cueing to circumvent dopamine dificits: a review of physical therapy treatment of gait disturbances in Parkinson's disease. Mov. Disord. 17, 1148–1160.

Rutherford, O.M., Jones, D.A., 1988. Contractile properties and fatiguability of the human adductor pollicis and first dorsal interosseus: a comparison of the effect of two chronic stimulation patterns. J. Neurol. Sci. 85, 319–331.

Sackley, C.M., Lincoln, N.B., 1996. Physiotherapy treatment for stroke patients: a survey of current practice. Physiother. Theory Pract. 12, 87–96.

Schrepfer, M.S., 2007. Aquatic Therapy. In: Kisner, C., Colby, L.A. (Eds.), Therapeutic Exercise Foundations and Techniques. FA Davis Co, Philadelphia, pp. 273–294.

Scott, O.M., Vrbová, G., Hyde, S.A., et al., 1986. Effects of electrical stimulation on normal and diseased human muscle. In: Nix, W.A., Vrbová, G. (Eds.), Electrical Stimulation and Neuromuscular Disorders. Springer-Verlag, Berlin, pp. 125–131.

Schultz-Krohn, W., Royeen, C.B., McCormack, G., Pope-Davis, S.A., Jourdan, J.M., 2006. Traditional sensorimotor approaches to intervention. In: Pendleton, H.M., Schultz-Krohn, W. (Eds.), Pedretti's Occupational Therapy: Practice Skills for Physical Dysfunction. Mosby, St Louis, pp. 726–768.

Seib, T., Price, R., Reyes, M.R., et al., 1994. The quantitative measurement of spasticity: effect of cutaneous electrical stimulation. Arch. Phys. Med. Rehabil. 75, 746–750.

Shacklock, M., 2005. Clinical Neurodynamics: a new system of

musculoskeletal treatment. Elsevier Butterworth-Heinemann, Edinburgh.

Sharmann, S.A., 2002. Movement Impairment Syndromes. Mosby, St Louis.

Shepherd, G.M., 1994. Neurobiology. Oxford University Press, New York.

Singer, B.J., Dunne, J.W., Singer, K.P., Jegasothy, G.M., Allison, G.T., 2004. Non surgical management of ankle contracture following acquired brain injury. Disabil. Rehabil. 26, 335–345.

Sonde, L., Kalimo, H., Viitanen, M., 2000. Stimulation with high-frequency TENS – effects on lower limb spasticity after stroke. Adv. Physiol. Educ. 2, 183–187.

Stokes, M.J., Blythe, G.M., 2001. Muscle Sounds – in Physiology, Sports Science and Clinical Investigation: Applications and History of Mechanomyography. Medintel Publications, Oxford.www.oxmedic.com.

Stokes, M., Cooper, R., 1989. Muscle fatigue as a limiting factor in functional electrical stimulation; a review. Physiotherapy Practice 5, 93–190.

Sullivan, K.J., Brown, D.A., Klassen, T., Mulroy, S., Ge, T., Azen, S.P., et al., 2007. Effects of task-specific locomotor and strength training in adults who were ambulatory after stroke: results of the STEPS randomized clinical trial. Phys. Ther. 87, 1580–1602.

Sullivan, S.J., Williams, L.R.T., Seaborne, D.E., et al., 1991. Effects of massage on alpha motorneurone excitability. Phys. Ther. 71, 555–560.

Suzuki, T., Fujiwara, T., Yase, Y., et al., 1995. Electrophysiological study of spinal motor neurone function in patients with cerebrovascular diseases – characteristic appearances of the H-reflex and F-wave. In: Proceedings of 12th International Congress of World Confederation for Physical Therapy. Washington, DC, p. 798.

Tardieu, C., Lespargot, A., Tabary, C., et al., 1988. For how long must the soleus muscle be stretched each day to prevent contracture? Dev. Med. Child Neurol. 30, 3–10.

Turton, A., Britton, E., 2005. A pilot randomized controlled trial of a daily muscle stretch regime to prevent contractures in the arm after stroke. Clin. Rehabil. 19, 600–612.

Twist, D., 1985. Effects of a wrapping technique on passive range of motion in a spastic upper extremity. Phys. Ther. 65, 299–304.

Umphred, D.A., Byl, N.N., Lazaro, R.T., 2007a. Roller ML Interventions for clients with movement disorders. In: Umphred, D.A. (Ed.), Neurological Rehabilitation. Mosby, St Louis, pp. 187–281.

Umphred, D.A., Bottomley, J.M., Davis, C.M., Galantino, M.L., West, T.M., 2007b. Alternative and complementary therapies: beyond traditional approaches to intervention in neurological diseases, syndromes, and disorders. In: Umphred, D.A. (Ed.), Neurological Rehabilitation. Mosby, St Louis, pp. 1138–1192.

Van, D., Jannink, M., Hermens, H., 2005. Effect of augmented feedback on motor function of the affected upper extremity in rehabilitation patients: a systematic review of randomized controlled trials. J. Rehabil. Med. 37, 202–211.

Vang, M.M., Coleman, K.A., Gardner, M.P., et al., 1995. Effects of functional electrical stimulation on spasticity. In: Proceedings of 12th International Congress of World Confederation for Physical Therapy, Washington, DC, p. 574.

Voss, D.E., Ionta, M., Meyers, B., 1985. Proprioceptive Neuromuscular Facilitation: Patterns and Techniques. Harper & Row, New York.

Wallen, M., Mackay, S., 1995. An evaluation of the soft splint in the acute

management of elbow hypertonicity. Occup. Ther. J. Res. 15, 3–16.

Wallen, M., O'Flaherty, S., 1991. The use of the soft splint in the management of spasticity of the upper limb. Aus. Occup. Ther. J. 38, 227–231.

Wang, R., 1994. Effect of proprioceptive neuromuscular facilitation on the gait of patients with hemiplegia of long and short duration. Phys. Ther. 74, 1108–1115.

Wang, C., Collet, J.P., Lau, J., 2004. The effect of tai chi on health outcomes in patients with chronic conditions: a systematic review. Arch. Intern. Med. 164, 493–501.

Whalley Hammell, K., 1995. Spinal Cord Injury Rehabilitation. Chapman & Hall, London.

Whittaker, J., Teyhen, D., Elliott, J., Cook, K., Langevin, H., Dahl, H., et al., 2007. Rehabilitative ultrasound imaging: understanding the yechnology and its applications. J. Orthop. Sports Phys. Ther. 37 (8), 435–449.

Whittle, M.W., 2007. Gait Analysis: An Introduction. Edinburgh, Butterworth-Heinemann.

Williams, P.E., 1990. Use of intermittent stretch in the prevention of serial sarcomere loss in immobilised muscle. Ann. Rheum. Dis. 49, 316–317.

Williams, P.E., Catanese, T., Lucey, E.G., et al., 1988. The importance of stretch and contractile activity in the prevention of connective tissue accumulation in muscle. J. Anat. 158, 109–114.

Wolf, S.L., 2007. Revisting constraint-induced movement therapy: are we too smitten with the mitten? Is

all nonuse "learned" and other quandries. Phys. Ther. 87, 1212–1223.

Woodford, H., Price, C., 2007. EMG biofeedback for the recovery of motor function after stroke. Cochrane Database Syst. Rev. 2, CD004585.

Wu, H.M., Tang, J.L., Lin, X.P., Lau, J.T.F., Leung, P.C., Woo, J., et al., 2006. Acupuncture for stroke rehabilitation. Cochrane Database Syst. Rev. 3, CD004131.

Wunderer, K., Schabrun, S.M., Chipchase, L.S., 2008. The effect of whole body vibration in common neurological conditions – a systematic review. Phys. Ther. Rev. 13, 434–442.

Young, T., Nicklin, C., 2000. Lower limb casting in neurology practical guidelines. Royal Hospital for Neuro-disability, London.

Yozbatiran, N., Donmez, B., Kayak, N., Bozan, O., 2006. Electrical stimulation of wrist and fingers for sensory and functional recovery in acute hemiplegia. Clin. Rehabil. 20, 4–11.

Zachazewski, J.E., Eberle, E.D., Jefferies, M., 1982. Effect of tone-inhibiting casts and orthoses on gait: a case report. Phys. Ther. 62, 453–455.

Zupan, A., Gregoric, M., 1995. Long-lasting effects of electrical stimulation upon muscles of patients suffering from progressive muscular dystrophy. Clin. Rehabil. 9, 102–109.

Chapter | 13 |

Vestibular rehabilitation

Dara Meldrum, Rory McConn Walsh

The overwhelming vertigo, the awful sickness and the turbulent eye movements – all enhanced by the slightest movement of the head, combine to form a picture of helpless misery that has few parallels in the whole field of injury and disease.

Cawthorne, 1945

INTRODUCTION

Normal postural control, or 'balance' as it is commonly known, is fundamental to activities of daily living. Visual, vestibular and somatosensory systems all have important and integrated roles to play in the maintenance of balance and the neurological patient can present with problems in any or all of these components.

This chapter will focus on the assessment and treatment of patients who have a primary problem in the vestibular system. Vestibular dysfunction is characterized by a number of signs and symptoms, including vertigo, gait and balance impairment, nausea and nystagmus (Table 13.1).

Patients with such dysfunction present the physiotherapist with specific problems and require specialized assessment and treatment techniques, collectively referred to as vestibular rehabilitation. Vestibular rehabilitation has its roots in the empirical work of Cawthorne and Cooksey who, in the 1940s, first documented the important role of exercise in recovery after a vestibular injury (Cooksey, 1945).

Table 13.1 Signs and symptoms of vestibular disorders

PRIMARY SYMPTOMS AND SIGNS	ASSOCIATED PROBLEMS
Vertigo	Neck and back pain
Dizziness/light-headedness	Physical deconditioning
Nausea and vomiting	Agoraphobia
Oscillopsia	Hyperventilation
Nystagmus	Falls
Disequilibrium/impaired balance	Hearing loss/tinnitus
Panic/anxiety	
Gait abnormality	
Fatigue	

There is now a moderately strong evidence base to support the role of physiotherapy in the management of patients with vestibular disorders (Hillier & Holohan, 2007; Hilton & Pinder, 2004) and vestibular rehabilitation is recognized as a specialist area within physiotherapy.

KEY POINT

Vertigo is defined as the sensation of motion when no motion is occurring relative to the Earth's gravity (Monsell et al., 1997). The sensation can be of the patient moving in relation to the environment or the environment moving in relation to the patient. It is generally accepted that true vertigo involves a spinning sensation and usually indicates inner-ear pathology (Blakley & Goebel, 2001). The word 'dizziness' is used to describe non-rotatory vertigo. These definitions should be considered when taking the patient's history as they will give clues to the underlying pathology.

INCIDENCE AND PREVALENCE OF DIZZINESS AND BALANCE DISORDERS

The prevalence of dizziness has been estimated to be one in five in the 18–64 age group with 50% of these reporting postural unsteadiness (Yardley et al., 1998b). Prevalence rises to one in three in the over-65s (Colledge et al., 1994) and dizziness is the most common complaint of patients presenting to primary care in those aged over 75 (Sloane, 1989). However, approximately 40% of patients with a complaint of dizziness do not consult their general practitioner, demonstrating a probable underestimation of the problem (Yardley et al., 1998b). There is a very low prevalence of dizziness in the under-25s and women are more likely to experience dizziness. Dizziness rarely results in hospitalization and the majority of patients are managed at primary care level with medication (Sloane, 1989).

NORMAL ANATOMY AND PHYSIOLOGY

The anatomy and physiology of the vestibular system are extremely complex and the reader is referred to Cohen (1999) and (Schubert & Minor, 2004) for a detailed description. A brief organizational overview is shown in Figure 13.1. The vestibular system has both sensory and motor functions and is generally divided into peripheral and central components. The peripheral system consists of the vestibular end organ and the vestibular nerve up to and including the dorsal root entry zone. The central system includes the vestibular nuclei in the brainstem and their central connections.

Peripheral vestibular system

The vestibular end organ includes the semicircular canals (SCC) and the otoliths (utricle and saccule). There are three SCCs on each side (horizontal, anterior and posterior) and they are oriented at approximately 90° angles to each other (Figure 13.1). Each canal is coupled functionally with a canal in the opposite end organ, i.e. both horizontal canals are coupled, as are the left anterior and right posterior, and the right posterior and left anterior canals. Specialized sensors known as hair cells are located in the semicircular canals in a region known as the cupula (Figure 13.1) and respond to angular velocity of head movement in different planes. Each canal responds best to movement in its own plane. For example, if the head turns to the right, the hair cells in the right horizontal SCC increase their firing rate and those in the left horizontal SCC decrease their firing rate (Figure 13.2). Thus the central nervous system (CNS) gains information relating to the velocity and direction of head movement.

The otoliths have different hair cells in a region known as the macula, and these are covered by a layer of calcium carbonate crystals called otoconia. They respond to the force of gravity and thus can provide the CNS with information on head tilt and linear acceleration (i.e. going up and down in a lift or going forwards or backwards in a car).

The peripheral system is a tonically active system, i.e. it always has a certain firing level (about 70–100 spikes per

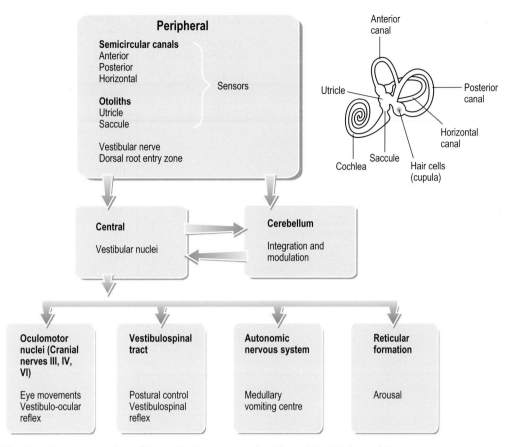

Figure 13.1 Functional organization of the vestibular system and vestibular labyrinth (top right).

second), which will increase or decrease with head movement. The CNS interprets any asymmetry in the firing rate as movement. This fact is of utmost importance when considering a patient who has loss of vestibular function on one side (i.e. decrease or absence of firing) since there will be a relative increase of firing on the intact side even when the head is not moving (Figure 13.2). This asymmetry and the resultant disturbance in cortical spatial orientation are thought to form the basis of vertigo (Brandt, 2000a). Afferent nerve fibres arising from hair cells collect to form the vestibular nerve, which enters the brain at the pontomedullary junction.

Central vestibular system

The vestibular nerve sends fibres to two main areas: the vestibular nuclei (in the pons and the medulla) and the cerebellum (Figure 13.1). The vestibular nuclei are responsible for integrating information received from the vestibular end organ with that received from other sensory systems and the cerebellum. Vestibular nuclei send fibres to the oculomotor nuclei, vestibulospinal tracts,

contralateral vestibular nuclei, reticular formation, thalamus, cerebellum, autonomic nervous system and the cortex. The parietal and insular areas of the cortex appear to be a specialized vestibular area (Brandt et al., 2002). The symptoms of nausea, vomiting and anxiety associated with vestibular disorders are thought to be a result of abnormal activation of the autonomic and reticular pathways respectively (Figure 13.1).

Vestibulo-ocular reflex and vestibulospinal reflex

The motor functions of the vestibular system include the vestibulo-ocular reflex (VOR) and the vestibulospinal reflex (VSR). The function of the VOR is to maintain stable vision when the head is moving. A good example of this is being able to focus on an object when walking. If the eyes moved with the head as it goes up and down when walking it would be impossible to see clearly. The VOR enables the eyes (through activation of the appropriate ocular muscles) to move in the opposite direction and at an equal velocity to the head. The image of the object

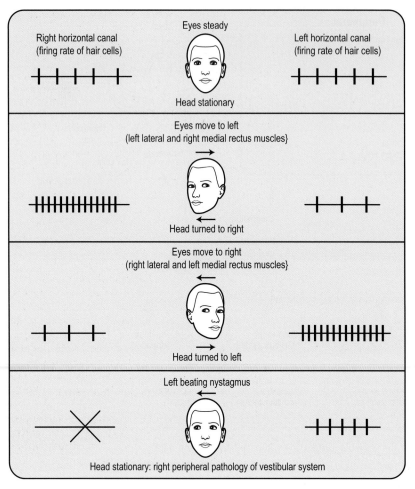

Figure 13.2 Function of the horizontal canals in generating a vestibulo-ocular reflex (VOR) during turning of the head and effect of loss of hair cell function. With loss of tonic firing on the right there is a relative increase in firing on the left; the brain interprets this as movement to the left (patient feels dizzy) and generates a VOR so that the eyes move to the right. The central nervous system corrects the eye movement with a saccadic movement to left, and a left-beating nystagmus is seen. (Firing rate for illustrative purposes only.)

thus remains stable on the retina. For the VOR to function normally, the velocity of eye movement must be equal to and in the opposite direction from the head movement. This is known as the 'gain' of the VOR. Patients who have problems with the vestibular system have impairment of the gain of the VOR and therefore demonstrate problems with gaze stability. They often describe that during self-motion stationary objects seem as if they are moving. The function of the VSR is primarily to maintain and regain postural control and this is achieved through activation of monosynaptic and polysynaptic vestibulospinal pathways.

CLASSIFICATION AND CAUSES OF VESTIBULAR DISORDERS

Vestibular disorders are classified anatomically into peripheral or central, depending on which area the pathology affects. Common peripheral and central vestibular

disorders are shown in Table 13.2. It is important to note that dizziness is not always caused by pathology affecting the vestibular system; there may be many other causes, including postural hypotension, cardiac disorders, psychiatric disorders and hyperventilation, and these should be evaluated prior to referral to physiotherapy. The exact cause of dizziness frequently remains uncertain and a trial of vestibular rehabilitation may be suggested in the absence of a specific diagnosis. The pathologies of disorders that can affect the central vestibular system (particularly cerebrovascular accidents, traumatic brain injury and multiple sclerosis) are considered in other chapters.

Peripheral disorders

Vestibular neuritis

This condition is also called neuronitis and is a common peripheral vestibular problem thought to be caused by a virus. It results in hair cell loss and unilateral vestibular paresis (or hypofunction). Patients present with an acute

Table 13.2 Peripheral and central vestibular disorders

PERIPHERAL	CENTRAL
Viral – vestibular neuritis/labyrinthitis	Ischaemia, e.g. lateral medullary syndrome (Wallenburg's syndrome)
Benign paroxysmal positional vertigo (BPPV)	
Perilymph fistula	Vertebrobasilar insufficiency
Ménière's disease	Infection
Vascular occlusion	Head injury
Iatrogenic (ototoxic drugs, surgery)	Degenerative disease, e.g. multiple sclerosis
Head injury	Friedreich's ataxia
Acoustic neuromas (may have a central component)	Base-of-skull abnormalities, e.g. Arnold–Chiari malformation
	Tumours of the cerebellopontine angle
	Drugs
	Epilepsy
	Migraine

onset of vertigo, nausea and vomiting that is severely incapacitating and worsened by head and eye movements. On examination a spontaneous horizontal nystagmus can be seen, the fast phase of which beats away from the involved side. This is due to the asymmetrical tonic firing of the vestibular nerves (Figure 13.2). Balance and gait abnormalities are also evident. Hearing is not generally affected; if it is, the condition is called labyrinthitis. These symptoms generally resolve over a period of 2–6 weeks.

Benign paroxysmal positional vertigo

Benign paroxysmal positional vertigo (BPPV) is the commonest cause of vertigo in peripheral vestibular disorders. It has a lifetime prevalence of 2.4% (Marom et al., 2009) and is more common in females (Baloh et al., 1987). Its aetiology is unknown in many cases but it can occur as a result of an earlier vestibular neuritis or head trauma. The name encompasses the following associated features:

- Benign – the prognosis for recovery is favourable
- Paroxysmal – the associated vertigo is short-lived, generally less than 1 minute
- Positional – the vertigo is provoked by head positioning
- Vertigo – a spinning sensation is experienced.

BPPV is thought to be caused by detached utricular otoconia entering one of the SCCs and either floating free in the canal (canalithiasis; Epley, 1980) or adhering to the cupula (cupulolithiasis; Epley, 1980). This has the effect of making the SCC with the displaced otoconia in it responsive to gravity when normally it is not. The SCCs usually respond to head movement in their respective planes and increase or decrease their firing rate during head movement, returning to normal tonic firing level when the head has stopped moving. However, the displaced otoconia are heavier, continue to move in the canal and stimulate the hair cells in the canal to continue firing. The central vestibular system interprets this as further movement and generates a VOR for that canal, and the patient develops nystagmus and vertigo.

This nystagmus, following movement into the provoking position, has a latency of 1–50 seconds, is generally transient in nature (it stops when the otoconia come to a resting position) and is most commonly torsional towards the affected ear. If the patient repeatedly moves into the provoking position the vertigo and nystagmus will decrease due to habituation of the response (Baloh et al., 1987).

The diagnosis of BPPV is generally made using the Hallpike–Dix manoeuvre (Figure 13.3, Table 13.3) in which the head is moved into a provocative position. BPPV is most commonly caused by canalithiasis affecting the posterior SCC, but can also affect the anterior and, very rarely, the horizontal canal (Baloh et al., 1993; De la Meilleure et al., 1996).

Patients with BPPV complain of vertigo associated with certain head movements, i.e. rolling over in bed, looking up, bending down, and will usually avoid these movements. BPPV is more common in older patients.

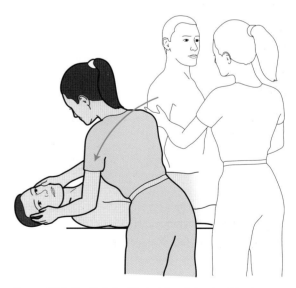

Figure 13.3 The Hallpike-Dix test for diagnosis of benign paroxysmal positional vertigo (BPPV).

Table 13.3 Oculomotor and positional tests of the vestibular patient

OCULOMOTOR EXAMINATION	DETAILS AND EXPECTED FINDINGS

Spontaneous nystagmus
  Room light (visual fixation)
  Frenzel lenses (no visual fixation)
	For the first four tests the patient is asked to hold the head stationary. Patient looks straight ahead. The eyes are observed for a nystagmus and the direction is noted. Frenzel lenses both remove visual fixation and magnify the eyes (Figure 13. 9). Nystagmus due to an acute unilateral peripheral vestibular disorder will have a fast phase away from the side of the lesion (Figure 13.2) and will be suppressed by visual fixation (i.e. focusing on something). Thus it is unlikely to be seen without Frenzel Lenses.

*Gaze evoked nystagmus**	Patient is asked to watch examiner's finger as it moves from left to right (about 30°) stopping at 30°. Normally the eyes will remain steady on the examiner's finger. If abnormal the eyes will make saccadic movements in an effort to remain on the examiner's finger.
*Smooth pursuit**	Ability to track examiners moving finger, from side to side and up and down with the eyes when the head is stationary. Normally the eyes make smooth movements, abnormalities include slow or saccadic movements of the eyes.
*Saccades**	The examiner holds two objects and asks the patient to look from one to the other (left to right, right to left, up to down and down to up starting from a mid position and moving about 30°). An abnormal response would be that the eyes over or under shoot the target
*VOR cancellation**	Ability to suppress the vestibulo-ocular reflex and move the eyes in phase with the head. Patient is asked to follow a moving target as the examiner moves the head in the same direction

Vestibulo-Ocular reflex- Halmagyi head thrust test (Halmagyi & Curthoys, 1988; Halmagyi et al., 2001)
  Slow head movement
  Fast head movement
	A normal VOR is when the eyes are able to stay fixated on a stationary target when the head moves. The patient is asked to keep their eyes steady on a target (usually the examiner's nose) whilst the examiner moves patient's head in a small range of movement (about 30°) from side to side and then up and down slowly. This is repeated with faster movements of the head. Patients with vestibular deficits are unable to keep the eyes steady and may use a saccadic movement to return their eyes to the target. For example in right vestibular hypofunction, if the head is moved to the right, the eyes may make a saccadic movement to the left. Abnormalities are more often seen with faster head movements.

Fukuda Step Test (Fukuda, 1959)	Also known as Unterberger's test. The patient is asked to close their eyes and march with high steps on the spot for 50 steps which they count themselves. The examiner stands behind the patient to ensure patient safety. The patient is observed for rotation and/or progression forwards from the start position. It is considered abnormal if the patient rotates more than 30° or progresses forwards more than 50 cm
Dyanmic Visual Acuity (Tian et al., 2002)	Tests visual acuity when the head is moving and is an indicator of VOR function. The patient is first asked to read a Snellen chart and static visual acuity is ascertained. The examiner then moves the head from side to side at a frequency of 1-2hz (using a metronome) and the patient then is asked to read a Snellen chart again. If visual acuity changes by more than 3 lines, acuity during head movement is considered impaired.
Positional tests *Hallpike-Dix test (Figure 13.3)*	The patient is long sitting on plinth with eyes open. The head is turned 45° to the side that is being tested. The patient is brought quickly into a lying position by the examiner until the cervical spine is in 30° of extension. This position is maintained for 50 seconds and the presence, duration and direction of nystagmus is noted. Symptoms are also noted. This test is diagnostic for BPPV. A positive finding is nystagmus (most commonly torsional towards the tested side) that comes on with a latency, may stay or disappear, and attenuates with repeated testing:

*Abnormality detected during these tests is indicative of central nervous system pathology.

Ménière's disease

The cause of Ménière's disease is an increase in volume and a problem with absorption of the endolymph (one of the fluids in the inner ear). This results in dilation of the endolymphatic spaces (endolymphatic hydrops). This happens episodically and an attack is characterized by a complaint of a fullness in the ear, reduction of hearing and tinnitus (a ringing sound in the ear). This is followed by vertigo, vomiting and postural imbalance and nystagmus is observed. The episodes may last from 30 minutes to 72 hours and then the patient gradually improves. Episodes are generally managed with medication, diet and rest, but in severe cases surgery may be indicated (see below). Although it was formerly thought vestibular rehabilitation was not indicated in patients with Ménière's, as attacks remit spontaneously, there is now some evidence to suggest it has a role in those patients who present with complaints of impaired balance between attacks (Gottshall et al., 2005).

Bilateral vestibular hypofunction

This condition can be caused by infections, e.g. meningitis, tumours (e.g. bilateral acoustic neuromas in neurofibromatosis), Ménière's disease, autoimmune diseases and ototoxic drugs (e.g. aminoglycoside antibiotics). In some cases the cause is unknown. Patients with bilateral vestibular hypofunction do not usually complain of vertigo when vestibular loss is symmetrical. Their main problems include balance and gait impairments and decreased gaze stability due to loss of VOR function. They complain that they cannot see clearly during head movements and describe their surroundings as bouncing or jumping. This is termed oscillopsia.

RECOVERY FROM VESTIBULAR PATHOLOGY: VESTIBULAR COMPENSATION

In most cases, the symptoms of patients with a unilateral vestibular loss spontaneously ameliorate over a period of weeks. The process by which the patient recovers is called vestibular compensation. The spontaneous nystagmus disappears by 2–3 days (static compensation) and the symptoms associated with movement (vertigo, visual blurring and postural unsteadiness) by 6 weeks (dynamic compensation). Hair cells have not been shown to regenerate in humans; therefore the patient must recover by other means.

Research has shown that plastic changes occur in the CNS in response to peripheral vestibular pathology and these changes are responsible for vestibular compensation (Curthoys, 2000; Zee, 2000). Three processes are thought to contribute:

1. Initially, the cerebellum *inhibits* firing of the vestibular nuclei of the *unaffected* side, probably to reduce the asymmetry produced by the lesion. The vestibular nucleus of the affected side begins spontaneously to fire tonically again, probably due to neurochemical changes produced by the loss of input (denervation supersensitivity; Curthoys, 2000).

2. The second process is known as sensory substitution. In this process the CNS reorganizes to substitute or utilize inputs more efficiently from intact systems, including vision and somatosensory and cervical proprioceptive systems. For example in slower head movements, saccadic movement of the eyes can be recruited to assist a poor VOR to help maintain stable vision (Schubert et al., 2008). An increase in muscle spindle input from the neck proprioceptors has also been demonstrated (Strupp et al., 1998a). The intact vestibular end organ is able to compensate somewhat for loss on the other side, as both sides respond to head movement in any direction. It is important to note also that if there is some remaining vestibular function on the pathological side, the CNS will utilize it.

3. Lastly, the process of habituation is thought to play a role in vestibular compensation. Habituation is generally defined as a reduction in response over time with repeated exposure to a specific stimulus. This is the process thought to underpin improvement with the Cawthorne Cooksey exercises (see below), in which the patient repeatedly performs head and/or eye movements that provoke symptoms of vertigo.

The reasons why some patients fail to compensate are not always clear, but may be a result of abnormality in the CNS, visual, somatosensory or musculoskeletal systems. Animal studies have shown that compensation is delayed by immobilization, reduced or absent visual inputs and is promoted by exercise (Courjon et al., 1977; Lacour et al., 1997). It is thought that the CNS needs to experience the error signals in order for vestibular compensation to occur. Certain medications, including those used in the treatment of vestibular problems, can delay compensation (Zee, 1985). An intact CNS is vitally important for the process of vestibular compensation and thus patients with central vestibular problems will have a slower and more incomplete recovery (Rudge & Chambers, 1982). In bilateral vestibular loss, there may be no remaining VOR function with which to compensate, so the process of sensory substitution plays a major role in the recovery of these patients and recovery will always be incomplete.

KEY POINT

Most patients with unilateral peripheral vestibular pathology spontaneously recover over a period of a few weeks through a process known as vestibular compensation. Patients who do not spontaneously recover present for treatment and may benefit from vestibular rehabilitation.

Multidisciplinary team

Patients with vestibular problems can be seen by a variety of members of the multidisciplinary team, including the physiotherapist, and communication between them facilitates optimum management. Diagnosis can be made at the level of primary care and it must be emphasized that the majority of patients are managed at this level as vestibular problems are generally associated with a favourable prognosis and spontaneous resolution. Patients who continue to experience problems are generally referred to ear, nose and throat specialists (also known as otologists or neurotologists), neurologists or neurosurgeons. Audiologists and audiological scientists carry out vestibular function testing and are involved in vestibular rehabilitation in some centres. Psychiatrists and psychologists are involved in the management of psychological problems associated with vestibular problems.

Medical and surgical management

Diagnosis/investigations

- Hearing tests (pure tone audiogram/speech discrimination): certain conditions that cause dizziness may also result in hearing loss. These include Ménière's disease, ototoxic medications, head trauma, acoustic neuromas and previous middle-ear surgery. A hearing test will provide valuable information on the inner ear (cochlea) and middle-ear function of these patients.
- Caloric/oculomotor testing: the caloric test is the most commonly used test of peripheral vestibular function and provides a separate, quantitative measure of lateral SCC function in each inner ear (Savundra & Luxon, 1997). This is performed by measuring the response of the VOR (nystagmus) to the instillation of cold and warm water down the external canal. As well as assessing peripheral vestibular function, oculomotor testing can also detect oculomotor disturbance (abnormal saccades, smooth pursuit) suggestive of a central disorder.
- Magnetic resonance imaging (MRI): any patient who presents with dizziness that is persistent or progressive should have an MRI scan (preferably with gadolinium enhancement) of the brain and cerebellopontine angle to exclude lesions such as a brain tumour, acoustic neuroma, multiple sclerosis or embolic/haemorrhagic events.
- Posturography (Figure 13.4): this provides a quantitative measure of certain functional aspects of dynamic equilibrium (Savundra & Luxon, 1997). It therefore has a role to play in the assessment of the disabled dizzy patient and can also be used in monitoring rehabilitation. To date, however, it has mainly been used as a research tool.

Medications

The acute rotatory vertigo suffered during an acute peripheral vestibular upset is due to sudden asymmetry in vestibular input to the CNS. Vestibular sedatives are a group of drugs that have a well-established record of controlling such attacks. These drugs have variable anticholinergic, antiemetic and sedative properties. They include phenothiazines (e.g. prochlorperazine, perphenazine), antihistamines (e.g. cinnarizine, dimenhydrinate, promethazine, meclizine) and benzodiazepines (e.g. diazepam, lorazepam; Moffat & Ballagh, 1997). These drugs are of particular value in the management of acute vertigo and they can be administered by intramuscular or intravenous injection, suppository, buccal absorption or orally, depending on the individual drug. However, they should be avoided in the management of chronic peripheral labyrinthine disorders as they may suppress central vestibular activity and thereby delay compensation and symptomatic recovery.

Betahistine and thiazide diuretics have been advocated in the management of Ménière's disease. Betahistine is a vasodilator that works directly on the inner ear and is thought to improve its microcirculation. Thiazide diuretics are thought to work in Ménière's disease by reducing the endolymphatic pressure by means of a systemic diuretic effect. However, much of the data reported regarding the efficacy of these drugs in Ménière's disease is conflicting.

Surgical management

Ménière's disease

In those patients with unilateral Ménière's disease that is symptomatic for 6 months to 1 year despite conservative management (betahistine, thiazide diuretic, salt/caffeine restriction), then surgery should be considered (Moffat & Ballagh, 1997). The type of surgery is dependent on the level of hearing in the affected ear.

If the hearing is not serviceable or useful (50% speech discrimination score, 50% speech reception threshold), then a labyrinthectomy is the preferred choice. This entails a mastoidectomy and drilling out the three SCCs under general anaesthesia. This is very effective at treating the vertiginous episodes by destroying all peripheral vestibular function, although all residual hearing is destroyed.

If the hearing is useful, then the surgery should attempt to preserve the remaining hearing. This can be done by means of topical gentamicin ablation therapy, endolymphatic sac decompression or by vestibular neurectomy. Topical gentamicin therapy involves the transtympanic instillation of gentamicin solution into the middle ear (Nedzelski et al., 1992). The gentamicin then diffuses into the inner ear across the round window membrane where it selectively destroys vestibular and not cochlear hair cells. Success rates of over 80% have been reported. The main disadvantage is that there is a risk of sensorineural hearing loss.

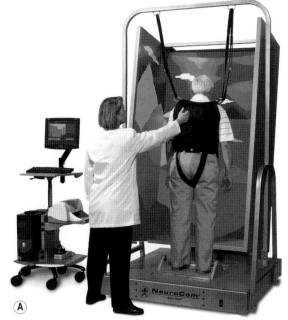

Sensory organization test (SOT) – Six conditions

	Condition		Sensory systems
1		Normal vision	👁
			🫘
		Fixed support	👣
2		Absent vision	
			🫘
		Fixed support	👣
3		Sway-referenced vision	👁
			🫘
		Fixed support	👣
4		Normal vision	👁
			🫘
		Sway-referenced support	👣
5		Absent vision	
			🫘
		Sway-referenced support	👣
6		Sway-referenced vision	👁
			🫘
		Sway-referenced support	👣
Visual input 👁		Red denotes 'sway-referenced' input. Visual surround follows subject's body sway, providing orientationally inaccurate information	
Vestibular input 🫘			
Somatosensory input 👣		Red denotes 'sway-referenced' input. Support surface follows subject's body sway, providing orientationally inaccurate information	

Figure 13.4 Computerized posturography. A. The Equitest system which consists of force platform and visual surround both of which can be sway referenced (move in tandem with postural sway). B. Postural sway under six conditions is generally tested in the sensory organization test (right hand side). Reprinted with permission from Equitest®, NeuroCom® International, Inc.

Endolymphatic sac decompression entails a mastoidectomy with removal of all bone over the endolymphatic sac/duct and possibly inserting a drain into it (Moffat, 1994). The sac is the proposed site of obstruction of endolymphatic reabsorption in Ménière's disease and this procedure enables the sac to expand during the active disease process. Vestibular neurectomy entails transecting the vestibular nerves in the posterior cranial fossa. The main disadvantages are damage to the facial and cochlear nerves together with intracranial complications. Vestibular rehabilitation is important following these procedures.

Persistent benign paroxysmal positional vertigo

Cases of intractable (1 year) and incapacitating BPPV can be treated by occlusion of the posterior semicircular canal (PSCC) (Parnes & McClure, 1990). This involves a mastoidectomy with isolation, and then occlusion of the PSCC. This is a safe and effective operation with success rates of over 90–95% (Walsh et al., 1999). Prior to this operation, singular neurectomy was advocated, but this is a technically more demanding operation with a risk of sensorineural hearing loss.

Acoustic neuromas

There are currently three methods of managing acoustic neuromas. These include conservative management, surgery (combined ear, nose and throat and neurosurgery) and stereotactic radiosurgery. Conservative management is reserved for small tumours that are not growing or for patients who are unfit or express a desire not to have surgery (Walsh et al., 2000). In those tumours that are growing and are causing symptoms, and those tumours greater than 1–2 cm in diameter, surgery should be considered. The aim of surgery is to remove the tumour without traumatizing the facial nerve, and, when indicated, to preserve hearing. Three surgical approaches are possible (translabyrinthine, retrosigmoid and middle cranial fossa) and the type depends on the level of remaining hearing. If the hearing is not serviceable or useful then a translabyrinthine approach is performed (House & Hitselberger, 1985). The main advantage of this technique is that there is minimal brain retraction and the access is excellent, although all remaining hearing is sacrificed.

If the hearing is useful, then the tumour is approached either via a retrosigmoid or a middle cranial fossa approach in an attempt to preserve the hearing (Sekhar et al., 1996). The main disadvantage of the former is that there is cerebellar retraction while the latter is technically demanding.

Stereotactic radiosurgery entails the accurate application of radiotherapy from an external source to the site of the acoustic neuroma with minimal surrounding tissue damage (Kondziolka et al., 1998). This is a relatively new technique that is currently undergoing rigorous evaluation.

Physical management

Physiotherapy assessment of the vestibular patient

The assessment of the vestibular patient is a crucial prerequisite to any treatment. Although many aspects of the examination are similar to that of any physiotherapy assessment, there are specific tests that should be performed. The patient should be made aware that aspects of the examination often provoke symptoms and leave the patient feeling unwell. A detailed history is taken of the present complaint, the nature, severity, duration and irritability of the problem, aggravating and alleviating factors. True vertigo (i.e. rotatory or spinning sensation) should be differentiated from dizziness, light-headedness, giddiness and disequilibrium.

A history should also be taken of any other associated symptoms (Table 13.1). It should be ascertained how long the patient has had the symptoms, and what was the initial presentation. Any previous episodes and their outcomes should be explored. Pertinent past medical history includes problems with vision, other neurological or musculoskeletal problems and any previous vestibular surgery.

The effects of the problem on the patient's occupational and leisure activities should also be noted. Medications, type, dosage and effect, and plans for cessation should also be discussed. Results of any investigations should be noted.

Physical examination

The examination of the vestibular patient includes assessment of posture, tone, power, sensation, proprioception, coordination and reflexes. Specific oculomotor and positional tests are also carried out (Table 13.3 and Figure 13.3). The cervical spine is always assessed prior to the oculomotor examination and a musculoskeletal examination is carried out on the lumbar spine and extremities if indicated. Gait and balance are then assessed (Table 13.4). Gait changes that might be observed are shown in Table 13.5. Acute vestibular patients will deviate to the side of their lesion if asked to walk slowly with eyes closed. This deviation reduces if they are asked to walk at a faster pace, or run, possibly due to an inhibition of vestibular function during highly automated movement (Brandt, 2000b).

Outcome measures

Outcome measures can include measures of balance and gait (Table 13.4). Several questionnaires have been developed which allow patients to rate their symptoms and the resultant effect on daily life. These include the Vertigo Handicap Questionnaire, the Vertigo Symptom Scale (Yardley et al., 1992), the Dizziness Handicap Inventory (Jacobson & Newman, 1990) and the Activites-specific Balance Confidence (ABC) scale (Jarlsater & Mattsson, 2003; Legters et al., 2005; Powell & Myers, 1995; Whitney et al., 1999). Recently, a new questionnaire, the Vestibular

Table 13.4 Balance assessment and outcome measures

Balance and gait outcome measures	
	Balance tests are timed for a period of up to 30 seconds and the best of three attempts is recorded for assessment of change over time.
Romberg (Black et al., 1982)	Patient stands with feet close together and eyes closed. This test can also be performed with eyes open in very severely impaired patients.

Tandem Romberg
    Eyes open
    Eyes closed
	Patient stands heel to toe with preferred foot in front.

One leg stance (Bohannon et al., 1984)
    Eyes open
    Eyes closed
	Patient is asked to stand on one leg with eyes open and then closed.

Tandem walking	Patient is asked to walk heel to toe on a line for a distance of 3 ft and the number of steps off the line are counted.
Fregly & Graybiel's Ataxia Test Battery (Fregly & Graybiel, 1968; Fregly et al., 1973)	Timed balance scores including Romberg (see above), Sharpened Romberg (Standing heel-to-toe), Walk a (12 ft) line eyes closed, and stand on one leg (SOL). Tests performed with eyes open and closed. Normal values available.
Functional reach test (Duncan et al., 1990; Mann et al., 1996)	This is the furthest distance that the patient can reach without moving their feet.
Berg Balance Scale (Berg et al., 1989) Tinetti's Balance Performance Assessment (Tinetti, 1986)	A 14 item functional balance assessment. A 13 item functional balance assessment and a nine item gait assessment.
Clinical test for sensory interaction in balance (CTSIB) (Shumway-Cook & Horak, 1986; Cohen et al., 1993) 1. Stand with feet together eyes open 2. Stand with feet together eyes closed 3. Stand with feet together and visual conflict dome 4. Stand on foam eyes open 5. Stand on foam eyes closed 6. Stand on foam with visual conflict dome	A six item test of balance involving manipulation of visual, vestibular and somatosensory systems. The visual conflict dome is a modified Japanese lantern placed over the patient's head which gives erroneous information about the vertical and thus reduces the ability of the patient to use visual cues for balance. This test has been modified to contain items 1,2,4,5.
Dynamic Gait Index (Shumway-Cook & Woollacott, 1995; Marchetti et al., 2008)	This scale measures mobility function and dynamic balance. The eight tasks of this scale include walking, walking with head turns, pivoting, walking over objects, walking around objects and going up stairs. The performance is rated on a 4-point scale. Eight different gait tasks: walking, walking at different speeds, walking with head movement in pitch and yaw planes, walking over and around obstacles, turning and stopping, stairs. The first four of these have been shown to effectively screen vestibular patients for gait dysfunction.
Four Square Step Test (Whitney et al., 2007)	Subject is timed as they walk over a series of four squares laid out on the floor with two canes.
Posturography (Fig 13.4)	Computerized system using a specialized forceplate and visual surround which measures postural sway in conditions similar to the CTSIB.

Continued

Table 13.4 Balance assessment and outcome measures—cont'd

Balance Evaluation Systems Test (BESTest) (Horak et al., 2009)	Recently developed, preliminary validity and reliability, patient is examined on six components of balance; Biomechanical constraints Stability limits/verticality Anticipatory postural adjustments Postural responses Sensory orientation Stability in gait Maximum score is 108
Activities Specific Balance Confidence Scale (Legters et al., 2005; Whitney et al., 1999; Powell & Myers, 1995; Jarlsater & Mattsson, 2003)	Subjective 16 item scale testing in which subjects rate their confidence during physical functioning.

Table 13.5 Common gait changes in vestibular patients (Marchetti et al., 2008; Mamoto et al., 2002; Whitney et al., 2009 a&b)

Cadence	Decreased
Step length	Decreased
Gait speed	Decreased
Step width	Increased
Time spent in double support	Increased
Head pitch rotation (as in nodding)	Increased
Walking with head movement up and down (pitch)/side to side (yaw)	Increased step length variability–difficulty performing when compared with normals

Rehabilitation Benefits Questionnaire (Morris et al., 2009) has been developed which provides additional information on quality of life.

Physiotherapy management of vestibular disorders

Vestibular rehabilitation aims to:

- educate the patient
- maximize vestibular compensation, thus reducing vertigo, dizziness and nausea
- improve balance and gait
- reduce or alleviate secondary problems such as physical deconditioning and neck or back pain.

Patient groups that benefit most from vestibular rehabilitation are shown in Box 13.1 and there are now many texts on this subject alone (Herdman, 2007; Luxon, Davies, 1997; Shepard & Telian, 1996).

A vestibular rehabilitation programme can involve treating many impairments and possible components of a programme are summarized in Box 13.2. Patients often report that they think their symptoms are too severe to

---

Box 13.1 **Patient groups that benefit from vestibular rehabilitation (Shepard & Telian, 1995)**

Patients with non-compensated peripheral vestibular disorders
Benign paroxysmal positional vertigo (BPPV)
Stable central vestibular lesions or mixed central and peripheral lesions (e.g. head injury)
Multifactorial balance abnormalities (e.g. elderly)
Postablative surgery (e.g. acoustic neuroma resection, labyrinthectomy)
Mèniére's disease

Box 13.2 **Components of a vestibular rehabilitation programme**

Assessment
Education
Habituation exercises
Adaptation exercises
Balance and gait re-education
Particle-repositioning manoeuvres (e.g. Epley's; see Figure 13.7)
Physical conditioning
Relaxation
Breathing exercises
Treatment of neck and back pain
Correction of postural abnormalities

have a benign cause and fear a more sinister pathology (most commonly a brain tumour), despite the latter being excluded by the medical team. The first encounter with the patient thus usually requires education and reassurance about the problem.

It is essential that the patient receives an explanation about the principles of vestibular compensation and the importance of movement for this process as patients have usually been avoiding symptom-provoking movements and postures.

Vestibular paresis/hypofunction

The patient with unilateral vestibular hypofunction who has failed to compensate usually has three main problems:

1. Decreased gain of the VOR, leading to decreased gaze stability during head movement
2. Vertigo or associated symptoms at rest or during head/self-movement (often termed motion sensitivity)
3. Impaired balance and gait.

Each of these require separate treatment approaches. Gaze stability is promoted with eye–head coordination exercises, also called adaptation exercises (Herdman et al., 1995; Szturm et al., 1994). For example, the patient is asked to look at a stationary object (this could be a letter pinned to a wall) and move the head from side to side and then up and down, keeping the object in focus. The patient is instructed to do the exercise for a minute. The speed and duration of the exercise are increased as tolerated and the exercise can be made more difficult by having the object move out of phase with the head. The patient moves an object he or she is holding to the left and the head to the right, keeping the eyes on the object at all times, and then performs the opposite movement (Figure 13.5).

Motion sensitivity is decreased by exercises that aim to habituate the patient to movement (Johansson et al., 2001; Norre & Beckers, 1989; Norre & De Weerdt, 1980). The Cawthorne Cooksey exercises, or modifications of them (Luxon & Davies, 1997) can be taught. An example of a Cawthorne Cooksey exercise programme is shown in Figure 13.6. It is first determined what head, eye or body movements bring on the patient's symptoms. Patients are

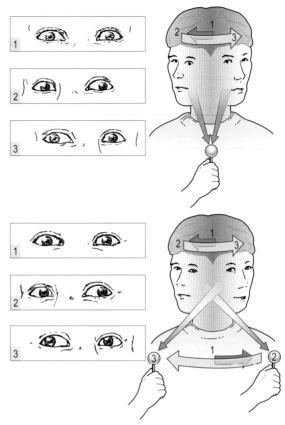

Instructions for vestibular adaptation exercises

Tape a business card on the wall in front of you so that you can read it

Move your head back and forth sideways, keep the words in focus

Move your head faster but keep the words in focus. Continue to do this for 1 or 2 minutes without stopping

Repeat the exercise moving your head up and down

Repeat the exercises using a large pattern such as a checkerboard (full-field stimulus)

Initially, this exercise can be performed in a sitting position. To increase the difficulty of the exercise and to work on static postural stability, this exercise can be performed while standing. Initially start with your feet apart, and gradually work toward standing with one foot in front of the other

Figure 13.5 Adaptation exercises. The patient focuses on a target (e.g. a letter on a page) that is either held by them or attached to a wall at varying distances away. While keeping the letter in focus they move their head from side to side and then up and down, stopping when sensations of vertigo or dizziness commence and/or the target goes out of focus. Speed and duration are gradually increased and the exercises can be practiced in sitting, standing, while walking, standing on one leg, standing in tandem stance, etc. To further increase complexity the target (held in the patient's hand) can be moved out of phase with the head. From Johnson & Griffith, Current Topics in Neurological Disease, 4th edition, 1993, published by Mosby, reprinted with permission of Elsevier Publishers.

Cawthorne Cooksey Exercises

			Start date	One month	Two months	Three months
Eyes	Movement of your eyes, keeping your head still 1) up and down, then side to side following your finger 2) focusing on your finger moving 3 feet to 1 foot from your face.	1 2				
Head Eyes open Eyes closed	3) bending forwards and backwards 4) turning from side to side 5) bending forwards and backwards 6) turning from side to side	3 4 5 6				
Trunk Eyes open Eyes closed	Eyes and head must follow the object 7) from standing, bend forwards to pick up an object from the floor and back up to standing 8) from standing, bend forwards to pick up object from floor, turn to left to place object behind, leave object, turn to right to pick up object, now place object back in front 9) from standing, drop shoulders and head, sideways to left and then right 10) from standing, reach with object up into the air to left then right 11) from standing, pick object from floor and reach high into the air 12) change sit to standing, turning one way sit down, stand up, turn opposite way, sit down 13) turning on spot to left and right 14) from standing, bend forward to touch floor and back to standing 15) from standing, bend forwards to touch floor, turn to left touch chair behind, turn to right to touch chair, back to the front 16) from standing, drop shoulders and head, sideways to left and then right 17) from standing, touch floor, reach high into the air 18) change sit to standing, turning one way sit down, stand up, turn opposite way sit down 19) turning on spot to left and right	7 8 9 10 11 12 13 14 15 16 17 18 19				
Lying down Eye open Eyes closed	If possible do not use a pillow 20) rolling head from side to side 21) rolling whole body from side to side 22) sitting up straight forwards 23) from lying, roll onto your side, sit up over edge of bed, lie down on opposite side and roll onto your back 24) rolling head from side to side 25) rolling whole body from side to side 26) sitting up straight forwards 27) from lying, roll onto your side, sit up over edge of bed, lie down on opposite side and roll onto your back	20 21 22 23 24 25 26 27				

Figure 13.6 Cawthorne Cooksey exercises. A Cawthorne Cooksey exercise programme is tailored to the patient. At the first assessment the patient is asked to perform each exercise five times and rate symptoms on a scale (0 = no symptoms, 1 = mild symptoms, 2 = moderate symptoms, 3 = severe symptoms). The patient is then given a home exercise programme doing only the exercises that cause mild to moderate symptoms. The exercises are then progressed as tolerated over time (see text for more details). (From Luxon L, Davies RA. Handbook of vestibular rehabilitation. London, Whurr Publishers, 1997. Reproduced with permission of Wiley-Blackwell Publishers.)

then instructed to carry out these movements three to four times a day. Each movement or exercise is repeated just to the point where symptoms begin to come on. Gradually over time the patient habituates to the movement and either the duration or the complexity of the exercise can be increased. It is very important that patients are warned that they should not feel excessively symptomatic after performing the exercises, as this may decrease compliance. Exercises should be graded gently and performed only as tolerated. In the early stages, patients may only be able to perform one exercise at a time.

Balance and gait re-education

Balance exercises are customized to the patient, depending on the findings of the balance assessment, and are included in the home exercise programme. For example, if a patient has a particular dependence on vision and it is known that there is some remaining vestibular function, the therapist might choose to include exercises that minimize visual inputs in order for the patient to utilize and strengthen remaining vestibular function. Exercises with eyes closed and/or on an unstable surface (such as a foam cushion) would be included in such a programme.

Balance exercises can be graded by progressively decreasing the area of the base of support, increasing the height of the centre of gravity from the supporting surface or manipulation of the environment by the removal or alteration of visual (for example, eyes closed or head moving) or somatosensory (for example, on foam or on an uneven surface) cues. The complexity of balance tasks is progressively increased over time as the patient improves. For example, when a patient is able to walk on the flat with good postural control, he or she can be asked to walk at a faster pace, walk on an incline or walk while talking or moving the head up and down or from side to side. Care should be taken in the initial stages to avoid falls. This is best achieved by having a relative or friend supervise or by having a supportive surface such as a wall or chair nearby.

Balance has been shown to improve with exercise in several randomized, controlled studies (Horak et al., 1992; Mruzek et al., 1995; Strupp et al., 1998b; Yardley et al., 1998a). Gait and postural re-education is also important. Retraining can include use of verbal and visual feedback. Gait aids may be necessary in the acute stages. The patient with a central vestibular loss requires a similar therapeutic approach but recovery will be slower and more incomplete (Furman & Whitney, 2000; Shepard & Telian, 1995).

The mainstay of treatment of the patient with bilateral vestibular loss is to encourage substitution of visual and proprioceptive systems for vestibular function (Krebs et al., 1993). It is thought that these patients may be able to substitute pursuit and saccadic eye movements (generated by the CNS) and the cervico-ocular reflex to maintain gaze stability (Bronstein & Hood, 1986). Thus, balance exercises and functional activities incorporating

saccadic and pursuit eye movements are included in programmes for these patients (Herdman, 2000). However, it has been shown that these patients may not improve with time and more research is needed in this area (Zingler et al., 2008).

Management of benign paroxysmal positional vertigo

The management of the patient with BPPV is based on manoeuvres or exercises which remove the otoconia responsible for the vertiginous episodes from the involved canal back into the utricle (Harvey et al., 1994; Herdman et al., 2000; Hilton & Pinder, 2004; Steenerson & Cronin, 1996). For canalithiasis (the otoconia are free-floating), Epley's manoeuvre or a modified version is commonly used (Figure 13.7). The head is moved through different positions so that the otoconia move out of the involved SCC. In 90% of cases one manoeuvre will alleviate symptoms, but a small number of patients will require it twice or three times. Recurrence of symptoms can occur with reports of anywhere between 3 and 21% of patients (Benyon, 1997). Patients can be taught to self-perform the manoeuvre.

If treatment is not successful or cupulolithiasis (i.e the otoconia are adherent to the cupula) is thought to be the problem, the Brandt and Daroff (1980) exercises can be performed (Figure 13.8). These exercises aim to free the otoconia from the cupula and disperse them back into the otolith. They are repeated every three waking hours until the vertigo subsides and terminated after two consecutive vertigo-free days. It has been found that patients with BPPV can also have balance impairment (Blatt et al., 2000), if so balance re-education should also form a part of rehabilitation for BBPV.

Secondary problems

Patients will often complain of neck pain and, less commonly, back pain associated with vertigo. Stiffness of the cervical spine caused by avoidance of head movements is frequently observed and these patients often benefit from joint mobilizations, electrotherapy and heat therapy. Cervical spine symptoms may be severe enough to interfere with habituation exercises and therefore should be treated. Habituation exercises that avoid cervical spine movement, such as eye movements or whole-body movements, may be performed until cervical spine symptoms improve.

Physical deconditioning can also occur as patients understandably limit any activity that causes an increase in their symptoms. Promoting exercise through a graduated walking programme is usually the easiest and most acceptable way for patients to increase their exercise tolerance again. Walking is also a functional and relevant context for the patient (as opposed to a static exercise bike, for example) and head movements and visual stimulation during walking probably assist the process of vestibular compensation. As patients improve they should be

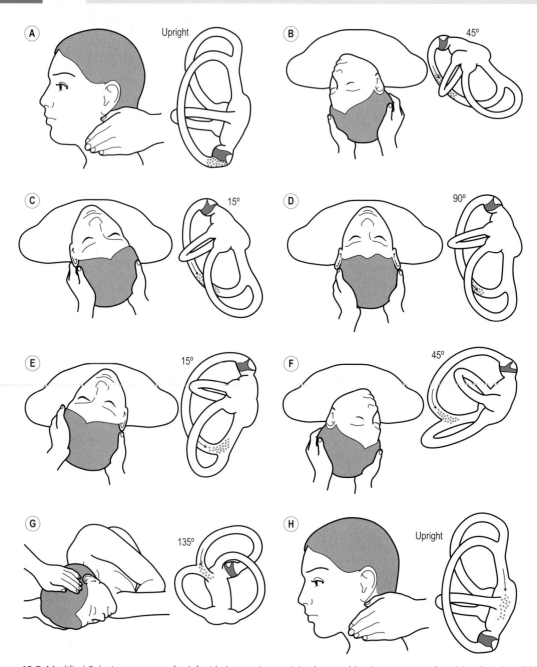

Figure 13.7 Modified Epley's manoeuvre for left-sided posterior semicircular canal benign paroxysmal positional vertigo (BPPV). The patient is brought into the left Hallpike position (A, B). The head is then slowly rotated in a stepwise position to the opposite side (C–F). As this is happening, the patient turns onto the right side so that the head has turned a total of 135° (G). The head is maintained in 30° extension throughout the manoeuvre. The patient is then brought up into sitting (H). (Reproduced from Harvey SA, Hain TC, Adamiac LC. Modified liberatory maneuver: effective treatment for benign paroxysmal positional vertigo. In: The Laryngoscope, 1994; 104. Reprinted with permission of Lippincott, Williams and Wilkins.)

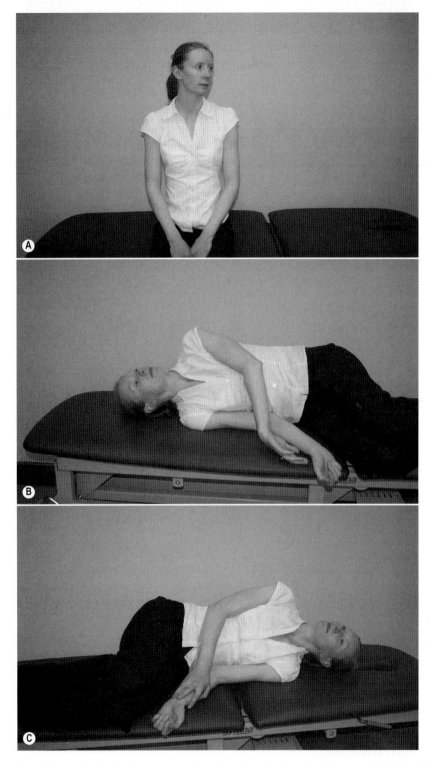

Figure 13.8 Brandt-Daroff exercises for benign paroxysmal positional vertigo (BPPV). A. The patient is instructed to sit in the middle of the bed and turn the head 45° away from the affected side (right side in this example). This places the right posterior semicircular canal in the coronal plane. B. The patient is then instructed to lie down quickly on to the affected side, keeping the head in the same position, and wait until vertigo develops and subsides (approximately 30 seconds). C. The patient is then instructed to sit up and, after any further vertigo settles, lie down in the mirror-image head position. The exercises are repeated every 3 hours for typically 10-20 repetitions.

encouraged to resume their normal sporting or leisure activities as tolerated.

The physiotherapist can also intervene in the symptoms of anxiety and hyperventilation. Simple education on breathing, control of breathing (breathing exercises), the adverse effects of hyperventilation on cerebral blood flow and the recognition of hyperventilation can help the patient recognize and control the problem. Relaxation classes or tapes can be used to teach the patient control of anxiety and associated muscular tension. Where significant anxiety exists or the patient complains of agoraphobia, psychological evaluation and treatment are indicated.

EVIDENCE BASE FOR VESTIBULAR REHABILITATION

Two recent systematic reviews which conducted meta-analyses have confirmed the safety and efficacy of vestibular rehabilitation (VR) programmes (Hillier & Holohan, 2007; Hilton & Pinder, 2004). For those with unilateral vestibular impairment, it was concluded that VR programmes are superior to sham or no treatment in reducing subjective complaints of dizziness and in improving gait and balance (Hillier & Holohan, 2007). However, no one treatment approach has been shown to be superior to another. It is also unclear whether programmes specifically customized for patients (Shepard & Telian 1995; Szturm et al., 1994) are needed or a less intensive approach, such as a one-off demonstration of exercises session combined with a booklet (Yardley et al., 2004), is appropriate. It is pertinent to note that an exercise only VR programme was shown to significantly reduce anxiety in one study (Teggi et al., 2009).

Hilton and Pinder (2004) concluded that Epley's manoevre is superior to sham or no treatment in the short-term resolution of BPPV. However, they cautioned that due to inadequate follow-up in studies, there is not sufficient evidence to confirm its benefit over the long term.

Newer treatments such as simulator-based rehabilitation (for example, focusing on a point on a large patterned disk while it rotates, sitting stationary in an enclosed black and white rotating optokinetic drum) or using computerized visual displays have shown some added benefit in VR (Pavlou et al., 2004, Viirre, Sitarz, 2002). The use of virtual reality systems is also being investigated (Whitney et al., 2009).

SPECIALIST CENTRES AND SUPPORT GROUPS

There are now many centres worldwide that specialize in vestibular rehabilitation and in the UK a physiotherapy clinical interest group, the Association of Physiotherapists with an Interest in Vestibular Rehabilitation (ACPIVR), has a database of physiotherapists who have specialized in vestibular rehabilitation (contact the Chartered Society of Physiotherapy (www.csp.org.uk) for details). The Royal National Institute for Deaf People (www.rnid.org.uk) and British Brain and Spine Foundation (www.bbsf.or.uk) both produce patient information leaflets on different aspects of vestibular and hearing problems. The Ménière's Society also provides support. See the Appendix for contact details of these organizations.

CONCLUSION

Vestibular rehabilitation is a developing area in physiotherapy. It is important that patients with vestibular problems are given access to this effective evidence-based treatment.

CASE HISTORIES

Case 1: Peripheral vestibular neuritis

History

Mr V., a 68-year-old, presented with a 6-month history of vertigo that was aggravated by walking, bending down, looking up and turning around. He described that his head constantly felt 'all mixed up and muzzy'. His symptoms began with a sudden onset of severe vertigo, vomiting and unsteadiness. He was then unable to walk unaided and was confined to bed for 4 days. Over the following few weeks his symptoms gradually decreased in severity but remained problematic.

Investigations

An MRI was normal. Hearing was normal. Electronystagmography (ENG) showed no positional nystagmus and all tests of smooth pursuit and saccades were normal. Caloric testing demonstrated a 100% right canal paresis with an 88% directional preponderance to the left. A diagnosis of a right peripheral vestibular neuritis was made.

Medications

Betahistine (Serc) and prochlorperazine (Stemetil) b.i.d.

Past medical history

Prostate surgery 2 years ago. No previous history of vertigo.

Social history

Mr V. was a retired accountant and was unable to pursue his usual hobbies of gardening and walking since the onset of his symptoms.

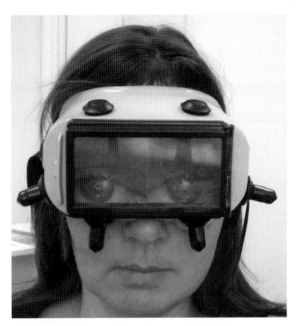

Figure 13.9 Frenzel lenses, used to remove visual fixation and magnify the eyes for ease of observation (see Table 13.3).

Physiotherapy assessment

Findings were normal on examination of tone, power, sensation, proprioception, reflexes and coordination. There were no cervical spine symptoms and the range of movement of the cervical spine was pain free and within normal limits. On oculomotor examination there was no spontaneous nystagmus (in room light or with Frenzel lenses on; Fig 13.9). Smooth pursuit and saccadic eye movements were normal. The VOR cancellation test was normal. VOR testing revealed a catch-up saccadic movement of the eyes to the left during a right Halmagyi head thrust test. Positional tests (Hallpike–Dix test) were negative bilaterally. A normal gait pattern was observed. The Romberg test was normal. Mr V. was unable to maintain tandem Romberg with his eyes closed. One-leg stance (OLS) test times were normal with eyes open but were decreased with eyes closed (left OLS: 3s/right OLS: 2s). He could tandem walk a 1-m line, but took four steps off the line. Mr V. had difficulty with item 5 (he was only able to maintain the position for 5 seconds) of the clinical test for sensory interaction in balance (CTSIB).

Assessment of motion sensitivity

When Mr V. performed repeated tracking movements with his eyes he reported moderate vertigo. He also reported severe vertigo with repeated head movements in all planes with eyes open and closed, bending down to touch the floor and turning on the spot.

Physiotherapy treatment

Mr V. was firstly given an explanation of why he was experiencing his symptoms and the process of vestibular compensation. He agreed that his main problems were motion sensitivity (i.e. vertigo provoked by movement) and balance impairment. His treatment programme aimed to increase the gain of the VOR through adaptation exercises and to decrease motion sensitivity.

Mr V. carried out an exercise programme four times daily. Initially exercises consisted of focusing on a business card in his hand whilst moving his head from side to side and then up and down at a speed that kept the letters in focus. He also carried out habituation exercises. These included visually tracking his own thumb as he moved it from side to side and then up and down while keeping his head steady. Other exercises included head and cervical spine movements (rotation and flexion and extension), which were performed with his eyes open and closed. Each exercise was only performed until vertigo began to develop. Over 4 months the speed, complexity and duration of exercises were gradually increased as symptoms lessened. Mr V. was also provided with a balance exercise programme that he performed daily. He was encouraged to discuss cessation of betahistine and prochlorperazine with his doctor and decrease use over time. He had discontinued all use of vestibular medications 2 months later.

Mr V. steadily improved and had five sessions of treatment over 6 months. Two months into treatment he developed a common cold and reported that his symptoms temporarily worsened. At his final visit he reported he felt '85% of normal'. His vertigo symptom scale and vertigo handicap questionnaire scores demonstrated a significant improvement. His balance had improved, demonstrated by an increase in time on balance tests. He had resumed his hobbies.

Case 2: Benign paroxysmal positional vertigo

History

Ms R., a 36-year-old, presented with a 2-week history of episodic vertigo which came on one morning after getting up. She described the vertigo as a severe spinning sensation associated with severe nausea. Due to the intensity of the symptoms she had been admitted to hospital for 2 days. Since the initial onset she reported several episodes of vertigo, which typically lasted 3–4 seconds and were associated with head movement, particularly rolling over in bed from right to left or bending down. She also described feeling unsteady and tired. Her symptoms were worse in the morning.

Investigations

A computed tomographic scan was normal. No vestibular function tests had been performed.

Medications

Prochlorperazine (Stemetil) prescribed on admission to hospital but discontinued after a week.

Social history

Ms R. was a secretary and had a sedentary lifestyle.

Past medical history

Appendectomy, tonsillectomy.

Physiotherapy assessment

Findings were normal on examination of tone, power, sensation, proprioception, reflexes and coordination. There were no cervical spine symptoms. Oculomotor examination was unremarkable except for the left Hallpike–Dix test. This reproduced the spinning sensation and was accompanied by a rotary nystagmus (beating up and towards the left ear) which came on with a latency of 10 seconds and lasted for 15 seconds. Gait was normal. On balance testing, there was impairment of the left and right OLS tests performed with eyes closed. All other balance tests were normal. Symptoms were consistent with a diagnosis of left posterior SCC BPPV.

Physiotherapy treatment

Following explanation of the likely cause of the symptoms and treatment, a modified Epley's manoeuvre was performed for the left posterior SCC (Figure 13.7). The patient was instructed to try and maintain the head upright for 10 minutes (i.e. avoid bending). Balance exercises were prescribed to perform at home.

A week later Ms R. reported she had been completely symptom-free since the first visit. The left Hallpike–Dix test was normal (no nystagmus or vertigo). Ms R. was advised to continue with her balance exercises and to contact the department if there were any recurrences of vertigo.

ACKNOWLEDGEMENTS

Dara Meldrum would like to acknowledge the expert teaching of Dr Susan Herdman and Dr Ronald Tusa (Emory University, Atlanta, Georgia, USA).

REFERENCES

Baloh, R.W., Honrubia, V., Jacobson, K., 1987. Benign positional vertigo: clinical and oculographic features in 240 cases. Neurology 37, 371–378.

Baloh, R.W., Jacobson, K., Honrubia, V., 1993. Horizontal semicircular canal variant of benign positional vertigo. Neurology 43, 2542–2549.

Benyon, G.J., 1997. A review of management of benign paroxysmal vertigo by exercise therapy and by repositioning manoeuvres. Br. J. Audiol. 31, 11–26.

Berg, K., Wood-Dauphinee, S., Williams, J.I., Gayton, D., 1989. Measuring balance in the elderly: preliminary development of an instrument. Physiother. Can. 41, 304–311.

Black, F.O., Wall 3rd, C., Rockette Jr., H. E., Kitch, R., 1982. Normal subject postural sway during the Romberg test. Am. J. Otolaryngol. 3, 309–318.

Blakley, B.W., Goebel, J., 2001. The meaning of the word "vertigo". Otolaryngol. Head Neck Surg. 125, 147–150.

Blatt, P.J., Georgakakis, G.A., Herdman, S.J., Clendaniel, R.A., Tusa, R.J., 2000. The effect of the canalith repositioning maneuver on resolving postural instability in patients with benign paroxysmal positional vertigo. Am. J. Otol. 21, 356–363.

Bohannon, R.W., Larkin, P.A., Cook, A.C., Gear, J., Singer, J., 1984. Decrease in timed balance test scores with aging. Phys. Ther. 64, 1067–1070.

Brandt, T., 2000a. Management of vestibular disorders. J. Neurol. 247, 491–499.

Brandt, T., 2000b. Vestibulopathic gait: you're better off running than walking. Curr. Opin. Neurol. 13, 3–5.

Brandt, T., Daroff, R.B., 1980. Physical therapy for benign paroxysmal positional vertigo. Arch. Otolaryngol. 106, 484–485.

Brandt, T., Glasauer, S., Stephan, T., Bense, S., Yousry, T.A., Deutschlander, A., et al., 2002. Visual-vestibular and visuovisual cortical interaction: new insights from fMRI and pet. Ann. N. Y. Acad. Sci. 956, 230–241.

Bronstein, A.M., Hood, J.D., 1986. The cervico-ocular reflex in normal subjects and patients with absent vestibular function. Brain Res. 373, 399–408.

Cawthorne, T., 1945. Vestibular Injuries. Proc. R. Soc. Med. 39, 270–273.

Cohen, H., Blatchly, C.A., Gombash, L.L., 1993. A study of the Clinical Test of Sensory Interaction and Balance... including commentary by Di Fabio RP with author response. Phys. Ther. 73, 346–354.

Cohen, H., 1999. Special Senses 2: The vestibular System. In: Cohen, H. (Ed.), Neuroscience for Rehabilitation. second ed. Williams, Wilkins, Philadelphia, Lippincott.

Colledge, N.R., Wilson, J.A., Macintyre, C.C., MacLennan, W.J., 1994. The prevalence and characteristics of dizziness in an elderly community. Age Ageing 23, 117–120.

Cooksey, F., 1945. Rehabilitation in vestibular injuries. Proc. Royal Soc. Med. 39, 273–278.

Courjon, J.H., Jeannerod, M., Ossuzio, I., Schmid, R., 1977. The role of vision in compensation of vestibulo ocular reflex after hemilabyrinthectomy in the cat. Exp. Brain Res. 28, 235–248.

Curthoys, I.S., 2000. Vestibular compensation and substitution. Curr. Opin. Neurol. 13, 27–30.

De la Meilleure, G., Dehaene, I., Depondt, M., Damman, W., Crevits, L., Vanhooren, G., 1996. Benign paroxysmal positional vertigo of the horizontal canal. J. Neurol. Neurosurg. Psychiatry 60, 68–71.

Duncan, P.W., Weiner, D.K., Chandler, J., Studenski, S., 1990. Functional reach: a new clinical measure of balance. J. Gerontol. 45, M192–M197.

Epley, J.M., 1980. New dimensions of benign paroxysmal positional vertigo. Otolaryngol. Head Neck Surg. 88, 599–605.

Fregly, A.R., Graybiel, A., 1968. An ataxia test battery not requiring rails. Aerosp. Med. 39, 277–282.

Fregly, A.R., Smith, M.J., Graybiel, A., 1973. Revised normative standards of performance of men on a quantitative ataxia test battery. Acta Otolaryngol. 75, 10–16.

Fukuda, T., 1959. The stepping test: two phases of the labyrinthine reflex. Acta Otolaryngol. 50, 95–108.

Furman, J.M., Whitney, S.L., 2000. Central causes of dizziness. Phys. Ther. 80, 179–187.

Gottshall, K.R., Hoffer, M.E., Moore, R.J., Balough, B.J., 2005. The role of vestibular rehabilitation in the treatment of Meniere's disease. Otolaryngol. Head Neck Surg. 133, 326–328.

Halmagyi, G.M., Aw, S.T., Cremer, P.D., Curthoys, I.S., Todd, M.J., 2001. Impulsive testing of individual semicircular canal function. Ann. N. Y. Acad. Sci. 942, 192–200.

Halmagyi, G.M., Curthoys, I.S., 1988. A clinical sign of canal paresis. Arch. Neurol. 45, 737–739.

Harvey, S.A., Hain, T.C., Adamiec, L.C., 1994. Modified liberatory maneuver: effective treatment for benign paroxysmal positional vertigo. Laryngoscope 104, 1206–1212.

Herdman, S.J., 2000. Vestibular Rehabilitation. F.A. Davis, Philadelphia.

Herdman, S.J., Blatt, P.J., Schubert, M.C., 2000. Vestibular rehabilitation of patients with vestibular hypofunction or with benign paroxysmal positional vertigo. Curr. Opin. Neurol. 13, 39–43.

Herdman, S.J., Clendaniel, R.A., Mattox, D.E., Holliday, M.J., Niparko, J.K., 1995. Vestibular adaptation exercises and recovery: acute stage after acoustic neuroma resection. Otolaryngol. Head Neck Surg. 113, 77–87.

Herdman, S.J., 2007. Vestibular Rehabilitation 3rd Edn. F.A. Davis, Philadelphia.

Hillier, S.L., Holohan, V., 2007. Vestibular rehabilitation for unilateral peripheral vestibular dysfunction. Cochrane Database Syst. Rev.

Hilton, M.P., Pinder, D.K., 2004. The Epley (canalith repositioning) manoeuvre for benign paroxysmal positional vertigo. Cochrane Database Syst. Rev.

Horak, F.B., Jones-Rycewicz, C., Black, F. O., Shumway-Cook, A., 1992. Effects of vestibular rehabilitation on dizziness and imbalance. Otolaryngol. Head Neck Surg. 106, 175–180.

Horak, F.B., Wrisley, D.M., Frank, J., 2009. The Balance Evaluation Systems Test (BESTest) to differentiate balance deficits. Phys. Ther. 89, 484–498.

House, W.F., Hitselberger, W.F., 1985. The neurotologist view of the surgical management of acoustic neuromas. Clin. Neurosurg. 32, 214–222.

Jacobson, G.P., Newman, C.W., 1990. The development of the Dizziness Handicap Inventory. Arch. Otolaryngol. Head Neck Surg. 116, 424–427.

Jarlsater, S., Mattsson, E., 2003. Test of reliability of the Dizziness Handicap Inventory and the Activities-specific Balance Confidence Scale for use in Sweden. Adv. Physiother. 5, 137–144.

Johansson, M., Akerlund, D., Larsen, H. C., Andersson, G., 2001. Randomized controlled trial of vestibular rehabilitation combined with cognitive-behavioral therapy for dizziness in older people. Otolaryngol. Head Neck Surg. 125, 151–156.

Kondziolka, D., Lunsford, L.D., McLaughlin, M.R., et al., 1998. Long-term outcomes after radiosurgery for acoustic neuromas. N. Eng. J. Med. 339, 1426–1433.

Krebs, D.E., Gill-Body, K.M., Riley, P.O., Parker, S.W., 1993. Double-blind, placebo-controlled trial of rehabilitation for bilateral vestibular hypofunction: preliminary report. Otolaryngol. Head Neck Surg. 109, 735–741.

Lacour, M., Barthelemy, J., Borel, L., Magnan, J., Xerri, C., Chays, A., et al., 1997. Sensory strategies in human postural control before and after unilateral vestibular neurotomy. Exp. Brain Res. 115, 300–310.

Legters, K., Whitney, S.L., Porter, R., Buczek, F., 2005. The relationship between the Activities-specific

Balance Confidence Scale and the Dynamic Gait Index in peripheral vestibular dysfunction. Physiother. Res. Int. 10, 10–22.

Luxon, L., Davies, R.A., 1997. Handbook of Vestibular Rehabilitation. Whurr Publishers, London.

Mamoto, Y., Yamamoto, K., Imai, T., Tamura, M., Kubo, T., 2002. Three-dimensional analysis of human locomotion in normal subjects and patients with vestibular deficiency. Acta Otolaryngol. 122, 495–500.

Mann, G.C., Whitney, S.L., Redfern, M.S., Borello-France, D.F., Furman, J.M., 1996. Functional reach and single leg stance in patients with peripheral vestibular disorders. J. Vestib. Res. 6, 343–353.

Marchetti, G.F., Whitney, S.L., Blatt, P.J., Morris, L.O., Vance, J.M., 2008. Temporal and spatial characteristics of gait during performance of the Dynamic Gait Index in people with and people without balance or vestibular disorders. Phys. Ther. 88, 640–651.

Marom, T., Oron, Y., Watad, W., Levy, D., Roth, Y., 2009. Revisiting benign paroxysmal positional vertigo pathophysiology. Am. J. Otolaryngol. 30, 250–255.

Moffat, D.A., 1994. Endolymphatic sac surgery: analysis of 100 operations. Clinical Otology 19, 261–266.

Moffat, D., Ballagh, R.H., 1997. Mèniére's disease. In: Booth, J.B. (Ed.), Scott Brown's Otolaryngology, vol. 3. Otology. Butterworth Heinemann, Oxford, pp. 1–50.

Monsell, E.M., Furman, J.M., Herdman, S. J., Konrad, H.R., Shepard, N.T., 1997. Computerized dynamic platform posturography. Otolaryngol. Head Neck Surg. 117, 394–398.

Morris, A.E., Lutman, M.E., Yardley, L., 2009. Measuring outcome fro vestibular rehabilitation, part II: Refinement and validation of a new self-report measure. Int. J. Audiol. 48:24–37.

Mruzek, M., Barin, K., Nichols, D.S., Burnett, C.N., Welling, D.B., 1995. Effects of vestibular rehabilitation and social reinforcement on recovery following ablative vestibular surgery... presented at the 97th Annual Meeting of the American Laryngological, Rhinological and Otological Society, Inc., Palm Beach, Fla, May 9, 1994. Laryngoscope 105, 686–692.

Nedzelski, J.M., Schessel, D.A., Bryce, G.E., et al., 1992. Chemical labyrinthectomy: local application of gentamicin for the treatment of unilateral Mèniére's disease. Am. J. Otol. 13, 18–22.

Norre, M.E., Beckers, A., 1989. Vestibular habituation training: exercise treatment for vertigo based upon the habituation effect. Otolaryngol. Head Neck Surg. 101, 14–19.

Norre, M.E., De Weerdt, W., 1980. Treatment of vertigo based on habituation. 2. Technique and results of habituation training. J. Laryngol. Otol. 94, 971–977.

Parnes, L.S., McClure, J.A., 1990. Posterior semicircular canal occlusion for intractable benign paroxysmal positional vertigo. Ann. Otol. Rhinol. Laryngol. 99, 330–334.

Pavlou, M., Lingeswaran, A., Davies, R. A., Gresty, M.A., Bronstein, A.M., 2004. Simulator based rehabilitation in refractory dizziness. J. Neurol. 251, 983–995.

Powell, L.E., Myers, A.M., 1995. The Activities-specific Balance Confidence (ABC) Scale. J. Gerontol. A Biol. Sci. Med. Sci. 50A, M28–M34.

Rudge, R., Chambers, B.R., 1982. Physiological basis for enduring vestibular symptoms. J. Neurol. Neurosurg. Psychiatry 45, 126–130.

Savundra, P., Luxon, L.M., 1997. The physiology of equilibrium and its application to the dizzy patient. In: Gleeson, M. (Ed.), Scott Brown's Otolaryngology, vol. 1. Basic Sciences. Butterworth Heinemann, Oxford, 4: pp. 1–65.

Sekhar, L.N., Gormley, W.B., Wright, D. C., 1996. The best treatment for vestibular schwannoma (accoustic neuroma): microsurgery or radiosurgery? Am. J. Otol. 17, 676–689.

Schubert, M.C., Migliaccio, A.A., Clendaniel, R.A., Allak, A., Carey, J.P., 2008. Mechanism of dynamic visual acuity recovery with vestibular rehabilitation. Arch. Phys. Med. Rehabil. 89, 500–507.

Schubert, M.C., Minor, L.B., 2004. Vestibulo-ocular physiology underlying vestibular hypofunction. Phys. Ther. 84, 373–385.

Shepard, N.T., Telian, S.A., 1995. Programmatic vestibular rehabilitation. Otolaryngol. Head Neck Surg. 112, 173–182.

Shepard, N.T., Telian, S.A., 1996. Practical Management of the Balance Disorder Patient. Singular, San Diego, CA.

Shumway-Cook, A., Horak, F.B., 1986. Assessing the influence of sensory interaction of balance. Suggestion from the field. Phys. Ther. 66, 1548–1550.

Shumway-Cook, A., Woollacott, M., 1995. Motor Control: Theory and Practical Applications. Williams and Wilkins, Baltimore.

Sloane, P.D., 1989. Dizziness in primary care. Results from the National Ambulatory Medical Care Survey. J. Fam. Pract. 29, 33–38.

Steenerson, R.L., Cronin, G.W., 1996. Comparison of the canalith repositioning procedure and vestibular habituation training in forty patients with benign paroxysmal positional vertigo. Otolaryngol. Head Neck Surg. 114, 61–64.

Strupp, M., Arbusow, V., Dieterich, M., Sautier, W., Brandt, T., 1998a. Perceptual and oculomotor effects of neck muscle vibration in vestibular neuritis. Ipsilateral somatosensory substitution of vestibular function. Brain 121 (Pt 4), 677–685.

Strupp, M., Arbusow, V., Maag, K.P., Gall, C., Brandt, T., 1998b. Vestibular exercises improve central vestibulospinal compensation after vestibular neuritis. Neurology 51, 838–844.

Szturm, T., Ireland, D.J., Lessing-Turner, M., 1994. Comparison of different exercise programs in the rehabilitation of patients with chronic peripheral vestibular dysfunction. J. Vestib. Res. 4, 461–479.

Teggi, R., Caldirola, D., Fabiano, B., Recanati, P., Bussi, M., 2009. Rehabilitation after acute vestibular disorders. J. Laryngol. Otol. 123, 397–402.

Tian, J.R., Shubayev, I., Demer, J.L., 2002. Dynamic visual acuity during passive and self-generated transient head rotation in normal and unilaterally vestibulopathic humans. Exp. Brain Res. 142, 486–495.

Tinetti M.E., 1986. Performance-oriented assessment of mobility problems in elderly patients. J. Am. Geriatr. Soc. 34(2):119–126.

Viirre, E., Sitarz, R., 2002. Vestibular rehabilitation using visual displays: preliminary study. Laryngoscope 112, 500–503.

Walsh, R.M., Bath, A.P., Cullen, J.R., et al., 1999. Long-term results of posterior semicircular canal occlusion for intractable benign paroxysmal positional vertigo. Clin. Otolaryngol. Allied Sci. 24, 316–323.

Walsh, R.M., Bath, A.P., Bance, M.L., et al., 2000. The role of conservative management of vestibular schwannomas. Clin. Otolaryngol. Allied Sci. 25, 28–39.

Whitney, S.L., Marchetti, G.F., Morris, L.O., Sparto, P.J., 2007. The reliability and validity of the Four Square Step Test for people with balance deficits secondary to a vestibular disorder. Arch. Phys. Med. Rehabil. 88, 99–104.

Whitney, S.L., Hudak, M.T., Marchetti, G.F., 1999. The activities-specific balance confidence scale and the dizziness handicap inventory: a comparison. J. Vestib. Res. 9, 253–259.

Whitney, S.L., Marchetti, G.F., Pritcher, M., Furman, J.M., 2009a. Gaze stabilization and gait performance in vestibular dysfunction. Gait Posture 29, 194–198.

Whitney, S.L., Sparto, P.J., Alahmari, K., Redfern, M.S., Furman, J.M., 2009b. The use of virtual reality for people with vestibular disorders: the Pittsburgh Experience. Phys. Ther. Rev. 14:299–306.

Yardley, L., Beech, S., Zander, L., Evans, T. Weinman, J., 1998b. A randomized controlled trial of exercise therapy for dizziness and vertigo in primary care. Br. J. Gen. Pract. 48, 1136–1140.

Yardley, L., Donovan-Hall, M., Smith, H. E., Walsh, B.M., Mullee, M., Bronstein, A.M., 2004. Effectiveness of primary care-based vestibular rehabilitation for chronic dizziness. Ann. Intern. Med. 141, 598–605.

Yardley, L., Masson, E., Verschuur, C., Haacke, N., Luxon, L., 1992. Symptoms, anxiety and handicap in dizzy patients: development of the vertigo symptom scale. J. Psychosom. Res. 36, 731–741.

Yardley, L., Owen, N., Nazareth, I., Luxon, L., 1998a. Prevalence and presentation of dizziness in a general practice community sample of working age people. Br. J. Gen. Pract. 48, 1131–1135.

Zee, D.S., 1985. Perspectives on the pharmacotherapy of vertigo. Arch. Otolaryngol. 111, 609–612.

Zee, D.S., 2000. Vestibular Adaptation. In: Herdman, S.J. (Ed.), Vestibular Rehabilitation. FA Davis, Philadelphia.

Zingler, V.C., Weintz, E., Jahn, K., Mike, A., Huppert, D., Rettinger, N., et al., 2008. Follow-up of vestibular function in bilateral vestibulopathy. J. Neurol. Neurosurg. Psychiatry 79, 284–288.

Chapter | **14** |

Physical management of altered tone and movement

Cherry Kilbride, Elizabeth Cassidy

CONTENTS

INTRODUCTION

The term *muscle tone* describes the normal resistance felt when moving a limb passively through range (Burke, 1988). Muscle tone is an integral part of movement and posture but following neurological insult may present in a variety of altered states (Table 14.1). The importance of tone alterations remains the subject of debate, at both a physiological level and within the wider discussion of

Table 14.1 Definitions of normal and altered tone

Normal muscle tone	'The resistance of the limb to passive stretch determined by the physical inertia of the limb as well as the passive mechanical properties of the soft tissues because in a normal, relaxed muscle, there is no neural response to the stretch' (Burke, 1988).
Hypertonia	'An increase in stiffness with resistance to stretch in one direction' (Ada & Canning, 2009, p. 81). There may be neural (e.g. spastic dystonia) and non-neural (e.g. contracture) contributory impairments. The term hypertonia should not be used interchangeably with spasticity because it is inaccurate and confusing (Ada & Canning, 2009).
Hypotonia	'Less than normal resistance to passive movement' (Ada & Canning, 2009).

KEY POINTS

- Muscle tone is an integral part of movement and function.
- Tone may be altered as a result of neuropathology.
- Both peripheral and central components of tone need to be considered in overall treatment and management.
- Consistent terminology should be used when describing altered presentations of tone.

OVERVIEW OF UPPER MOTOR NEURONE SYNDROME

The upper motor neurone syndrome (UMNS) occurs following a lesion affecting part or all of the long descending tracts that control tone and movement, and which have a direct or indirect influence on the excitability of the motor neurone pool (Barnes, 2008). The clinical picture following an upper motor neurone (UMN) lesion depends on the site and size of the lesion and how much neural adaptation has taken place since the lesion occurred (Sheean, 2002).

Impairments arising from nervous system lesions were originally classified into two groups described as either 'positive' or 'negative' (Jackson, 1958). This classification is still used, particularly with reference to UMNS (see Table 14.2). This system has good clinical utility and provides a helpful structure for the assessment of the underlying causes of activity limitations and their relative contribution to the overall clinical picture (Ada & Canning, 2009; Carr & Shepherd, 2003).

Positive features

Positive features describe exaggerations of normally occurring motor activity, e.g. hyperreflexia. These impairments are further classified into two groups (Sheean, 2008):

1. **Afferently** driven features mediated by hyperactive spinal reflexes, only observed in response to peripheral stimulation, e.g. spasticity
2. **Efferently** driven features mediated by increased supraspinal drive onto the motor neurone pool and observed on movement, e.g. spastic dystonia.

Negative features

Negative features refer to a loss or reduction in normal activity, e.g. weakness. The functional significance of the negative features in terms of their contribution to disability cannot be underestimated (Ada & Canning, 2009; Barnes, 2008; Canning et al, 2004; Landau, 1980). For example,

its relevance to physiotherapists treating neurological patients (Boyd & Ada, 2008). Furthermore, secondary changes within the peripheral tissues are known to contribute to and complicate the clinical picture (O'Dwyer & Ada, 1996). Irrespective of the underlying cause, physiotherapists manage the effects of tone alterations using their skills of clinical reasoning to judge whether tone changes enable or inhibit an individual's function. For example, patients may use extensor spasticity to stand and transfer; conversely, muscle spasms may be so disabling that they hinder comfortable seating (Thompson et al., 2005). Movement disorders that include dysfunction of muscle tone are complex and challenge the interpretation and identification of which component primarily contributes to the movement dysfunction. Currently within clinical practice there is inconsistent use of terminology to describe tonal alterations and peripheral adaptations, which hinders effective decision-making and communication between healthcare professionals. Drawing upon recent literature, this chapter defines the most commonly used terms (Tables 14.1–14.4) and places the physical management of these manifestations within the International Classification of Functioning, Disability and Health (ICF) (World Health Organization (WHO), 2001).

In addition to the above, appropriate intervention and management of movement dysfunction, irrespective of underlying cause, requires a broad knowledge of different areas, which include:

- motor control
- neuroscience
- neuropathology
- kinesiology
- learning theory
- anatomy.

Table 14.2 Features of upper motor neurone syndrome (Sheean, 2002, 2008)

Positive features	Afferent drive: in response to peripheral stimulation	
(additional or exaggerated phenomena: muscle overactivity)	Proprioceptive stretch reflexes:	
		Spasticity Clonus Tendon hyperreflexia with irradiation Positive support reaction
	Nociceptive reflexes:	
		Flexor spasms
	Cutaneous reflexes:	
		Extensor spasms Extensor plantar response (positive Babinski)
	Efferent drive: supraspinal activity, observed during movement	
		Spastic dystonia Associated reactions
	Disordered control of voluntary movement:	
		Reduced reciprocal inhibition leading to pathological (spastic) co-contraction Excessive reciprocal inhibition leading to apparent weakness
Negative features		
(loss or reduction of phenomena)		Weakness Fatiguability Loss of dexterity Acute hypotonia
Adaptive features		
(soft tissue)	Non-neural contributions (biomechanical component)	Stiffness and shortening of peripheral soft tissue structures
	Neural contributions (overactive muscle contraction)	
		Spasticity Spastic dystonia Hyperreflexia

most of the rehabilitation effort for recovery of functional movement for people with cerebral lesions (e.g. stroke) is usually directed towards the negative features because of their proportionally greater contribution to the prevailing activity limitations and participation restrictions (Carr & Shepherd, 2003). This is not to say that the positive features do not have functional consequences, but that simply reducing impairment like spasticity will not necessarily improve function unless the negative and adaptive features are also addressed (Boyd & Ada, 2008).

Adaptive features

Adaptive features are secondary impairments that develop as adaptations to the primary impairments (the positive and negative features); their combined effects have a profound influence on functional performance (e.g. the effect of shortening of gastrocnemius/soleus on walking and sit to stand) such that the adaptive features are usually considered alongside the positive and negative features as part of the clinical

291

Table 14.3 Definitions of the positive features of upper motor neurone syndrome

Positive features	
Spasticity	'A motor disorder characterised by a velocity-dependent increase in tonic stretch reflexes with exaggerated tendon jerks resulting from hyperexcitability of the stretch reflex as one component of the upper motor neurone syndrome' (Lance, 1980, 485).
Clasp knife phenomenon	The response of a muscle with spasticity to passive stretch – a rapid stretch to the muscle elicits a velocity dependent tonic stretch reflex. The resistance produced by the reflex contraction of the muscle slows the movement thereby reducing the stimulus eliciting the stretch reflex to below threshold and the resistance to the passive movement melts away. As the stretch continues, a second mechanism comes into play which suggests that as the muscle continues to lengthen the sensitivity to stretch reduces, indicating that the tonic stretch reflex is length – as well as velocity – dependent (Burke, 1988; Sheean, 2008).
Clonus	A rhythmical contraction of a muscle in response to a brisk stretch, maintained. Often seen in the gastrocnemius/soleus as the heel hangs off the footplate of a wheelchair and stretches the back of the calf. The stretch of the calf elicits a stretch reflex causing gastrocnemius/soleus to contract, plantarflexing the ankle and eliminating the stretch. If the relaxation is rapid and the stretch is maintained, another stretch reflex will be elicited and the ankle will plantarflex, again setting up the cycle for a sustained rhythmic contraction. This will continue as long as the stretch is maintained (Burke, 1988; Sheean, 2008).
Hyperreflexia	A greater than normal reflex response (e.g. the presence of reflex responses when a relaxed muscle is stretched at the speed of normal movement (Boyd & Ada, 2008, p. 80).
Positive support reaction	A response of the lower limb, evoked by the foot coming into contact with the ground and eliciting a proprioceptive stretch of the intrinsic foot muscles and an exteroceptive stimulus, caused by pressure on the sole of the foot during attempted weight bearing. It produces plantar flexion and inversion of the ankle, and sometimes knee extension (Bobath, 1990).
Flexor spasms	Usually lower limb spasms that are probably distorted flexor withdrawal reflexes. Caused by nociceptive (e.g. pressure sores), cutaneous (e.g. bed sheets moving across the legs) or visceral (e.g. distended bladder or bowel) stimuli (Sheean, 2008).
Extensor spasms	Extension of the lower limb usually evoked by cutaneous stimulation of the groin, buttock, or back of the leg or following a sudden stretch to the iliopsoas and thus evoking the extensor component of the crossed extensor reflex (Burke, 1988; Sheean, 2008).
Extensor plantar response (Babinski sign)	Upward movement (dorsiflexion/extension) of the great toe with ankle dorsiflexion in response to a non-painful cutaneous stimulation on the plantar aspect of the foot moving from a lateral to medial direction; a disinhibited flexor withdrawal reflex. A normal Babinski test would produce flexion of the great toe and plantar flexion of the ankle (Burke, 1988; Sheean, 2008).

Continued

Table 14.3 Definitions of the positive features of upper motor neurone syndrome—cont'd

Spastic dystonia	'Continuous muscle contractions that occur in the apparent absence of voluntary contraction and of any sensory feedback from the periphery (proprioceptive, cutaneous or nociceptive)' (Sheean, 2002, p. 7). Thought to be due to tonic supraspinal drive to the alpha motor neurones, e.g. the hemiplegic posture (Sheean, 2008). Spastic dystonia can be altered by changes in posture (Denny-Brown (1966) cited in Sheean, 2008) and through stretch modulation via proprioceptive or vestibular mechanisms (Burke, 1988).
Associated reactions	An involuntary activation of muscles remote from those normally engaged in the task, e.g. upper limb flexion during sit to stand. The amount of activation and movement is usually in proportion to the effort expended in executing the task. Thought to be due to tonic efferent drive of alpha motor neurones and may be due to a failure to inhibit spread of motor activity through propriospinal pathways in addition to soft tissue adaptation (Sheean, 2002, 2008).
	Reciprocal innervation (coordination): Task dependent control of agonists and antagonists minimising the number of commands sent to individual muscles mediated by the Ia inhibitory interneurone (Gordon, 1991). Reciprocal inhibition: Inhibition of antagonists which would otherwise inhibit voluntary movement; enhances speed and efficiency of movement by making sure that prime movers are not opposed by antagonists (Gordon, 1991). Co-contraction: The simultaneous contraction of agonist and agonist, e.g. around the wrist during a gripping activity (Gordon, 1991).
Disordered reciprocal inhibition	Disruption to the descending excitatory and inhibitory signals from the major descending pathways converging on the Ia inhibitory interneurone, causing difficulty with reciprocal co-ordination and shifting between co-contraction and reciprocal inhibition and impairing reciprocal innervation and the task-dependent coordination of agonists and antagonists. The clinical picture may be complicated by soft tissue adaptation and remains a topic of debate in the literature (Sheean, 2008).
Reduced reciprocal inhibition	Pathological (spastic) co-contraction, e.g. elbow flexors are not inhibited as the elbow extends due to simultaneous activation of the flexors and extensors (Sheean, 2008).
Excessive reciprocal inhibition	Sustained activation of one muscle group causing inability to activate the antagonist when required, e.g. activation of soleus during the gait cycle which is sustained during swing phase and results in inhibition of tibialis anterior; often attributed to weakness in tibialis anterior (Sheean, 2008).

assessment (Carr & Shepherd, 2003). Adaptive changes result in an increased resistance to passive movement termed hypertonia. In UMNS, hypertonia should be understood simply as an increased resistance to passive movement. Further assessment should help determine whether the resistance is principally due to neural influences, e.g. hyperreflexia, or non-neural influences (local or peripheral adaptation of soft tissue structures) or a combination of the two. This is an important distinction because stiffness and contracture may exist in the absence of neural influences (O'Dwyer et al., 1996) or may be primarily due to neural activity or a combination of both (O'Dwyer & Ada, 1996). As the treatment for the neural component differs from that of the non-neural component, further clinical investigation will be required to identify the most appropriate intervention (O'Dwyer & Ada, 1996).

The characteristic features of UNMS are outlined in Table 14.2. Tables 14.3 and 14.4 provide definitions for each of the impairments.

Table 14.4 Definitions of the negative features of upper motor neurone syndrome

Negative features	
Weakness	An inability to generate, sustain and synchronize the necessary voluntary force for effective motor behaviour (Landau, 1988) causing disorganization of motor behaviour inappropriate to the task and context (Carr & Shepherd, 2003). Mechanisms involve: (a) disrupted descending input onto the motor neurone pool; (b) decreased number of motor units activated; (c) decreased motor unit discharge rate; and (d) disrupted motor unit recruitment (Gemperline, et al., 1995; Rosenfalck & Andreassen, 1980).
Fatiguability	Combined influence of disuse and deconditioning, as well as an increase in the proportion of functionally slow motor units which result in poor endurance for sustained voluntary force output (Carr & Shepherd, 1998).
Loss of dexterity	An inability or difficulty in performing actions quickly and skilfully using independent movements of any part of the body (particularly loss of fractionation – independent movement of individual fingers, e.g. typing or manipulating objects), spatial and/or temporal inaccuracies due to slow production of force and an inability to rapidly alter the degree of contraction in specific muscles or muscle groups during task performance, resulting in a loss of flexibility of motor control with respect to the changing environment or task demands (Ada & Canning, 2009).
Acute hypotonia *(neural shock)*	Suppression of spinal reflexes for a variable amount of time (depending on the site of the lesion), the return of spinal reflex behaviour suggests that mechanisms of neuronal plasticity may be involved (Sheean, 2002).

The primary impairments of UMNS result from disruption of the supraspinal control of descending pathways that normally control excitatory and inhibitory influences on proprioceptive, cutaneous and nociceptive spinal reflexes (Sheean, 2008). These reflexes become hyperactive and account for the majority of the positive features of UMNS (Sheean, 2008). It is likely that the positive features emerge due to a combination of diminished descending cortical control in addition to plastic reorganization at spinal cord and cortical level (Sheean, 2008).

As stated previously, the clinical picture of UMNS depends primarily on the location of the lesion; the signs and symptoms of cortical UMN lesions are very different from those associated with spinal cord UMN lesions. To understand the range of clinical features that arise following UMN lesions, knowledge of the organization and function of specific descending pathways is required. The following describes the inhibitory and excitatory systems involved in spinal reflex activity.

The inhibitory system

Corticoreticular fibres, which travel with, but are separate from, the corticospinal tract, facilitate an inhibitory area in the medulla called the ventromedial reticular formation. This area gives rise to the dorsal reticulospinal tract which is located in the dorsolateral funiculus (a column of fibres in the spinal cord). The main influence of the dorsal reticulospinal tract, which acts weakly with the corticospinal tract, is inhibitory to stretch reflexes and flexor reflexes (Sheean, 2008) (see Figure 14.1A).

The excitatory system

This system is slightly more diffusely organized in the brain stem and is not under tight cortical control; the bulbopontine tegmentum is the most important area because it gives rise to the medial reticulospinal tract. This tract, acting weakly with the vestibulospinal tract, is excitatory to stretch reflexes and extensor reflexes but, like the inhibitory system, is also inhibitory to flexor reflexes (Sheean, 2008) (see Figure 14.1A).

It is already possible to see from the above how disruption to one or all of the descending pathways will disrupt the balance of the excitatory and inhibitory inputs to the spinal motor neurones. The critical features of the descending system are therefore identified by Sheean (2008) as:

a. the corticoreticular drive to the inhibitory system
b. the anatomical separateness of the inhibitory and excitatory tracts
c. both excitatory and inhibitory tracts inhibit flexor reflexes.

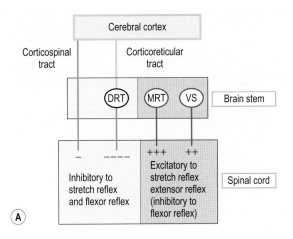

Normal situation

Dynamic control of spinal neurones influencing normal spinal reflex activity. The inhibitory system (corticospinal tract and the dorsoreticulospinal tract acting under the influence of the corticoreticular tract) and the excitatory system (medial reticulospinal tract acting weakly with the vestibulospinal tract) are in dynamic balance, able to adjust the level of inhibition acting on spinal cord reflexes (Sheean 2008) depending on the task and environmental demands.

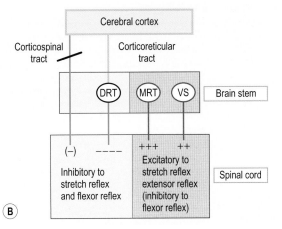

Discrete corticospinal tract lesion

The main excitatory and inhibitory systems remain intact maintaining the dynamic control of excitation and inhibition on spinal reflex behaviour. Clinical features include mild weakness, tendon hyperreflexia and an extensor plantar response. There are no other signs of muscle over-activity (Sheean 2008).

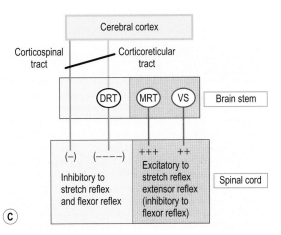

Internal capsule lesion

Additional interruption of the corticoreticular pathway that normally facilitates the dorsoreticulospinal tract of the inhibitory system. Lesions are often partial and lead to some loss of inhibition to stretch reflexes and flexor reflexes. Positive features of UMNS remain mild. The excitatory system is more dominant facilitating extensor reflex activity and stretch reflexes but inhibiting flexors. Thus cortical strokes lead to mild positive features; mild spasticity and hyperreflexia and mild clonus; no flexor spasms (Sheean 2008).

Figure 14.1 Clinical presentations resulting from lesions to different anatomical locations of the descending tracts. DRT, dorsoreticulospinal tract; MRT, medial reticulospinal tract; VS, vestibulospinal tract.; + excitatory pathway; - inhibitory pathway

Continued

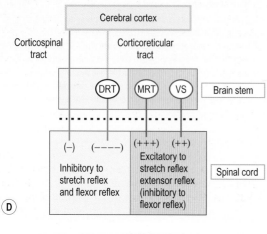

Incomplete spinal cord lesion

Positive features will depend on the site and extent of the spinal cord lesion. If the lesion exclusively involves the inhibitory system then there would be a loss of inhibitory drive and unopposed excitatory drive to the stretch reflex and extensor reflex and partial inhibition of the flexor reflexes. The clinical picture in this case may be one of extension with spasticity, extensor spasms and hyperreflexia (Sheean 2008).

Complete spinal cord lesion

Loss of supraspinal control; spinal reflexes are unopposed and become hyperactive. As both flexor and extensor reflexes are disinhibited then people with complete spinal cord transection may experience flexor and extensor spasms. The net effect of all the afferent inputs at one time tip the scales one way or another; for example if a patient develops a pressure sore the increased input to the spinal reflex system from the flexor reflex afferents (see Box 14.1) might push the overriding spinal reflex activity towards flexion (Sheean 2008).

Figure 14.1—cont'd

Figure 14.1 A–E explains the origin of the clinical presentations resulting from lesions to different anatomical locations of the descending tracts, after Sheean (1998, 2008). Figure 14.1E refers to flexor reflex afferent (FRA) reflexes, which are described in more detail in Box 14.1.

It is essential that the neuro-physiotherapist has a thorough understanding of the pathophysiology of different neurological conditions, as the clinical presentation of the patient is influenced by the site of the lesion(s). As such, the selection of the appropriate intervention or management strategy should be critically informed by this knowledge. The remainder of this chapter reviews a range of interventions and outcome measures that may be appropriate for people with neurological impairments.

Box 14.1 What are flexor reflex afferent (FRA) reflexes?

FRA reflexes are multi-connected spinal reflex pathways that are normally tightly controlled by supraspinal activity in both the excitatory and inhibitory systems (Sheean, 2008). FRA reflexes carry information from the skin, fascia, muscle, bone, capsule, bursa and gastrointestinal tract. Their activity can result in either facilitation of flexor activity, flexor inhibition or excitation of extensor activity (Sheean, 2008). It is thought that under normal conditions supraspinal control determines which pathways are activated according to the functional task (Burke, 1988). In UMNS with extensive spinal lesions (e.g. multiple sclerosis) the activity of the FRAs is no longer controlled by descending input. Therefore, constipation or pressures sores for example, may increase the input from flexor reflex afferents to the spinal cord and tip the reflex activity towards flexor dominance reflected clinically as flexor spasms or paraplegia in flexion (Sheean, 2008).

PHYSICAL MANAGEMENT OF POSITIVE, NEGATIVE AND ADAPTIVE FEATURES

Limitations in activities and restrictions in participation from loss of movement can arise from the combined effect of positive (i.e. spasticity), negative (i.e. weakness) and adaptive features (i.e. contractures) (Ada et al., 2006b). Interventions include manual (hands on), specific adjuncts to treatment and education.

Use of movement

Manual techniques are amongst the principle means available to the physiotherapists in the treatment and management of the altered tone seen post neurological insult. The importance of afferent inputs and their effects on muscle tone and postural/biomechanical alignment have been well documented in the literature (Rothwell, 1994; Shumway-Cook & Woollacott, 2007). Changes in cortical representations have been shown to accompany functional gains after rehabilitation (Johansson, 2000; Richards et al., 2008). Such studies help to provide direct evidence that altering passive or active sensory input can drive motor output; therapeutic movement and handling is a means of altering afferent input to the patient. An understanding of the basic principles that affect neural plasticity is key to enhancing motor recovery after neurological insult (Kleim & Jones, 2008).

The main aims of physical interventions are:

- maintenance of soft tissue length and underlying structures
- modulation of muscle tone
- re-education of movement.

Maintenance of soft tissue length

The need for prevention of soft tissue changes in people with neurological impairments as a prerequisite to the prevention of contractures is widely acknowledged (Bovend'Eerdt et al., 2008; Katalinic et al., 2008). Without full range of motion, peripheral changes cause muscle imbalance and can compound any central motor dysfunction (Fitzgerald & Stokes, 2004). The physiotherapist must be able to make an in-depth analysis of posture and movement patterns as a basis for clinical reasoning and deciding upon primary problems and secondary compensations (Meadows & Williams, 2009). Stretching is widely used as an intervention to prevent or minimize contracture formation.

Stretching, assisted and passive movements

When handling a patient, the therapist must be ready to adapt to any changes in the response of the muscle to the afferent input from the movement. The aim of stretch interventions is to maintain or increase range of movement in soft tissues and can be carried out by the therapist or by the patient. Stretching can have immediate and lasting effects; the former being related to changes in the viscous properties whereas the mechanism behind longer lasting effects is still not fully understood but thought to be connected to changes in sarcomeres; Katalinic et al. (2008) and Bovend'Eerdt et al. (2008) provide detailed overviews. Changes in the muscle itself include thixotrophy (Vattanaslip et al., 2000) and even where there is no neurological damage, the normal resistance to movement is the result of such things as muscle, tendon and connective tissue inherent stiffness.

The length of time required to prevent contracture formation also remains an area of debate; the literature suggests intervals from 30 minutes to 6 hours (Tardieu et al, 1988; Williams, 1990). Discussion continues in clinical practice as to the effectiveness of applying stretch and remains an active area of research (Katalinic et al., 2008).

Changes in the motor and sensory systems can be expected even when movement is passive (Lotze et al., 2003) or, indeed, if physical movements are cognitively rehearsed (mental practice; Page et al., 2009). The importance of carrying out active/assisted or passive movements through their full range is paramount and attention should be paid to muscles that cross two or more joints. Movements should be performed with care, confidence and variety, and the patient should be taken out of his or her preferred posture. Movement should not be vigorous, and never forced, as this could be a causative factor in heterotopic ossification (HO), although the underlying mechanism remains poorly understood (Chua & Kong, 2003). However, movement can prevent the development of HO and should be carefully encouraged even when HO is present (Knight et al., 2003).

Modulation of muscle tone

Therapeutic movement and alteration in alignment of body parts are thought to be able to influence muscle tone in other areas indirectly. The trunk, head and shoulder and pelvic girdles have been proposed to be particularly influential in altering muscle tone (Meadows et al., 2009). Schmit et al. (2000) found that repeated joint movements had beneficial, albeit short-term, effects on spastic hypertonia at the elbow. This alteration of muscle tone may be augmented by presynaptic inhibition from the periphery, leading to neuroplastic adaptation (Rothwell, 1994). Additional preliminary findings around therapeutic touch, such as slow stroking on hypertonic muscles in multiple sclerosis, has indicated a reduction in alpha-motor neuron excitability (Brouwer & de Andrade, 1995). The use of rotation is also thought to be important in modulating tone (Proske et al., 2000) and the additional components of traction and compression can likewise be used (Rosche et al., 1996). Mayston (2002) also suggests that therapists alter tone at a non-neural level by affecting muscle length and range, which gives an improved alignment as a prerequisite for better movement.

Re-education of movement

As movement dysfunction arises from a combination of positive, negative and adaptive impairments, the clinical reasoning process and interventions subsequently selected should reflect this balance. Many therapists believe that a higher quality of movement translates directly to greater functional ability (Davidson & Waters, 2000) but this relationship has yet to be proven empirically. Reduction of tone should be only part of a treatment so as not to affect function inadvertently for those who rely upon positive features for the achievement of motor goals, e.g. transfers. Other factors such as practice, specificity of training, transfer of training and feedback need to be considered as part of the overall framework of therapeutic practice (Lennon & Bassile, 2009). Treatment can be based on one or more of the various models of motor control and some of these treatment approaches are discussed in Chapter 12, as well as in the chapters on specific conditons (Chs 2–10).

Weight-bearing

Therapeutic standing is a way of maintaining length in the soft tissues, modulating tone and encouraging extensor activity. To be most effective it should be dynamic to promote tonal changes (Massion, 1994), activating the extensor muscles whilst reciprocally inhibiting the flexors via the vestibuar system (Markham, 1987; Brown, 1994). Standing can be effective in modulating tone and reducing the frequency of spasms, whilst maintaining joint range (Bohannon, 1993). A pilot study looking at the efficacy and feasibility of a therapeutic standing programme for people with multiple sclerosis showed increased range of movement in wheelchair-dependent subjects and a downward trend in spasticity and spasms was noted (Baker et al., 2007). A decrease in motor neuron excitability in patients with spastic hemiparesis was also noted after a single session of standing on a tilt table for 30 minutes (Tsai et al., 2001). Tilt tables can be used to stand medically stable patients in the early stages of rehabilitation, even if they are still unconscious; wedges under the feet can be used as required to increase the stretch on the calf musculature. Alternatively, in the more awake patient, backslabs (Carter & Edwards, 2002) or electrical standing frames may be used (Figure 14.2). With the current emphasis on risk management it is recommended that, where possible and practicable, equipment should be used to minimize the manual handling risk (Chartered Society of Physiotherapy (CSP), 2008). The use of standing hoists can allow patients to weight-bear regularly in a normal functional task and so should be encouraged (Figure 14.3).

Weight-bearing with specific alignment can also be achieved through the upper limbs to maintain length and influence tone, but must be performed with extreme care. Normal biomechanical alignment is maintained by external rotation at the shoulder and the wrist joint should not be overstretched (Champion & Barber, 2009).

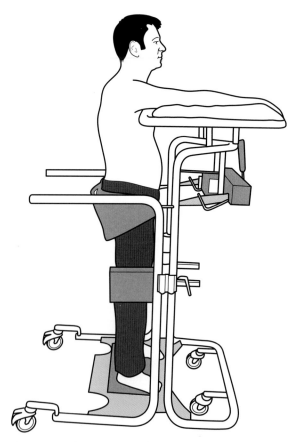

Figure 14.2 Electric standing frames can enable patients to stand for long periods, providing weight-bearing, stretching and promoting activity in the trunk.

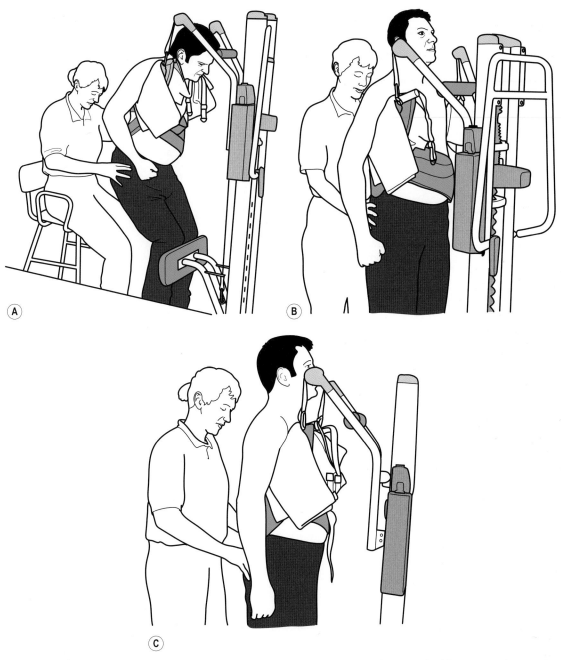

Figure 14.3 A patient progressing from sit to stand in a standing hoist (A–C). Physiotherapists should encourage the use of a standing hoist for suitable patients, as they provide weight-bearing in a functional activity.

KEY POINTS

♦ Movement dysfunction arises from a combination of positive, negative and adaptive features.
♦ Interventions aimed solely at the reduction of positive features do not necessaily lead to improvements in activity and participation.
♦ Weight-bearing should be dynamic and involve movement whenever possible.
♦ Alignment of limbs must be maintained.

ADJUNCTS TO PHYSICAL MANAGEMENT

This section covers the various approaches to physical management, including specific treatment techniques and the use of equipment.

Positioning and seating

Therapeutic positioning and seating is underpinned by the premise of providing sufficient external support to enable a person to cope better with the effects of gravity, and to maintain postural alignment without using undue muscular activity; the reader is referred to Pope (2007) for a detailed review of posture and seating.

KEY POINTS

Effective positioning and seating is essential to:
♦ maximize function
♦ promote socialization
♦ reduce sustained postures
♦ prevent pressure sores
♦ maintain soft tissue length
♦ reduce discomfort and noxious stimuli.

The relationship between positioning and outcome is still the subject of debate, with research evidence, whilst not conclusive, showing limited effectiveness (de Jong et al., 2006; Fox et al., 2000; Gustafsson & McKenna, 2006). However, there remains a consensus view in the literature advocating the importance of positioning and the need for multidisciplinary team involvement (Pope, 2007; Intercollegiate Stroke Working Party (ISWP), 2008). Where possible, positioning should be integrated into functional activities in a normal daily routine (Figure 14.4) and appropriate manual handling equipment and techniques always considered

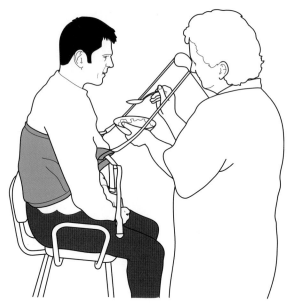

Figure 14.4 This patient uses a perching chair to sit and eat his breakfast, which encourages development of trunk stability and weight-bearing through his lower limbs, whilst carrying out a functional activity.

(CSP, 2008). Standard positioning charts are useful to promote consistency across the team and can be personalized, for example drawing on additional pillows to illustrate adjustment for specific postural needs; alternatively, photographs obtained with informed consent can be used.

Positioning in bed

Optimal positioning of a patient in supine can present a variety of challenges for the therapist. For example, patients with predominantly negative impairments may all too readily accept the supportive surface and be at risk of loss of range, whereas those with positive or indeed adaptive impairments may not be able to adapt their posture to the base provided. The use of pillows, wedges and T-rolls can assist in altering limb and body postures and help provide appropriate support (Figure 14.5). Profiling electrical beds can also be utilized to help maintain different postural alignment, likewise side-lying can be used for introducing change and breaking up any predominant tonal patterns or preferred postures. Positioning a patient in prone can be beneficial for some but its use must be considered carefully, for instance those with tracheotomies or severe contractures may be unable to achieve this position. As the head, shoulders, thighs and knees are the main load-bearing areas in prone, the introduction of a wedge can facilitate function by moving the fulcrum of movement to the pelvis (Pope,

Figure 14.5 The use of a T-roll to prevent lower-limb extension and adduction.

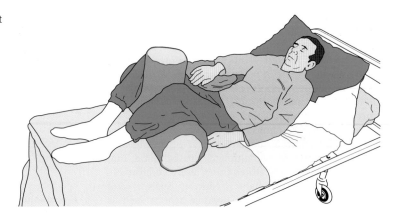

2007) or a commercially produced beanbag can also be tried to encourage head extension and shoulder protraction (Figure 14.6).

Mattresses

All patients should have a mattress that matches his or her pressure and positoning needs; a recent Cochrane Review by McInnes et al. (2008) provides comprehensive evaluation of the different support surfaces for pressure ulcer prevention. Physiotherapists should collaborate with nursing staff to facilitate optimal prescription for function. For example, the use of *overlays* on a standard mattress may be sufficient for pressure care yet affect transfers, as it increases the overall bed height so only a standing hoist can be used with taller patients. A replacement mattress that is the same height as a standard mattress but has higher pressure relieving properties may be preferable in terms of rehabilitation, although it is more costly. Overhead hoists may have to be used for air-filled mattresses. Findings from the PRESSURE Trial Group (Nixon et al., 2006) indicated that more than one-third of patients reported difficulties associated with movement in bed, and getting in and out of bed with overlays.

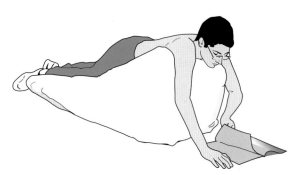

Figure 14.6 The use of a bean bag to induce a comfortable prone position.

For acute head injuries where intracranial pressure (ICP) is a concern, electronic pressure beds can offer an effective way to achieve weight transference and positive effects on respiratory function. For patients with uncontrolled movements (e.g. Huntington's disease, see Ch. 7), reduced sensation, or cognitive or perceptual deficits, the use of cot sides, or placing the mattress on the floor, should be considered to reduce the risk of injury to the patient from falling out of bed.

Sitting

Being able to sit well not only is central to an effective posture management system, but it can also help with respiration, eating and communication whilst promoting social interaction. The position of the pelvis is the keystone for building a framework of postural support, whereas hips, knees and feet should be at 90°, and consideration given to the provision of head and arm support (Pope, 2007). Ideally hospitals and rehabilitation units should have a range of wheelchairs and seating systems, e.g. tilt in space, available for short-term loan where the needs of the acute patient may change rapidly. Pressure care and postural support cushions should be considered in conjunction with MDT colleagues. Collins (2007) details a practical guide to cushions, however, in practice, ward chairs often have to be adapted with everyday items such as towels and pillows to help achieve optimum postures. If patients have severe prolonged difficulties with seating a referral to a specialist seating service should be considered.

Electric and self-propelled wheelchairs

Appropriate wheelchair provision can promote independence and improve quality of life (Devitt et al., 2004). However, debate remains in clinical practice over encouraging self-propulsion in the early stages of rehabilitation with Cornall (1991) stating it increases spasticity, whereas more recent studies have shown no adverse effects (Barrett et al., 2001; Pomeroy et al., 2003). A wide variety of manual or electric wheelchairs, including indoor/outdoor electrically powered chairs (EPIOC) are available through either the NHS or privately and the introduction of a voucher scheme has helped to increase choice (www.direct.gov.uk). However, findings from a qualitative study of people with severe disability from multiple sclerosis found that whilst tilt-in-space wheelchairs were more comfortable than standard wheelchairs, reducing spasms and improving posture, they had negative aspects such as their bulky size and lack of manoeuvrability (Dewey et al., 2004).

Whilst electric wheelchairs provide an alternative to manual chairs, cognitive and perceptual difficulties can limit a person's ability to use one, but it should nonetheless not be ruled out automatically before the individual is assessed (Dawson & Thornton, 2003). Some wheelchairs offer the facility of helping the person into a near-standing position, which is helpful for maintaining range of movement in joints and for pressure care (O'Connor & Smith, 2008).

KEY POINTS

- Collaborative teamwork is essential in the management of altered tone.
- Effective seating and posture systems are like 'silent therapists'.
- There is no one correct position; varying posture as part of the 24 hour management programme is essential.

Splinting/casting*

The best approach to contractures remains prevention yet in some patients, despite proactive intervention, adaptive impairments still occur. Altered tone has long been implicated in the development of contractures and without intervention affected areas are at risk of losing range from soft-tissue changes (Goldspink & Williams, 1990). Results from a recent study showed for the first time that spasticity can cause contracture in the first 4 months post stroke, but authors noted that thereafter muscle weakness became the main reason for limitations in activities (Ada et al., 2006b). Patients who show no functional recovery in muscle activity 2 to 4 weeks after stroke have been shown to be at high risk of developing contractures (Pandyan et al., 2003).

---

*The terms are used interchangeably.

KEY POINTS

Patients most at risk of developing contractures are those who:
- are unconscious
- are immobile and have altered tone
- show evidence of shortening with current intervention
- have fractures or pressure sores
- score 9 or less on the Glasgow Coma Scale
- are not able to be stood (medically unstable).

If positioning and regular movement are ineffective in preventing loss in range of motion, then splinting the affected body part may be undertaken as part of therapy.

Whilst the mechanism behind this intervention remains not fully understood it is thought to have a neurophysiological and biomechanical basis (Lannin et al., 2007b; Mortenson & Eng, 2003; Moseley et al., 2008).

Taking the decision to cast a limb requires careful clinical reasoning and discussion with colleagues in the MDT. Splinting may be precluded if the condition of the patient's skin or vascular system is poor as there is a risk of pressure sores and tissue damage. If the patient is demonstrating challenging behaviour the splint may present a danger to the patient or others. Incontinence will need to be managed in conjunction with the nursing staff; if the cast becomes wet or soiled it will require removal and replacing. The use of a synthetic/fibreglass-based material instead of plaster is preferable in these types of situations as it is more durable, lighter and dries more rapidly. The development of new materials has given rise to more techniques, e.g. the ability to combine 'soft and hard' sections means that areas can be selectively reinforced as required. Details about application procedures are outside the scope of this text and the reader are referred to Edwards and Charlton (2002), although, as pointed out by Lannin et al. (2007b) in a recent systematic review, there is little consensus in practice for casting protocols.

Main forms of splinting

Splinting in neurology broadly falls into the following categories: preventative, corrective and dynamic.

Preventive splinting

Preventive splinting (Stoeckmann, 2001) may be necessary for patients who exhibit a number of the identified risk factors. Mortenson and Eng (2003) carried out a systematic review of the use of casts in adults with joint hypomobility and hypertonia following brain injury and a grade B on the hierarchy of evidence scale was given to the use of casting to increase range of motion or to prevent its loss. Reduction of spasticity is cited as a goal of casting in neurological patients (Fess et al., 2005). Barnard et al. (1984) reported a decrease in this positive impairment after using plaster boots, whereas King (1982) noted less spasticity in the elbow flexors following casting. Robichaud and Agostinucci (1996) hypothesized that this effect might be due to the reduction in input to tactile, proprioceptive and temperature receptors from wearing the cast. They suggested that the cast promotes total contact, even pressure and warmth, thus decreasing the excitability of the alpha or gamma motor neurones in the spinal cord. This hypothesis was further supported by Childers et al. (1999), who used electromyography (EMG) to look at the use of inhibitory casting to decrease spasticity in the upper limb and found a reduction in the vibratory inhibition index. This correlated with a decrease in motor neurone excitability in the hypertonic upper limb. However, in the absence of activity and function, any gains in movement achieved may be difficult to maintain, particularly in the presence of persistent tonal changes (Hill, 1994). In early rehabilitation after stroke, a night splint has been found to be as effective as standing on a tilt table for 30 minutes in maintaining range of movement at the ankle joint (Robinson et al., 2008).

An alternative to casting is pressure splints (Johnstone, 1995) which may be used for short periods of the day. Pizzi et al. (2005) examined the effects of reflex inhibitory splinting (using a volar static splint) in 40 people with post stroke spasticity of the upper limb. The authors found that during the 3 months of the study the splint, which was worn for 90 minutes a day, was well tolerated with a reduction in elbow spasticity and significant gains in wrist passive range of movement (extension more than flexion). Its use was recommended as part of an integrative approach to maintenance.

Corrective splinting or serial casting

Corrective splinting is used to increase range of movement in the presence of contracture, although the lasting effects of any gains achieved may be transient and difficult to maintain (Moseley et al., 2008). However, there is good evidence (level 1b) supporting the use of casting to gain range of elbow extension in adults following brain injury (Lannin et al., 2007b).

Two common methods of serial casting are cyclinders or drop out casts. The advantage of drop out casts is that active movement can still be encouraged and function is less compromised. Electrical stimulation can also be applied to the appropriate muscle (Stoeckmann, 2001). Frequency of changing corrective casts and the amount of stretch applied varies within clinical practice (Edwards & Charlton, 2002; Lannin et al., 2007b). With lower limb casting a platform should be built under the toes to prevent clawing and shortening of the toe flexors. Cyclinders made from synthetic material can be 'zipped' with a cut down the length of the splint to effectively bivalve it. This approach has a number of benefits; it is easy to remove to check the skin with high-risk patients; it can be held in place with bandages for prolonged periods, but removed for therapy or personal hygeine.

Cast braces with adjustable hinges can be used for slowly correcting contracted joints, especially at the elbow or knee when the contracture is 90° or more and serial casting is difficult. A risk factor may be swelling around the elbow or knee. Orthoses with a sprung hinge can assist in stretching out contractures (Farmer & James, 2001). Interesting results have been noted in five patients, who were described as having chronic spastic hemiparesis secondary to stroke, and who wore simple wrist splints made of mesh material during the daytime for 8 weeks. They had significant increases in the active range of shoulder flexion and finger extension with a decrease in muscle tone (Fujiwara et al., 2004). Contrary to these findings, Lannin et al. (2007a) in a study of 63 adults post stroke concluded that splints that held the wrist in either neutral or extension and were worn overnight for 4 weeks did not reduce wrist contracture. The authors concluded, therefore, that the practice of *routine* wrist splinting after stroke should be stopped, a claim that has been countered in the literature by Marossezky et al. (2008) who suggest the conclusion could be restated as 'splinting does not prevent contracture in patients at minimal risk of contracture'. Clinicians thus need to consider the merits of each individual case and not routinely carry out any intervention, including splinting, without clinical reasoning.

With patients with established contractures, surgery should be considered. A conservative approach should always be considered if handling the limb alters tone, if movement is felt or observed, or if there is a soft end feel. A preliminary cast should be applied if there is any doubt about the approach. If casting is going to be successful, a gain in range is usually evident after the removal of the first splint. An X-ray should be taken to exclude HO, where clinical assessment indicates this may be present.

Dynamic splinting

Dynamic or functional splinting aims to facilitate recovery and assist stability for improved function (Fess et al., 2005). Examples are ankle–foot orthoses (de Wit et al., 2004; Pohl & Mehrholz, 2006) and hinged ankle-foot orthoses (Tyson & Thornton, 2001). A recent study by Tyson and Rogerson (2009) describes how non-ambulant patients undergoing rehabilitation felt their walking, confidence and safety improved with the use of assistive walking devices. They were also satisfied with the appearance and comfort of the splints; walking impairments remained unchanged.

Strapping is an alternative short-term method, can be applied to virtually any joint and is particularly useful for the ankle and shoulder joints. Strapping is gaining in popularity in conjunction with musculoskeletal muscle imbalance treatment approaches (see Ch. 12). In the presence of mild hypertonia, strapping may suffice, in particular for the prevention of hemiplegic shoulder pain (Griffin & Bernhardt, 2006). Hangar et al. (2000) found that where patients had their shoulders strapped they had a trend towards less pain and better arm and hand function on final assessment. The short-term effect of using dynamic Lycra splints on the upper limb with neurological impairments suggests some benefits in function (Gracies et al., 2000; Watson et al., 2007).

Orthotic insoles

The use of orthotic insoles should be explored with the podiatry department. A primary goal of foot orthoses is to aid the maintenance and redistribution of weight-bearing patterns (Edwards & Charlton, 2002). In cases where the alignment is good and there is minimal shortening, the authors have clinical experience of using orthotic insoles to 'walk out' contracture.

Targeted strength training

Targeted strength training is an important aspect of neurological rehabilitation (Ch. 18). Previous concerns that such intervention would lead to an increase of positive features has not been bourne out by the research evidence (Flansbjer et al., 2008; ISWP, 2008). Indeed, the increasing recognition of negative impairments such as muscle weakness, which is a cardinal feature post stroke (Cramp et al., 2006), has translated to changes in clinical practice, with therapists incorporating task-specific muscle strengthening exercises into treatment programmes (Ada et al., 2006a; Bale & Strand, 2008). However, the wider effects of strengthening on improving participation in societal roles remain unknown (Morris et al., 2004). Chapter 18 discusses the role of muscle strengthening in different neurological disorders and outlines the need for further clinical research.

Exercise

Evidence suggests that exercise does not result in increased positive features and indeed can help to address negative and adaptive changes (see Ch. 18). Nevertheless, neurological impairments can bring challenges to maintaining an active lifestyle in keeping with health-related fitness, but exercise programmes can be designed to increase cardiovascular conditioning (Kilbreath & Davis, 2005; Pang et al., 2005; White & Dressendorfer, 2004). For example, people with moderate disability post stroke have been involved in fitness programmes including aerobic and strength components lasting from 30 to 90 minutes (Duncan et al., 2003). Dawes et al. (2000) found that high-intensity cycling did not lead to any increase in tone. This finding was further supported by Lee et al. (2008) who looked at the effects of aerobic cycle training and progressive resistance training on walking ability post stroke, and found that both musculoskeletal and cardiovascular impairments were still modifiable some years after stroke with selected robust exercise. The use of partial-body-weight support treadmill training has likewise produced positive outcomes on functional mobility (Hesse, 2008) and aerobic treadmill training has been noted for its potential to reduce effort and fatigue in people with multiple sclerosis (Newman et al., 2007).

Hydrotherapy and swimming

Hydrotherapy and swimming can provide freedom and challenge of movement to people with neurological impairments that are often not available to them on land (Cook, 2007). During hydrotherapy the water has a dual role, providing support and warmth, and has a global effect on muscle activity; it can be utilized to alter tone and joint range prior to treatment on dry land. Cook (2007) provides a comprehensive overview of the muscular, cardiovascular, haematological, renal and respiratory effects of immersion. Although the published evidence for hydrotherapy in neurological conditions is sparse, beneficial effects have been noted in people with spasticity following spinal injury (Kesiktas et al., 2004), stroke (Taylor et al., 1993) and multiple sclerosis (Peterson, 2001). The Halliwick concept is one well recognized approach for people of all ages which emphasizes ability rather than disability (Skinner & Thomson, 2008).

Electrical stimulation

Electrical stimulation is used in a number of different formats by physiotherapists in the treatment of positive and negative impairments with mixed results. A systematic review of electrical stimulation for shoulder pain found no significant effect on upper limb spasticity, but some improved range of passive lateral rotation noted (Price & Pandyan, 2001), whereas electrical stimulation combined with Bobath therapy in a randomized controlled trial (RCT; $n=40$) helped reduce plantarflexor spasticity in a cohort of stroke patients (Bakhtiary & Fatemy, 2008). Another study using a home programme of neuromuscular and sensory amplitude electrical stimulation on 10 people with chronic stroke had mixed results; four showed a reduction in spasticity yet others had an increase in tone that Sullivan and Headman (2007) attributed to subjects having to travel to the testing site in extreme cold weather. Krause et al. (2008) found that functional electrical stimulation along with cycling interventions in five people with spinal cord injury led to a reduction in spastic muscle tone. Results from a randomized single blind crossover trial of 32 people with multiple sclerosis that looked at the effect of transcutaneous electrical nerve stimulation (TENS) on spasticity suggest it does not appear to be effective with spasticity, but that longer applications (8 hours per day) may be useful with pain and muscle spasm (Miller et al., 2007).

Electrical stimulation has also been recommended by the National Institute for Health and Clinical Excellence (NICE) (2009) for use with *drop foot*, a negative impairment of central neurological origin. EMG triggered FES has been studied in the rehabilitation of wrist and finger extensors in later stage stroke and has shown positive changes in the ability to grasp small objects and maintain muscle activity (Hara et al., 2006).

Biofeedback

Evidence regarding the use of biofeedback in neurological rehabilitation is mixed. Hiraoka (2001) reported an increased functional ability in the hemiplegic upper limb following the use of EMG biofeedback, whereas a Cochrane Review by Woodford and Price (2007) on standard physiotherapy plus EMG feedback only indicated possible positive effects at the shoulder. Moreland et al. (1998) found it had a beneficial effect on improving the strength of ankle dorsiflexors. Van Peppen et al. (2006) reported no significant difference with the use of visual feedback in balance or walking ability, yet an earlier study by Sackley and Lincoln (1997) found visual feedback seemed linked to recovery of balance. Cheng et al. (2004) described improved weight transference with biofeedback.

Medication

The therapist needs a basic understanding of the pharmacological means of controlling altered tone (see chapters on specific neurological conditions). Physiotherapists' skills in assessing tone, over time, can also play a valid role in evaluating the effectiveness of drugs and when they should be administered. Medication may be appropriate where physical means are inadequate, but consideration needs to be given to their use (Thompson et al., 2005). Pain increases spasticity and so the use of analgesia should be considered; however, not all patients can communicate effectively to request analgesia.

It is essential to establish if the presentation of spasticity is generalized, regional or focal. The treatment options are then clearer. For generalized spasticity, oral medication may be a first approach. For focal spasticity, injections of botulinum toxin may be a useful adjunct to therapy or, where more permanent paralysis is required, phenol nerve blocks can be used. Guidelines for the use of botulinum toxin have been produced and emphasize the need for a multidisciplinary team approach (Royal College of Physicians, 2009). Intrathecal baclofen may be used where spasticity is a major problem; functional benefit may be gained if it unmasks underlying motor control previously hidden by the positive impairment or alleviates pain from muscle spasms (Kofler et al., 2009).

Continuous passive movement

Whilst continuous passive movement (CPM) machines are common in orthopaedics they can also be beneficial in neurological physiotherapy. For example, CPM can be used to help improve range of movement in head-injured patients with contractures (Macfarlane & Thornton, 1997); it is thought to assist in the breakdown of abnormal cross-bridge attachments, which have been shown to contribute to abnormal stiffness during lengthening (Carey & Burghardt, 1993). However, unless combined with active movement, it is likely to require repeated use to prevent the reformation of anomalous attachments (Singer et al., 2001). Furthermore, Lynch et al. (2005) compared the use of CPM with self-range motion exercise in 32 stroke patients and found a positive trend for CPM towards improved shoulder joint stability but no differences in motor impairment, disability, pain or tone.

Thermal treatments

Ice can have a temporary effect in reducing tone, although it is usually applied as an adjunct and only in a specific area. The application of ice to spastic quadriceps muscle has been demonstrated to lead to an objectively measured reduction in spasticity (Brown et al., 1993). Cooling has also been shown to have some benefits to patients with an essential tremor (Cooper et al., 2000). Two studies (Feys et al., 2005; Quintern et al., 1999) reported significant reductions in tremor following cooling of the upper limb in people with MS that could have important functional implications when performing discrete functional activities such as intermittent self-catheterization or taking a meal. However, the effect of cold in people with MS can be variable, exacerbating symptoms in some people (see Ch. 5).

The application of heat packs can help to increase range of motion (Funk et al., 2001) by altering the properties of connective tissue that can be affected in movement dysfunction (Hardy & Woodall, 1998).

Acupuncture

The use of acupuncture in the treatment of neurological conditions remains the subject of debate. The National Clinical Guideline for Stroke (ISWP, 2008), in drawing upon key evidence from two Cochrane Systematic Reviews (SR) by Wu et al. (2006) and Zhang et al. (2005), recommends acupuncture should only be used in the context of ongoing clinical trials. Results of these SRs show acupuncture to be safe in the stroke population post 30 days, but evidence of benefit remains lacking, requiring more methodologically sound research to be carried out. Yet in a small RCT ($n=7$) conducted by Mukherjee et al. (2007), a significant decrease in spasticity in wrist flexors was noted when using electroacupuncture combined with strengthening exercises. Sonde et al. (2000) likewise reported a decrease in spasticity in the lower limb following the use of high-frequency TENS to stimulate acupuncture points. Donnellan and Shanley (2008) examined the use of acupuncture in people with secondary progressive multiple sclerosis and raised the possibility it may provoke lower limb muscle spasms in those with spasticity. Overall, they concluded that there was preliminary evidence to suggest acupuncture is safe in this population, but advised that the risk of increasing spasms should be raised with individuals.

KEY POINTS

- ♦ Prevention remains the best approach for contractures.
- ♦ For established contractures, the full range of techniques and approaches should be considered before surgical intervention.
- ♦ Effective intervention will include both treatment and management.
- ♦ Adjuncts should be used to support physical means and not used in isolation.
- ♦ Increasing evidence is emerging for the use of muscle-strengthening and aerobic exercise, even in the presence of tonal changes.

Education of patients and carers

Management of altered tone requires a 24-hour approach and education is an essential component. Education needs to be tailored to the patient's abilities and desire to know and must be given in a way that is understandable. Allison et al. (2008) found that health professionals' use of language was often a barrier to patient and carer understanding. The physiotherapist must try to judge what information to provide and when to provide it, but it is the patient who decides when or if he/she uses this information. Research indicates that information is best delivered in a way that actively involves patients and carers and allows them to have repeated opportunities to ask questions and to feel empowered about making decisions (Reynolds, 2005a; Smith et al, 2008; also see Ch. 11).

Patients need education to be able to identify possible triggers of increased spasms. Nociceptive stimuli, such as those from skin, bladder and bowel (even tight clothing and wrinkled seat cushions), can exacerbate spasticity

through stimulating flexor reflex afferent (FRA) activity (Sheean, 2008). With patients who have difficulty communicating or who are in a comatose state, increasing spasticity can be a sign that there is another problem, such as infection or constipation.

Patients may be able to learn to exhale and breathe through spasms to help prevent further tensing and worsening the spasm (Livingstone, 1998). Some patients will be able to gain further cognitive control over their spasms. If clonus is a problem, patients can be taught to push down through the long axis of the lower leg via the knee, giving a prolonged stretch to inhibit overactivity in the affected muscles.

A home programme may be incorporated into the overall management of tone, and compliance may be increased if exercises are included as part of everyday life, e.g. standing up against a wall whilst brushing teeth. Even if the person is unable to carry out all the exercises or stretches independently, he or she should direct a carer and thus retain responsibility. In some cases the spouse or partner may not see this as part of his or her role and the wish to maintain the partner and not the carer role should be respected (Courts et al., 2005). All carers should have their needs assessed separately (ISWP, 2008). Relevant information about support groups or networks (see Appendix) can also be provided.

KEY POINTS

- ♦ Patients must be empowered in decision-making and so be given clear information that is easy to understand and be offered repeated opportunities to seek clarification.

FACTORS INFLUENCING DECISION-MAKING IN THE MANAGEMENT OF ALTERED MUSCLE TONE

Factors that influence decision-making include:

- the neurological condition
- physical and cognitive abilities of the patient
- carryover of treatment into everyday activities
- severity of tonal alteration
- current and previous function
- presence of additional pathologies.

A holistic view of the patient should be taken when making decisions about the management of tonal difficulties; Thompson et al. (2005) and Barnes (2008) provide useful algorithms to assist clinical decision-making. Details of the patient's previous lifestyle should be considered, as well as his or her aspirations for the future. Quality of life is both personal and subjective; the individual must be consulted and goals set jointly (see next section and Ch. 11). The views of family and friends should be sought if it is not possible to communicate with the patient.

Diagnosis and prognosis

The approach to the management of tonal impairment will depend on the patient's diagnosis. For the patient with a rapidly deteriorating condition, such as a primary brain tumour or motor neurone disease, the priorities would be aimed at increasing activities and participation, with an emphasis on management and monitoring. Importance would be placed on the provision of equipment, and timely advice to carers regarding transfers and positioning as appropriate. Impairment focused goals would only be appropriate to address problems such as pain.

Prediction of outcome is multifactorial and individual, although there are some common factors linked to a more positive prognosis (Counsell et al., 2004; Jiang et al., 2002). In acute head injury where the prognosis is difficult to predict and the patient is at particular risk of developing contractures, emphasis is often placed on respiratory problems and insufficient attention given to potential adaptive impairments. The physiotherapist should advocate on behalf of the patient and be proactive in their approach to rehabilitation until factors indicate otherwise.

The ability to learn

The response to physical rehabilitation cannot be seen in isolation from perception, cognition, motivation, premorbid ability, behavioural difficulties and communication dysfunction. Motor learning is described as a complex perception–cognition–action process (Shumway-Cook & Woollacott, 2007). This area is covered in more detail in Chapter 17 on psychological management. Motivation is described by the WHO as a global mental function that can be both a conscious or unconscious drive that leads to an incentive to act (WHO, 2001) and is key in rehabilitation.

Potential for physical change

When handling a patient, certain signs indicate a potentially favourable outcome for physical change. These include:

- a change in tone in response to handling or positioning
- the ability of the patient to actively engage in the movement
- the presence of any active movement.

Altered tone may not be constant and the wider picture should be sought through a full assessment, preferably over

at least two sessions at different times of the day. However, it is important to remember that, in the absence of movement, preventing deterioration is an extremely valid reason for active intervention, especially in the early stages of rehabilitation and for people with progressive conditions.

Carryover and teamwork

Carryover can be described as the extent to which treatment gains are maintained and used functionally between treatment sessions. Management of physical impairments requires a 24-hour approach for maximum effectiveness and it is essential the whole rehabilitation team works towards common goals and has the knowledge and skills necessary to provide a coordinated approach (Thompson et al., 2005). For example, the speech and language therapist could undertake treatment while the patient is in a standing frame, or a perching stool could be used to encourage a more extended posture during activities in other therapies. Regular communication between staff including joint goals and treatment sessions, meetings, multidisciplinary notes and training may assist professions to work together effectively (Kilbride et al., 2005; Reynolds, 2005b).

KEY POINTS

- A holistic view of the patient should be taken when making decisions about the management of physical impairments.
- Physiotherapy intervention needs to ensure it is not based purely on the physical presentation of the patient, but also on the diagnosis and prognosis, and psychosocial factors.
- Teamwork is critical in the treatment and management of patients.

MEASURING EFFECTS OF INTERVENTIONS

Altered tone and movement patterns from the singular or combined effects of positive, negative or adaptive impairments can affect the individual at the various levels of body function/structure, activity and participation (WHO, 2001). When selecting an outcome measure to assess the impact of an intervention consideration should be given as to what level is affected; see Table 14.5 for examples of different scales that can be utilized. Ideally, selected outcome measures should be a combination of impairment and activity to ensure interventions remain patient centred.

Please note there can be some areas of overlap between categories; issues of reliability and validity should also be

Table 14.5 Commonly used outcome measures (Wade, 1992)

ICF LEVEL	EXAMPLES OF OUTCOME MEASURES
Body functions and structure	Ashworth Scale, Modified Ashwoth Scale, Tardieu Scale, Glasgow Coma Scale, Fugl Meyer, Visual Assessment Scale, Stroke Impact Scale (SIS) (impairment section), Motor Assessment Scale (MAS), Nine Hole Peg Test, MRC Measure of Power, Timed Walk
Activity	Motor Assessment Scale, FIM, FAM, Nottingham ADL, Barthel Index, SIS activity section, 10 metre walk, 6 minute walk, Action Research Arm Test, EDSS (Kurtzke Expanded Disability Scale), Timed Up & Go, Berg Balance scale
Participation	SIS partcipation section, Quality of Life SF 36, Nottingham Health Profile, Stroke-Adated Sickness Impact profile (SA-SIP-30)

(From Wade, DT, 1992. Measurement in neurological rehabilitation. By permission of Oxford University Press.)

taken into account (Stokes, 2009). Nevertheless, it is recognized that the measurement of tone at the level of impairment in the practice setting is challenging. Measurement is often based on the assessment of resistance to passive movement of the limb, but the limitation in movement may be from a combination of impairments (Ada et al., 2006b). Levin et al. (2009) also raised an important point that many outcome measures are not sensitive enough to differentiate how a task is accomplished, for example the quality of movement; without attention to quality it is not possible to tell if compensatory movements have been utilized or if there has been recovery of motor patterns. The authors (*ibid*) propose a solution within the framework of the ICF model (WHO, 2001).

Commonly used scales are the Ashworth Scale (AS) (Ashworth, 1964), the Modified Ashworth Scale (MAS) (Bohannon & Smith, 1987), which has greater reliability in the upper limb (Pandyan et al., 1999) and the Tardieu Scale (Tardieu et al., 1954). The Tardieu Scale is said to be able to identify the presence of spasticity in upper and lower limb muscles more effectively than the AS and distinguish between spasticity and contracture (Patrick & Ada, 2006). The Modified Tardieu Scale has also been shown to be more reliable than the MAS in patients with severe brain injury (Mehrholz et al., 2005). The Motor

Assessment Scale (Carr et al., 1985) also includes a measurement of tone as well as activity items. There is yet to be developed a widely available clinical tool with good validity and reliability that can distinguish between neural and non-neural components, although some early work on a novel approach to objectively measuring tone and biomechanical properties in the clinical setting using a non-invasive hand-held device called a Myoton®, (www.myoton.com) has been documented (Ianieri et al., 2008).

Other clinical measures

A paper walkway (Tyson & Thornton, 2001) can give useful information in the absence of a gait laboratory (i.e. stride length, step width and length). Painted footprints allow changes in weight distribution to be recorded and are a useful way of documenting the realignment of the foot complex. Similarly, periodic photographs allow comparison over time (Tyson & DeSouza, 2003). The procedure needs to be standardized to ensure that the same perspective and distance are used each time. Video recordings are an excellent means of documenting change in posture and movement (Wiles et al., 2003). It is possible to use frequency of events, e.g. spasms (Snow et al., 1990) to assess the outcome of intervention.

Goal setting and goal attainment scaling

Goal setting is the key to good practice in rehabilitation and should actively involve patients in the process wherever possible; if the patient is not able to participate, appropriate family members or a patient advocate should be included (ISWP, 2008). However, in practice, goal setting varies and a recent postal survey found that patients need to be given more opportunities to be engaged in the process but 'the shift from the patient role to one of partnership in care is developing slowly' (Holliday et al., 2005, p.231).

Goals should be SMART:
S = specific
M = measurable
A = achievable
R = realistic
T = timely

Cott & Finch, 1990

The goal attainment scale (GAS), a mathematical way to quantify achievement of goals, was first described in the 1960s (Kiresuk & Sherman, 1968); Turner-Stokes (2009) provides up to date practical guidance for its use in rehabilitation. For patients with severe and complex disabilities, goals may be divided into *passive* or *active* function, where passive is related to ease of caring for the individual and active represents a gain in independent activity (Ashford & Turner-Stokes, 2006).

KEY POINTS

◆ Measurement of outcome is essential and must relate to the aims of treatment
◆ Measurement of tone is difficult to achieve reliably in the clinical setting.

MOVEMENT DISORDERS AND TONAL CHANGES

Parkinson's disease

Physiotherapy is unlikely to influence the cardinal signs of Parkinson's disease, therefore rehabilitation is primarily concerned with the treatment and management of the functional consequences of these primary impairments (Stack, 2009), see Chapter 6 and Table 14.6.

Ataxia

Ataxia is a general term used to describe the decomposition of movement (Rothwell, 1994). Ataxia is characterized by errors in the rate, range, direction and force of movement (Ada & Canning, 2009) and, in general terms, movement is characterized as being uncoordinated. Ataxia is the principle symptom of cerebellar disorder, but is also noted in sensory ataxia (Lindsay & Bone, 2004). Ataxia presents with various movement disorders, see Table 14.7 and Chapter 5 on MS.

A systematic review of physiotherapy for people with cerebellar ataxia (Martin et al., 2009) concluded there is modest evidence for the effectiveness of physiotherapy to improve gait, trunk control and activity limitations. Further guidance by Cassidy et al. (2009) on physiotherapy interventions can be found at www.ataxia.org.uk. In vestibular ataxia, habituation exercises should be used, and can lead to a decrease in symptoms (Herdman & Whitney, 2000; see also Ch. 13). In sensory ataxia, the use of compensation strategies for function (Figure 14.7) and advice are essential to prevent injury or skin damage.

Other movement disorders and alterations in muscle tone

This section describes and provides definitions for other movement disorders and alterations in muscle tone that the physiotherapist may see infrequently, but nonetheless will need to be aware of and be able to identify (Tables 14.8, 14.9). Physiotherapy will have no direct effect on these impairments, but interventions should focus on preventing secondary complications.

Table 14.6 Cardinal signs of Parkinson's disease

Bradykinesia	Slowness of movement (Berardelli, et al., 2001)
Akinesia	Inability to initiate or prolonged initiation of movement due to difficulty selecting and/or activating motor pathways in the central nervous system (Berardelli, et al., 2001), may result in 'freezing' episodes (motor blocks) during the execution of complex movement (Morris, 2000), e.g. turning may provoke freezing; it is worse during the simultaneous performance of more than one task, e.g. walking and talking (Bloem, et al., 2001). Akinesia also describes the poverty of movement seen in Parkinson's disease, e.g. in facial expression or arm swing during walking (Berardelli, et al., 2001).
Hypokinesia	Small amplitude movements, e.g. producing micrographia, i.e. small writing (Berardelli, et al., 2001) or slowed movement.
Rigidity	Increased resistance to passive movement, bidirectional, not velocity dependent and does not involve hyperexcitable tendon reflexes. Resistance felt throughout movement is referred to as 'lead pipe' rigidity. When a tremor is superimposed on rigidity it is termed 'cog-wheel' rigidity (Sanger, et al., 2003).
Resting tremor	See Table 14.9

CASE HISTORIES

For each case history, a certain point in the patient's rehabilitation has been described. The aim of these presentations is to give an overview, not to provide detailed descriptions of treatment.

Steve

Steve, a 24-year-old man, suffered a head injury from a climbing accident. Initially he was admitted to a neurosurgical unit at a specialist hospital where he underwent a craniotomy and removal of a haematoma from the frontoparietal region. Scanning revealed widespread contusions. He was intubated and ventilated for a week and bilateral prophylactic below knee casts were applied as he had considerable extensor activity and was at risk of losing full range of dorsiflexion in both lower limbs. He

Table 14.7 Movement disorders seen in cerebellar ataxia

Dysmetria	Excessive movement or overshooting (hypermetria) or a deficient extent of movement or undershooting (hypometria). Seen as an inaccurate amplitude of movement and misplaced force, reflecting impaired timing of force generation.
Rebound	Problem with braking of movement. Demonstrated by asking the individual to flex the elbow isometrically against the examiner's resistance. When resistance is suddenly released, the person is unable to stop the resultant movement, the limb overshoots and rebounds excessively.
Dysdiadochokinesia	Difficulty performing rapidly alternating movements, e.g. pronation and supination, which worsens with repeated attempts.
Tremor	See Table 14.9 intention tremor
Dyssynergia	Lack of coordination between agonists and antagonists and other synergists resulting in absence of smooth sequential performance of muscle action, e.g. heel to shin test.
Hypotonia	Diminished resistance to passive movement, although the mechanism behind this remains unclear.

(From Carr J, Shepherd R. Neurological Rehabilitation: Optimising Motor Performance. Oxford, Butterworth Heinemann, 1998. Reprinted with permission of Elsevier Ltd.)

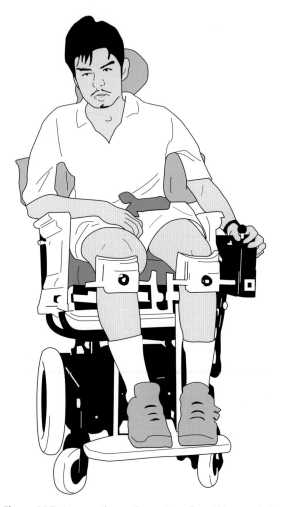

Figure 14.7 A supportive seating system allows this very ataxic young man to be able to drive a powered wheelchair.

developed a flexion contracture of his right arm, which could not be splinted due to a large abrasion. Four weeks later he was transferred to a surgical ward in his local general hospital.

Problems identified

Steve was nasogastrically fed due to the risk of aspiration from dysphagia. He had marked extensor activity in the lower limbs. His left arm was functional but his right arm was flexed and contracted with no useful movement. He was unable to sit independently and had attention-seeking behaviour.

Clinical decision-making

Regular team meetings were arranged and the family was invited to therapy sessions and to a case conference where the team identified a requirement for long-term rehabilitation to maximize Steve's functional recovery; he was referred to a specialist rehabilitation centre.

Action taken

It was decided to give Steve a percutaneous endoscopic gastrostomy (PEG) in liaison with the speech and language therapist, dietician and surgeon. A joint session with the occupational therapist provided him with a temporary supportive seating package. The below knee casts were taken off and, with daily standing and the use of

Table 14.8 Definitions of other movement disorders	
Dyskinesia	An umbrella term that means difficulty moving (see Appendix 1, Glossary)
Myoclonus	Brief, shock like jerks of a limb or body parts that may be restricted to one part of the body (focal myclonus) or generalized (generalized myoclonus) (Delgado & Albright, 2003)
Ballismus	From the Greek meaning jumping about. Violent, large amplitude involuntary, flailing movement of the limbs, sometimes affecting one side of the body (hemiballismus) (Delgado & Albright, 2003)
Chorea	From the Greek khoreia meaning dance. An involuntary hyperkinetic movement disorder characterized by random, quick jerks that move from one joint to another (Delgado & Albright, 2003). A feature of Huntington's disease (see Ch. 7).
Dystonia	Sustained contraction of muscle groups, resulting in twisting movements and unusual postures (Albanese, et al., 2006). Classification of dystonia is made by: (a) cause, e.g. whether dystonia is the only clinical sign or combined with other neurological features; (b) age at onset (early or late); and (c) distribution (e.g. focal, generalized). Treatment is primarily pharmacological (e.g. Botulinum toxin) or surgical (e.g. deep brain stimulation) (Albanese, et al., 2006)
Tremor	See Table 14.9 for detailed definitions.

removable night splints, range of movement was maintained. A series of drop-out casts were applied to his right arm to increase range. Staff tried to ignore inappropriate behaviour and socially reward good behaviour. The nurses and physiotherapist undertook a joint risk assessment and a standing hoist was used on the ward for transfers. He was transferred to the rehabilitation unit after 2 months.

Evaluation of outcome

Steve's range of flexion at the elbow and ankles was measured. Baseline charts were kept to monitor periods of attention-seeking behaviour. Functional and behavioural goals were set jointly by Steve, his family and the team. He achieved the functional goals of independent sitting and dressing his upper body.

Jenny

Jenny, a 26-year-old single mother, had been diagnosed with multiple sclerosis resulting in a partial paraplegia. She was referred for outpatient physiotherapy by a neurologist, following a relapse. Jenny had been a wheelchair user for 3 years and presented in low mood and with social isolation. She had fears about losing her 4-year-old daughter if she approached social services for any help. Her wheelchair was small, the canvas sagged, and she found it difficult to propel for long distances.

Problems identified

On examination, Jenny was found to have a weak trunk, with overactivity and moderate contractures of the hip flexors and adductors. She compensated by using her arms for support in a flexed internally rotated position. She was unable to stand and spent all day sitting. Her flexor spasms were becoming worse, and she had only flickers of activity in her lower limbs. She was very emotional on assessment and cried when asked about how she managed with daily tasks.

Decision-making

Worsening spasms concerned Jenny as they were affecting her function. Prompt action was needed to prevent this interfering with her transfers. There was also reduced range of motion in the hips and knees. On examination she had more activity in her trunk than she was currently using. It appeared that she had developed habitual postures resulting from her relapse. She also had psychosocial needs.

Action taken

Jenny kept a diary detailing when she had a spasm and why it happened. Active treatment included teaching Jenny to relax through spasms and to be much more aware of what triggered them. Therapists made backslabs to enable her to stand with alignment of trunk on pelvis and gain activation of her trunk muscles whilst carrying out activities with her upper limbs. After a risk assessment and trial period with a standing frame, Jenny was provided with one for use at home and began daily standing. She was given a perching stool for use in the kitchen. She was referred to her local wheelchair clinic for a review of her seating needs. Once the relationship between Jenny and her physiotherapist was established, she agreed to visit her general practitioner's counsellor and to attend the local multiple sclerosis support group.

Table 14.9 Definitions of tremor (Deuschl, et al., 1998)

Tremor	A rhythmic, involuntary movement of a limb or body part, classified into the following categories.
Resting tremor	Occurs at rest when the limb is relaxed and fully supported, e.g. Parkinson's disease and is known as 'pill-rolling'.
Action tremors: occur during movement, i.e. produced by voluntary contraction of muscle	*Postural tremor:* occurs when voluntarily maintaining a position against gravity, e.g. holding an arm out straight.
	Isometric tremor: tremor as a result of muscle contraction against a solid stationary object, e.g. making a fist.
	Kinetic tremor: occurs during any type of voluntary movement, further subdivided into: i Simple kinetic tremor: occurs during voluntary movements that are not target-directed, e.g. flexion/extension or pronation/supination ii Intention tremor: occurs during target directed, visually guided movements (e.g. finger-nose test); the tremor worsens as the target is approached in the terminal phase of the movement.
	Task-specific tremor: tremor that is exacerbated during specific activities, e.g. writing.

Reprinted with permission of John Wiley & Sons.

Evaluation of outcome

The frequency of spasms was monitored and by discharge they had declined significantly and Jenny was aware of triggers. She was going out regularly and subjective assessment suggested that her mood had improved substantially. Following discussions with Jenny and other team members, it was organized for her daughter to attend a nursery in the morning, giving Jenny some free time to manage the household tasks. Instead of giving her a prescribed exercise programme, the emphasis was on incorporating activities such as standing into her daily life and adopting different postures that would maintain her abilities.

REFERENCES

Ada, L., Canning, C.G., 2009. Common motor impairments and their impact on activity. In: Lennon, S., Stokes, M. (Eds.), Pocketbook of Neurological Physiotherapy. Churchill Livingstone, Elsevier, Edinburgh, pp. 73–93.

Ada, L., Dorsch, S., Canning, C., 2006a. Strengthening interventions increase and improve activity after stroke: a systematic review. Aust. J. Physiother. 52, 241–248.

Ada, L., O'Dwyer, N., O'Neill, E., 2006b. Relation between spasticity, weakness and contracture of the elbow flexors and upper limb activity after stroke: an observational study. Disabil. Rehabil. 28, 891–897.

Albanese, A., Barnes, M.P., Bhatia, K.P., et al., 2006. A systematic review on the diagnosis and treatment of primary (idiopathic) dystonia and dystonia plus syndromes: report of an EFNS/MDS-ES Task Force. Eur. J. Neurol. 13, 433–444.

Allison, R., Evans, P.H., Kilbride, C., 2008. Secondary prevention of stroke: using the experiences of patients and carers to inform the development of an educational resource. Fam. Pract. 25, 355–361.

Ashford, S., Turner-Stokes, L., 2006. Goal attainment for spasticity management using botulinum toxin. Physiother. Res. Int. 11, 24–34.

Ashworth, B., 1964. Preliminary trial of carisoprodal in multiple sclerosis. Practioner 192, 540–542.

Baker, K., Cassidy, E., Rone-Adams, S., 2007. Therapeutic standing for people with multiple sclerosis: Eficacy and feasibility. Int. J. Ther. Rehabil. 14, 104–109.

Bale, M., Strand, L.I., 2008. Does functional strength training of the leg in subacute stroke improve physical performance? A pilot randomized controlled trial. Clin. Rehabil. 22, 911–921.

Bakhtiary, A.H., Fatemy, E., 2008. Does electrical stimulation reduce spasticty after stroke? A randomized controlled study. Clin. Rehabil. 22, 418–425.

Barnard, P., Dill, H., Eldredge, P., et al., 1984. Reduction of hypertonicity by early casting in a comatose head-injured individual. A case report. Phys. Ther. 64, 1540–1542.

Barnes, M.P., 2008. An overview of the clinical management of spasticity. In: Barnes, M.P., Johnson, G.R. (Eds.), Upper motor neurone syndrome and spasticity: clinical management and neurophysiology. Cambridge University Press, Cambridge, pp. 1–8.

Barrett, J.A., Watkins, C., Plant, R., et al., 2001. The COSTAR wheelchair study: a two-centred pilot study of self-propulsion in a wheelchair in early stroke rehabilitation. Clin. Rehabil. 15, 32–41.

Berardelli, A., Rothwell, J.C., Thompson, P.D., Hallett, M., 2001. Pathophysiology of bradykinesia in Parkinson's disease. Brain 124, 2131–2146.

Bloem, B.R., Valkenburg, V.V., Slabbekoorn, M., van Dijk, J.G., 2001. The multiple task test. Strategies in Parkinson's disease. Exp. Brain Res. 137, 478–486.

Bobath, B., 1990. Adult Hemiplegia Evaluation and Treatment. Butterworth Heinemann, Oxford.

Bohannon, R.W., 1993. Tilt table standing for reducing spasticity after spinal cord injury. Arch. Phys. Med. Rehabil. 74, 1121–1122.

Bohannon, R.W., Smith, M.B., 1987. Interrater reliability of a modified Ashworth scale of muscle spasticity. Phys. Ther. 67, 206–207.

Bovend'Eerdt, T.J., Newman, M., Barker, K., et al., 2008. The Effects of Stretching in Spasticity: A Systematic Review. Arch. Phys. Med. Rehabil. 89, 1395–1406.

Boyd, R.N., Ada, L., 2008. Physiotherapy management of spasticity. In: Barnes, M.P., Johnson, G.R. (Eds.), Upper motor neurone syndrome and spasticity: clinical management and neurophysiology. Cambridge University Press, Cambridge, pp. 79–98.

Brouwer, B., de Andrade, V.S., 1995. The effects of slow stroking on spasticity in patients with multiple sclerosis; a pilot study. Physiother. Theory Pract. 11, 13–21.

Brown, P., 1994. Pathophysiology of spasticity – editorial. J. Neurol. Neurosurg. Psychiatry 57, 773–777.

Brown, R.A., Holdsworth, L., Leslie, G.C., et al., 1993. The effects of time after stroke and selected therapeutic techniques on quadriceps muscle tone in stroke patients. Physiother. Theory Pract. 9, 131–142.

Burke, D., 1988. Spasticity as an adaptation to pyramidal tract injury. In: Waxman, S.G. (Ed.), Functional Recovery in Neurological Disease. Advances in Neurology, vol. 47. Ravenpress, New York, pp. 401–423.

Canning, C.G., Ada, L., Adams, R., O'Dwyer, N.J., 2004. Loss of strength contributes more to physical disability after stroke than loss of dexterity. Clin. Rehabil. 18, 300–308.

Carey, J.R., Burghardt, T.P., 1993. Movement dysfunction following central nervous system lesions: a problem of neurologic or muscular impairment? Phys. Ther. 73, 538–547.

Carr, J.H., Shepherd, R.B., Nordholm, L., et al., 1985. Investigation of a new motor assessment scale for stroke patients. Phys. Ther. 65, 175–176.

Carr, J., Shepherd, R., 1998. Neurological Rehabilitation: Optimising Motor Performance, Butterworth Heinemann, Oxford.

Carr, J., Shepherd, R., 2003. Stroke Rehabilitation: guidelines for exercise and training to optimise motor skill, Butterworth Heinemann, Oxford.

Carter, P., Edwards, S., 2002. General principles of treatment. In: Edwards, S. (Ed.), Neurological Physiotherapy. Churchill Livingstone, London, pp. 121–153.

Cassidy, E., Kilbride, C., Holland, A., 2009. Guidance for Physiotherapy Intervention for People with Ataxia. Available from www.ataxia.org.uk.

Champion, J., Barber, C., 2009. Recovery of the upper limb. In: Meadows, L., Raine, S., Lynch-Ellerington, M. (Eds.), Bobath Concept: Theory and Clinical Practice in Neurological Rehabilitation. Wiley-Blackwell, Oxford.

Chartered Society of Physiotherapy, 2008. Guidance on Manual Handling in Physiotherapy, third ed. The Chartered Society of Physiotherapy, London.

Cheng, P.T., Chin-Man, W., Chai-Ying, C., 2004. Effects of visual feedback rhythmic weight-shift training on hemiplegic stroke patients. Clin. Rehabil. 18, 747–753.

Childers, M.K., Biswass, S.S., Petroski, G., et al., 1999. Inhibitory casting decreases a vibratory inhibition index of the h reflex in the upper limb. Arch. Phys. Med. Rehabil. 80, 714–716.

Chua, K.S.G., Kong, K.H., 2003. Acquired heterotopic ossification in the settings of cerebral anoxia and alternative therapy: two cases. Brain Inj. 17, 535–544.

Collins, F., 2007. A practical guide to wheelchair cushions. Int. J. Ther. Rehabil. 14, 557–561.

Cook, B., 2007. Hydrotherapy. In: Pope, P.M. (Ed.), Severe and Complex Neurological Disability. Management of the Physical Condition. Butterworth Heinemann Elsevier, Edinburgh, pp. 216–229.

Cooper, C., Evidente, V.G.H., Hentz, J.G., et al., 2000. The effect of temperature on hand function in patients with tremor. J. Hand Ther. 13, 276–288.

Cornall, C., 1991. Self propelling wheel chairs: the effects on spasticity in hemiplegic patients. Physiother. Theory Pract. 7, 13–21.

Cott, C., Finch, E., 1990. Goal setting in physical therapy practice. Physiother. Canada 43, 19–22.

Counsell, C., Dennis, M., McDowall, M., 2004. Predicting fucntional outcome in acute stroke: comparison of a simple six variable model with other predictive systems and informal clinical prediciton. J. Neurol. Neurosurg. Psychiatry 75, 401–405.

Courts, N.F., Newton, A.N., McNeal, L.J., 2005. Husbands and wives living with multiple sclerosis. J. Neurosci. Nurs. 37, 20–27.

Cramp, M.C., Greenwood, R.J., Gill, C., et al., 2006. Low intensity strength training for ambulatory stroke patients. Disabil. Rehabil. 28, 883–889.

Davidson, I., Waters, K., 2000. Physiotherapists working with stroke patients: a national survey. Physiotherapy 86, 69–80.

Dawes, H., Bateman, A., Wade, D., et al., 2000. High intensity cycling exercise after stroke: a single case study. Clin. Rehabil. 14, 570–573.

Dawson, J., Thornton, H., 2003. Can Patients with Unilateral Neglect following Stroke drive Electrical Powered Wheelchairs? Br. J. Occup. Ther. 66, 49–54.

De Jong, L.D., Nieuwboer, A., Aufdemkampe, G., 2006. Contracture preventive positioning of the hemiplegic arm in subacute stroke patients: a pilot randomized controlled trial. Clin. Rehabil. 20, 656–667.

Delagdo, R.M., Albright, A.L., 2003. Movement disorders in children: definitions, classifications and grading systems. J. Child Neurol. 18, S1–S8.

Denny Brown, D., 1966. The Cerebral Control of Movement. Liverpool University Press, Liverpool, cited in Sheean, G. 1998 Pathophysiology of Spasticity. In: Sheean, G. (Ed.), Spasticity Rehabilitation. Churchill Communications Europe Limited, London, pp. 287–295.

Deuschl, G., Bain, P., Brin, M., an Ad Hoc Scientific Committee, 1998. Consensus statement of the movement disorder society on tremor. Mov. Disord. 13 (Suppl. 3), 2–23.

Devitt, R., Chau, B., Jutai, J.W., 2004. The Effect of Wheelchair Use on the Quality of Life of Persons with Multiple Sclerosis. Occup. Ther. Health Care 17, 63–79.

Dewey, A., Rice-Oxley, M., Dean, T., 2004. A Qualitative Study Comparing the Experiences of Tilt-in-Space Wheelchair Use and Conventional Wheelchair Use by Clients Severely Disabled with Multiple Sclerosis. Br. J. Occup. Ther. 67, 65–74.

de Wit, D.C., Buurke, J.H., Nijlant, et al., 2004. The effect of an ankle-foot orthosis on walking ability in chronic stroke patients: a randomized controlled trial. Clin. Rehabil. 18, 550–557.

Donnellan, C.P., Shanley, J., 2008. Comparison of the effect of two types of acupuncture on quality of life in secondary progressive multiple sclerosis: a preliminary single randomised controlled trial. Clin. Rehabil. 22, 195–205.

Duncan, P., Studenski, S., Richards, L., et al., 2003. Randomized clinical trial of therapeutic exercise in subacute stroke. Stroke 34, 2173–2180.

Edwards, S., Charlton, P., 2002. Splinting and the use of orthoses in the management of patients with neurological disorder. In: Edwards, S. (Ed.), Neurological Physiotherapy. Churchill Livingstone, London, pp. 219–254.

Fess, E., Gettle, K.S., Philips, C.A., et al., 2005. Splinting for Patients with Upper Extremity Spasticity. In: Fess, E., Gettle, K.S., Philips, C.A. et al., (Eds.), Hand and Upper Extremity Splinting. Principles and Methods, third ed. Elsevier Mosby, Missouri, pp. 517–536.

Farmer, S., James, M., 2001. Contractures in orthopaedic and neurological conditions: a review of causes and treatment. Disabil. and Rehabil. 23, 549–558.

Feys, P., Helsen, W., Liu, X., et al., 2005. Effects of peripheral cooling on intention tremor in multiple sclerosis. J. Neurol. Neurosurg. Psychiatry 76, 373–379.

Fitzferald, D., Stokes, M., 2004. Muscle imbalance in neurological conditions. In: Stokes, M., (Ed.), Physical Management in Neurological Rehabilitation, second ed. Elsevier Mosby, Edinburgh, pp. 501–516.

Flansbjer, U.B., Miller, M., Downham, D., et al., 2008. Progressive resistance training after stroke: effects on muscle strength, muscle tone, gait performance and perceived participation. J. Rehabil. Med. 40, 42–48.

Fox, P., Richardson, J., McInnes, B., et al., 2000. Effectiveness of a Bed Positioning Program for Treating Older Adults With Knee Contractures Who Are Institutionalised. Phys. Ther. 80, 363–372.

Fujiwara, T., Liu, M., Hase, K., et al., 2004. Electrophysiological and clinical assessment of a simple wrist-hand splint for patients with chronic spastic hemiparesis secondary to stroke. Electromyogr. Clin. Neurophysiol. 44, 423–429.

Funk, D., Swank, A.M., Adams, K.J., et al., 2001. Effects of moist heat pack application over static stretching on hamstring flexibility. J. Strength Cond. Res. 15, 123–126.

Gemperline, J.J., Allen, S., Walk, D., Rymer, W.Z., 1995. Characteristics of motor unit discharge in subjects with hemiparesis. Muscle Nerve 18, 1101–1114.

Goldspink, G., Williams, P.E., 1990. Muscle fibre and connective tissue changes associated with use and disuse. In: Ada, L., Canning, C. (Eds.), Key Issues in Neurological Physiotherapy. Butterworth Heinnemann, London, pp. 20–50.

Gordon, J., 1991. Spinal Mechanisms of Motor Coordination. In: Kendel, E.R., Schwartz, J.H., Jessell, T.M. (Eds.), Principles of Neuroscience. Appleton Lange Norwalk, Connecticut, pp. 581–595.

Gracies, J.M., Fitzpatrick, R., Wilson, L., et al., 2000. Short term effects of dynamic Lycra splints on upper limb in hemiplegic patients. Arch. Phys. Med. Rehabil. 81, 1547–1555.

Griffin, A., Bernhardt, J., 2006. Strapping the hemiplegic shoulder prevents development of pain during rehabilitation: a randomized controlled trial. Clin. Rehabil. 20, 287–295.

Gustafsson, L., McKenna, K., 2006. A programme of static positional stretches does not reduce hemiplegic shoulder pain or maintain shoulder range of motion – a randomized controlled trial. Clin. Rehabil. 20, 277–286.

Hanger, H.C., Whitewood, P., Brown, G., et al., 2000. A randomised controlled trial of strapping to prevent post stroke shoulder pain. Clin. Rehabil. 14, 370–380.

Hara, Y., Ogawa, S., Muraoka, Y., 2006. Hybride power-assisted functional electrical stimulation to improve hemiparetic upper-extremity function. Am. J. Phys. Med. Rehabil. 85, 977–985.

Hardy, M., Woodall, W., 1998. Therapeutic effects of heat, cold and stretch on connective tissue. J. Hand Ther. 11, 148–156.

Herdman, S.J., Whitney, S.L., 2000. Assessment and management of central vestibular disorders. In: Herdman, S. (Ed.), Vestibular Rehabilitation, second ed. FA Davis, Philadelphia.

Hesse, S., 2008. Treadmill training with partial body weight support after stroke. A review. NeuroRehabilitation 23, 55–65.

Hill, J., 1994. The effects of casting on upper extremity motor disorders after brain injury. Am. J. Occup. Ther. 48, 219–223.

Hiraoka, K., 2001. Rehabilitation effort to improve upper limb extremity function in post-stroke patients: a meta-analysis. J. Phys. Ther. 13, 5–9.

Holliday, R.C., Antoun, M., Playford, D., 2005. A Survey of Goal-Setting Methods Used in Rehabilitation. Neurorehabil. Neural Repair 19, 227–231.

Ianieri, G., Ranieri, M., Marvulli, R., et al., 2008. The approach to rehabilitation in post-traumatic spasticity. Abstracts Toxins 51, 29.

Intercollegiate Stroke Working Party, 2008. National clinical guideline for stroke, third ed. Royal College of Physicians, London.

Jackson, H.J., 1958. Evolution and dissolution of the nervous system speech and various papers, addresses and lectures. In: Taylor, J., Holmes, G., Walshe, F.M.R. (Eds.), John Hughlings Jackson Selected Writings, vol. 2. Arts and Boeve Nijmegen.

Jiang, J.-Y., Gao, G.-Y., Li, W.-P., et al., 2002. Early Indicators of Prognosis in 846 Cases of Severe Traumatic Brain Injury. J. Neurotrauma 19, 869–874.

Johansson, B.B., 2000. Brain plasticity and stroke rehabilitation: the Willis lecture. Stroke 31, 223–230.

Johnstone, M., 1995. Restoration of Normal Movement after Stroke. Churchill Livingstone, Edinburgh.

Katalinic, O.M., Harvey, L.A., Herbert, R.D., et al., 2008. Stretch interventions for contractures. Cochrane Database Syst. Rev. (4), CD 007455.

Kesiktas, N., Erdogan, N., Gulsen, G., et al., 2004. The Use of Hydrotherapy for the Management of Spasticity. Neurorehabil. Neural Repair 18, 268–273.

Kilbreath, S.L., Davis, G.M., 2005. Cardiorespiratory fitness after stroke. In: Refshauge, K., Ada, L., Ellis, E. (Eds.), Science-Based Rehabilitation. Theories into Practice. Elsevier Butterworth Heinemann, Edinburgh, pp. 131–158.

Kilbride, C., Meyer, J., Flatley, M., et al., 2005. Stroke Units: the implementation of a complex intervention. Educational Action Research 13, 479–503.

King, T.I., 1982. Plaster splinting as a means of reducing elbow flexor spasticity: a case study. Am. J. Occup. Ther. 36, 671–673.

Kiresuk, T., Sherman, R., 1968. Goal attainment scaling: a general method of evaluating comprehensive mental health programmes. Community Ment. Health J. 4, 443–453, cited in Turner-Stokes, L., 2009. Goal attainment scaling (GAS) in rehabilitation: a practical guide. Clin. Rehabil. 23, 362–370.

Kleim, J.A., Jones, T.A., 2008. Principles of experience-dependent neural plasticity: implications for rehabilitation. American Journal of Speech Hearing and Language Research 51, 225–239.

Knight, L.A., Thornton, H.A., Turner-Stokes, L., 2003. Management of neurogenic heterotrophic ossification. Physiotherapy 89, 471–477.

Kofler, M., Quirbach, E., Schauer, R., et al., 2009. Limitations of Intrathecal Baclofen for Spastic Hemiparesis Following Stroke. Neurorehabil. Neural Repair 23, 26–31.

Krause, P., Szecsi, A., Straube, A., 2008. Changes in spastic muscle tone increase in patients with spinal cord injury using functional electrical stimulation and passive leg movements. Clin. Rehabil. 22, 627–634.

Lance, J.W., 1980. Symposium synopsis. In: Feldman, R.G., Young, R.R., Koella, W.P. (Eds.), Spasticity: Disordered Motor Control. Year Book Medical Publishers, Chicago, pp. 485–494.

Landau, W.M., 1980. Spasticity: what is it? What is it not? In: Feldman, R.G., Young, R.R., Koella, W.P. (Eds.), Spasticity: Disordered Motor Control. Year Book Medical Publishers, Chicago, pp. 17–24.

Landau, W.M., 1988. Clinical Neuromythology II, parables of palsy pills and PT pedagogy. A spastic dialectic. Neurology 38, 1496–1499.

Lannin, N.A., Cusick, A., McCluskey, A., et al., 2007a. Effects of splinting on wrist contracture after stroke: a randomized controlled trial. Stroke 38, 111–116.

Lannin, N.A., Novak, I., Cusick, A., 2007b. A systematic review of the upper extremity casting for children and adults with central nervous system motor disorders. Clin. Rehabil. 21, 963–976.

Lee, M.J., Kilbreath, S.L., Singh, M.F., et al., 2008. Comparison of effect of aerobic cycle training and progressive resistance training on walking ability after stroke: a randomized sham exercise-controlled trial. J. Am. Geriatr. Soc. 56, 976–985.

Lennon, S., Bassile, C., 2009. Guiding principles for neurological physiotherapy. In: Lennon, S., Stokes, M. (Eds.), Pocketbook of Neurological Physiotherapy. Churchill Livingstone Elsevier, Edinburgh, pp. 97–111.

Levin, M.F., Kleim, J.A., Wolf, S.L., 2009. What Do Motor "Recovery" and "Compensation" Mean in Patients Following Stroke? Neurorehabil. Neural Repair 23, 313–319.

Lindsay, K.W., Bone, I., 2004. Neurology and Neurosurgery Illustrated, fourth ed. Churchill Livingstone, Edinburgh.

Livingstone, L., 1998. Coping with labour: what are the options? In: Sapsford, R., Bullock-Saxton, J., Markwell, S. (Eds.), Women's Health. A Textbook for Physiotherapists. WB Saunders, London.

Lotze, M., Braun, C., Birbaumer, N., et al., 2003. Motor learning elicited by voluntary drive. Brain 126, 866–872.

Lynch, D., Ferraro, M., Krol, J., et al., 2005. Continuous passive motion improves shoulder joint integrity following stroke. Clin. Rehabil. 19, 594–599.

Macfarlane, A., Thornton, H.A., 1997. Solving the problem of contractures – throw out the recipe book? Physiother. Res. Int. 2, 1–6.

Markham, C.H., 1987. Vestibular control of muscular tone and posture. Can. J. Neurol. Sci. 14, 493–496.

Marossezky, J.E., Gurka, J.A., Baguley, I.J., 2008. Splinting Poststroke: the Jury Is Still Out. Stroke 39, e46.

Martin, C.L., Tan, D., Bragge, P., 2009. Effectiveness of physiotherapy for adults with cerebellar dysfunction: a systematic review. Clin. Rehabil. 23, 15–26.

Massion, J., 1994. Postural control system. Curr. Opin. Neurobiol. 4, 877–887.

Mayston, M., 2002. Problem solving in neurological physiotherapy – setting the scene. In: Edwards, S. (Ed.), Neurological Physiotherapy. Churchill Livingstone, London, pp. 3–19.

McInnes, E., Bell-Syer, S.E., Dumville, J.C., et al., 2008. Support surfaces for pressure ulcer prevention. Cochrane Database Syst. Rev. 4, CD001735.

Meadows, L., Raine, S., Lynch-Ellerington, M. (Eds.), 2009. Bobath Concept: Theory and Clinical Practice in Neurological Rehabilitation. Wiley-Blackwell, Oxford.

Meadows, L., Williams, J., 2009. An Understanding of Functional Movement as a Basis for Clinical Reasoning. In: Meadows, L., Raine, S., Lynch-Ellerington, M. (Eds.), Bobath Concept: Theory and Clinical Practice in Neurological Rehabilitation. Wiley-Blackwell, Oxford.

Mehrholz, J., Wagner, K., Meißner, M., et al., 2005. Reliability of the Modified Tardieu Scale and the Modified Ashworth Scale in adult patients with severe brain injury: a comparison study. Clin. Rehabil. 19, 751–759.

Miller, L., Mattison, P., Paul, L., et al., 2007. The effects of transcutaneous electrical nerve stimulation (TENS) on spasticity in multiple sclerosis. Clin. Rehabil. 13, 527–533.

Moreland, J.D., Thompson, M.A., Fuoco, A.R., 1998. Electromyographic biofeedback to improve lower extremity function after stroke; a meta-analysis. Arch. Phys. Med. Rehabil. 79, 134–140.

Morris, M., 2000. Movement disorders in peoplw with Parkinson's disease: a model for physical therapy. Phys. Ther. 80, 578–597.

Morris, S.L., Dodd, K.J., Morris, M.E., 2004. Outcomes of progressive resistance strength training following stroke: a systematic review. Clin. Rehabil. 18, 27–39.

Mortenson, P.A., Eng, J., 2003. The Use of Casts in the Management of Joint Mobility and Hypertonia Following Brain Injury in Adults. A Systematic Review. Phys. Ther. 83, 648–658.

Moseley, A., Hassett, L.M., Leung, J., et al., 2008. Serial casting versus positioning for the treatment of elbow contractures in adults with traumatic brain injury: a randomized controlled trial. Clin. Rehabil. 22, 406–417.

Mukherjee, M., McPeak, L.K., Redford, J.B., et al., 2007. The effect of electro-acupuncture on spasticity of the wrist joint in chronic stroke survivors. Arch. Phys. Med. Rehabil. 88, 159–166.

National Institute for Health and Clinical Excellence, 2009. Functional electrical stimulation for drop foot of central origin. Accessed 22.04.09 from http://www.nice.org.uk/nicemedia/pdf/IPG278Guidance.pdf.

Newman, M.A., Dawes, H., van den Berg, M., et al., 2007. Can aerobic treadmill training reduce the effort of walking and fatigue in people with multiple sclerosis: a pilot study. Mult. Scler. 13, 113–119.

Nixon, J., Nelson, E.A., Cranny, G., et al., 2006. Pressure relieving support surfaces: a randomised evaluation. Health Technol. Assess. 10, iii–iiv, ix–ix, 1–163.

O'Connor, R., Smith, R., 2008. Wheelchair and Special Seating for Neurological Conditions. Advances in Clinical Neurosciences and Rehabilitation 8, 18–22.

O'Dwyer, N., Ada, L., 1996. Reflex hyperexcitability and muscle contracture in relation to spastic hypertonia. Curr. Opin. Neurol. 9, 451–455.

O'Dwyer, N., Ada, L., Neilson, P., 1996. Spasticity and muscle contracture following stroke. Brain 119, 1737–1749.

Page, S.J., Szaflarski, J.P., Eliassen, J.C., et al., 2009. Cortical Plasticity Following Motor Skill Learning During mental Practice in Stroke. Neurorehabil. Neural Repair 23, 382–388.

Pandyan, A.D., Cameron, M., Powell, J., et al., 2003. Contractures in the post-stroke wrist: a pilot study of its time course of development and its association with upper limb recovery. Clin. Rehabil. 17, 88–95.

Pandyan, A.D., Johnson, G.R., Price, C.I.M., et al., 1999. A review of the properties and limitations of the Ashworth and modified Ashworth scales as measures of spasticity. Clin. Rehabil. 13, 373–383.

Pang, M.Y.C., Eng, J.J., Dawson, A.S., et al., 2005. A community-based Fitness and Mobility Exercise (FAME) program for older adults with chronic stroke: A randomized controlled trial. J. Am. Geriatr. Soc. 53, 416–423.

Patrick, E., Ada, L., 2006. The Tardieu Scale differentiates contracture from spasticity whereas the Ashworth Scale is confounded by it. Clin. Rehabil. 20, 173–182.

Peterson, C., 2001. Exercise in 94 degree F water for a patient with multiple sclerosis. Phys. Ther. 81, 1049–1058.

Pizzi, A., Carlucci, G., Falsini, C., et al., 2005. Application of a volar splint in poststroke spasticity of the upper limb. Arch. Phys. Med. Rehabil. 86, 1855–1859.

Pohl, M., Mehrholz, J., 2006. Immediate effects of an individually designed functional ankle-foot orthosis on stance and gait in hemiparetic patients. Clin. Rehabil. 20, 324–330.

Pomeroy, V., Mickelborough, J., Hill, E., et al., 2003. A hypothesis: self propulsion in a wheelchair early after stroke might not be harmful. Clin. Rehabil. 17, 174–180.

Pope, P.M., 2007. Severe and Complex Neurological Disability. Management of the Physical Condition. Butterworth Heinemann Elsevier, Edinburgh.

Price, C.I.M., Pandyan, A.D., 2001. Electrical stimulation for preventing and treating post stroke shoulder pain: a systematic Cochrane review. Clin. Rehabil. 15, 5–19.

Proske, U., Wise, A.K., Gregory, J.E., 2000. The role of muscle receptors in the detection of movements. Prog. Neurobiol. 60, 85–96.

Qunitern, J., Immisch, I., Albrecht, H., et al., 1999. Influence of visual and propriocpetive afferences on upper limb ataxian patients with mulitple sclerosis. J. Neurol. Sci. 163, 61–69.

Reynolds, F., 2005a. Patient education and empowerment. In: Reynolds, F. (Ed.), Communication and Clinical Effectiveness in Rehabilitation. Elsevier Butterworth Heinemann, Edinburgh, pp. 169–201.

Reynolds, F., 2005b. Teamwork in the rehabilitation setting. In: Reynolds, F. (Ed.), Communication and Clinical Effectiveness in Rehabilitation. Elsevier Butterworth Heinemann, Edinburgh, pp. 205–225.

Richards, L.G., Stewart, K.C., Woodbury, M.L., et al., 2008. Movement-dependent stroke recovery: a systematic review and meta-analysis of TMA and fMRI evidence. Neuropsychologia 46, 3–11.

Robichaud, J.A., Agostinucci, J., 1996. Air–splint pressure effect on soleus muscle alpha motoneuron reflex excitability in subjects with spinal cord injury. Arch. Phys. Med. Rehabil. 77, 778–782.

Robinson, W., Smith, R., Aung, O., et al., 2008. No difference between wearing a night splint and standing on a tilt table I preventing ankle contracture early after stroke: a randomised trial. Aust. J. Physiother. 54, 33–38.

Rosche, J., Rub, B., Niemann-Delius, B., et al., 1996. Effects of physiotherapy on F-wave amplitudes in spasticity. Electromyogr. Clin. Neurophysiol. 36, 509–511.

Rosenfalck, A., Andreassen, S., 1980. Impaired regulation of force and firing pattern of single motor units in patients with spasticity. J. Neurol. Neurosurg. Psychiatry 43, 907–916.

Rothwell, J.C., 1994. Control of Human Voluntary Movement, second ed. Chapman & Hall, London.

Royal College of Physicians, 2009. British Society of Rehabilitation Medicine. Chartered Society of Physiotherapy et al. Spasticity in adults: management using botulinum toxin. National Guideline. Royal College of Physicians, London.

Sackley, C.M., Lincoln, N.B., 1997. Single-blind randomised controlled trial of visual feedback after stroke: effects on stance and symmetry and function. Disabil. Rehabil. 19, 536–546.

Sanger, T.D., Delgardo, M.R., Gaebler-Spira, D., et al., 2003. Classification and definition of disorders casuing hypertonia in childhood. Paediatrics 111, e89–e97.

Schmit, B.D., Dewald, J.P., Rymer, W.Z., 2000. Stretch reflex adaptation in elbow flexors during repeated passive movements in unilateral brain-injured patients. Arch. Phys. Med. Rehabil. 81, 269–278.

Sheean, G., 1998. Pathophysiology of Spasticity. In: Sheean, G. (Ed.), Spasticity Rehabilitation. Churchill Communications Europe Limited, London, pp. 287–295.

Sheean, G., 2002. The Pathophysiology of Spasticity. Eur. J. Neurol. 9 (Suppl. 1), 3–9.

Sheean, G., 2008. Neurophysiology of Spasticity. In: Barnes, M.P., Johnson, G.R. (Eds.), Upper Motor Neurone Syndrome and Spasticity: Clinical Management and Neurophysiology. Cambridge University Press, Cambridge, pp. 9–63.

Shumway-Cook, A., Woollacott, M., 2007. Motor control: translating research into clinical practice, third ed. Lippincott Williams & Wilkins, Philadelphia.

Singer, B., Dunne, J., Allison, G., 2001. Clinical evaluation of hypertonia in the triceps surae muscles. Phys. Ther. Rev. 6, 71–80.

Skinner, A., Thomson, A., 2008. Aquatics Therapy and the Halliwick Concept. Exceptional Parent 38, 76–77.

Smith, J., Forster, A., House, A., et al., 2008. Information provision for stroke patients and their caregivers. Cochrane Database Syst. Rev. (2), CD001919.

Snow, B.J., Tsui, J.K.C., Bhatt, M.H., et al., 1990. Treatment of spasticity with Botulinum toxin: a double blind study. Ann. Neurol. 28, 512–515.

Sonde, L., Kalimo, H., Viitanen, M., 2000. Stimulation with high frequency TENS – effects on lower limb spasticity after stroke. Advances in Physiotherapy 2, 183–187.

Stack, E., 2009. The patient with degenerative disease: Parkinson's disease. In: Lennon, S., Stokes, M. (Eds.), Pocketbook of Neurological Physiotherapy. Churchill Livingstone, Elsevier, Edinburgh, pp. 175–190.

Stoeckmann, T., 2001. Casting for the person with spasticity. Top. Stroke Rehabil. 8, 27–35.

Stokes, E., 2009. Outcome measurement. In: Stokes, M., Lennon, S. (Eds.), Pocketbook of Neurological Physiotherapy. Churchill Livingstone Elsevier, Edinburgh, pp. 191–201.

Sullivan, J.E., Headman, L.D., 2007. Effects of home-based sensory and motor amplitude electrical stimulation on arm dysfunction in chronic stroke. Clin. Rehabil. 21, 142–150.

Tardieu, C., Lespargot, A., Tabary, C., et al., 1988. How long must the soleus muscle be stretched each day to prevent contracture? Dev. Med. Child Neurol. 30, 3–10.

Tardieu, G., Shentoub, S., Delarue, R., 1954. A la recherche d'une technique de mesure de la spasticite. Review Neurol 91, 143–144.

Taylor, E.W., Morris, D., Shaddeau, S., et al., 1993. Effects of water walking on hemiplegic gait. Aquatic physical therapy. Journal of the Aquatic Section of the American Physical Therapy Association 1, 10–13.

Thompson, A.J., Jarrett, L., Lockley, L., et al., 2005. Clinical management of spasticity. J. Neurol. Neurosurg. Psychiatry 76, 459–463.

Thornton, H., Kilbride, C., 2004. Physical management of abnormal tone and movement. In: Stokes, M. (Ed.), Physical Management in Neurological Rehabilitation, second ed. Elsevier Mosby, Edinburgh, pp. 431–450.

Tsai, K.H., Chun-Yu, Y., Chang, H.Y., et al., 2001. Effects of a Single Session of Prolonged Muscle Stretch on Spastic Muscle of Stroke Patients. Proc. Natl. Sci. Counc. Repub. China B 25, 76–81.

Turner-Stokes, L., 2009. Goal attainment scaling (GAS) in rehabilitation: a practical guide. Clin. Rehabil. 23, 362–370.

Tyson, S.F., DeSouza, L.H., 2003. A clinical model for the assessment of posture and balance in people with stroke. Disabil. Rehabil. 25, 120–126.

Tyson, S.F., Rogerson, L., 2009. Assistive walking devices in nonambulant patients undergoing rehabilitation after stroke: the effects on functional mobility, walking impairments and patients' opinion. Arch. Phys. Med. Rehabil. 90, 475–479.

Tyson, S.F., Thornton, H.A., 2001. The effect of a hinged ankle foot orthosis on hemiplegic gait: objective measures and users' opinions. Clin. Rehabil. 15, 53–58.

Van Peppen, R.P.S., Kortsmit, M., Lindeman, E., et al., 2006. Effects of Visual Feedback Therapy on Postural Control in Bilateral Standing after Stroke: A Systematic Review. J. Rehabil. Med. 38, 3–9.

Vattanaslip, W., Ada, L., Crosbie, J., 2000. Contribution of thixotrophy, spasticity, and contracture to ankle stiffness after stroke. J. Neurol. Neurosurg. Psychiatry 69, 34–39.

Wade, D.T., 1992. Measurement in neurological rehabilitation. Oxford University Press, Oxford.

Watson, M.J., Crosby, P., Matthew, M., 2007. An evaluation of the effects of a dynamic lycra splint orthoses on arm function in a late stage patient with acquired brain injury. Brain Inj. 21, 753–761.

White, L.J., Dressendorfer, R.H., 2004. Exercise and Multiple Sclerosis. Sports Med. 34, 1077–1100.

Wiles, C.M., Newcombe, R.G., Fuller, K.J., et al., 2003. Use of videotape to assess mobility in a controlled randomized crossover trial of physiotherapy in chronic multiple sclerosis. Clin. Rehabil. 17, 256–263.

Williams, P.E., 1990. Use of intermittent stretch in the prevention of serial sarcomere loss in immobilised muscle. Ann. Rheum. Dis. 49, 3–16.

Woodford, H., Price, C., 2007. EMG biofeedback for the recovery of motor function after stroke. Cochrane Database Syst. Rev. (2), CD004585.

World Health Organization, 2001. International Classification of Functioning and Disability. WHO, Geneva. Available online at http:/www.who.int/classification/icf.

Wu, H.M., Tang, J.L., Lin, X.P., et al., 2006. Acupuncture for stroke rehabilitation. Cochrane Database Syst. Rev. (3), CD004131.

Zhang, S.H., Liu, M., Asplund, K., et al., 2005. Acupuncture for acute stroke. Cochrane Database Syst. Rev. (2), CD003317.

Chapter | **15** |

Respiratory management in neurological rehabilitation

Anne Bruton

INTRODUCTON

Respiratory problems are not confined to respiratory patients. Every patient has the potential to develop respiratory dysfunction. This is particularly true for patients with neurological disorders. As well as problems with reduced central drive or neuromuscular weakness associated with pathology and trauma, many neurological patients are susceptible to respiratory infections through immobility or aspiration (see Table 15.1). As respiratory dysfunction can be life-threatening, it makes sense for every physiotherapist to be competent to conduct an assessment of the respiratory system, to be aware of the common problems with which patients present, and to have a basic toolkit of interventions designed to manage such problems. This chapter will cover the areas of respiratory assessment, problem recognition and respiratory physiotherapy management in neurological patients.

RESPIRATORY ASSESSMENT

A comprehensive respiratory assessment as outlined in Box 15.1 is only possible in a patient in a stable situation. If any 'red flags' are noticed (see Box 15.2), the assessment may need to be adapted and shortened. Although it is generally recognized that neurological disease may result in respiratory dysfunction, its presentation in such patients may be atypical, because of wider effects of the underlying condition (Polkey et al., 1999). The tests starred (*) in Box 15.1 will now be described further in relation to neurological patients.

Arterial blood gases

Arterial blood gas (ABG) sampling is performed to obtain accurate measures of arterial oxygen (PaO_2), arterial carbon dioxide ($PaCO_2$), and blood acidity/alkalinity (pH); these variables combined with body temperature allow for calculation of bicarbonate (HCO_3) and arterial oxygen saturation (SaO_2). Both PaO_2 and $PaCO_2$ can be affected by respiratory muscle weakness. Mild weakness leads to slight hypoxaemia (low oxygen, i.e. PaO_2 <8 kPa/<60 mmHg)

Table 15.1 Clinical course for some neurological conditions commonly associated with respiratory problems

DISORDER	CLINICAL COURSE	PREVALENCE OF RESPIRATORY INVOLVEMENT
CNS		
Multiple sclerosis	Relapsing	Pulmonary function impaired in 63%; respiratory failure or infection causes death in 5%
Parkinson's disease	Slowly progressive	Pneumonia accounts for 20% of deaths, possibly from bulbar or upper airway muscle involvement and impaired cough
Spinal cord		
Trauma	Permanent	High lesions (C1–3) usually require long-term ventilation
Motor neurone		
Postpolio syndrome	Very slowly progressive	Respiratory impairment usually only in those with initial respiratory muscle involvement
Motor neurone disease	Progressive	Death almost uniformly due to respiratory complications
Motor nerves		
Guillain-Barré syndrome	Slowly reversible	Respiratory failure in 28%
Charcot–Marie–Tooth	Very slowly progressive	96–100% have prolonged phrenic nerve conduction; 30% have vital capacity <80% predicted
Neuromuscular junction		
Myasthenia gravis	Reversible	Aspiration pneumonia gives rise to crises with 6% mortality
Botulism	Slowly reversible	8% mortality due to respiratory failure
Muscle		
Duchenne muscular dystrophy	Progressive	Respiratory failure is major cause of death

(Adapted from Aboussouan 2005, with permission.)

Box 15.1 **Elements of a respiratory assessment**

General end-of-bed observations:
Breathing pattern, cyanosis, distress, accessory muscle use, swallowing, speech pattern, posture.

History (from patient/relatives/friends):
Past medical history, history of present complaint, recent symptoms (cough/sputum/chest tightness/breathlessness), smoking history, environmental exposures (pollution/occupational), family health history, travel history, social history, drug history.

Clinical examination:
Inspection – hands (finger clubbing, tremor, temperature); chest shape; breathing rate, depth, frequency, symmetry (left:right) and regularity; sputum (quantity, colour, smell); cough competence

Palpation checking for – tracheal centrality; chest pulsations/tenderness/depressions/bulges/movements/scars; tactile/vocal fremitus

Percussion – to detect chest resonance/dullness

Auscultation – to listen for presence/absence normal or added lung sounds.

Current general status:
Body temperature, blood pressure, pulse rate, fluid balance, blood chemistry, intracranial pressure.

Respiratory bedside/laboratory testing:
Chest X-rays/other imaging, sputum culture, arterial blood gases (ABGs)*, pulse oximetry and capnometry*, lung function tests (e.g. vital capacity)*, peak cough flow*, inspiratory/expiratory pressures* (mouth/sniff/transdiaphragmatic).

*Tests described in text (see page 319, 'Respiratory Assessments')

and hypocapnia (low carbon dioxide, i.e. $PaCO_2 < 4.7$ kPa/<35 mmHg); severe weakness causes hypercapnia (high carbon dioxide, i.e. $PaCO_2 > 6$kPa/>45 mmHg), but only when muscle strength is $<40\%$ predicted (ATS 2002). However, ABG derangement is a late feature in neuromuscular disease, so normal results are compatible with significant weakness of the respiratory muscles (Hutchinson & Whyte, 2008). Patients with established respiratory failure from neuromuscular weakness will show hypoxaemia and a compensated respiratory acidosis (raised $PaCO_2$ and HCO_3 with a normal or mildly reduced pH).

Pulse oximetry and capnometry

Pulse oximetry and capnometry provide non-invasive measures of blood oxygenation and alveolar carbon dioxide. Transcutaneous pulse oximetry estimates oxygen saturation (SpO_2) of *capillary* blood, based on the absorption of light from light-emitting diodes positioned in a finger clip or adhesive strip probe. SpO_2 indicates the oxygen bound to haemoglobin, while PaO_2 indicates the oxygen dissolved in the plasma. Normal SpO_2 is 95–98%, but patients with very low levels of haemoglobin (normal $=11$–18 g/dl) can have 100% saturation. Pulse oximetry can help to identify problems such as atelectasis and pneumonia; however, it only measures oxygenation, not ventilation. It is possible to have normal oxygen saturation while carbon dioxide is rising. Capnometry measures carbon dioxide at the end of expiration, known as end-tidal carbon dioxide ($ETCO_2$). It is expressed as a percentage or in kPa/mmHg. In patients with normal lungs and normal ventilation/perfusion ratios, $ETCO_2$ equates to $PaCO_2$. Normal values are around 5–6%, which equates to 4.7–6.0 kPa (35–45 mmHg). Both pulse oximetry and capnometry permit continuous monitoring

(e.g. overnight). This can be useful because patients with respiratory muscle weakness may develop nocturnal hypoventilation, leading to elevated carbon dioxide levels not initially detectable during the day.

Vital capacity

Vital capacity (VC) is the volume change at the mouth between full inspiration and complete expiration (see Figure 15.1). VC can be measured using conventional spirometers or recorded from equipment used to measure static lung volumes and their subdivisions. Guidelines for measurement have been published by the American Thoracic Society/European Respiratory Society task force (Wanger et al., 2005).

Ideally, the VC manoeuvre is performed with the patient using a mouthpiece and wearing a nose clip. In patients with neuromuscular weakness, assistance may be required to provide a seal around the mouthpiece, or a facemask may be substituted. It is important that patients understand they must completely fill and empty their lungs. The largest value from at least three acceptable manoeuvres (with a rest of ≥ 1 minute between manoeuvres) is used.

Normal values are calculated from the patient's age, height and gender. A normal VC, with no significant fall when supine, means that respiratory muscle weakness is unlikely. However, muscle weakness in conditions such as myasthenia gravis can fluctuate significantly. Generally, it is only when muscle force is reduced to less than 50% of predicted that a decrease in VC can be observed. A fall in VC by more than 15–20% when the patient lies supine specifically suggests weakness of the diaphragm.

In *acute* neuromuscular disorders the VC and oxygen saturation should be rechecked at frequent intervals. A VC <1 L in an adult (<15 mL/kg), a fall in VC by more than 50% on serial testing, or onset of bulbar palsy are

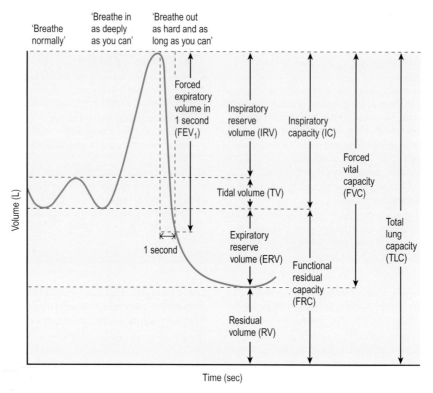

'Breathe normally'

'Breathe in as deeply as you can'

'Breathe out as hard and as long as you can'

Forced expiratory volume in 1 second (FEV₁)

Inspiratory reserve volume (IRV)

Inspiratory capacity (IC)

Forced vital capacity (FVC)

Tidal volume (TV)

Total lung capacity (TLC)

1 second

Expiratory reserve volume (ERV)

Functional residual capacity (FRC)

Residual volume (RV)

Volume (L)

Time (sec)

Figure 15.1 Lung volumes and capacities in neurological disease. (From Aboussouan LF. Respiratory disorders in neurologic diseases. Cleve Clin J Med 2005; 72:511–520. Reprinted with permission. Copyright © 2005 Cleveland Clinic. All rights reserved.)

all indications to involve the intensive care unit (Hutchinson & White, 2008). In *chronic* neuromuscular disorders, monitoring can be less frequent, but a serial fall in VC (particularly a fall below 1.2–1.5 L or <40–50% of predicted) indicates a need for further respiratory assessment (Hutchinson & Whyte, 2008).

Peak cough flow

A normal cough requires the ability to generate sufficient inspiratory and expiratory power and a functional glottis. Ability to cough effectively is therefore compromised by either inspiratory or expiratory muscle weakness. However, expiratory muscle weakness has greater impact as mild to moderate expiratory muscle weakness can result in a weak cough, even if inspiration is normal (Boitano, 2006). In some neurological disorders, such as bulbar type motor neurone disease (MND; see Ch. 8), a functional glottis may be absent. Formal cough assessment requires the insertion of gastric balloons and is conducted in specialized laboratories, but cough strength can be assessed at the bedside using peak cough flow (PCF). PCF is a measure of maximal airflow generated during a cough manoeuvre. It provides a global indicator of cough strength that correlates well with the ability to clear secretions.

The recent joint guidelines from the British Thoracic Society (BTS) and Association of Chartered Physiotherapists in Respiratory Care for respiratory physiotherapy (Bott et al., 2009), include a guide for recording PCF in patients with neuromuscular weakness. It can be measured through either a mouthpiece or face mask attached to a peak flow meter and expressed in litres/minute or litres/second. The patient should be instructed to breathe in as deeply as possible and cough hard into the device. PCF is expected to be higher than peak expiratory flow, but in patients with bulbar dysfunction, this difference is not seen – potentially offering a way to monitor the onset of bulbar involvement (Boitano, 2006).

PCF is dependent on effort and lung volume, with cooperation being essential. The largest value from at least three acceptable attempts is usually recorded. Normal PCF is around 360 to 840 L/minute (Hutchinson & Whyte, 2008). Airway clearance becomes impaired and the risk of serious infection increases when PCF<160 L/minute, so in chronic progressive conditions, airway clearance techniques should be taught before these levels are approached (Tzeng & Bach, 2000). It has been suggested that any neuromuscular patients with a PCF<270 L/minute should be considered at risk of respiratory complications.

Inspiratory/expiratory pressures

Guidelines for testing the respiratory muscles have been published by the American Thoracic Society (2002). Inspiratory and expiratory pressures are recorded to assess respiratory muscle strength, but should be viewed as indices of global respiratory muscle output rather than as direct measures of their contractile properties (ATS, 2002). Mouth and nasal pressures can be recorded at the bedside using hand-held pressure meters. These volitional bedside tests are simple, portable and inexpensive; but their accuracy and reliability has been questioned because of their dependence on maximal effort and their significant learning effect. Non-volitional tests such as phrenic nerve stimulation are more reliable, but are expensive and confined to specialist centres.

Measurement of the maximum static inspiratory pressure generated at the mouth (PImax), or the maximum static expiratory pressure (PEmax), are the classic volitional tests of respiratory muscle strength. PImax can be more sensitive to respiratory muscle weakness than VC, because decreases in respiratory muscle strength occur before decreases in lung volume can be identified.

Patients are normally seated and noseclips are not required. Careful instruction and encouraged motivation are essential. Measurements require maximal inspiratory or expiratory efforts against a quasi occlusion. The pressure must be maintained for at least 1.5 seconds, so that the maximum pressure sustained for 1 second can be recorded. The maximum value of three manoeuvres that vary by less than 20% is usually recorded, but some authors have recommended that more measures are needed to reach a true maximum, and even low variability between measures may not guarantee that maximal efforts have been made (Aldrich & Spiro, 1995). Although simple in principle, the manoeuvres are difficult for many patients and require a good seal around the mouthpiece. Low values may therefore be due to true muscle weakness, or a submaximal effort, or air leaks, e.g. in the case of facial muscle weakness. The sniff is an alternative manoeuvre that is more natural and easier for most patients (see section on Sniff test).

The normal ranges for PImax and PEmax are wide, so that values in the lower quarter of the normal range are compatible both with normal strength and with mild or moderate weakness. In adults a PImax of more than 80 cmH$_2$O in males, or 70 cmH$_2$O in females, excludes clinically significant respiratory muscle weakness (Hutchinson & Whyte, 2008).

Sniff test

A sniff is a short, sharp voluntary inspiratory manoeuvre involving contraction of the diaphragm and other inspiratory muscles. Sniff nasal inspiratory pressure (SNIP) has been proposed as a volitional, non-invasive measure of inspiratory muscle strength. Peak nasal pressure is measured in one occluded nostril during a maximal sniff, performed from relaxed end-expiration through the other open nostril. Portable commercial systems are available for measuring SNIP at the bedside. Patients should be encouraged to make maximal efforts, with a rest between sniffs. Most patients achieve a plateau within 5–10 attempts. A sniff test is not suitable in patients with nasal congestion, which leads to falsely low values (Fitting, 2006). The sniff is easily performed by most patients, requires little practice and is relatively reproducible. It is therefore a useful voluntary test for evaluating diaphragm strength in the clinical setting, giving equal or greater pressures than PImax. However, SNIP and PImax are not interchangeable and should be considered as complementing one another for the assessment of inspiratory muscle strength.

There are reference values for SNIP in adults (Uldry & Fitting, 1995) and children (Rafferty et al., 2000). Surprisingly, SNIP is similar in children and adults, despite a large difference in respiratory muscle mass. Values of maximal SNIP greater than 70 cmH$_2$O (males) or 60 cmH$_2$O (females) are unlikely to be associated with significant inspiratory muscle weakness (Hutchinson & Whyte, 2008). The SNIP test appears particularly suited to neuromuscular weakness because it obviates the use of a mouthpiece and because it is easily mastered by most patients. However, assessment of severe muscle weakness should not rely on SNIP alone, but should include other tests such as PImax, vital capacity, nocturnal oximetry or ABGs (Fitting, 2006).

RESPIRATORY PROBLEMS ASSOCIATED WITH NEUROLOGICAL CONDITIONS

At a simplistic level, the mechanics of the respiratory system function as a pump to drive air into the body, analogous to the heart pumping blood around the body. The four essential elements of the pump are intact central neurological drive, neural pathways, thoracic cage and respiratory muscles. The respiratory system is only effective when there is a balance between the load on the system and the capacity of the respiratory pump to overcome this load (Polkey et al., 1995). Respiratory load is determined by the lung, thoracic and airway mechanics; respiratory capacity is the neuromusculoskeletal competence. Problems arise either from an increase in load (e.g. excessive secretions or bronchoconstriction) or from a decrease in capacity (e.g. neuromuscular pathology) or from a combination of both. Common relevant neurological problems are reduced airway protection and respiratory muscle weakness:

- Reduced airway protection (through reduced consciousness or bulbar/upper airway weakness) –

Table 15.2 Primary respiratory muscles and their level of innervations

RESPIRATORY MUSCLES	SPINAL LEVEL
Sternomastoids	C1–C3
Diaphragm	C3–C5
Scalenes	C3–C8
Parasternal intercostals	T1–T5
Interosseus intercostals	T1–T11
External/internal abdominal obliques	T6–T12
Transversus abdominis	T7–L1

may lead to aspiration and/or infection, which in turn can lead to *breathlessness/dyspnoea, sputum retention* and *atelectasis* (literally 'airlessness', collapse of lung tissue preventing alveolar gas exchange)

- Respiratory muscle weakness (see Table 15.2) or fatigue (through original pathology, immobility or acquired disorders) – may lead to inability to ventilate and/or inability to cough which in turn can lead to *breathlessness/dyspnoea, sputum retention, atelectasis, hypoventilation* (inadequate ventilation, often related to reduced rate or depth of respiration) and *respiratory failure.*

Some of these problems will be discussed further in the next section on physiotherapy management.

Physiotherapy management of specific problems

Problem 1: Breathlessness/dyspnoea

Dyspnoea occurs with mismatching of muscular effort relative to ventilation. It is a subjective sensation that is poorly related to objective tests of respiratory function. Dyspnoea occurs in airways obstruction, increased neural effort relative to muscular function (as occurs in neuromuscular weakness), and excessive breathing response relative to metabolic demand. Dyspnoea can be an unreliable symptom, but marked dyspnoea only when lying flat is typical of isolated diaphragm paralysis, as is breathlessness on immersion in water.

Once any treatable cause for breathlessness has been identified, appropriate action by the multidisciplinary team needs to be taken to relieve that cause where practicable (e.g. antibiotics for a respiratory infection, chest drain for pneumothorax). Symptom relief can be achieved through physiotherapy management of the breathless patient as described in Hough (2001). Techniques in

current physiotherapy practice include: positioning, relaxation and various forms of breathing retraining (e.g. pursed lip breathing, Papworth breathing, Buteyko breathing) as well as complementary therapies such as acupuncture; however, there is a lack of evidence for effectiveness of any of these techniques in neurological patients. An overview of dyspnoea in neurological conditions has recently been published (Murtagh et al., 2006).

Oxygen therapy for dyspnoea

Even in patients with primary respiratory conditions, the use of oxygen to relieve breathlessness is controversial. In patients with neuromuscular weakness, although low flow oxygen is commonly prescribed and may relieve some symptoms and hypoxia, it usually results in a further increase in arterial CO_2 and may therefore aggravate other symptoms. It should therefore be avoided or used with *extreme caution* in this group (Bott et al., 2009).

Problem 2: Sputum retention and atelectasis

In patients with neurological disorders, an ineffective cough is the main reason for sputum retention. Recent evidence-based guidelines on airway clearance techniques gave 10 recommendations for various patient populations (McCool & Rosen, 2006). However, only three of these recommendations related specifically to patients with neuromuscular weakness (i.e. manual cough assist (MCA), mechanical cough assist and expiratory muscle strength training) and none were supported by any robust evidence (Haas et al., 2007).

Box 15.3 provides the indicators of atelectasis or respiratory infection. Airway clearance therapy can be divided into techniques: to augment inspiration, to augment expiration/cough, and to mobilize/remove secretions (see Box 15.4 for a list of techniques in common clinical use).

Augmenting inspiration

Inspiration can be augmented through thoracic expansion exercises in those who can perform them voluntarily, or by 'air stacking' which can be achieved under volition by glossopharyngeal breathing (see Bott et al., 2009 for a description), or by the use of a manual resuscitator bag or ventilator. Its effectiveness depends on ability to

---

Box 15.3 **Indicators of atelectasis or infection**

Rising	Falling
Temperature	Vital capacity
Pulse rate	Peak cough flow
Anxiety	
Secretion quantity/viscosity	
Breathlessness	

Box 15.4 Techniques for managing sputum retention and/or atelectasis

Abdominal binder	Intrapulmonary percussive
Active cycle of	ventilation
breathing	Manual hyperinflation and
techniques	suction (intubated patients)
Assisted cough	Manual physiotherapy
Autogenic drainage	techniques
BiPAP/CPAP/IPPB*	Nebulizers/humidifiers
Bronchoscopy	Physical exercise
ELTGOL**	Positioning/postural drainage
Glossopharyngeal	Positive pressure devices (e.g.
breathing	PEP mask)
Incentive spirometry	Respiratory muscle training
In-exsufflator	Suction

*Bilevel positive airways pressure, continuous positive airways pressure, intermittent positive pressure breathing
**Slow expiration with the glottis open in a lateral posture known as ELTGOL (from the French: Expiration Lent Totale avec la Glotte Ouverte in infraLateral)

achieve glottis closure (Gauld, 2009). The aim is to increase volume so that expiratory flow can be increased and a cough is more effective. No barotrauma or complications have ever been reported from air stacking.

Augmenting expiration/cough

This can be achieved through forced expiratory techniques in those who can perform them or through MCA, mechanical cough assist using an in-exsufflator (which augments both inspiration and expiration), or expiratory muscle training. These are described below.

Manual cough assist

This involves using an abdominal thrust or a thoracic compression to augment the patient's own cough – usually after augmented inspiration. The abdominal thrust is like a well-known manoeuvre to prevent choking, the Heimlich manoeuvre (Heimlich, 1975), which involves an upward thrust below the ribcage, so this technique should not be performed if the patient has a full stomach. Many patients prefer a thoracic squeeze, but its effectiveness is limited if there is decreased chest wall compliance, as is common in Duchenne muscular dystrophy (DMD; see Ch. 10) and scoliosis. When performing an abdominal thrust it is important to stabilize the chest wall and be careful not to injure abdominal organs or cause gastric reflux (Finder et al., 2004). Various hand placements can be used to provide costal lateral compression. Evidence for benefits of MCA is not high level, but it has consistently been found to increase peak cough flow. Its use is limited by severe scoliosis, orthopaedic or abdominal abnormalities, abdominal surgery, or the presence of

abdominal/pelvic catheters. MCA should not be used in patients with Greenfield filters (filter in inferior vena cava to prevent pulmonary emboli) (Boitano, 2006). Recent research has reported that best cough improvement results from a combination of breathstacking plus MCA and that most benefit is derived by patients with VC >340 mL and PEmax < 34 cmH$_2$O, but that MCA seems to interfere with spontaneous cough in patients with stronger cough and PEmax >34 cmH$_2$O (Toussaint et al., 2009).

Mechanical cough assist (insufflation-exsufflation)

Devices such as the CoughAssist (Figure 15.2) provide mechanical insufflation-exsufflation (MIE) via a face mask and promote maximum lung inflation during inspiration with the use of positive pressure. A normal cough is simulated when inflation is followed by an abrupt switch to negative pressure in the upper airway. The device can also be used in patients with tracheostomy or endotracheal tubes.

MIE is indicated when inspiratory, expiratory and bulbar muscles are dysfunctional, but the latter are not completely paralysed and glottic closure is still possible (as is the case for most patients with neuromuscular diseases). Potential contraindications include a history of bullous emphysema (abnormal increase in size of air spaces arising from destruction of airway walls), susceptibility to pneumothorax (air in the pleural space causing collapse of lung tissue), or recent pulmonary barotrauma (damage to the lung from rapid or excessive pressure changes). If bulbar function is intact, MIE is not needed because cough flow can be greatly increased by abdominal thrusts following air stacking. MIE has been in use for secretion clearance since its first description in 1954. Despite increasing acceptance for airway clearance in

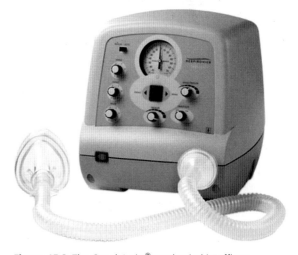

Figure 15.2 The CoughAssist® mechanical insufflator-exsufflator. Photograph reproduced with kind permission from Philips Respironics.

patients with neuromuscular disease, there remains a lack of agreement on settings, with pressure settings ranging from 15 cmH$_2$O to 45 cmH$_2$O (insufflation and exsufflation pressures). Fauroux et al. (2008) demonstrated greater efficacy at higher settings (up to peak pressures of 45 cmH$_2$O). During periods of acute illness the settings may need to change as lung mechanics change (Finder et al., 2004). Bach (2003) believes that mechanical insufflation/exsufflation is critical for avoiding hospitalizations, pneumonias, episodes of respiratory failure, and tracheostomy for patients with DMD, spinal muscular atrophy, and non-bulbar ALS.

Expiratory muscle training (see Respiratory muscle training section)

Mobilizing/removing secretions

In patients with neurological disorders manual physiotherapy techniques may be impossible due to chest wall or spinal deformities, or osteoporosis (Haas et al., 2007). Research in this group has focused on using mechanical devices such as the intrapulmonary percussive ventilator (IPV) or high frequency chest wall oscillator/compressor (HFCWO/C). HFCWO/C is administered via an external device (a commercially available vest) that delivers rapid small compressions to the thorax and generates high flows in small airways, to mobilize secretions from smaller airways to larger airways. Results for the use of HFCWO/C in neurological conditions have been inconsistent, so that although the technique is well tolerated and may be beneficial in some patients, it is not possible to recommend its use at present. IPV vibrates the airways internally, via the mouth, while the patient breathes spontaneously. Insufficient research has been conducted to judge its value in patients with neurological disorders. According to Haas (2007) when faced with a neurological patient with problems clearing secretions, and trying to choose which therapy to apply, the physiotherapist should ask four questions:

- Is there a pathophysiological rationale for using this therapy?
- What is the potential for adverse effects?
- What is the cost of the equipment needed?
- What are the patient's preferences?

Problem 3: Hypoventilation

Hypoventilation occurs when ventilation is reduced, so it does not match the patient's rate of oxygen consumption and carbon dioxide production, resulting in hypercapnia. Hypoventilation may be secondary to several mechanisms, including central respiratory drive depression, neuromuscular disorders, chest wall abnormalities, obesity hypoventilation and chronic obstructive pulmonary disease (COPD). Neuromuscular diseases that can cause

> **Box 15.5 Common signs and symptoms of respiratory muscle weakness/fatigue**
>
> - Unexplained breathlessness – disproportionate on exercise, worse on immersion in water, worse/only in supine
> - Ineffective cough – unable to clear secretions, repeated chest infections
> - Poor chest expansion – may be bilateral or unilateral
> - Abnormal breathing rate – may be fast or slow
> - Use of accessory muscles at rest
> - Abnormal movement of ribcage and abdomen – lack of normal synchronicity
> - Mental confusion or somnolence – due to arterial blood gas derangement.

alveolar hypoventilation include myasthenia gravis, MND, Guillain-Barré syndrome, and muscular dystrophy. Central respiratory drive is maintained in patients with neuromuscular disorders, so hypoventilation is secondary to respiratory muscle weakness in these patients.

In the absence of significant respiratory muscle weakness, it may be possible to correct hypoventilation through strategies such as positioning to improve diaphragm mechanics, thoracic expansion exercises, respiratory muscle training or general physical exercise. In patients with significant respiratory muscle weakness, some form of non-invasive ventilation is often recommended – see section on respiratory failure below. Box 15.5 provides the signs and symptoms of respiratory muscle weakness or fatigue. Paradoxical (inward) inspiratory movement of the abdominal wall signifies respiratory strength reduced to at least about 30% of normal (Polkey et al., 1999).

Respiratory muscle training

The respiratory muscles are physiologically, structurally and biochemically similar to other skeletal muscles, and it is therefore generally accepted that they will respond to appropriate strength and endurance training programmes in a similar manner (see Ch. 18). The controversy surrounds the issue of whether an increase in respiratory muscle strength or endurance confers any significant health benefit. There are a number of commercial devices available, but as with skeletal muscle training, there is a lack of consensus as to the optimal training programme (i.e. load, repetitions, frequency).

Although RMT has been studied extensively in some respiratory conditions, there is currently little evidence for use in patients with neurological conditions beyond spinal cord injury (SCI; see Ch. 4). According to a recent systematic review by Sheel et al. (2008), there are insufficient data to recommend the use of either exercise training or inspiratory muscle training for improved respiratory function in people with SCI. From another systematic review by Van Houtte et al. (2006) it was concluded that respiratory muscle training in SCI tended to improve *expiratory* muscle strength, vital capacity and residual volume. Insufficient data were available to make conclusions concerning the effects on *inspiratory* muscle strength, respiratory muscle endurance, quality of life, exercise performance or respiratory complications.

There is some limited evidence of benefit from the use of RMT in multiple sclerosis (MS; see Ch. 5) and DMD and currently a Cochrane review by Eagle and Chatwin (2006) is underway (online protocol updated 14/01/2009), which aims to assess the benefit and risk of RMT in children and adults with neuromuscular disease.

Problem 4: Respiratory failure

Acute respiratory failure

Acute respiratory failure has many causes and develops over minutes to hours. It is characterized by changes in ABGs and acid–base status and there are two types:

- Type I or hypoxaemic respiratory failure – a PaO_2 of <8 kPa (60 mmHg) with normal or low $PaCO_2$
- Type II or ventilatory/hypercapnic respiratory failure – a $PaCO_2$ of >6.7 kPa (50 mmHg) usually accompanied by a fall in pH <7.3, in addition to hypoxaemia.

Guillain-Barré and myasthenia gravis account for the majority of cases of acute respiratory failure associated with neuromuscular disease in the developed world (Mehta, 2006). To avoid emergency intubation and ventilation it is essential to monitor patients regularly for signs and symptoms of impending failure (see Box 15.6).

Chronic respiratory failure

Chronic respiratory failure associated with neuromuscular disease develops over several days or weeks and may initially have few symptoms. A history of fatigue, lethargy, difficulty concentrating, poor sleep and daytime sleepiness, and morning headache (indicating hypercapnia) suggest possible chronic ventilatory failure. Neuromuscular conditions in which this type of respiratory failure occurs in the late stages include muscular dystrophy, MND, MS, other progressive neuropathies and myopathies, and spinal cord injury (tetraplegia).

Management of respiratory failure

The management of respiratory failure will primarily be medical as invasive mechanical ventilation may be required and if the patient has impaired bulbar or upper airway muscle function a tracheostomy is likely to be needed. See the section on care of the brain injured patient for more information on physiotherapy during invasive ventilation.

Non-invasive ventilation

In some institutions non invasive ventilation (NIV) is managed by physiotherapists. NIV is effective in providing intermittent, often nocturnal, support in various neuromuscular diseases and should be considered the standard of care for patients with MND who develop respiratory muscle weakness with PImax of <60% predicted or hypercapnia (Lechtzin, 2006). It is inappropriate for acute respiratory failure unless upper airway function is well

---

Box 15.6 **Signs and symptoms of *impending* acute respiratory failure in neuromuscular disease**

General warning signs

Increasing generalized weakness

Dysphagia

Dysarthria

Dyspnoea on exertion and at rest

Impaired gag reflex

Rapid progression of symptoms

Subjective assessment

Rapid shallow breathing

Tachycardia

Weak cough

Inability to talk in complete sentences

Accessory muscle use

Abdominal paradox

Orthopnoea

Weakness of trapezius and neck muscles (inability to lift head)

Single breath count* <15

Cough after swallowing

Objective assessment

VC<20 mL/kg or serial VC drop by 30%**

PImax <30 cmH$_2$O

PEmax <40 cmH$_2$O

Nocturnal oxygen desaturation

Daytime hypercapnia (PaCO$_2$ >6 kPa /45 mmHg)

(Adapted from Mehta, 2006.)

*Performed by asking the patient to count after a maximal inspiratory effort. Normal = 50

**VC may be less reliable in myasthenia gravis due to fluctuating nature of disease

preserved (Mehta, 2006) and therefore there is limited evidence to support its use in Guillain-Barré or myasthenia gravis.

NIV can be delivered via volume limited or pressure limited ventilators. Volume limited units are used mainly for long-term invasive ventilation. Pressure limited ventilators often allow the setting of both inspiratory and expiratory pressures (i.e. bilevel). Pressures are set according to patient tolerance, but Boitano (2006) suggests that 'wide-span' bilevel airway pressure (BiPAP) support, in which the difference between inspiratory and expiratory pressures is $\geq$ 10 cmH$_2$O, most effectively augments ventilation. Typical pressures would, therefore, be approximately 12–14 cmH$_2$O for inspiration and 2–4 cmH$_2$O for expiration. A minimal expiratory pressure is better tolerated by patients with neuromuscular disease provided upper airway patency remains good during sleep. A spontaneous timed rate of 12–16 breaths per minute is necessary to provide back-up support during REM sleep when diaphragm weakness may preclude ability to trigger a breath. Interfaces vary, but nasal masks are the most common. Some patients with mouth weakness struggle to prevent air leakage around the mouth, in which case a chin strap or full face mask may be needed. If a mask fails to fit well or is too uncomfortable, a nose plug interface may be used, although this may not work as effectively. Hess (2006) has written a review of NIV equipment and its application in neuromuscular disease.

A Cochrane review into the use of nocturnal ventilation for hypoventilation in neuromuscular disorders has concluded that current evidence about any therapeutic benefit is weak, but consistent, suggesting alleviation of the symptoms of chronic hypoventilation in the short term. In three small studies survival was prolonged mainly in participants with MND. With the exception of MND, they recommended that further larger randomized trials are needed to confirm long-term beneficial effects of nocturnal mechanical ventilation on quality of life, morbidity and mortality, to assess its cost–benefit ratio in neuromuscular and chest wall diseases and to compare the different types and modes of ventilation (Annane et al., 2007).

RESPIRATORY PHYSIOTHERAPY MANAGEMENT POST BRAIN INJURY

Respiratory dysfunction is the most frequent medical complication in patients with brain injury (see Ch. 3). About 20–50% of neurosurgical patients develop pulmonary complications (such as aspiration of gastric contents or pneumonia), which significantly worsen neurological outcome and increase mortality. In traumatic brain injury the Brain Trauma Foundation (2000) recommends prevention of hypoxia by maintaining PaO2 >8 kPa (60

mmHg) and arterial oxygen saturation of greater than 90%. However, use of high levels of oxygen is not recommended and a SaO$_2$ of 91–94% is considered optimal in neurosurgical patients. In patients with brain injury PaO$_2$ is believed to be less important than brain tissue partial pressure (PbtO$_2$). Normal values for PbtO$_2$ are 2.13 kPa (16 mmHg) +/- 5.32 kPa (40 mmHg). A PbtO$_2$ <0.67 kPa (5 mmHg) is associated with severe brain injury and a low chance of brain survival.

Hypocapnia (low CO$_2$) is a potent cerebral vasoconstrictor, effectively reducing intracranial pressure (ICP), so short periods of hyperventilation to induce hypocapnia to PaCO$_2$ of 4.66 kPa (35 mmHg), and even of 3.33 kPa (25 mmHg) may be used acutely in the treatment of increased ICP (Rozet & Domino, 2007). However, hypocapnia may exacerbate brain ischaemia in patients with brain injury, although the degree of ischaemia remains controversial. It is suggested that lowering the PaCO$_2$ produces vasoconstriction of the blood vessels, thus reducing blood flow and, ultimately, brain oxygen delivery.

The goals of respiratory management in brain injury patients are therefore to attain normocapnia and prevent hypoxia. The same physiotherapy techniques described earlier may be used to achieve these goals in a spontaneously breathing patient, but invasive mechanical ventilation will frequently be needed (see Box 15.7).

Management of brain injury patients requiring invasive ventilation

Care of the ventilated patient with brain injury is a complex area, and respiratory physiotherapy will be aimed primarily at minimizing secretion retention, maximizing oxygenation, and re-expanding atelectatic lung segments. Techniques include those already described with the addition of more specialized techniques such as manual hyperinflation, suction and rotational therapy (see Stiller, 2000 for a full description). Some patients will require a

---

Box 15.7 **Indicators of need for intubation/ ventilation in the neurosurgical patient**

- Inability to protect the airway or clear secretions
- Need to reduce ICP by control of ventilation
- PaO$_2$ <8 kPa (60 mmHg) in spite of supplemental oxygen (by mask)
- PaCO$_2$ >6.67 kPa (50 mmHg), and /or pH <7.2
- Respiratory rate >40/minute or <10/minute
- Muscle fatigue
- Haemodynamic instability

(Adapted from Rozet & Domino, 2007.)

tracheostomy, the detailed management of which is described in Jones and Moffatt (2002). A tracheostomy is a surgical procedure to create a direct airway through an opening in the trachea which facilitates secretion removal and protects the airway. It may be carried out for patients requiring prolonged invasive ventilation or for patients breathing spontaneously. It is therefore possible for a tracheostomy to remain in situ after a patient has been weaned from invasive ventilation. Physiotherapists are frequently involved with decisions relating to timing of weaning from mechanical ventilation and removal of tracheostomy tubes.

According to Olson et al. (2007) aggressive respiratory care in brain injury patients who require ventilation is essential to promote recovery without respiratory complications. However, although there is comparatively strong evidence for physiotherapy as the treatment of choice in acute lobar atelectasis, the evidence for the role of the physiotherapist in preventing respiratory complications (rather than treating them), is less strong. The need to avoid excessive stimulation of patients at risk of intracranial hypertension is often cited as a reason for avoiding some techniques in these patients, but there is a lack of conclusive evidence supporting the hypothesis that the techniques negatively impact ICP (Olson et al., 2007). Sogame et al. (2008) recommend daily respiratory physiotherapy and the use of a protocol to optimize early ventilator withdrawal for all ventilated neurosurgical patients. Recent guidelines for physiotherapy in the critically ill have been published (Gosselink et al., 2008), however their recommendations are not specific to brain injury patients, for whom minimal handling may be best practice. When managing a brain-injured patient via mechanical ventilation, the physiotherapist must make a clinical judgement based on the balance between potential positive and negative effects of interventions.

REFERENCES

Aboussouan, L.S., 2005. Respiratory disorders in neurologic diseases. Cleveland Clinic Journal of Medicine 72 (6), 511–520.

Aldrich, T.K., Spiro, P., 1995. Maximal inspiratory pressure: does reproducibility indicate full effort? Thorax 50, 40–43.

Annane, D., Orlikowski, D., Chevret, S., et al., 2007. Nocturnal mechanical ventilation for chronic hypoventilation in patients with neuromuscular and chest wall disorders. Cochrane Database Syst. Rev. (4) CD001941.

ATS, 2002. ATS/ERS Statement on respiratory muscle testing. Am. J. Respir. Crit. Care Med. 166 (4), 518–624.

Bach, J.R., 2003. Mechanical insufflation/exsufflation: has it come of age? A commentary. Eur. Respir. J. 21 (3), 385–386.

Boitano, L.J., 2006. Management of airway clearance in neuromuscular disease. Respir. Care 51 (8), 913–922.

Bott, J., Blumenthal, S., Buxton, M., et al., 2009. Guidelines for the physiotherapy management of the adult, medical, spontaneously breathing patient. Thorax 64 (Suppl. 1), i1–i51.

The Brain Trauma Foundation. The American Association of Neurological Surgeons. The Joint Section on Neurotrauma and Critical Care, 2000. Resuscitation of blood pressure and oxygenation. J. Neurotrauma 17 (6–7), 471–478.

Eagle, M., Chatwin, M., 2006. Respiratory muscle training in children and adults with neuromuscular disease (Protocol). Cochrane Database Syst. Rev. (3) CD006155. DOI:10.1002/14651858.CD006155.

Fauroux, B., Guillemot, N., Aubertin, G., et al., 2008. Physiologic benefits of mechanical insufflation-exsufflation in children with neuromuscular diseases. Chest 133 (1), 161–168.

Finder, J.D., Birnkrant, D., Carl, J., et al., 2004. Respiratory care of the patient with Duchenne muscular dystrophy: ATS consensus statement. Am. J. Respir. Crit. Care Med. 170 (4), 456–465.

Fitting, J.W., 2006. Sniff nasal inspiratory pressure: simple or too simple? Eur. Respir. J. 27 (5), 881–883.

Gauld, L.M., 2009. Airway clearance in neuromuscular weakness. Dev. Med. Child. Neurol.

Gosselink, R., Bott, J., Johnson, M., et al., 2008. Physiotherapy for adult patients with critical illness: recommendations of the European Respiratory Society and European Society of Intensive Care Medicine Task Force on Physiotherapy for Critically Ill Patients. Intensive Care Med. 34 (7), 1188–1199.

Haas, C.F., Loik, P.S., Gay, S.E., 2007. Airway clearance applications in the elderly and in patients with neurologic or neuromuscular compromise. Respir. Care 52 (10), 1362–1381.

Heimlich, H.J., 1975. A life-saving maneuver to prevent food-choking. JAMA 234 (4), 398–401.

Hess, D.R., 2006. Noninvasive ventilation in neuromuscular disease: equipment and application. Respir. Care 51 (8), 896–911.

Hough, A., 2001. Physiotherapy in Respiratory Care: an evidence-based approach to respiratory and cardiac management: A problem-solving approach. Nelson Thornes, Cheltenham, UK.

Hutchinson, D., Whyte, K., 2008. Neuromuscular disease and respiratory failure Practical Neurology 8, 229–237.

Jones, M., Moffatt, F., 2002. Cardiopulmonary physiotherapy. Informa Healthcare .

Lechtzin, N., 2006. Respiratory effects of amyotrophic lateral sclerosis: problems and solutions. Respir. Care 51 (8), 871–881.

McCool, F.D., Rosen, M.J., 2006. Nonpharmacologic airway clearance therapies: ACCP evidence-based clinical practice guidelines. Chest 129 (Suppl. 1), 250S–259S.

Mehta, S., 2006. Neuromuscular disease causing acute respiratory failure. Respir. Care 51 (9), 1016–1021.

Murtagh, F., Burman, R., Edmonds, P., 2006. Breathlessness in neurological conditions. In: Booth, S., Dudgeon, D. (Eds.), Dyspnoea in advanced disease. A guide to clinical management. Oxford University Press, Oxford, pp. 99–112.

Olson, D.M., Thoyre, S.M., Turner, D.A., et al., 2007. Changes in intracranial pressure associated with chest physiotherapy. Neurocrit. Care 6 (2), 100–103.

Polkey, M.I., Lyall, R.A., Moxham, J., et al., 1999. Respiratory aspects of neurological disease. J. Neurol. Neurosurg. Psychiatry 66 (1), 5–15.

Polkey, M.I., Green, M., Moxham, J., 1995. Measurement of respiratory muscle strength. Thorax 50, 1131–1135.

Rafferty, G.F., Leech, S., Knight, L., et al., 2000. Sniff nasal inspiratory pressure in children. Pediatr. Pulmonol. 29 (6), 468–475.

Rozet, I., Domino, K.B., 2007. Respiratory care. Best Pract. Res. Clin. Anaesthesiol. 21 (4), 465–482.

Sheel, A.W., Reid, W.D., Townson, A.F., et al., 2008. Effects of exercise training and inspiratory muscle training in spinal cord injury: a systematic review. J. Spinal Cord Med. 31 (5), 500–508.

Sogame, L.C., Vidotto, M.C., Jardim, J.R., et al., 2008. Incidence and risk factors for postoperative pulmonary complications in elective intracranial surgery. J. Neurosurg. 109 (2), 222–227.

Stiller, K., 2000. Physiotherapy in intensive care: towards an evidence-based practice. Chest 118 (6), 1801–1813.

Toussaint, M., Boitano, L.J., Gathot, V., et al., 2009. Limits of effective cough-augmentation techniques in patients with neuromuscular disease. Respir. Care 54 (3), 359–366.

Tzeng, A.C., Bach, J.R., 2000. Prevention of pulmonary morbidity for patients with neuromuscular disease. Chest 118 (5), 1390–1396.

Uldry, C., Fitting, J.W., 1995. Maximal values of sniff nasal inspiratory pressure in healthy subjects. Thorax 50 (4), 371–375.

Van Houtte, S., Vanlandewijck, Y., Gosselink, R., 2006. Respiratory muscle training in persons with spinal cord injury: a systematic review. Respir. Med. 100 (11), 1886–1895.

Wanger, J., Clausen, J.L., Coates, A., et al., 2005. Standardisation of the measurement of lung volumes. Eur. Respir. J. 26 (3), 511–522.

Chapter | **16** |

Pain management in neurological rehabilitation

Paul Watson

CONTENTS

INTRODUCTION

Neuropathic pain is defined as 'Pain arising as a direct consequence of a lesion or disease affecting the somatosensory system' (Treede et al., 2008). It is commonly seen following specific trauma to a nerve following injury or surgery but this chapter will focus mainly on the pain which develops as a result of neurological conditions. However, as the pathophysiology is often common between trauma-induced pain and that from disease processes, literature from a cross section will be reviewed and included.

The diagnosis of neuropathic pain can be very difficult as it commonly exists with other painful conditions and is frequently missed by practitioners who do not specialize in pain. The diagnosis allows the underlying pathology, peripheral or central, to be treated more effectively.

Central or peripheral?

It should be remembered that the patient's report of pain, the nature and severity, does not always distinguish between central and peripheral neuropathic pain; to the patient it feels the same irrespective of the location. Some tools can be used to distinguish neuropathic pain from non-neuropathic pain, which have usually been developed and tested on patients with peripheral neuropathic pain (Bennett et al., 2007) and have not been established in patients with central neuropathic pain with the exception of multiple sclerosis (MS) (Rog et al., 2007). Careful examination, quantitative testing and response to prior treatments can help elucidate the possible cause.

It is perhaps useful to refresh some of the definitions which are important in neuropathic pain (Merskey & Bogduk, 1994):

International Association for the Study of Pain definitions

Allodynia – pain caused by a generally non-noxious stimulus
Anaesthesia dolorosa – pain in an area which is anaesthetic

Dysaesthesia – an abnormal unpleasant sensation
Hyperalgesia – an exaggerated painful response to a
normally painful sensation
Hyperesthesia – increased sensitivity to stimulation
Hyperpathia – an abnormally painful reaction to a
stimulus, especially a repetitive stimulus
Parasthesia – abnormal sensation, spontaneous or
evoked.

Occasionally the sensations the patient reports might
seem bizarre and may not fit the common definition of
'pain'; this is immaterial to the patient. Some sensations
can be extremely distressing even if we might not describe
them as pain *per se*. We should also remember that
patients with central neuropathic pain who usually have
functional impairment, grossly altered biomechanics and
ongoing secondary changes associated with neurological
damage, are more likely to have co-existing pathologies
and musculoskeletal pain problems. Each patient should
be considered individually and the pain problem can be
very complex. It should also be remembered that neuropathic pain may be persistent, paroxysmal (come and go
without explanation), evoked (dependent on a stimulus)
or any combination or all of these. Some peripheral neuropathic pains may start with a relatively trivial injury and
the patient may have had trouble convincing health-care
professionals of the veracity of their condition and consequently the condition goes undiagnosed for some time. A
careful examination of the area is essential.

Central neuropathic pain

Central neuropathic pain can arise from primary injury or
dysfunction within the central nervous system (CNS)
(Merskey & Bogduk, 1994) and can arise at any level or
even from more than one level. The recently suggested
prerequisites for a diagnosis of the condition are:

- the pain is in a neuroanatomically plausible pain
  distribution
- a history of a relevant lesion of a disease affecting the
  central somatosensory system
- negative or positive sensory signs confined to the
  somatotopic representation of the body within the
  CNS
- a diagnostic test explaining the presence of
  neuropathic pain (Treede et al., 2008).

It is important to distinguish the changes which may
occur as a result of neuroplastic changes after damage to
the peripheral nervous system (PNS) or which may occur
in chronic pain states which may begin with an injury in
another part of the body other than the CNS. In these
conditions the dysfunction of the CNS is considered to
be secondary to ongoing nociception rather than from a
primary source in the CNS.

Central neuropathic pain states can be usefully classified into three main groups: (1) pain associated with

progressive neurological conditions, e.g. MS; (2) pain
following stroke; and (3) pain following spinal cord
injury. Another group which does not necessarily fall
into these is neuropathic pain associated with HIV infection. This may be due to damage caused by the HIV virus
itself or by neuropathy as a result of the antiretroviral
treatment (Cox & Rice, 2008). This last group will not
be considered here.

The prevalence of pain for all causes in MS has been
estimated at between 43% and 70% (Moulin et al.,
1988; Solaro et al., 2004). One of the best estimates for
the presence of central neuropathic pain is that over
27% of patients report the condition (Osterberg et al.,
2005). It is commonly widespread with an increased prevalence in the lower limbs and a variable clinical picture
but a low report of paroxysmal pain. A small proportion
of patients report pain at the onset of their MS but in general the incidence for central neuropathic pain syndrome
(CNPS) is reported to be higher in the early years. However, this may be an artefact of diagnosis, as additional
musculoskeletal pain and pain associated with spasticity
may predominate in the later stages of the disease masking the true prevalence of neuropathic pain. The actual
cause of CNPS in MS is difficult to determine owing to
the disseminated nature of the disease. Using MRI, Osterberg et al. (2005) demonstrated hyperintensity of activity
in the lateral and medial thalamic regions in one-third
of MS patients with CNPS and concluded that, although
there is an indication that the cause of the pain may share
some similarities with central stroke pain, they could not
conclude that lesions in the thalamus were the cause of
the pain and postulated that lesions in the spinal cord,
particularly the spino- and quintothalamic pathways, are
likely to be the cause. A previous hypothesis also suggested the importance of lesions in the neospinothalamic
pathway, which may become hyperexcitable following
lesioning.

Pain is also seen in Parkinson's disease but the exact
reason for this is yet to be determined. It is suspected that
the basal ganglia and dopaminergic systems are involved
in the processing of nociception to higher centres (see
Ch. 6).

Post-stroke pain is the commonest CNPS seen in the
population because of the common occurrence of stroke.
Andersen et al. (1995) followed 207 new stroke patients
who survived for 6 months and were able to participate
in a quantitative sensory testing protocol. In this study
abnormal sensory signs were common (47%) and 8% of
patients were diagnosed with post-stroke pain. There does
not appear to be a higher prevalence in either ischaemic
or haemorrhagic strokes, but because more people sustain
ischaemic strokes CNPS is more commonly seen in this
group of patients in clinical practice (Andersen et al.,
1995).

The original description of a possible cause of post-
stroke pain was made over one hundred years ago

(Dejerine & Roussy, 1906) and since that time the role of lesions of the thalamus in 'thalamic pain' has been well documented. The literature on the importance of lesions in and around the thalamus has grown. Lateral medullary infarctions are more likely to result in damage to the spinothalamic and trigeminothalamic pathways and have the highest incidence in the development of CNPS (MacGowan et al., 1997). The incidence of pain following damage to the thalamus is also high. In an MRI study of people with post-stroke pain a high proportion of them had thalamic lesions (>60%), but multiple lesions were seen in almost all of the patients and no thalamic involvement was demonstrated in others, so the specificity of the location is difficult to demonstrate (Bowsher et al., 1998).

Pain following spinal cord injury

About two-thirds or more of people who sustain a spinal cord injury report persistent pain, but this can be due to a number of reasons, not all of which are due to CNPS (Siddall et al., 2002). A proposed classification for spinal cord injury pain describes two broad groups: nociceptive and neuropathic. Nociceptive is further broken down into musculoskeletal and visceral (Siddall et al., 2002). Neuropathic is subdivided into:

- pain below the level of lesion (spinal cord trauma or ischaemia)
- pain at the level of lesion (nerve root compression, syringomyelia, spinal cord trauma/ischaemia), i.e. at level neuropathic pain
- pain above the lesion (compressive neuropathies, complex regional pain syndromes) (Siddall et al., 2002), the latter may not always be specific to the spinal cord injury.

In a 5-year follow-up of 73 patients with spinal cord injury Siddall et al. found 81% of patients reported pain; of these 41% had neuropathic pain at the level of the lesion and 34% had neuropathic pain below the level of lesion. Most patients reported more than one type of pain with musculoskeletal pain being the commonest (59%), although the least severe (Siddall et al., 2003).

At level neuropathic pain corresponds to the segmental level of the injury often involving two dermatomes above or below. At level neuropathic pain can be a result of damage to the nerve roots or the spinal cord and is characterized by allodynia and hyperalgesia in the affected dermatomes. The physiology is the same as by which peripheral neuropathic pain develops following damage or constriction of peripheral nerve roots in the affected area.

Below level pain is purported to be caused by changes in the spinal cord in or near the area of injury as described above and also as a result of what is sometimes termed a 'supraspinal generator'. A loss of neurological input to higher centres, especially the thalamus, may result in abnormal activity, in particular spontaneous activity. However, the nature of the pain, which is often persistent without the spontaneous outburst of pain, suggests that there is more than one area of the brain implicated as a supraspinal generator.

MECHANISM OF NEUROPATHIC PAIN

Much of the information on the cause of neuropathic pain comes from animal studies on peripheral nerve injury in experimental conditions. It can be argued whether such studies can reliably replicate the experience of pain in human subjects. However, such animal models allow a careful analysis of the physiological processes involved, which have informed pharmacological innovations for humans. By the nature of the experiments performed the information on the changes in the peripheral nerves, dorsal root ganglion (DRG) and the spinal cord is much greater than the information on the physiological changes which occur in the brain. Such experiments are also time limited to a few weeks, whereas neuropathic pain patients may have symptoms for months before consulting and often have had the condition for many years when seen in pain clinics. The long-term consequences of neuropathic pain cannot be investigated in these types of laboratory experiments, although new animal models are being developed.

The physiological changes following a nerve injury which lead to neuropathic pain have been grouped into peripheral and central phenomena (Wallace & Rice, 2008).

Peripheral physiological changes

- Sensitization and spontaneous activity in sensory neurones
- Abnormal ion channel expression
- Altered neuronal biochemistry
- Sensory neurone cell death
- Immune/neurological interactions
- Loss of trophic support for neurones.

Central physiological changes

- Central sensitization
- Spinal reorganization
- Changes in inhibitory systems
- Glial cell activation
- Alterations in descending modulation
- Cortical reorganization.

Following nerve injury an increase in DRG activity has been observed caused by spontaneous electrical activity or activity following low-intensity stimulation of the injured nerve. This increased activity is associated with hyperalgesia and parasthesia. Neurones may also demonstrate repetitive changes or oscillations in the resting potential also giving rise to hyperalgesia and spontaneous outbursts of pain. This also might explain the unpredictable nature of the condition, the variable response and dysesthesia.

Following injury, Wallarian degeneration occurs in myelinated neurones (Wallace & Rice, 2008). Activity or spontaneous activity in these may result in depolarization of adjacent uninjured unmyelinated neurones. Should this occur in mechanoreceptors, for example, stimulation of these through touch or movement may result in allodynia and hyperalgesia.

Key to the pathophysiology of neuropathic pain are the changes which take place in the ion channels of the nerve cell following nerve damage (Wallace & Rice, 2008). Perhaps the most important, or at least the best understood, is the alteration in the activation of sodium channels which alter the action potential of the cell membrane (Wallace & Rice, 2008). Much of the effectiveness of pharmacological treatment is attributed to the action of the drugs in producing sodium channel blockade (e.g. lidocaine, carbamazepine, tricyclic antidepressants). There are many different sodium channels in the DRG and the relevance of all is not understood. Some appear to increase in activity, whereas others reduce; some increase in number and others appear to change location on the cell. There are two main groups of channels classified by their sensitivity to tetrodoxin (TTX), a neurotoxin found in fish which binds to some voltage-gated channels; receptors are classified as sensitive (TTX-s) or resistant (TTX-r). TTX-s channels are found predominantly on A fibres, whereas TTX-r are seen specifically in the smaller C-fibre nociceptive neurones.

TREATMENT OF NEUROPATHIC PAIN

The management of peripheral neuropathic pain is reasonably well researched but the management of central neuropathic pain comes mainly from low-quality evidence based on prospective and retrospective case series and some cohort studies. The few randomized controlled trials conducted are often under-powered.

Treatment for neuropathic pain should not be seen in isolation. Pain is often present in association with other co-morbidities including, depression, insomnia or poor sleep and anxiety, and in association with considerable social and economic consequences all of which affect the patient's ability to cope with the condition and their tolerance of the pain.

A careful and full explanation of the cause of neuropathic pain is essential. The nature of neuropathic pain makes it very difficult for patients to understand. Why should there be pain in an area they cannot feel? What

causes impulse pains? Why is an area so excruciating to touch? Why is there pain if the damage is over and done? These are all questions the patient finds particularly difficult. A careful understanding of the pain and how the medication and treatments fit with each component reduces distress and can enhance treatment adherence.

Recent reviews on the management of both central and peripheral neuropathic pain have reached a good level of consensus guidelines for the pharmacological management of neuropathic pain (Dworkin et al., 2007) and it is worthwhile considering the recent National Institute for Health and Clinical Excellence (NICE) guidelines for the pharmacological management of neuropathic pain (NICE, 2010).

NICE guidelines on pharmacological therapies for neuropathic pain

Recent recommendations regarding the use of pharmacological agents in the management of neuropathic pain have been developed by NICE (2010). They describe three lines of possible pharmacological treatment for people with neuropathic pain. Patients with diabetic neuropathy should be treated specifically with duloxetine. It recommends all neuropathic pain from all other causes should be treated according to the guidelines.

The main classes of drugs used in the management of neuropathic pain are antidepressants, topical applications (capsaicin and lidocaine plasters) opioids and anticonvulsant medications. With the exception of duloxetine for the treatment of painful diabetic neuropathy, there is little evidence of condition-specific effects for these drugs.

Some of the drugs currently used in the management of neuropathic pain are not licensed in the UK for this use (e.g. amitriptyline and nortriptyline) and patients might often be confused why such medications are prescribed when pain is not explicitly described as an indication for prescription on the accompanying medical information. It is essential that the reason for prescription of these medications is made clear to the patient. Failure to receive appropriate information about medication may result in non-compliance with drug therapy.

The first line of treatment should be either the antiepileptic pregabalin or the tricyclic antidepressant amitriptyline. The dose of pregabalin starts at 150 mg/day divided into two or three equal doses, increasing to an effective dose or maximum tolerated dose to no more than 600 mg/day. Amitriptyline commences at 10 mg/day and increases to no more than 75 mg/day according to effect and patient tolerance. Because of the sedating effects of amitriptyline this is taken some time before going to bed. The dose of amitriptyline may be increased further but only in consultation with a pain specialist. If amitriptyline proves to be effective but the adverse effects (typically drowsiness and dry mouth) prove intolerable the patient may be trialled on nortriptyline or imipramine, which may be tolerated better. There is some evidence of cardiac toxicity from amitriptyline and so high doses should be avoided in people with an increased cardiac risk. The possibility of causing falls in elderly or unsteady people should also be considered.

If the first-line treatment fails to provide sufficient effect at the maximum tolerated dose, pregabalin can be added to or substituted for amitriptyline, and vice versa, following the above guidance on dosage. Both pregabalin and gabapentin are calcium channel α2-δ ligands which bind to the α2-δ component of the calcium channels reducing the release of glutamate, norepinephrine (noradrenaline) and substance P. Both pregabalin and gabapentin have been seen to improve sleep. Dizziness, somnolence and cognitive impairment are the main side effects.

The NICE guidance does not recommend the use of opioids as a first-line treatment for neuropathic pain and only recommends them in coordination with a referral to a specialist pain service. The drug of choice in this situation is tramadol; a μ-opioid which also blocks the reuptake of serotonin. This is given as either a monotherapy in place of the first- and second-line therapies or in conjunction with the treatments described above. In either case a referral to a specialist pain service is recommended. The side effects of tramadol are the same as other opioids; constipation, somnolence and nausea. The NICE guidelines do not recommend the use of other opioid therapies without the opinion of a specialist pain service.

These guidelines reflect the management recommended by non-pain specialists and do not cover all the pharmacological options available. For example a previous review of the literature recommended the use of cannabinoids as a second-line therapy in the management of neuropathic pain associated with MS, although concerns about the long-term safety and the risk of precipitating psychosis may have been a factor in not recommending them in the NICE guidance.

Injectable drugs

Sustained infusions into the blood stream (parenteral therapy) or directly into the space surrounding the spinal cord (intrathecal injections) have been performed with positive effects on central stroke pain. Parenteral injections of lidocaineanticonvulsants, the N-methyl-D-aspartic acid (NMDA) antagonist ketamine (Eide et al., 1995) and the opioid alfentanil (Eide et al., 1995) have all been demonstrated to be effective in randomized controlled trials. Intrathecal injections of morphine combined with clonidine have been demonstrated as useful in combination but not alone. The anti-spasticity drug Baclofen, a derivative of gamma-aminobutyric acid, has been demonstrated to provide pain relief, but this may be mainly due to its effect on musculoskeletal pain (Loubser & Akman, 1996), although one RCT has demonstrated a central effect on neuropathic pain (Herman et al., 1992).

Intrathecal injections are not without problems. They might be technically difficult to insert in the correct place, especially in people with spinal cord injuries, and the risk of infections associated with indwelling cannulae can be a significant concern. The difficulty with all injection therapies is that they do not represent a long-term solution to the problem, but might be helpful in allowing rehabilitation or providing relief during severe episodes of pain.

Mirror box therapy

For patients with chronic regional pain syndrome of a single limb, rehabilitation using the unaffected limb reflected in a mirror to 'trick' the brain into seeing the limb moving without pain has been developed (Moseley et al., 2008). Patients with neuropathic pain frequently experience severe pain on movement and tactile stimulation of the affected limb. Mirror box therapy allows the patient to observe the impression that the affected limb is moving or being touched. The mechanism for this remains speculative but seeing the limb being touched activates the visual or visuotactile cells in the secondary somatosensory cortex (SII) which facilitates SI neurones and promotes inhibition, and probably facilitates inhibition at the thalamic level. Giving a sense of normalization of sensory input may promote neural reorganization which leads to an improvement in tactile acuity and a reduction in pain (Moseley et al., 2008).

A recent review concluded that there was good evidence to support the use of mirror box therapy combined with a graded motor imagery programme and recommended its use be included in future guidelines (Daly & Bialocerkowski, 2009) for chronic regional pain syndrome. There is little evidence thus far to support its use in central neuropathic conditions. One study on a limited number of subjects with pain following spinal cord injury demonstrated that using a mirror and back projection of walking legs to give and impression the patient was walking led to a reduction in pain on a single exposure which was greater than imagined activity or watching a film. A further mean reduction in pain was observed over 3 weeks of daily exposure to the visual illusion of walking. However, this study used only five patients and one had to withdraw due to distress on the first exposure to the visual illusion (Moseley, 2007).

Cognitive behavioural therapy

Pain management programmes base on the principles of cognitive behavioural therapy are one of the mainstays of the management of chronic intractable pain. There are only limited data on the role of pain management programmes in the management of pain in neurological conditions. Traditionally pain management programmes run with a heterogeneous group of patients, the assumption being that the difficulties faced by people with chronic pain are common irrespective of the cause or nature of their condition. This has been questioned recently and there do appear to be subtle differences in the way in which people with a neuropathic pain problem deal with their pain when compared to those with low back pain, the commonest reason for referral to pain management (Daniel et al., 2008). The most notable difference is that those with neuropathic pain are more likely to report their pain is as a result of damage. Pain management programmes often try to avoid the term damage as it is unhelpful and focus on causes of pain that do not focus on tissue damage. However, reference to the role of previous damage as a cause of the onset of pain and to explain the continuance of pain as a consequence of damage in the past rather than ongoing injury might be useful in explaining pain to those with neuropathic pain.

Persistent pain has significant physical, social and psychological consequences. Often those patients with pain from a neurological condition may have additional physical or cognitive difficulties compounding their condition.

It is important to understand that pain management is not delivered as an alternative to medical treatments but the two should be delivered in a complimentary way.

The main aims of a pain management approach (Watson, 2004) are to:

- assist the patient in altering their belief that their problems are unmanageable and beyond their control
- inform patients about their condition
- assist patients to move from a passive to an active role in the management of their conditions
- enable patients to become active problem solvers to help them cope with their pain through the development of effective ways of responding to pain, emotion and the environment
- help patients to monitor thoughts emotions and behaviours, and to identify how these are influenced by internal and external events
- give patients a feeling of competence in the execution of positive strategies in the management of their condition
- help patients to develop a programme of paced activity to reduce the effects of physical deconditioning (see Ch. 18)
- assist patients in developing coping strategies which can be developed once contact with the clinician has ended.

The main outcomes of a pain management programme are:

- improved physical fitness
- reduced disability
- reintegration into work or meaningful activities
- increased effective problem solving
- reduced pain-related fear
- reduced depression.

Note that a reduction in pain is not listed above as an outcome. However, a reduction in pain is reported in the literature as a common outcome (Eccleston et al., 2009; Morley et al., 2008), although the effects are modest and not as large as the effects on mood.

Pain management requires a full biopsychosocial assessment of the patient. This will include a physical examination to guide any specific physical exercises required to address specific deconditioning and dysfunction as part of the programme. The patient's understanding of their condition and their beliefs about it and how this affects their current behaviour is assessed. The current coping strategies are identified to help elucidate both helpful and unhelpful behaviours. The role of significant others is also assessed. For a full account of the assessment at management of chronic pain see specific texts such as Main et al. (2008).

Education

Information helps to underpin the changes in cognition and behaviour which are the aims of the programme. Patients may have surprisingly little understanding of their condition even years after onset and continued contact with health-care professionals. This is important in such a complicated condition such as neuropathic pain. Education in normally provided in written form supplemented by group or individual discussions. Providing information in itself is of little importance unless this is understood and ultimately results in changes in the way in which a person views their condition and the behaviour they engage in as a result of this information. Providing the ability to test out new information successfully will enhance retention.

Goal setting and pacing

Patients with neuropathic pain may have limited activity as a consequence of the initial cause of the pain, as in the case of stroke or spinal cord injury. Limited physical capacity, due to inactivity, and lowered pain tolerance also restrict function. Engaging in certain activities often increases pain and this increase may remain for some time after the activity has ceased. Some people restrict their activity so much that they become more restricted over time due to the effects of physical deconditioning. Although there is much debate about the effect or even the fact of deconditioning, many people with neuropathic pain are severely limited in their physical activity in the affected body part and frank deconditioning and degeneration of physical abilities are often seen at the local level.

Resumption of physical activity is a mainstay of pain management programmes, but the effects attributed to physical activity alone are very modest and recent authors have suggested a more systematized approach of activity scheduling (Main et al., 2008; Sullivan, 2008). Appropriate scheduling of activity has been demonstrated to result in reductions in fear of pain, disability and depression, although none of the data relates specifically to patients with pain from neurological conditions. It involves identifying avoided activities, setting a baseline for participation (time and intensity) and allocating time during the day to perform the activity. These activities are typically activities of daily living rather than just specific physical exercises. The patient only discontinues the activity after the agreed goal has been completed regardless of the level of pain. If the goals are chosen well it should be unlikely that the patient will discontinue the activity due to intolerable pain.

The goals are chosen so that the patient participates in desired and valued activities. Setting and achieving goals in valued activities helps to mitigate the effect of interference of pain on lifestyle and reduces pain- and disability-associated depression (Morley & Sutherland, 2008).

Physical exercise and increasing fitness are common goals for pain management and can be useful to offset specific problems as a result of the pain or those associated with the primary condition. It is most useful if the majority of exercises used are those which the patients will be able to practice without the help of the therapist. Therapist contact time is limited and the establishment of a self-help programme is an essential aim of pain management (Watson, 2004).

Cognitive restructuring

A cognitive-behavioural model of pain and disability assumes that the way a person thinks about their condition can influence how they behave and feel. Common unhelpful thinking styles or cognitive distortions include catastrophizing (thinking the worst), overgeneralization (relating negative events to unconnected experiences), personalization (perceiving self is at fault) and selective abstraction (identifying negative experiences and ignoring positive ones). Once these are identified and the way in which they influence emotion and ultimately how this affects the way in which the person behaves towards their pain and disability, the therapist can help them identify the problems which stem from unhelpful thoughts, challenge these and identify different ways of helping them appraise situations and experiences (Thorn & Kahajda, 2006). Thought monitoring is an important component whereby the patient tries to distance themselves from their own behaviour and emotions and tries to rationalize it, identifying unhelpful thoughts and the emotional effect they have on them. In this way they can check themselves and try an alternative appraisal.

Maintenance

Chronic pain is characterized by periods of 'flare-up' with an accompanying restriction of physical activity, low mood and repeated health-care consultation. It is important that the lessons learned in the pain management programme are put into practice in the patient's own environment. This is done with a combination of homework and practice and behavioural experimentation where the patient is asked to engage in specific behaviours they might find challenging – for example lifting objects with the affected limb. They then monitor and appraise the experience challenging their unhelpful beliefs. Eventually the patient is likely to become less fearful of the activity and increase activity. Specific paradigms to challenge fear of activity have been developed in musculoskeletal pain (Vlaeyen et al., 2002), but the evidence of their effectiveness in neurological conditions remains to be established.

Using diaries or getting the patient to report back on their use and the relative success or otherwise of strategies is useful, not only in identifying what works and readdressing problems, but also in identifying patients who are finding it hard to do what is required.

The involvement of the patient's family also is an important factor in maintenance. The family should be aware of the aims of the programme and be instructed in how best to support the patient. It has been well documented how the behaviour of significant others can impact on the disability and distress of the patient. However, research in this area remains sketchy and how family members can help to best effect requires further attention.

Staff adherence to cognitive behavioural management is something which is not often addressed but is vitally important. All staff should be encouraged to understand the aims of such a programme and actively support the aims of treatment. All must share the same approach to therapy and present the same explanations about the condition to the patient and how it may help their condition.

CONCLUSION

Pain in neurological conditions is complex. This chapter has highlighted the main approaches to the management of pain of a neurological origin; in doing so the other causes of pain have not been directly addressed. Pain in such conditions may arise from more than one source requiring multiple approaches from health-care practitioners with different perspectives. It is important that all of these perspectives put the patient centre stage. The very nature of pain in those with a damaged nervous system often means they will have pain permanently and will need to develop strategies to cope with it beyond the use of medication and invasive procedures. Physiotherapists with their close contact with these patients and their rehabilitation perspective are pivotal in helping people to come to terms with pain and to enable them to get the best possible function despite the pain.

REFERENCES

Andersen, G., Vestergaard, K., Ingeman-Neilsen, M., Jensen, T., 1995. Incidence of central post-stroke pain. Pain 61, 187–193.

Bennett, M., Attal, N., Backonja, M., Baron, R., Bouhassira, D., Freynhagen, R., et al., 2007. Using screening tools to identify neuropathic pain. Pain 127, 199–203.

Bowsher, D., Leijon, G., Thuomas, K.A., 1998. Central poststroke pain: correlation of MRI with clinical pain characteristics and sensory abnormalities. Neurology 51, 1352–1358.

Cox, S., Rice, A., 2008. HIV and AIDS. In: Wilson, P., Watson, P.J., Haythornthwaite, J.A., Jensen, T. (Eds.), Clinical Pain Management: Chronic Pain. 2nd edition. Hodder-Arnold, London, pp. 352–361.

Daly, A.E., Bialocerkowski, A.E., 2009. Does evidence support physiotherapy management of adult Complex Regional Pain Syndrome Type One? A systematic review. Eur. J. Pain 13 (4), 339–353.

Daniel, H.C., Narewska, J., Serpell, M., Hoggart, B., Johnson, R., Rice, A.S.C., 2008. Comparison of psychological and physical function in neuropathic pain and nociceptive pain: implications for cognitive behavioral pain management programs. Eur. J. Pain 12 (6), 731–741.

Dejerine, J., Roussy, G., 1906. La syndrome thalamique. Rev. Neurol. (Paris) 14, 521–532.

Dworkin, R.H., O'Connor, A.B., Backonja, M., Farrar, J., Finnerup, N., Jensen, T., et al., 2007. Pharmalogical management of neuropathic pain: Evidence based recommendations. Pain 132, 237–251.

Eccleston, C., Williams, A.C.D.C., Morley, S., 2009. Psychological therapies for the management of chronic pain (excluding headache) in adults. Cochrane Database Syst. Rev. (2), CD007407.

Eide, P., Stubhaug, A., Stenehjem, A., 1995. Central dysesthesia pain after traumatic spinal cord injury is dependent on N-Methyl-D-aspartate receptor activation. Neurosurgery 37, 1080–1087.

Herman, R., D'Luzansky, S., Ippolito, R., 1992. Intrathecal Baclofen suppressed central pain in patients with spinal cord injury. Clin. J. Pain 8, 338–345.

Loubser, P., Akman, N., 1996. Effects of intrathecal Baclofen on chronic spinal cord injury pain. J. Pain Symptom Manage. 12, 241–247.

MacGowan, D., Janal, M., Clark, W., 1997. Central post-stoke pain and Wallenberg's lateral medullary infarction: frequency character and determinants in 63 patients. Neurology 49, 120–125.

Main, C., Sullivan, M.J.L., Watson, P.J., 2008. Pain Management: Practical applications of the biopsychosocial perspective in clinical and occupational settings. Edinburgh, Churchill Livingstone.

Merskey, H., Bogduk, N., 1994. Classification of chronic pain: descriptions of chronic pain syndromes and definitions of pain terms. IASP Press, Seattle.

Morley, S., Sutherland, R., 2008. Self-pain enmeshment: future possible selves, sociotropy, autonomy and adjustment to chronic pain. Pain 137, 366–377.

Morley, S., Williams, A.C.D.C., Hussain, S., 2008. Estimating the clinical effectiveness of cognitive behavioural therapy in the clinic: evaluation of a CBT informed pain management programme. Pain 137, 670–680.

Moseley, G.L., 2007. Using visual illusion to reduce at-level neuropathic pain in paraplegia. Pain 130, 294–298.

Moseley, G.L., Gallace, A., Spence, C., 2008. Is mirror therapy all it is cracked up to be? Current evidence and future directions. Pain 138, 7–10.

Moulin, D., Foley, K., Ebers, G., 1988. Pain syndromes in Multiple Sclerosis. Neurology 38, 1830–1834.

NICE, 2010. Neuropathic pain: the pharmacological management of neuropathic pain in adults in non-specialist settings. National Institute for Health and Clinical Excellence, London.

Osterberg, A., Boivie, J., Thuomas, K.A., 2005. Central pain in multiple sclerosis - prevalence and clinical characteristics. Eur. J. Pain 9, 531–542.

Rog, D., Nurmikko, T., Freide, T., Young, C., 2007. Validation and reliability of the Neuropathic Pain Scale (NPS) in multiple sclerosis. Clin. J. Pain 23, 473–481.

Siddall, P., McClelland, J., Rutkowski, S., Cousins, M., 2003. A longitudinal study of the prevalence and characteristics of pain in the first 5 years following spinal cord injury. Pain 103, 249–257.

Siddall, P., Yezierski, R., Loeser, J.D., 2002. Taxonomy and epidemiology of spinal cord injury pain. In: Yezierski, R. (Ed.), Spinal cord injury pain: assessment, mechanisms, management. Progress in pain research and management, IASP Press, Seattle.

Solaro, C., Brichetto, G., Amato, M., 2004. The prevalence of pain in Multiple Sclerosis: A Multicentre cross-sectional study. Neurology 63, 919–921.

Sullivan, M.J.L., 2008. Toward a biopsychomotor conceptualization of pain: implications for research and intervention. Clin. J. Pain 24 (4), 281–290.

Thorn, B., Kahajda, M., 2006. Group cognitive therapy for chronic pain. J. Clin. Psychol. 62, 1355–1366.

Treede, R., Jensen, T., Campbell, J., 2008. Neuropathic pain: redefinition and a grading system for clinical and research purposes. Neurology 70, 1630–1635.

Vlaeyen, J.W.S., De Jong, J., Geilen, M., Heuts, P., Van Breukelen, G., 2002. The treatment of fear of movement/(re)injury in chronic low back pain: Further evidence on the effectiveness of exposure in vivo. Clin. J. Pain 18 (4), 251–261.

Wallace, V., Rice, A., 2008. Applied physiology: neuropathic pain. In: Wilson, P., Watson, P., Haythornthwaite, J.A., Jensen, T. (Eds.), Clinical Pain Management: Chronic Pain. 2nd edition. Hodder-Arnold, London, pp. 3–23.

Watson, P.J., 2004. Managing chronic pain. In: Boyling, J., Jull, G. (Eds.), Grieve's Modern Manual Therapy: the vertebral column. Churchill-Livingston, Edinburgh, pp. 551–566.

Chapter | 17 |

Clinical neuropsychology in rehabilitation

J. Graham Beaumont

CONTENTS

INTRODUCTION

The field of clinical psychology that is concerned with neurological disorders has now become known as clinical neuropsychology. Although in the UK there is no formal definition of a clinical neuropsychologist, developments are currently under way which will result in the establishment of professional qualifications in neuropsychology. In practice, clinical neuropsychologists are clinical psychologists registered with the UK Health Professions Council, with specialist experience and expertise in the field of neuropsychology, and often title themselves 'neuropsychologists'.

Whilst clinical neuropsychology is only now emerging as an independent area of professional psychology, it has a history as long as that of modern scientific psychology. From the end of the last century, psychologists have investigated the behavioural effects of lesions to the brain, not only for the light this study could shed on the operation of normal brain processes but also from a genuine desire to alleviate the distress and disability resulting from neurological injury and disease.

Clinical neuropsychology was given an inevitable stimulus by the two world wars of the twentieth century, the study of missile wounds proving a fertile ground for the association of specific psychological deficits with defined regions of the brain. This research carried significant implications for a debate, inherited from nineteenth-century neurology which occupied at least the first half of the twentieth century, about the nature of the representation of psychological functions in the brain. Put rather crudely, the opposite poles of the debate argued either for the highly localized and specific representation of functions, or for a mass action view whereby psychological functions are distributed across the entire cerebral cortex. This debate has never been finally resolved, but the position that most clinical neuropsychologists now adopt is one of relative localization: that many functions are localized to regions of the cortex but cannot be more finely localized. This is often qualified by a tertiary model of cortical function in that the primary cortex, subserving sensation and discrete motor control, is quite highly localized; the secondary cortex, subserving perception and the control of movements, is rather less localized; and the tertiary or association cortex, supporting all higher-level functions, is much less clearly localized. However, current developments in connectionist theory, which point to radical models for neuropsychological processes, are starting to modify these views. For a fuller discussion, see Beaumont (1996, 2008) and for illustrations see Code et al. (1996, 2001).

Only within the last three decades has rehabilitation become an active focus of interest for clinical neuropsychology. Before that time clinicians saw their role as primarily one of assessment, either in the context of diagnosis or of vocational adjustment. The widespread introduction of modern neuroimaging greatly diminished the contribution of neuropsychology to diagnosis and as a result the embarrassing period of neglect of rehabilitation, both in terms of research and of practical interventions, came to an end. Rehabilitation is now the central focus of neuropsychology and assessment is understood, quite properly, as only a significant stage in the planning of rehabilitation and management.

APPROACHES IN CLINICAL NEUROPSYCHOLOGY

Clinical psychological management involves detailed assessment, which is discussed prior to reviewing interventions.

Neuropsychological assessment

Neuropsychological assessment should be understood as the essential precursor to the planning and implementation of rehabilitation. It is not an end in itself, but is designed to provide a description in psychological terms of the client's current state with respect to the clinical problems being addressed. Such a description should provide an insight into the processes which are no longer functioning normally in that individual, and so provide the rationale upon which the intervention is based. Subsequent reassessments allow progress to be monitored and interventions to be adjusted, according to the client's current state. Rehabilitation should never proceed without an adequate assessment having been undertaken.

The three traditions

There are historically three traditions in clinical neuropsychology. The first, most eloquently expressed in the work of Luria (see Christensen, 1974), is based upon behavioural neurology, although it is a much more sophisticated extension of it. The approach is based upon the presentation of simple tasks, selected in a coherent way from a wide variety of tests available, which any normal individual can be expected successfully to complete without difficulty. Any failure on the task is a pathological sign and the pattern of these signs, in skilled hands, allows a psychological description to be built up.

The second tradition, associated with work in North America, is a psychometric battery-based approach, most notably expressed in the Halstead–Reitan and Luria Nebraska Neuropsychological Test Batteries (any apparent theoretical link with the approach of Luria is quite illusory). In this approach a standard, and often large, battery of tests is administered to all clients and the resulting descriptions arise out of a psychometric analysis of the pattern of test scores.

The third approach, the normative individual-centred approach, has been dominant in Europe, particularly in the UK, but is now the leading international methodology. It relies upon the use of specific tests, associated wherever possible with adequate normative standardization, which are selected to investigate hypotheses about the client's deficits; testing these hypotheses permits the psychological description to be built up. Whilst requiring a high level of expertise, this neuropsychological detective work can be more efficient and provide a finer degree of analysis, when applied intelligently. In practice, many neuropsychologists employ a mixture of these approaches, although the normative individual-centred approach is generally becoming more dominant.

Cognitive functions

The greater part of neuropsychological assessment concentrates upon cognitive functions: perception, learning, memory, language, thinking and reasoning. This is a reflection of the principal interests of contemporary psychology. There is a bewildering variety of test procedures available to the clinical neuropsychologist, but most involve the presentation of standardized test materials in a controlled way; this can yield reliable scores which are then interpreted with respect to appropriate normative data. These norms may be more or less adequate for the clinical population under consideration, and there are certainly some excellent, some very good, and some rather inadequate tests.

Even a partial description of the most popular tests is outside the scope of this chapter, but a good introduction may be found in both Halligan et al. (2003) and Goldstein and McNeil (2004), and a more thorough account in Hobben and Milberg (2002), Lezak et al. (2004) and Spreen and Strauss (2006).

Behavioural assessment

Assessment of behaviour (as distinct from specifically cognitive performance), usually in relation to undesirable behaviours or defective interpersonal or social skills, relies more directly upon observational recording. Here the object is to identify the antecedents of the behaviour under investigation, and then to analyze the consequences of the behaviour for the individual. In this way an understanding can be gained of what 'causes' the behaviour, and what maintains the behaviour in the individual's repertoire. This information can be used to construct a programme designed to modify behaviour (see below) or simply to provide feedback for the client allowing him or her to gain the insight to modify his or her own behaviour.

Behavioural sampling—the regular observation and recording of relevant aspects of behaviour for fixed samples of time—is frequently employed, and carers may also be requested to maintain records or diaries of specific events. Video recording, sometimes with detailed analysis, may also be employed.

Affective states

Clinical neuropsychologists are also commonly asked to evaluate other aspects of behaviour: affective states, motivation, insight, adjustment to disability, pain and, often most difficult of all, the possible psychological basis of apparently organic neurological states. It is for this reason, amongst others, that a thorough training in clinical psychology is considered essential for neuropsychological practice. A certain number of standard questionnaires and rating scales are available to assist in this assessment, but the neuropsychologist must commonly rely upon clinical experience and expertise in forming a judgement.

Outcome measures and the quality of life

The political climate of health service changes in the UK has forced health-care providers to consider the outcome of their interventions, and this can only be to the advantage of clients. Psychologists, because of their expertise in the measurement of behaviour, have been prominent in the development of outcome measures. Within neuropsychological rehabilitation there is a variety of measures, of which the Barthel Index (Wade, 1992) is widely used, and FIM–FAM (Functional Independence Measure–Functional Assessment Measure; Cook et al., 1994; Ditunno, 1992) is growing in popularity as it can be linked to problem-oriented and client-centred rehabilitation planning. However, none of the available scales is adequate to assess the status of severely disabled clients (Stokes, 2009), and there is also a lack of good measures of the specific outcome of psychological interventions. Research is actively being undertaken to fill these gaps, and a discussion is to be found in Fleminger and Powell (1999).

Allied to the need to assess outcomes has been a growing interest in 'quality of life' (QoL), recognizing that consideration should be given not only to functional and physical status, but also to the individual's personal feelings and life experience. A central problem is that QoL is not a unitary concept and encompasses a range of ideas, from the spiritual and metaphysical to cognitions about health and happiness. What is clear is that QoL relates not in a direct, but in a very complex way to health status, physical disability and handicap, and that the precise nature of this relationship has yet to be clarified.

Cognitive neuropsychology

Cognitive neuropsychology should be understood as a distinct, and currently very fashionable, approach within neuropsychology. Of growing importance over the past decade, cognitive neuropsychology concentrates upon the single case and seeks to explain psychological deficits in terms of the components of cognitive information-processing models. Such models, which are now quite detailed in respect of functions, such as reading, spelling and face recognition, are based upon experimental data derived from normal individuals and from clinical investigations. These models are modular, and dysfunction can be understood in terms of the faulty performance of either the modules or the connections between them.

Cognitive neuropsychological analysis has been of enormous importance in developing our understanding of both normal and abnormal cognitive psychological functions within the brain but, partly because of the resources required to analyze a problem fully using this approach in the individual case, it has not made such a great impact upon the clinical practice of neuropsychologists.

Neuropsychological interventions

Management strategies include cognitive and behavioural interventions as well as psychotherapy.

Cognitive interventions

Cognitive interventions aim to reduce the impact of deficits in the areas of memory, learning, perception, language, and thinking and reasoning. How this is achieved depends in part upon the model of recovery that is adopted but, in general, requires either new learning or the development of strategies which bypass the abnormal components in the system. There are often a variety of routes by which an end result may be achieved. Perhaps trivially, consider how many ways 9 may be multiplied by 9 to achieve 81. There are in fact at least 9 ways. If you learnt the solution by rote learning, you may well find that your children have been taught a different method: 9 x 10 – 9, or the fact that the first digit of the solution is 9 – 1 and that the two digits of the answer sum to 9. These are different 'strategies' of finding the solution. If the previously available strategy has been lost, it may be more successful to teach a new strategy that relies upon different brain mechanisms.

Besides the explicit teaching of new strategies, appropriately structured training may be employed; this is often based upon 'error-free learning', which has been shown to be most effective following head injury. Aids to performance, which may be either external (such as diaries to aid memory) or internal (mnemonics), may also be successfully employed. These interventions are more fully developed in some areas than others, and have been used most extensively in the rehabilitation of memory (Baddeley et al., 2002; Wilson & Moffat, 1992), but the basic principles can be applied in any area of cognitive function (see also Ponsford, 1995; Prigatano, 1999; Riddoch & Humphreys, 1994; Sohlberg & Mateer, 2002).

Behavioural interventions

Behavioural interventions are less widely employed, but may be appropriate to address the remediation of undesirable behaviours and in situations where the residual cognitive function of the individual is severely limited. These interventions are based upon psychological learning theory that, put rather simply, states that behaviour is determined by its consequences. Behaviour that leads to a 'good' outcome for the individual will increase in frequency; that which has an undesirable outcome for the individual will decrease in frequency. Behaviours that are desirable (from the perspective of the rehabilitation goals) can therefore be increased by ensuring that they are positively reinforced (given a good outcome for the individual), whilst undesirable behaviours do not receive such reinforcement. In laboratory situations, negative reinforcement (punishment) might be used to reduce the frequency of a behaviour, but in a clinical situation its use would be extremely exceptional (perhaps only in relation to a significant life-threatening behaviour and then only with informed consent); in practice, the lack of positive reinforcement is sufficient for the undesired behaviour to reduce in frequency.

The range of behavioural techniques is both wider and more sophisticated than this brief account might suggest, and in certain selected contexts these approaches may be highly effective (Wood, 1990). However, the demands on resources and staff skills are high, given that a behavioural programme must be applied consistently, contingently and continuously, often over a very protracted period. For this reason, behavioural approaches are less commonly employed outside specialist facilities, although they are perhaps unreasonably neglected within other rehabilitation contexts.

Psychotherapy; staff, team and organizational support; research

Psychologists in neuropsychological practice are also involved in a variety of more general clinical psychological issues. Amongst these is the provision of psychotherapy or counselling, which may follow one of a large variety of models and is often eclectic in nature, addressing issues of personal loss, life changes, and adjustment to disability. The psychotherapeutic techniques appropriate to neuropsychological disability are relatively underdeveloped, and are associated with a number of specific problems, such as cognitive limitations and impairment of memory.

Because of their specialist knowledge of human and social relations, and of organizational processes, psychologists will advise and provide practical support to the construction and functioning of clinical teams, besides giving staff support at an individual level. Staff stress is often high in the neurological care setting and the health and welfare of staff is important, not only as an end in itself, but also because it has consequences for the care of patients.

Psychologists, who have been trained in methods of research design and analysis, are also commonly active in research relating to neurodisability and in supporting the research of others, and regard it as an important aspect of their role.

NEUROPSYCHOLOGICAL CONSEQUENCES OF NEUROLOGICAL DISORDERS

The consequences and management of neuropsychological problems cannot be discussed in any detail in this chapter, but several useful texts exist (e.g. Beaumont, 2008; Beaumont et al 1996; Halligan et al., 2003; Kolb & Whishaw, 2003).

General considerations

The neuropsychological consequences of neurological disease depend upon a number of factors, not all of which are determined by the neurological aetiology.

Focal versus diffuse

Focal, relatively localized, lesions result in quite different effects from lesions which diffusely affect the cerebral cortex. Most specific neuropsychological deficits of cognitive function are associated with relatively focal lesions (following trauma, tumours, or surgical intervention), and these have generally been the area of study of neuropsychologists. By contrast, diffuse lesions (following infections, generalized degeneration or widespread closed head injury) tend to affect level of consciousness, attention, motivation and initiation and affect, rather than specific psychological functions.

Acute versus chronic

Acute lesions have greater effects than chronic lesions. In the acute period following the acquisition of a lesion there may be widespread disruption of psychological functions, together with changes in the level of consciousness, confusion and loss of orientation. Amnesia is common in the acute period, and the duration of post-traumatic amnesia, before continuous memory and full orientation return, is the best indicator of the severity of the lesion (see Ch. 3). Neuropsychological consequences diminish over time, most of the recovery occurring within the first 6–12 months, but with further improvements occurring over the next year or a little longer.

Progressive versus static; speed of development

Lesions that continue to develop, such as tumours and degenerative conditions, have a greater impact than lesions that are essentially static after the initial acute period, such as trauma, cerebrovascular accidents and surgical interventions. The assumption is that the brain accommodates more readily the presence of a static lesion, but must continue to adapt to a developing lesion.

Within progressive lesions, those that develop more rapidly will cause greater psychological disruption than those which develop more slowly. This effect is seen most clearly in the case of tumours, where slow-growing tumours such as meningiomas have much less effect than more rapidly growing tumours such as gliomas. Indeed, meningiomas may grow to a very considerable size before they cause sufficient interference with psychological function to come to medical attention; this is most unlikely to happen in the case of the more aggressive tumours, where a much smaller lesion will have dramatic behavioural consequences.

Site and lateralization

The site is obviously of relevance in the case of a focal lesion, and will determine the neuropsychological consequences within the principle of relative localization (see above). Lateralization, whether the lesion is primarily located in the left or right hemisphere of the cerebral cortex, is also of relevance as the psychological functions assumed by the two hemispheres are known to differ. There is an enormous literature on cerebral lateralization, which was the most prominent research topic of neuropsychology for the two decades from about 1960, and most functions show some degree of differential lateralization. The clearest case is speech, which is exclusively located in the left hemisphere of about 95% of right-handed individuals (Beaumont et al., 1996; Kolb & Whishaw, 2003).

Age of acquisition

The age at which a lesion is acquired may also be of relevance, as the effects are less in the younger patient and throughout the childhood years (the Kennard principle). This was previously attributed to an increased 'plasticity' of the developing brain, in that alternative regions could subsume the functions previously destined to be located in the area containing the lesion. However, there is now some doubt over this hypothesis, partly due to accumulating evidence for the continuing neural adaptability of the brain in adult life (DeFlna et al., 2009; Hoffman & Harrison, 2009; Stein & Hoffman, 2003). The explanation may lie at least as much in the cognitive flexibility of the developing psychological systems and the greater opportunities for alternative forms of learning in the pre-adult period.

Specific aetiologies

As stated above, it is not possible to describe the management of neuropsychological problems in the conditions mentioned in this section. As well as the psychology texts cited in this chapter, the reader is referred to a book on neurological rehabilitation which devotes sections to cognitive and behavioural problems (Greenwood et al., 2003).

Head injury

Head injury is the most common cause of neurodisability for which rehabilitation is undertaken (see Ch. 3). It affects young males more than any other group and effective intervention can result in a very favourable outcome. Head injuries range from very mild to very severe and profound, with dramatic differences in the behavioural consequences up to and including prolonged coma and vegetative states. The lesions associated with head injury are generally focal or multifocal, and static, although acceleration–deceleration closed head injuries may result in widespread and diffuse lesions across the cortex. An important consideration is that even apparently very mild head injuries associated with a brief period of concussion may sometimes have significant behavioural consequences in terms of anxiety, depression, changes in personality and subtle disorders of memory, with consequent effects upon occupational performance, social activity and personal relationships.

Stroke

Stroke, perhaps because it tends to occur in the more elderly, has received less attention than head injury. The effects of strokes and other cerebrovascular accidents will depend upon the area and proportion of the arterial distribution which is lost, ranging from the whole territory of one of the main cerebral arteries, which is a substantial proportion of the cortex, down to relatively discrete focal lesions associated with a distal portion of one of these arteries (see Ch. 2). Although the neuropsychological consequences depend primarily on the area of cortex affected, the picture is often complicated by the occurrence of further, perhaps minor, strokes that prevent the psychological condition being stable, and by associated arterial disease, which may result in more general and perhaps fluctuating insufficiency of the blood supply to the entire cortex.

Degenerative conditions

Interest in the degenerative conditions from a neuropsychological perspective has grown in recent years. Other than the dementias of later life, principally dementia of the Alzheimer type, which are clearly associated with deficits of cognitive function of a progressive nature, there are a number of other degenerative conditions which occur in adult life, but of which the neuropsychological consequences are only beginning to be understood. Multiple sclerosis, the most common neurological disease of the population, Parkinson's disease, Huntington's disease and motor neurone disease, sometimes referred to collectively as the subcortical dementias, are all associated with cognitive, affective and behavioural deficits in a significant proportion of those with the disease, and almost all those whose disease progresses to an advanced stage suffer psychological sequelae (see Chs 5–8). Disorders of memory, attention and affect are common as primary consequences of the disease in this group, and there are naturally significant psychological disturbances associated with being a sufferer of one of these diseases.

Spinal injuries

Spinal cord injury clearly differs from other neurological conditions in that the patient has suffered a disabling condition, but all neural systems supporting psychological functions are intact (see Ch. 4). The main issue is therefore one of adjustment to the disability, both in terms of the primary impairment dependent upon the spinal cord lesion, and the secondary consequences of handicap that follow from the disability. Amongst the primary disabilities are loss of mobility and other functional capacities (especially if the upper limbs are affected), together with loss of bladder and bowel control, and, most importantly for psychological health, sexual function may also be affected. Depression is very common following spinal injury, and the facilitation of insight and adjustment to the disability is a primary task for the neuropsychologist.

Neuropsychological disorders of movement

Apraxia

Apraxia refers to disorders of voluntary movement in the absence of sensory loss, paresis or motor weakness. It is normally demonstrated when the patient is asked to respond to a command, or to produce an action outside its normal context. It is therefore probably the intentional aspects of the task that are the root of the problem. A distinction is often drawn between ideomotor and ideational apraxia. Ideomotor apraxia is a disorder affecting the ability to produce simple gestures either on command or by imitation, while the ability to perform more complex tasks may be largely intact; that 'the patient knows what to do but not how to do it' is a helpful dictum. By contrast, ideational apraxia refers to the inability to perform actions requiring a well-ordered sequence of elements. However, while this is an important distinction in the literature there is still considerable debate about the dissociability of these two conditions. Both conditions are associated with lesions in the posterior cortical regions, especially the parietal lobe, and in the dominant hemisphere. An interesting feature of both conditions is that the relevant behaviours may be performed without difficulty in everyday life; the problem only appears when conscious attention is directed to the task. Dressing apraxia has been regarded as an independent form of apraxia, but there is some reason to believe that it is only the difficulty of this particular task which involves the integration of body elements with external space, and complex personal movements in relation to highly plastic objects that makes it appear a distinct entity. Constructional apraxia is, however, a distinct type of apraxia and involves a defect in the spatial aspects of a task in relationship to individual motor movements. The problem appears to lie in the integration of visuospatial information and voluntary motor acts, and may be apparent in drawing, or in the construction of 3D models. The disorder is also associated with lesions of parietal cortex and some believe that it may take a different form when the right hemisphere is involved affecting visuospatial perception, or the left hemisphere affecting motor execution.

Neglect

Unilateral neglect, or unilateral hemi-inattention, has attracted considerable research interest in recent years. Patients with this disorder act as if one side of space, more commonly the left side of space following right parietal lesion, did not exist. This is in the absence of any visual field defect. In extreme cases the patient may only eat food on the right half of their plate, dress the right side of their body and attend to visual events to their right. It can occur in relation to imagined scenes as to real stimuli. There is still considerable debate about whether the problem is one of disordered internal representations, or one of attentional deficit. It seems clear, however, that patients have some semantic access to the information appearing in the neglected space, but this information does not enter consciousness, or direct behaviour. Voluntary limb activation, out of sight and on the neglected side, has proved the most effective treatment approach to date.

Motor memory

Memory for motor acts, and in particular motor skills, has been shown to be distinct from memory for semantic or episodic information. It is noteworthy that even patients with a dense global amnesia, as in the amnesic syndrome, may retain the ability to perform previously learned motor skills. Their ability to acquire new motor skills may be less impaired than their ability to learn new semantic information or recall recent events. While disorders of motor memory are much less well researched than other aspects of memory, it is worth noting that even a serious impairment of memory will not necessarily prevent the learning of new motor tasks. We can conversely assume that there are specific disorders of motor memory in the absence of other memory problems, but these are little studied.

CONCLUDING ISSUES

Factors that influence psychological management and that need to be considered include the cognitive ability and psychological adjustment of the patient, and a collaborative team approach.

Cognitive ability

An important determinant of the psychological effects of neurological injury or disease is the cognitive status of the individual. Besides specific cognitive deficits, which may limit both psychological and functional adjustment to the disease, more general factors, such as attentional capacity, motivation, and the capacity for learning and the acquisition of skills, will all contribute to the eventual outcome.

Pre-morbid intellectual capacity will also be a factor; it is known that the best protective factor against dementia in advanced age is to be more intelligent as an adult, and the same principle applies to all neuropsychological deficits. The more you have, the less you will be affected by a given loss, and the more you have left with which to compensate. Nevertheless, those who functioned at a high intellectual level with a mentally demanding occupation before illness may also be more acutely aware of relatively subtle deficits in their ability and this may have a disproportionate effect upon their capacity to pursue a previous occupation.

Relatively intact cognitive abilities may contribute to the ability to benefit from rehabilitation interventions, and to gain insight and consequent adjustment to the disability, although in some severely affected individuals the lack of insight and memory for what has been lost may result in an unawareness which is in some respects protective, even if it cannot be regarded as psychologically healthy.

Psychological adjustment

Good psychological adjustment depends upon:

- satisfactory insight into the events and psychological changes that have occurred and a personal acceptance of these changes
- an appropriate adjustment of the perception of self
- a modification of beliefs and personal goals
- the acquisition of appropriate strategies to compensate as far as is possible for any residual handicap.

It implies not only psychological adjustment, but also the re-establishment of personal, family and social relationships, both intimate and more distant. It may also involve occupational adjustment and redefinition of personal roles in all these contexts. This is something that the psychologist must understand and have the skills to facilitate.

It should also be recognized that not all those who acquire neurological diseases had perfect psychological adjustment before the problem occurred; occasionally, the personality of a patient, as perceived by those close to him or her, has actually been improved by the condition. Not everyone who is neurologically intact is in good psychological health, and the goal of returning the client to this state may be confounded by circumstances quite unrelated to the neurological problem.

The process of care

Neuropsychologists generally work within a team, particularly in rehabilitation settings. They must contribute to the team not only by their support, but also by effectively playing the appropriate multidisciplinary role within the team. A psychologist who is privileged to work within an expert and committed team will respect the particular contributions made by other team members. They will come to realize that it is only by the collaborative efforts of the disciplines within the team that the optimal outcome will be achieved for the patient, and that the patient will have the best chance of a good psychological adjustment to his or her condition and obtain the best quality of life that is possible.

REFERENCES

Baddeley, A.D., Kopelman, M., Wilson, B.A. (Eds.), 2002. The handbook of memory disorders for clinicians. second ed. John Wiley, Chichester.

Beaumont, J.G., 2008. Introduction to neuropsychology. Guilford Press, New York.

Beaumont, J.G., 1996. Neuropsychology. In: Beaumont, J.G., Kenealy, P.M., Rogers, M.J.C. (Eds.), Blackwell dictionary of neuropsychology. Blackwell Publishers, Oxford, pp. 523–531.

Beaumont, J.G., Kenealy, P.M., Rogers, M.J.C. (Eds.), 1996. Blackwell dictionary of neuropsychology. Blackwell Publishers, Oxford.

Christensen, A.L., 1974. Luria's neuropsychological investigation. Copenhagen, Munksgaard.

Code, C., Wallesch, C.W., Lecours, A.R., Joanette, Y., 1996. Classic cases in neuropsychology. Psychology Press, Hove.

Code, C., Wallesch, C.W., Joanette, Y., Lecours, A.R., 2001. Classic cases in neuropsychology, vol. II. Psychology Press, Hove.

Cook, L., Smith, D.S., Truman, G., 1994. Using Functional Independence Measure profiles as an index of outcome in the rehabilitation of brain-injured patients. Arch. Phys. Med. Rehabil. 75, 390–393.

DeFlna, P., Fellus, J., Polito, M.Z., Thompson, J.W., Moser, R.S., DeLuca, J., 2009. The new neuroscience frontier: promoting neuroplasticity and brain repair in traumatic brain injury. J. Clin. Neuropsychol. 23 (8), 1391–1399.

Ditunno Jr., J.F., 1992. Functional assessment measures in CNS trauma. J. Neurotrauma 9 (Suppl. 1), S301–S305.

Fleminger, S., Powell, J. (Eds.), 1999. Evaluation of outcomes in brain injury rehabilitation. Psychology Press, Hove.

Goldstein, L.H., McNeil, J.E., 2004. Clinical neuropsychology: A practical guide to assessment and management for clinicians. John Wiley, Chichester.

Greenwood, R., Barnes, M.P., McMillan, T.M. et al. (Eds.), 2003. Handbook of neurological rehabilitation. Psychology Press, London.

Halligan, P.W., Kischka, U., Marshall, J.C. (Eds.), 2003. Handbook of clinical neuropsychology. Oxford University Press, Oxford.

Hobben, N., Milberg, W., 2002. Essentials of neuropsychological assessment. Wiley, New York.

Hoffman, S.W., Harrison, C., 2009. The interaction between psychological health and traumatic brain injury: a neuroscience perspective. J. Clin. Neuropsychol. 23 (8), 1400–1415.

Kolb, B., Whishaw, I.Q., 2003. Fundamentals of human neuropsychology, fifth ed. WH Freeman and Co., New York.

Lezak, M., Howieson, D.B., Loring, D.W., et al., 2004. Neuropsychological assessment, fourth ed. Oxford University Press, New York.

Ponsford, J., 1995. Traumatic brain injury; Rehabilitation for everyday adaptive living. Psychology Press, Hove.

Prigatano, G., 1999. Principles of neuropsychological rehabilitation. Oxford University Press, Oxford.

Riddoch, M.J., Humphreys, G.W., 1994. Cognitive neuropsychology and cognitive rehabilitation. Lawrence Erlbaum Assoc., Hove.

Sohlberg, M.M., Mateer, C.A., 2002. Cognitive rehabilitation: An integrative neuropsychological approach. Guilford Press, New York.

Spreen, O., Strauss, E.A., 2006. compendium of neuropsychological tests: Administration, norms and commentary, third ed. Oxford University Press, New York.

Stein, D.G., Hoffman, S.W., 2003. Concepts of CNS plasticity in the context of brain damage and repair. J. Head Trauma Rehabil. 18 (4), 317–341.

Stokes, E.K., 2009. Outcome measurement. In: Lennon, S., Stokes, M. (Eds.), Pocketbook of Neurological Physiotherapy. Edinburgh. Elsevier, Churchill Livingstone, pp. 191–201.

Wade, D.T., 1992. The Barthel ADL index: guidelines. In: Wade, D.T. (Ed.), Measurement in neurological rehabilitation. Oxford University Press, Oxford, pp. 177–178.

Wilson, B.A., Moffat, N., 1992. Clinical management of memory problems, second ed. Chapman & Hall, London.

Wood, R.L., 1990. Neurobehavioural sequelae of traumatic brain injury. Taylor & Francis, London.

Section | 3 |

Skill acquisition and learning

Chapter | **18**

Physical activity and exercise in neurological rehabilitation

Bernhard Haas, Amanda Austin

CONTENTS

TERMINOLOGY AND DEFINITIONS

- **Activity:** In general and related to the ICF classification, activity is defined as the 'performance of a task' (WHO, 2001).

- **Physical activity**: Body movements produced by skeletal muscles that results in a substantial increase over resting expenditure (Bouchard et al., 2007).
- **Physical fitness:** A set of attributes relating to the ability to perform physical activity and is comprised of skills-related, health-related and physiologic components (American College of Sports Medicine, 2006):
  - **Performance-related fitness**: Components of fitness necessary for optimal performance at work or sport (Bouchard et al., 2007).
  - **Health-related fitness**: Components of fitness that benefit from a physically active lifestyle and relate to health (Bouchard et al., 2007). These include cardiovascular endurance, muscular strength and endurance, flexibility and body composition (American College of Sports Medicine (ACSM), 2006).
- **Exercise:** Physical activity which involves planned, structured and repetitive movements with the aim to maintain or improve physical fitness (ACSM, 2006).
- Strength is the capacity of a muscle or a group of muscles to produce the force necessary for initiating, maintaining and controlling movement (Ng & Shepherd, 2000).

INTRODUCTION AND CONTEXT

Engaging in exercise and being physically active has shown substantial health benefits in the general population. There is now overwhelming evidence that active lifestyles reduce rates of hypertension, obesity, stroke, coronary artery disease, some cancers, diabetes and osteoporosis (Blair, 2007; Cluve, 2008). A change in lifestyle from inactivity to activity and participation in exercise is associated with a reduction in disease and reduced premature mortality. This suggests that for most of us it is never too late to start being active and change exercise behaviour because the benefits are achievable at any age (ACSM, 2006).

Individuals with neurological conditions are often challenged by movement difficulties and therefore adopt a more sedentary lifestyle with increasing muscle weakness and cardiovascular deconditioning. This exposes them to all the risk factors associated with inactivity, in addition to the risk factors that contributed to their conditions in the first place. A basic level of fitness is essential for carrying out activities of daily living. For example, light housework and carrying shopping requires approximately 40–50% of peak VO_2. Housework of lower workload intensity requires a minimum of 32% of peak VO_2 (Arnett et al., 2008). This chapter proposes that, just like the general population, individuals with neurological conditions also benefit from staying active and taking regular exercise. This chapter therefore provides an overview of activity and exercise in these patient groups and outlines the current evidence to support this aspect of patient management. Wherever possible, guidance for exercise prescription will be presented. Aerobic training, resisted muscle strengthening, constraint-induced movement therapy and treadmill training will be discussed in more detail. Also see 'Exercise and Movement' in Chapter 12.

BEING ACTIVE WITH A NEUROLOGICAL CONDITION

Most people know that being active has health benefits and yet the majority of the general population is not adequately active to benefit (Marcus et al., 2000). Levels of exercise adoption suggest that this is also true for people with neurological conditions. For example, peak oxygen consumption following stroke has been found to be as low as low as 50% of the capacity of age- and sex-matched sedentary controls (Pang et al., 2006). In many cases it may be the fact that a person has an impairment or disability which contributes to their inactivity. Serious life events, such as being diagnosed with a long-term condition, make it more difficult to adopt or maintain an adequate level of exercise (Oman & King, 2000). It is probably unrealistic to expect our patients to change typical behaviours of exercise after a stroke, acquired brain injury, or being diagnosed with Parkinson's disease. However, it appears that it is exactly this type of behaviour change that is required in most of our patients if they are to experience what we know are the benefits of exercise. Therefore, we are seriously challenged to identify the barriers to exercise adoption (also see 'Engagement with falls prevention' in Ch. 20). We will also need to be able to design more appropriate exercise service models and

prescribe specific exercises to meet the goals of the patient, or adapt more general exercise guidance to fit specific conditions.

Kang (2007) found that young people with disabilities face many barriers to participating in or maintaining exercise behaviour. Barriers most frequently cited were a lack of time and actual pain and discomfort during exercise. Others were lack of facilities to exercise with peers, adverse weather and misconceptions by non-disabled people about the ability of the patient to take part in exercise. A better understanding of exercise 'adherence models' therefore may help service provision in the long term. It has recently been suggested that it is predominantly the intentions from the outset, described as the 'Theory of Planned Behaviour' (Yardley & Donovan-Hall, 2007), that determine exercise adherence and, to a lesser extent, symptom experience during exercise and rehabilitation. Very specific support in the form of counselling has also improved exercise adherence (van der Ploeg et al., 2006). A recent study (Elsworth et al., 2009) reported that people with neurological conditions would enjoy being active and taking part in exercise, but that they are mostly put off by embarrassment and the lack of well-educated staff with detailed knowledge of individual conditions. Group participation with people with similar disabilities was preferred and supervision by professionals with appropriate expertise was seen as a priority. This chapter therefore outlines the barriers that can relate to the individual and their personal concerns, the professional and support staff and their expertise, the facilities and transport and the overall service provision (see Figure 18.1).

Overcoming barriers to leading an active life and participating in exercise is a key challenge for rehabilitation therapists and knowledge of reported barriers is the first step in rising to this challenge. The reader is at this stage also reminded that physical activity and participation in

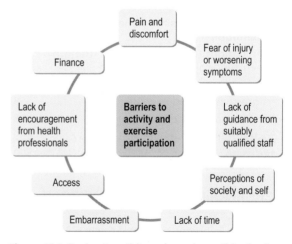

Figure 18.1 Barriers to activity and exercise participation in people with long-term conditions.

exercise fit into the ICF model and framework described by the World Health Organization (WHO, 2001). According to this classification model, barriers to being active and taking part in exercise may well be related to the impairments caused by a particular pathological process. In addition, attitudes of society, inappropriate environments and a lack of adequate transport may make it difficult for some people to take part in regular exercise.

Opening opportunities for participation in exercise is therefore a specific challenge and some recent developments utilizing internet technology may offer alternatives to the more traditional fitness centre or rehabilitation facility. A range of small-scale studies has investigated the feasibility and potential outcome of home-based community exercise supported by internet technology. Often referred to as 'telehealth' or 'telemedicine', this approach seems appropriate in certain circumstances and may be of particular interest to individuals who live in more rural communities. Van den Berg et al. (2006) investigated the internet-based delivery of a home exercise programme for people with rheumatoid arthritis. Whilst the findings may not directly translate to people with neurological conditions, it is worth considering the lessons learned from this trial. The study compared two internet-based exercise programmes. One programme was individualized to the participant with tailored exercises and e-mail correspondence. The other only contained general exercise advice. The group receiving individualized exercise guidance was significantly better in achieving recommended exercise amounts. Finkelstein et al. (2008) evaluated the acceptability and effectiveness of a home-based telemedicine exercise programme in a small group of people with multiple sclerosis (MS). Support and guidance by a telehealth team over the 12-week exercise period showed significant improvements in walking ability and balance scores. Patients were also very satisfied with the service.

Hartley (2009) investigated the use of an exercise therapy model, largely based on patient self-management. The study showed that a self-management exercise programme for people with early MS was effective in improving gait and quality of life.

MEASURING PHYSICAL ACTIVITY AND FITNESS IN NEUROLOGICAL REHABILITATION

Measurement and assessment of activity and physical fitness also fits into the ICF classification (WHO, 2001). Therapists are encouraged to choose appropriate assessment tools to capture the ability or difficulty of an individual to take part in physical activities. This may involve selecting either a global activity scale or, where available, a disease-specific measurement. Table 18.1 provides a selection of measurement scales to choose from. Guidance on a variety of rehabilitation measurements has been produced by Ainsworth (2009), Finch et al. (2002), Stokes (2009) and Bowling (2001).

More recently, a number of authors have evaluated the use of motion sensors in various patient groups, including some with neurological conditions. No comprehensive review on the use of these devices for people with neurological conditions currently exists and therefore there is yet no clear sense of the value of these instruments in neuro-rehabilitation. However, early signs suggest that these relatively simple and inexpensive devices may provide an objective measure of activity and therefore add to the often subjective nature of activity scales or patient recall. The group of motion sensors suggested for this purpose range from simple step counters to a variety of accelerometers. The technology has been evaluated in a group of older people by de Bruin et al. (2008)

Table 18.1 Activity measurement scales

ACTIVITY SCALE/ MEASUREMENT	REFERENCE	COMMENT
Barthel Index	Mahoney and Barthel, 1965	Has been used in stroke, spinal cord injuries, MS and older people; good reliability in stroke
Functional Independence Measure (FIM)	Keith et al., 1987	Has been used in MS, older people, stroke, head injury, Parkinson's disease; reliability variable between conditions
Rivermead Mobility Index	Collen et al., 1991	Developed for stroke patients and has shown reliability in this group
Baecke Activity Questionnaire	Voorips et al., 1991	Designed for use in older people; has been used in Parkinson's disease
Physical Activity Questionnaire (IPAQ)	Craig et al., 2003	The questionnaire can be administered in different forms (e.g. telephone or interview) and has shown reliability

Table 18.2 Measurements and tests for physical and health-related fitness

EXERCISE/ FITNESS MEASUREMENT	REFERENCE	COMMENT
Walking tests, e.g. • Timed up and go test • Self selected walking speed • 2, 6, 12 minute walk test • Self paced walk test • Shuttle walk test	Finch et al., 2002 Mudge and Stott, 2007	The various tests have been used with different patient groups. The reader is referred to Finch et al. (2002) or Mudge and Stott (2007) for a more detailed review
Physiological Cost Index	Danielsson et al., 2007	Measures energy expenditure during walking; reliable in normal subjects but not fully consistent in stroke
Rating of perceived exertion	Borg, 1998	Reliable and correlates well with heart rate and lactate thresholds
Graded exercise testing with metabolic test systems and protocols on treadmill or cycle ergometer	American College of Sports Medicine, 2006	Objective measure of exercise capacity and helps identify limiting factors Measurements can be reliable and have been used in various patient groups

and their findings suggest that the technology is available and improving in terms of device reliability. Acceptability for the wearer varies between devices and must be considered carefully. Accelerometers have also been used in activity assessment in young people with cerebral palsy (Van der Slot et al., 2007), stroke patients (Hale et al., 2008) and in Parkinson's disease (Skidmore et al., 2008). Common to all these studies was the relative ease of use and good reliability of measurements.

Measuring physical or health-related fitness requires a set of scales or tools, which will be different from activity measurements. Therapists or researchers are advised to consider carefully the nature of the impairment they may wish to evaluate and also the cost of measurement and the necessary skill required in conducting fitness measurements. A range of measurements and tools are available and Table 18.2 provides a selection of relevant fitness assessment tools. In many instances simple timed walking tests will provide a useful measure of walking-related fitness/ability which can be used to assess, review or screen patients. More complex measurements, particularly those that involve the measurement of metabolic systems, will of course provide an extensive range of information. However, conducting measurements of this nature requires specialist equipment and training, and may not add significantly to the patient assessment information. Therefore, therapists are advised to consider carefully what type of assessment information they require.

Graded exercise tests have an inherent risk of cardiac events and should only be conducted when appropriate facilities to deal with cardiac arrests are available. The following indicate when to terminate a graded exercise test:

• Onset of angina or angina-like symptoms
• Signs of poor perfusion (light-headedness, confusion, ataxia, pallor, cyanosis, nausea, cold and clammy skin)

• Failure of heart rate to increase with increased exercise intensity
• Noticeable change in heart rhythm
• Blood pressure rises to above 240/120 mmHg
• Physical or verbal manifestation of severe fatigue
• Failure of the testing or monitoring equipment
• Patient requests to stop.

EFFECTS OF EXERCISE AND PHYSICAL ACTIVITY

Evidence suggests that staying active and taking regular exercise has clear health benefits (Blair, 2007). There is now also a growing body of evidence showing that people with neurological conditions can benefit from exercise. There are now growing recommendations to include aspects of exercise training as part of the overall rehabilitation for people following spinal cord injury (Janssen & Hopman, 2005), stroke (Royal College of Physicians, 2004), MS (Rietberg et al., 2004), cerebral palsy (Rogers et al., 2008) and Parkinson's disease (Skidmore et al., 2008). The effects of exercise are usually described in terms of acute and chronic effects on the cardiorespiratory and neuromuscular system. Table 18.3 briefly summarizes some of these general effects of exercise. For further details, the reader is referred to exercise physiology textbooks, such as McArdle et al. (2006). It is important to note that the response to exercise in people with neurological conditions will vary and therapists are advised to take this into account when prescribing exercise.

The effects on the nervous system of exercise and its response have not undergone extensive research. However, it appears that this area would be of particular interest to patients with neurological conditions. A small body of

Table 18.3 Key effects and responses to exercise

EXERCISE RESPONSE AND EFFECT	COMMENT
Acute cardiorespiratory response	• HR increases linear to work-rate and oxygen uptake • HR increase depends on age, body composition, fitness, type of activity, illness, medications, environmental factors
Cardiorespiratory training effect	• Increase in VO_2max, cardiac output, blood volume, minute ventilation • Decrease in HRrest, HRsubmax
Acute response to resisted muscle training	• Motor unit activation dependent on amount of resistance and size principle • Type I (slow oxydative) first activated, then • Type II (fast glycolytic) for powerful action • Muscle soreness
Training effect of resisted muscle strengthening	• Hyperplasia (increase in number of muscle cells) • Muscle fibre size increase dependent on type of training • Strengthening of ligaments, tendons and bone • Metabolic changes (enzymatic adaptation, energy, capillary supply) • Increased neural drive

HR, heart rate; VO_2, maximal oxygen uptake

knowledge exists which suggests that there may be effects of exercise which go beyond conditioning of the cardiorespiratory and muscular system. These effects have so far been studied in animal models under a limited number of conditions. These studies suggest that taking part in regular aerobic exercise may have a neuroprotective effect. Smith & Zigmond (2003) investigated this possibility in an animal model of Parkinson's disease. Their study showed that forced physical activity in rats had a neuroprotective effect, believed to be due to a reduction in oxidative stress. Exercise may be able to slow the cognitive decline seen in Parkinson's disease and also in Alzheimer's disease (Dishman et al., 2006). Exercise enhances the calcium transport to the brain which in turn enhances dopamine synthesis. This may explain the potential for neuroprotection or restoration in Parkinson's disease and dementia (Sutoo & Akiyama, 2003). An intensive 12-week 'running' activity in rats after middle cerebral artery occlusion has resulted in reduced infarct volumes, mediated via increased nerve growth factor (Ang et al., 2003). The authors concluded that physical exercise may cause neuroprotection following stroke. These studies are restricted to animal models but they point towards an exciting potential role of exercise in rehabilitation. This role may go beyond increasing fitness and strength for the purpose of improving function and quality of life. Exercise may protect the brain from some chronic diseases, such as Parkinson's disease. Exercise may also have potential to facilitate brain plasticity following stroke. Basic research and clinical studies suggest that high intensity (i.e. high repetition, velocity and complexity) is a characteristic of exercise that may be important in promoting activity-dependent neuroplasticity of the injured brain (Nudo & Milliken, 1996).

AEROBIC EXERCISE TRAINING IN NEUROLOGICAL REHABILITATION

There is an increasing range of aerobic exercise options being accessed by people with neurological conditions. These range from aerobic exercise programmes (e.g. overground walking or treadmill training programmes) and an array of sporting and exercise classes to the use of technology (e.g. virtual reality training). These options, supported by the growing body of evidence, present the therapist and patient with the ability to select a programme for an individual, which is timely and can be carried out in an appropriate environment.

Aerobic exercise programmes

Walking, either overground or treadmill, is a task-orientated aerobic exercise programme that emerges from the literature as a firm favourite. Overground programmes have the additional advantage of being easily accessible and of low cost. Ada et al. (2003b) showed that a community-based programme incorporating treadmill training alongside an overground walking programme significantly improved walking speed and walking capacity, although effects on disability were less clear. Trials involving treadmills have also demonstrated improvements ranging from improved gait speed and capacity (Macko et al., 2005) to changes in corticomotor excitablity (Fisher et al., 2008). Further detail and guidance for the use of treadmill training can be seen later in this chapter.

Table 18.4 Guidance for aerobic exercise prescription in neurological rehabilitation

	STROKE/BRAIN INJURY	SPINAL CORD INJURY	MULTIPLE SCLEROSIS
Intensity	40–70% VO_2peak or 50–80% HRmax	50–80% HRpeak	50–70% VO_2peak or 60–85% HRpeak
Frequency	3–7 times/week	3–5 times/week	3 times/week
Duration	20–60 minutes or multiples of 10 minutes	20–60 minutes	30 minutes

HR, heart rate; VO_2, maximal oxygen uptake

Another common aerobic approach utilizes cycle ergometry with functional and health-related quality of life improvements being demonstrated in a range of conditions including MS (Kileff & Ashburn, 2005; Mostert & Kesselring, 2002); spinal cord injury (Ditor et al., 2003; Hicks et al., 2003); and stroke (Tang et al., 2009). Aquatic exercise programmes are also popular and research has shown improvements in peak workload and function (Chu et al., 2004; Pariser et al., 2006).

A combination of aerobic exercise, including walking, cycling and swimming, can result in positive treatment outcomes (Pang et al., 2006; Snook & Motl, 2009). Comprehensive guidance for prescribing aerobic exercise in neurological rehabilitation is currently incomplete and not fully based on high-quality evidence. Table 18.4 outlines some guidance for a number of conditions based on Gordon et al. (2004) and the ACSM (2003). The guidance is very broad and must be adapted to the individual after careful assessment.

Sports/exercise classes

Increasingly, a range of sporting options (e.g. swimming, athletics and wheelchair sports such as basketball, rugby or tennis) and exercise classes with some aerobic effects (e.g. tai chi, dance or yoga) are being undertaken by people with neurological conditions as part of rehabilitation and as activities following discharge from conventional rehabilitation. One reason for therapists to consider incorporating these types of exercise into their exercise recomendations is that these activities may not only improve physical function, but also increase levels of participation.

People with spinal cord injury participating in sports have reported effects on aspects of health-related quality of life as well as facilitation of community reintegration by, for example, improved social reintegration networks or peer support (Labronici et al., 2000; Tasiemski et al., 2005). It is worth noting that Tasiemski et al. (2000) found that levels of participation in sporting activities decreased significantly after injury in people with spinal cord injury and that barriers to participation in these activities remain a complex issue, as illustrated in Figure 18.1 previously.

Therapists should also consider the use of other exercise classes such as tai chi, yoga or ballroom dancing. In older adults with chronic conditions tai chi appears to be safe and effective in promoting balance control, flexibility and cardiovascular fitness, alongside the psychosocial benefits (Wang et al., 2004). Tai chi has been trialled with people with Parkinson's disease, but currently there is a lack of robust literature in this area (Lee et al., 2008). More recently yoga has been proposed as one of a range of mind–body therapies that could be of benefit to people with neurological conditions (Wahbeh et al., 2008). Researchers are also turning to innovative options such as dance, e.g. tango or American ballroom, which is showing promise in improving measures of walking, balance and quality of life measures in people with Parkinson's disease (Hackney & Earhart, 2009).

Virtual reality training

Advances in virtual reality technology mean that devices using computer and gaming technology, such as the Nintendo Wii ®, are now found in many people's homes. The potential of these types of adjuncts to maximize task-orientated practice and increase energy expenditure are beginning to be explored. The use of games using the Nintendo Wii ®, for example, has shown to increase energy expenditure in a group of asymptomatic participants (Graves et al., 2007; Lanningham-Forster et al., 2009). Research in individuals with neurological disorders, such as cerebral palsy, is beginning to emerge (Deutsch et al., 2008).

Treadmill training

The incentive to provide a challenging environment, in which there is an opportunity to practise repetitively the missing components of gait, has underpinned another task-specific activity. This involves using a treadmill for gait training and also for improvements in aerobic function. A harness can be used for individuals with significant functional limitations, and this also offers the opportunity to grade the amount of body weight support provided. Therapists help to facilitate alternating stepping and weight-bearing, and as many as three therapists may be required to assist with the complete gait cycle.

Shepherd and Carr (1999) argued that there are three reasons why treadmill training can support gait re-education:

- It allows a complete practice of the gait cycle
- It provides opportunity for gaining improvements in speed and endurance
- It optimizes aerobic fitness.

Recent work has also suggested that treadmill training may also have positive effects on upper limb function, cognitive function and social participation (Ploughman et al., 2008; Smith & Thompson, 2008). It is important to note that these findings are currently based on limited research work. The effects of treadmill training beyond walking may therefore be co-incidental.

The original work on the effects of treadmill training involved animal studies (Barbeau et al., 1999). Animals with transected spinal cords were able to generate activity in lower limb muscles and produce a stepping motion. Research carried out on humans with incomplete spinal cord injury also showed it was possible to elicit similar activity when the individual was suspended in a harness and stepping was facilitated on a treadmill (Dobkin, 1999). This served to support the theory that humans may possess specific neural circuitry in the lumbar spinal cord that may have the ability for motor learning. The mechanism for motor learning appears as a consequence of repeated sensory inputs into lumbosacral motoneurones and interneurones, which leads to long-term potentiation. Repeated practice of the gait cycle, involving alternating loading and unloading of the lower-limbs and hip extension, seems to be the main sensory drive to promote the motor activity (Hesse, 1999).

Task-specific training on a treadmill is likely to induce expansion of subcortical and cortical locomotion areas in individuals following stroke and spinal cord injury (Dobkin, 1999; Hesse, 1999). It is also important to note, however, that whilst treadmill training has the potential to improve gait function in a number of neurological conditions, this approach may not necessarily be superior to other methods of gait training. Dickstein (2008) compared treatment outcomes of various therapeutic interventions on gait speed following stroke. The comparison indicated that gait speed can be improved through a variety of interventions but treadmill training was not found to be superior in this patient group. The authors concluded that 'low-tech' techniques can be as effective in gait training following stroke as more expensive treadmill and robotic approaches.

Readers are also reminded that treadmill walking can differ from overground walking and this can have profound effects on gait rehabilitation. Treadmill walking can result in an increase in cadence and a shortening of step length compared to overground walking. Wearing a harness dampens vertical spinal acceleration and reduces trunk rotation. Applying a body-weight support reduces the need to oppose gravity and this again reduces not only vertical, but also anterior-posterior acceleration (Aaslund & Moe-Nilssen, 2008). The altered visual experience of walking across a moving ground may also be difficult to cope with for some individuals.

KEY POINTS

Treadmill training:
- can be used safely
- with added harness systems provides security
- offers task-specific practice of ambulation
- improves gait parameters
- has not been found to increase spasticity
- may not be superior to low tech approaches for gait training following stroke
- differs slightly from overground walking.

Gait rehabilitation using treadmill training with partial body-weight support offers the possibility for active and task-specific gait training following stroke, even with individuals with low levels of functional ability (Hesse et al., 1999). Hesse et al. (1995a, 1995b) investigated the use of treadmill training and partial body-weight support with individuals following chronic stroke. These early studies showed some encouraging results, with changes in gait parameters such as stride length, cadence and velocity following the intervention, even if treadmill training may not be superior to other low tech approaches. Figure 18.2 shows a man with incomplete spinal cord injury at C5–C6 using a treadmill with harness body-weight support.

Smith et al. (1998) found normalization of reflexive activity in some individuals by the end of their programme, implying that reductions in spasticity could also accompany the strength gains seen in treadmill training. This indicates that there is no evidence to support the fear that treadmill training increases mass synergistic activity in the weaker side. Forrester et al. (2006) investigated the effects of treadmill training on central motor excitability. They showed, through transcranial magnetic stimulation, that treadmill training has the potential to alter the responsiveness of the lower-extremity central motor pathways.

As well as people with stroke, treadmill training has also been used by people with spinal cord injury (Behrman & Harkema, 2000; Dobkin, 2004), cerebral palsy (Schindl et al., 2000), MS (Giesser et al., 2007) and Parkinson's disease (Fisher et al., 2008). Despite methodological limitations these studies suggest that treadmill training can be an effective tool for improving gait function in serveral neurological pathologies.

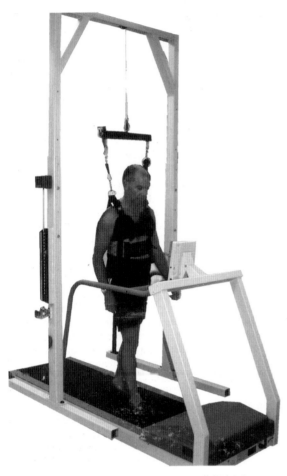

Figure 18.2 A man with incomplete spinal cord injury at C5–C6 using a treadmill with harness body weight support.

Behrman and Harkema (2000) described the range of sensory cues needed to induce a reasonably normal reciprocal gait pattern when using treadmill training following spinal cord injury. Listed below, they could just as easily be adopted as aims for any treadmill training programme attempting to normalize gait:

- Generation of speeds which induce normal stepping responses
- Applying a maximal sustainable load on the supporting limb during stance phase
- Maintaining upright trunk and head posture
- Obtaining near-normal ankle, knee and hip kinematics throughout gait cycle
- Synchronizing the timing of extension and loading of supporting limb, with simultaneous unloading of the contralateral limb
- Decreasing weight-bearing through handrails by encouraging arm swing.

Body-weight support and mechanized gait training

The optimum level of body-weight support seems to be that which allows maximum loading of the limb during the stance phase, whilst providing support for those individuals who are unable to maintain an upright posture independently. There is also agreement that as soon as an individual is progressing towards being able to balance independently whilst taking a step, the inclusion of practice of overground walking should be given more priority (Behrman & Harkema, 2000).

Hesse et al. (1997) suggested using a limit of 30% body-weight support; above this level heel strike and limb loading are compromised. Body-weight support has been shown to reduce double support time, and therefore may offer more scope to compensate for balance deficits, whilst maintaining an upright posture and producing a stepping motion (Barbeau et al., 1999).

The effort required by physiotherapists to assist with the gait cycle may be reduced with body-weight support systems, but still needs careful consideration. Training programmes often describe the involvement of three therapists for individuals with a spinal cord injury and two for stroke. One therapist stands astride the treadmill and behind the patient, facilitating lateral pelvic tilt and weight shift. The other one or two therapists crouch alongside the treadmill to lift and position the patient's lower-limb(s).

Understandable concerns about the effort required by therapists during the treatment has led researchers to look at developing other assistive devices, such as the mechanized gait trainer developed by Hesse et al. (1999, 2000) and, more recently, robotic devices to add to the treadmill set-up. Aoyagi et al. (2007) designed their robotic system with the aim of working alongside the therapists who would be able to facilitate certain elements of the gait cycle. The robotic device would then remove the need for several therapists to be involved in coordinating several tasks at the same time. This particular system reported good technical qualities, but the complexity of instruments of this nature, in terms of attachments and adjustments, may limit their use in clinical practice. Lo & Triche (2008) investigated the use of body-weight supported treadmill training with and without robotic assistance in two groups of people with MS. Gait measurements improved significantly in both groups but the differences between groups were not significant, suggesting that the robotic device may not add anything to the outcome of the intervention, but that it may ease the work input by therapy staff.

Regnaux et al. (2008) suggested that robotic devices impose additional mechanical constraints on the gait cycle and the impacts of these on gait training are not yet fully understood.

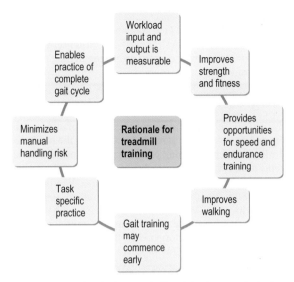

Figure 18.3 Rationale for treadmill training in neurological conditions.

It may be fair to conclude that new technology is being developed with the aim of easing the manual handling load of gait re-education, but at present there is no one system which seems to be able to address all necessary rehabilitation and therapy needs. Ultimately, it is unlikely that treadmill training will replace overground walking practice within neurorehabilitation. However, it clearly provides an addition to the repertoire of task-specific training programmes that have gained credibility. Figure 18.3 summarizes the rationale for using treadmill training in neurorehabilitation.

RESISTED STRENGTH TRAINING IN NEUROLOGICAL REHABILITATION

Interventions to improve muscle strength in neurological rehabilitation

There are a number of treatments available to therapists to improve muscle strength (Ada et al., 2006; Bohannon, 2007a; Dobkin, 2004), these include:

- resisted strength training
- progressive resisted exercise
- biofeedback
- electrical stimulation
- robotic therapies.

Meta-analysis of results from trials of these types of interventions in stroke has shown potential for improvements both at the impairment and activity levels (Ada et al., 2006).

Investigations into muscle weakness following stroke have concluded that there is reduced muscle strength in the limbs contralateral to the side of the brain lesion (Andrews & Bohannon, 2000; Bohannon, 1997b; Bohannon & Walsh, 1992; Sunnerhagen et al., 1999;). It must also be remembered that the limbs ipsilateral to the brain lesion are not 'normal', but also show signs of muscular weakness (Andrews & Bohannon, 2000; Harris et al., 2001). The trunk muscles, both contralateral and ipsilateral to the brain lesion, are weakened with all trunk movements being affected by the weakness (Bohannon, 1995; Bohannon et al., 1995; Tanaka et al., 1997). Lower limb paresis or weakness following a stroke is seen in about 4–15% of all strokes (Jungehulsing et al., 2008; Wandel et al., 2000). In those able to perform voluntary movements, lower limb strength may be reduced by 45% in the paretic side at the time they are discharged from rehabilitation (Andrews & Bohannon, 2000).

A minimum level of muscle strength is required to carry out physical activities and weakness can lead to substantial activity limitations. Brill et al. (2000) found evidence for this in the healthy population and studies of muscle strength of individuals with neurological conditions have reached similar conclusions (Bohannon, 2007b). Lower limb weakness has been correlated with a reduction in walking speed and endurance (Nakamura, 1988), a need for assistance with walking (Bohannon, 1988) and for assistance with transfers (Bohannon, 1989). Bohannon (2007a, 2007b) proposes that there are thresholds of force generation required to perform certain activities: for example, the achievement of sit to stand requires a minimum knee extensor force. The upper limb muscle weakness found in stroke contributes to reduced dexterity, hand grip and hand function (Canning et al., 2004; Ng & Shepherd, 2000). Contrary to common beliefs, flexor muscles in the upper limb are weaker than the extensor muscles (Andrews & Bohannon, 2000).

Two main causes of weakness are present following stroke; firstly, the ability to activate the muscle is compromised by poor descending motor control and, secondly, muscle weakness is related to disuse muscle atrophy after a period of decreased activity (Newsam & Baker, 2004). Central causes of weakness relate not only to the lack of descending drive, but also to changes in intrinsic motor neuron properties; these lead to lower motor unit firing rates, poor rate modulation and delayed recruitment (Ada et al., 2003a; Zijdewind & Thomas, 2003). Whilst stroke has been used as an example above, muscle weakness has also been demonstrated in other neurological pathologies such as: cerebral palsy (Maruishi et al., 2001), Parkinson's disease (Allen et al., 2009), spinal cord injury (Arnold et al., 2006) and multiple sclerosis (Freeman et al., 2008).

Understanding the causes of muscle weakness, how they change with time and are affected by interventions may allow clinicians to target treatment interventions appropriately. Interventions that, for example, help to predominately maintain or improve the peripheral component may not result in any large strength-related changes in function, as these would depend on the ability of the central nervous system to adequately activate the motor neuron pool (Landau & Sahrmann, 2002).

Strength measurements are not frequently used in stroke rehabilitation. However, Bohannon (1997a) and Bohannon and Walsh (1992) have established that, despite their limitations, strength measurements can give useful information and can be reliable, provided that standardized procedures are followed.

Resisted strength training

The use of resisted strengthening exercises in neurological rehabilitation has now been broadly accepted as best clinical practice and should be implemented with the aim to maintain or increase muscle strength and function. The National Clinical Guidelines for Stroke (Royal College of Physicians, 2004) clearly recommend strengthening programmes in targeted muscles.

Evidence from other neurogical conditions also points toward muscle weakness as an impairment which could be improved with resisted strengthening exercises. Individuals with cerebral palsy (Scianni et al., 2009), Parkinson's disease (Scandalis et al., 2001) and MS (de Boldt & McCubbin, 2002) have the potential to gain muscle strength and increase function.

Clear evidence-based guidance for the prescription of resisted strength training programmes have yet to be developed for the majority of neurological conditions. The following guidance is based on the ACSM (2003) and offers broad help for those who prescribe and monitor strengthening exercises to patients with neurological conditions (see Table 18.5). It is important to note that this guidance is broad and requires careful assessment and potential modification with individual patients.

In addition, researchers have tended to apply loads of about 60–85% of the muscle's force-generating capacity, which is measured at the beginning of the strengthening programme and then regularly throughout. Therefore, it is important to remember that strength training should be individualized and specific to the muscle groups that require strengthening. Free weights, resistance apparatus and isokinetic machines, as well as resistance arm and leg ergometers, can be used for strengthening exercise programmes.

Progressive resisted exercise

Evidence is growing to support the use of progressive resisted exercise, i.e. progressively increasing the resistance during a strength training programme to improve muscle-generating force in neurological conditions such as cerebral palsy (Dodd et al., 2003) and stroke (Morris et al., 2004), with promising trends evident for improvements in activity over and above those seen with resisted strength training alone. An increase in transient muscle soreness has been reported, but this is not unexpected with resisted exercise (Taylor et al., 2005).

Morris et al. (2004) suggest that there are three important factors to a progressive resisted exercise protocol:

- Sufficient load (resistance)
- Progressively increasing resistance as strength increases
- Performance of the exercises for a sufficient amount of time.

Taylor et al. (2005) stress the importance of allowing sufficient rest between each set of exercises. Body positioning during training may also be an important factor, such as training in functional positions or during functional tasks (Ada et al., 2004; Morris et al., 2004; Wolf et al., 2006, 2008). In less severely affected patients, training effects in such positions can be greater than those seen with resistance strength training (Winstein et al., 2004). Therefore, it is important to perform the training wherever possible in a functional position, for example, quadriceps-strengthening exercises during a sit to stand task.

Adjuncts to strength training

There are a range of adjuncts that can be used for strength training, which are increasingly being incorporated into neurological rehabilitation. These include biofeedback, electrical stimulation and robotic therapies.

Table 18.5 Guidance for resisted strengthening exercises in neurological rehabilitation

	STROKE/BRAIN INJURY	SPINAL CORD INJURY	MULTIPLE SCLEROSIS
Intensity	3 sets of 8–15 repetitions	2–3 sets of 8–15 repetitions	2–3 sets of 8–15 repetitions
Frequency	2 sessions/week	2–4 sessions/week	Not on same day as aerobic training

Notes: Strengthening programme should involve major muscle groups and use concentric as well as eccentric activities
Weaker individuals will benefit from reducing weights/resistance, so that they can perform more (i.e. 15) repetitions
Many patients will need supervision, feedback and clear guidance

Biofeedback using electromyographic (EMG) signals from muscles is commonly used in musculoskeletal and women's health by physiotherapists; the potential for this modality to aid in improving muscle strength in neurological rehabilitation is increasingly being proposed (Carr & Shepherd, 2006; Glinsky et al., 2007). However, evidence from robust clinical trials is still lacking (Scianni et al., 2009; Woodford & Price, 2007). A number of systematic reviews of controlled trials of *electrical stimulation* in a range of neurological conditions have highlighted its potential effects on strength (Ada & Foongchomcheay, 2002; Glanz et al., 1996; Glinsky et al., 2007; Kerr et al., 2004; Pomeroy et al., 2006; Singer, 1987). Although the majority of research is devoted to studies in the upper limb, there are promising studies in the lower limb where the majority of work has targeted the dorsiflexors to improve a known consequence of stroke: dropped foot (Burridge et al., 1997; Macdonnell et al., 1994; Merletti et al., 1978). The uptake of electrical stimulation in clinical practice remains low, which may relate to the lack of robust evidence and the lack of clinical guidelines for its use.

Robotic therapies are currently mostly confined to laboratory research. However, they are showing potential both for recovery of upper limb function following stroke (Prange et al., 2006) and lower limb function following stroke and spinal cord injury (see treadmill training above). Krebs et al. (2009) propose that the ability for robotic therapies to combine repetitive, intense, task-specific practice may be key to the neurological recovery seen with these modalities. Merholz et al. (2008) in their systematic review reported that improvements are more likely to be seen in muscle strength and arm motor function than in activities of daily living. Whether these therapies can be incorporated into day-to-day clinical practice remains untested.

The potential to combine principles from interventions to target muscle weakness warrants further investigation. For example, Newsam and Baker (2004) found that the combination of electrical stimulation and progressive resisted exercise showed strength improvements over and above that from progressive resisted exercise alone.

KEY POINTS

Muscle-strengthening programmes:
- can be used safely
- increase muscle strength
- improve a patient's activity level
- have not been found to increase spasticity.

Consider training in functional positions.
Consider training with adjuncts.

CONSTRAINT INDUCED MOVEMENT THERAPY

Programmes that incorporate an intensive therapy programme described as forced-use or constraint induced movement therapy (CIMT) have shown some of the most promising evidence thus far that motor recovery can be facilitated over and above the natural period of recovery after a stroke (Liepert et al., 2000). Indeed, this form of task-oriented training (Wolf et al., 2006, 2008) can result in functional improvements that, in less severely affected patients, can be greater than that seen with strength training (Winstein et al., 2004). Following any severe and sudden neurological insult there may be a period of shock or diaschesis; the threshold necessary for motor output then becomes elevated. It has been suggested that if successful motor output is not achieved, a conditioned suppression of activity may be the result (Sunderland & Tuke, 2005). Failure or difficulty in the attempt to move may then further suppress limb use, and this has been termed 'learned non use' (Taub et al., 1998).

After brain damage, such as that resulting from stroke, a complex pattern of neurological reorganization occurs (see Ch. 2). There have been reports of a reduction in motor cortex excitability, in the cortical representation of the paralysed muscles and an alteration in cortical activation (Liepert et al., 2001; Ward & Cohen, 2004). Non-invasive techniques for studying the human brain, such as transcranial magnetic stimulation and functional magnetic resonance imaging, are demonstrating the potential for CIMT to induce functionally relevant cortical reorganization (Levy et al., 2001; Sawaki et al., 2008).

Programmes using CIMT or modified CIMT focus attention towards the weaker limb and use repeated and extensive practice termed 'shaping' for up to 6 hours per day. The stronger arm is constrained in a sling and/or padded mitt. The motivation for motor output changes and subsequent accomplishment of a task then serves as a positive reinforcement for future attempts. Modified constraint or mCIMT, a variation of CIMT, is used to describe shorter periods of restraint over a longer intervention period and has also shown potential for improvements in motor control (Page et al., 2001).

Research in CIMT has demonstrated significant changes in measures of upper limb function in chronic (Page et al., 2004; Taub et al., 1993; Van der Lee et al., 1999; Wittenberg et al., 2003), subacute (Alberts et al., 2004; Page et al., 2002; Wolf et al., 2006) and acute stroke (Dromerick et al., 2000; Page et al., 2005). This body of evidence has resulted in CIMT being incorporated into the National Clinical Guidelines for Stroke (Royal College of Physicians, 2004). This recommends the use of CIMT with patients who have at least 10 degrees of active wrist and finger extension; who are more than 1 year post stroke; and are able to walk independently without an aid.

Some researchers and clinicians have questioned the suitability of all patients for CIMT. Inclusion criteria used in a number of studies were stringent and excluded a large proportion of stroke patients with significant impairments. Taub et al. (1998) discussed more relaxed criteria and more recently studies in patients outside these inclusion criteria have shown improvements in motor control (Bonifer et al., 2005; Page & Levin, 2007; Wu et al., 2007).

Tuke (2008), in a narrative review of CIMT, discussed the important elements for a CIMT programme:

- Type of CIMT, i.e. traditional or modified
- Restraint, e.g. sling, padded mitt
- Wear time, e.g. various times up to 90% of waking hours
- Excluded activities, e.g. those with balance or safety considerations
- Compliance, e.g. log book or instruction cards
- Shaping, i.e. therapy component of CIMT
- Shaping dosage, e.g. various times up to 6 hours a day
- Group vs individual treatment
- Environment, i.e. inpatient vs outpatient.

Therapists and patients have raised some concerns about the practicalities of administering such an intensive programme, questioning patients' ability to engage actively during the proposed hours of practice (Page et al., 2002). These concerns are being addressed by studies such as The EXCITE trial of CIMT, which showed significant improvements in motor function after a 2-week programme (Wolf et al., 2006) with functional improvements persisting at 1 and 2 years' post-intervention (Wolf et al., 2008). Concerns over safety for patients with balance deficits are also being addressed by the use of padded mitts and excluded activities such as tasks involving balance (Dromerick et al., 2000; Sterr & Freivogel, 2003). Taub & Uswatte (2006) summarized that some of the questions remaining to be answered include:

- how cost-effective is CIMT therapy?
- what are optimal training and other treatment parameters?
- what patient characteristics moderate the effects of CIMT therapy?

CONCLUSION

The evidence supports the need for therapists to create opportunities in which an individual is encouraged to persevere with tasks that are meaningful and at a level sufficient to induce changes in strength and fitness. Therapists require knowledge about how to help facilitate a change in exercise behaviour, so that activity is maintained long term to prevent secondary deconditioning. Therapists may need to think beyond the restraints of the neurogym, and consider more active and dynamic collaboration with agencies providing leisure and social pursuits. This could involve the use of a range of activities which can have wide-ranging effects, for example tai chi, sports, dance or yoga, as well as new technologies based on computer gaming technologies.

REFERENCES

Aaslund, M.K., Moe-Nilssen, R., 2008. Treadmill walking with body weight support: Effect of treadmill, harness and body weight support systems. Gait Posture 28, 303–308.

Ada, L., Foongchomcheay, 2002. Efficacy of electrical stimulation in preventing or reducing subluxation of the shoulder following stroke: a meta-analysis. Aust. J. Physiother. 48, 257–267.

Ada, L., Canning, C., Shau-Ling, L., 2003a. Stroke patients have selective muscle weakness in shortened range. Brain 126, (3), 724–731.

Ada, L., Dean, C.M., Hall, J.M., Bampton, J., Crompton, S., 2003b. A treadmill and overground walking program improves walking in persons residing in the community after stroke: a placebo controlled randomized trial. Arch. Phys. Med. Rehabil. 84, 1486–1491.

Ada, L., Dorsch, S., Canning, C., 2004. Strengthening interventions improve strength and improve activity after stroke: a systematic review. Aust. J. Physiother. 52, 241–248.

Ada, L., Dorsch, S., Canning, C.G., 2006. Strengthening interventions increase strength and improve activity after stroke: a systematic review. Aust. J. Physiother. 52, 241–248.

Ainsworth, B.E., 2009. How do I measure physical activity in my patients? Questionnaires and objective methods. Br. J. Sports Med. 43 (1), 6–9.

Alberts, J.L., Butler, A.J., Wolf, S.L., 2004. The effects of constraint induced therapy on precision grip: a preliminary study. Neurorehabil. Neural Repair 18, 250–258.

Allen, N.E., Canning, C.G., Sherrington, C., Fung, V.S., 2009. Bradykinesia, muscle weakness and reduced muscle power in parkinson's. Mov. Disord 24 (5), 1344–1351.

American College of Sports Medicine, 2003. Exercise Management for Persons with Chronic Diseases and Disability, vol. 2. Human Kinetics, Champaign.

American College of Sports Medicine, 2006. 2006 ACSM's Guidelines for Exercise Testing and Prescription, seventh ed. Lippincott Williams & Wilkins, Philadelphia.

Andrews, A.W., Bohannon, R.W., 2000. Distribution of muscle strength impairments following stroke. Clin. Rehabil. 14, 79–87.

Ang, E.T., Wong, P.T.H., Moochhalla, S., et al., 2003. Neuroprotection associated with running: is it a result of increased endogenous neurotrophic factors? Neuroscience 118, 335–345.

Aoyagi, D., Ichinose, W.D., Harkema, S. J., et al., 2007. A robot and control algorithm that can synchronously assist in naturalistic motion during body-weight-supported gait training following neurologic injury. IEEE Trans. Neural Syst. Rehabil. Eng. 15, 387–399.

Arnett, S.W., Laity, J.H., Agrawal, S.K., Cress, M.E., 2008. Aerobic reserve and physical functional performance in older adults. Age Ageing 37, 384–389.

Arnold, P.M., Filardi, T.Z., Strang, R.D., McMahon, J.K., 2006. Early neurologic assessment of the patient with spinal cord injury. Top. Spinal Cord Inj. Rehabil. 12, (1), 38–48.

Barbeau, H., Fung, J., Visintin, M., 1999. New approach to retrain gait in stroke and spinal cord injured subjects. Neurorehabil. Neural Repair 13, 177–178.

Behrman, A., Harkema, S., 2000. Locomotion training after human spinal cord injury: a series of case studies. Phys. Ther. 80, 688–699.

Blair, S.N., 2007. Physical inactivity: a mayor public health problem. Br. Nutri. Found. Nutr. Bull. 32, 113–117.

Bohannon, R., 1988. Determinants of transfer capacity in patients with hemiparesis. Physiother. Can. 40, 236–239.

Bohannon, R., 1989. Selected determinants of ambulatory capacity in patients with hemiplegia. Clin. Rehabil. 3, 47–53.

Bohannon, R.W., 1995. Recovery and correlates of trunk muscle strength after stroke. Int. J. Rehabil. Res. 18, 162–167.

Bohannon, R.W., 1997a. Reference values for extremity muscle strength obtained by hand-held dynamometry from adults aged 20–79 years. Arch. Phys. Med. Rehabil. 78, 26–32.

Bohannon, R.W., 1997b. Measurement and nature of muscle strength in patients with stroke. J. Neurol. Rehabil. 11, 115–125.

Bohannon, R., 2007a. Muscle strength and muscle training after stroke. J. Rehabil. Med. 39, 14–20.

Bohannon, R., 2007b. Knee extension strength and body weight determine sit to stand independence after stroke. Physiother. Theory. Pract. 23 (5), 291–297.

Bohannon, R.W., Cassidy, D., Walsh, S., 1995. Trunk muscle strength is impaired multidirectionally after stroke. Clin. Rehabil. 9, 47–51.

Bohannon, R., Walsh, S., 1992. Nature, reliability and predictive value of muscle performance measures in patients with hemiparesis following stroke. Arch. Phys. Med. Rehabil. 73, 721–725.

Bonifer, N.M., Andersen, K.M., Arcieniegas, D.B., 2005. Constraint induced movement therapy after stroke: efficacy for patients with minimal upper extremity motor ability. Arch. Phys. Med. Rehabil. 86, 1867–1873.

Borg, G., 1998. Borg's Perceived Exertion and Pain Scales. Human Kinetics, Illinois.

Bowling, A., 2001. Measuring Disease, second ed. Open University Press, Buckingham.

Bouchard, C., Blair, S.N., Haskell, W.L., 2007. Physical Activity and Health. Human Kinetics, Champaign.

Brill, P.A., Macera, C.A., Davis, D.R., et al., 2000. Muscular strength and physical function. Med. Sci. Sports Exerc. 32, 412–416.

Burridge, J., Taylor, P., Hagan, S., Wood, D., Swain, I., 1997. The effects of common peroneal nerve stimulation on the effort and speed of walking: a randomized controlled trial with chronic hemiplegic patients. Clin. Rehabil. 11, 201–210.

Canning, C., Ada, L., Adams, R., O'Dwyer, N., 2004. Loss of strength contributes more to physical disability after stroke than loss of dexterity. Clin. Rehabil. 18, 300–307.

Carr, J.H., Shepherd, R.B., 2006. The changing face of neurological rehabilitation. Revista Brasileira de Fisioterapia 10 (2), 147–156.

Chu, K.S., Eng, J.J., Dawson, A.S., Harris, J.E., Ozkaplan, A., Gylfadottir, S., 2004. Water-based exercise for cardiovascular fitness in people with chronic stroke. Arch. Phys. Med. Rehabil. 85, 870–874.

Cluve, A., 2008. Exercise and glycemic control in diabetes. Benefits, challenges, and adjustments to pharmacotherapy. Phys. Ther. 88, 1297–1321.

Collen, F.M., Wade, D.T., Robb, G.F., et al., 1991. The Rivermead Mobility Index: A further development of the Rivermead Motor Assessment. Int. Disabil. Stud. 10, 61–63.

Craig, C.L., Marshall, A.L., Sjostrom, M., et al., 2003. International Physical Activity Questionnaire: 12-Country Reliability and Validity. Med. Sci. Sports Exerc. 35, 1381–1395.

Danielsson, A., Willén, C., Sunnerhagen, K.S., 2007. Measurement of energy cost by the physiological cost index in walking after stroke. Arch. Phys. Med. Rehabil. 88, 1298–1303.

de Bolt, L., McCubbin, J., 2004. The effects of home based resistance exercises on balance, power and mobility in adults with multiple sclerosis. Arch. Phys. Med. Rehabil. 85, 290–297.

de Bruin, E.D., Hartmann, A., Uebelhart, D., et al., 2008. Wearable systems for monitoring mobility-related activities in older people: a systematic review. Clin. Rehabil. 22, 878–895.

Deutsch, J.E., Borbely, M., Filler, J., Huhn, K., Guarrera-Bowlby, P., 2008. Use of a low cost, commercially available gaming console (Wii) for rehabilitation of and adolescent with cerebral palsy. Phys. Ther. 88 (10), 1196–1207.

Dickstein, R., 2008. Rehabilitation of gait speed after stroke: A critical review of intervention approaches. Neurorehabil. Neural Repair 22, 649–660.

Dishman, R.K., Berthoud, H.R., Booth, F. W., et al., 2006. Neurobiology of Exercise. Obesity 13, 345–356.

Ditor, D.S., Latimer, A.E., Ginis, M.K., Arbour, K.P., McCartney, N., Hicks, A.L., 2003. Maintenance of exercise participation in individuals with spinal cord injury: effects on quality of life, stress and pain. Spinal Cord 41, 446–450.

Dobkin, B.H., 1999. An overview of treadmill locomotor training with partial body weight support: a neurologically sound approach whose time has come for randomized clinical trials. Neurorehabil. Neural Repair 13, 157–165.

Dobkin, D., 2004. Strategies for stroke rehabilitation. Lancet Neurol. 3, 528–536.

Dodd, K.J., Taylor, N.F., Graham, H.K., 2003. A randomized clinical trial of strength training in young people with cerebral palsy. Dev. Med. Child Neurol. 45, 652–657.

Dromerick, A., Edwards, D., Hahm, M., 2000. Does the application of constraint induced movement therapy during acute rehabilitation reduce arm impairment after stroke? Stroke 31, 2984–2988.

Elsworth, C., Dawes, H., Sackley, C., et al., 2009. A study of perceved facilitators to physical activity in neurological conditions. Int. J. Ther. Rehabil. 16, 17–23.

Finch, E., Brooks, D., Stratford, P.W., et al., 2002. Physical Rehabilitation Outcome Measures, vol. 2. Lippincott, Toronto.

Finkelstein, J., Lapshin, O., Castro, H., et al., 2008. Home-based physical telerehabilitation in patients with multiple sclerosis: A pilot study. J. Rehabil. Res. Dev. 45, 1361–1374.

Fisher, B.E., Wu, A.D., Salem, G.J., et al., 2008. The effect of exercise training in improving motor performance and corticomotor excitability in people with early parkinsons disease. Arch. Phys. Med. Rehabil. 89, 1221–1229.

Forrester, L.W., Hanley, D.F., Macko, R.F., 2006. Effects of Treadmill Exercise on Transcranial Magnetic Stimulation-Induced Excitability to Quadriceps After Stroke. Arch. Phys. Med. Rehabil. 87, 229–234.

Freeman, J.A., Porter, B., Thompson, A.J., 2008. Neurorehabilitation in multiple sclerosis. Top. Spinal Cord Inj. Rehabil. 14 (2), 63–75.

Giesser, B., Beres-Jones, J., Budovitch, A., et al., 2007. Locomotor training using body weight support on a treadmill improves mobility in persons with multiple sclerosis: a pilot study. Mult. Scler. 13, 224–231.

Glanz, M., Klawansky, S., Stason, W., Berkey, C., Chalmers, T., 1996. Functional electrostimulation in poststroke rehabilitation: a meta analysis of the randomized controlled trials. Arch. Phys. Med. Rehabil. 77, 549–553.

Glinsky, J., Harvey, L., Van Es, P., 2007. Efficacy of electrical stimulation to increase muscle strength in people with neurological conditions: a systematic review. Physiother. Res. Int. 12 (3), 175–194.

Gordon, N.F., Gulanick, M., Costa, F., et al., 2004. Physical activity and exercise recommendations for stroke survivors: An American Heart Association scientific statement from the Council on Clinical Cardiology, Subcommittee on Exercise, Cardiac Rehabilitation, and Prevention; the Council on Cardiovascular Nursing, the Council on Nutrition, Physical Activity and Metabolism and the Stroke Council. Circulation 109, 2031–2041.

Graves, L., Stratton, G., Ridgers, N.D., Cable, N.T., 2007. Comparison of energy expenditure in adolescents when playing new generation and sedentary computer games: cross sectional study. BMJ 335 (7633), 1282–1284.

Hackney, M.E., Earhart, G.M., 2009. Effects of dance on movement control in Parkinsons disease: a comparison of argentine tango and American ballroom. J. Rehabil. Med. 41 (6), 475–481.

Hale, L.A., Pal, J., Becker, I., 2008. Measuring free-living physical activity in adults with and without neurologic dysfunction with a triaxial accelerometer. Arch. Phys. Med. Rehabil. 89, 1765–1771.

Harris, M.L., Polkey, M.I., Bath, P.M.W., et al., 2001. Quadriceps muscle weakness following acute hemiplegic stroke. Clin. Rehabil. 15, 274–281.

Hartley, S., 2009. Developing a self-management and exercise model for people with multiple sclerosis. Int. J. Ther. Rehabil. 16, 34–42.

Hesse, S., Bertelt, C., Jahnke, M., et al., 1995a. Treadmill training with partial body weight support compared with physiotherapy in nonambulatory hemiparetic patients. Stroke 26, 976–981.

Hesse, S., Malezic, M., Schaffrin, A., et al., 1995b. Restoration of gait by combined treadmill training and multichannel electrical stimulation in non-ambulatory hemiparetic patients. Scand. J. Rehabil. Med. 27, 199–204.

Hesse, S., Helm, B., Krajnick, J., 1997. Treadmill training with partial body weight support: influence of body weight release on the gait of hemiparetic patients. J. Neurol. Rehabil. 11, 15–20.

Hesse, S., Uhlenbrock, D., Sarkodie-Gyan, T., 1999. Gait pattern of severely disabled hemiparetic subjects on a new controlled gait trainer as compared to assisted treadmill walking with partial body weight support. Clin. Rehabil. 13, 401–410.

Hesse, S., Uhlenbrock, D., Werner, C., et al., 2000. A mechanized gait trainer for restoring gait in nonambulatory subjects. Arch. Phys. Med. Rehabil. 81, 1158–1161.

Hicks, A.L., Martin, K.A., Ditor, D.S., et al., 2003. Long-term exercise training in persons with spinal cord injury: effects on strength, arm ergometry performance and psychological well being. Spinal Cord 41, 34–43.

Janssen, T.W.J., Hopman, M.T.E., 2005. Spinal Cord Injury. In: Skinner, J.S. (Ed.), Exercise Testing and Exercise Prescription for Special Cases. third ed. Lippincott Williams & Wilkins, Philadelphia.

Jungehulsing, G., Muller-Nordhorn, J., Nolte, C., et al., 2008. Prevalence of stroke and stroke symptoms: a population-based survey of 28,090 participants. Neuroepidemiology 30 (1), 51–57.

Kang, M., Zhu, W., Ragan, B.G., Frogley, M., 2007. Exercise barrier severity and perseverance of active youth with physical disabilities. Rehabil. Psychol. 52, 170–179.

Keith, R.A., Granger, C.V., Hamilton, B.B., et al., 1987. The Functional Independence Measure: A new tool for rehabilitation. In: Eisenberg, M.G., Grzesiak, R.C. (Eds.), Advances in Clinical Rehabilitation. Springer, Berlin.

Kerr, C., McDowell, B., McDonough, S., 2004. Electrical stimulation in cerebral palsy: a review of effects on strength and motor function. Dev. Med. Child Neurol. 46, 205–213.

Kileff, J., Ashburn, A., 2005. A pilot study of the effect of aerobic exercise on people with moderate disability multiple sclerosis. Clin. Rehabil. 19, 165–169.

Krebs, H.I., Volpe, B., Hogan, N., 2009. A working model of stroke recovery from rehabilitation robotics practitioners. J. Neuroeng. Rehabil. 25 (6), 6.

Labronici, R.H., Cunha, M.C., Oliviera, A., Gabbai, A.A., 2000. Sport as integration of the physically handicapped in our society. Arq. Neuropsiquiatr. 50 (4), 1092–1099.

Landau, W.M., Sahrmann, S., 2002. Preservation of directly stimulated muscle strength in hemiplegia due to stroke. Arch. Neurol. 59 (9), 1453–1457.

Lanningham-Foster, L., Foster, R.C., McCrady, S.K., Jensen, T.B., Mitre, N., Levine, J.A., 2009. Activity promoting video games and increased energy expenditure. J. Pediatr. 154 (6), 819–823.

Lee, M.S., Lam, P., Ernst, E., 2008. Effectiveness of tai chi for parkinsons disease : a critical review. Parkinsonism Relat. Disord. 14, 589–594.

Levy, C.F., Nichols, D.S., Schmalbrock, P.M., Keller, P., Chakeres, D., 2001. Functional MRI evidence of cortical reorganization in upper limb stroke hemiplegia treated with constraint induced movement therapy. Am. J. Phys. Med. Rehabil. 80 (1), 4–12.

Liepert, J., Bauder, H., Miltner, W.H., Taub, E., Weiler, C., 2000. Treatment-induced cortical reorganization after stroke in humans. Stroke 31, 1210–1216.

Liepert, J., Uhde, I., Graf, S., Leidner, O., Weiller, C., 2001. Motor cortex plasticity during forced use therapy in stroke patients: a preliminary study. J. Neurol. 248 (4), 315–321.

Lo, A.C., Triche, E.W., 2008. Improving gait in Multiple sclerosis using robot-assisted, body weight supported treadmill training. Neurorehabil. Neural Repair 22, 661–671.

Macdonnell, R., Triggs, W.W., Leikauskas, J., Bourque, M., Robb, K., Day, B., 1994. Functional electrical stimulation to the affected lower limb and recovery after cerebral infarction. J. Stroke Cerebrovas. Funct. 4, 155–160.

Macko, R.F., Ivey, F.M., Forrester, L.W., 2005. Task-orientated aerobic exercise in chronic hemiparetic stroke: training protocols and treatment effects. Top. Stroke Rehabil. 12 (1), 45–57.

Mahoney, F.I., Barthel, D.W., 1965. Functional evaluation: the Barthel index. Md. State. Med. J. (February), 61–65.

Marcus, B.H., Dubbert, P.M., Forsyth, L. H., et al., 2000. Physical activity behaviour change: issues in adoption and maintenance. Health Psychol. 19, 32–41.

Maruishi, M., Mano, Y., Sasaki, T., et al., 2001. Cerebral palsy in adults: independent effects of muscle strength and muscle tone. Arch. Phys. Med. Rehabil. 82, 637–641.

McArdle, W.D., Katch, F.I., Katch, V.L., 2006. Exercise Physiology, sixth ed. Lippincott Williams &Wilkins, Baltimore.

Merholz, J., Platz, T., Kugler, J., Pohl, M., 2008. Electromechanical and robot assisted arm training for improving arm function and activities of daily living after stroke. Cochrane Database Syst. Rev. (4) CDE006876.

Merletti, R., Selasci, F., Latella, D., et al., 1978. A control trial of muscle force recovery in hemiparetic patients during treatment with functional electrical stimulation. Scand. J. Rehabil. Med. 10, 147–154.

Morris, S., Dodd, K., Morris, M., 2004. Outcomes of progressive resistance training following stroke: a systematic review. Clin. Rehabil. 18, 27–38.

Mostert, S., Kesselring, J., 2002. Effects of a short-term exercise training programme on aerobic fitness, fatigue, health perception and activity level of subjects with multiple sclerosis. Mult. Scler. 8, 161–168.

Mudge, S., Stott, S., 2007. Outcome measures to assess walking ability following stroke: a systematic review of the literature. Physiotherapy 93, 198–200.

Nakamura, R., Handa, T., Watanabe, S., Morohashi, I., 1988. Walking cycle after stroke. J. Exp. Med. 154, 241–244.

Newsam, C., Baker, L., 2004. Effect of an electric stimulation facilitation program on quadriceps motor unit recruitment after stroke. Arch. Phys. Med. Rehabil. 85, 2040–2045.

Ng, S.S.M., Shepherd, R.B., 2000. Weakness in patients with stroke: implications for strength training in neurorehabilitation. Phys. Ther. Rev. 5, 227–238.

Nudo, R.J., Milliken, G.W., 1996. Reorganization of movement representation in primary motor cortex following focal ischaemia infarcts in adult squirrel monkeys. J. Neurophysiol. 75, 2144–2149.

Oman, R.F., King, A.C., 2000. The effect of life events and exercise program format on the adoption and maintenance of exercise behaviour. Health Psychol. 19, 605–612.

Page, S.J., Levine, P., 2007. Modified constraint induced therapy in patients with chronic stroke exhibiting minimal movement ability in the affected arm. Phys. Ther. 87, 872–878.

Page, S.J., Levine, P., Leonard, A.C., 2005. Modified constraint-induced therapy in acute stroke: a randomised controlled pilot study. Neurorehabil. Neural Repair 19, 27–32.

Page, S., Levine, P., Sisto, S., Bond, Q., Johnston, M.V., 2002. Stroke patients and therapist opinion of constraint induced movement therapy. Clin. Rehabil. 16, 55–60.

Page, S.J., Sisto, S.A., Johnston, M.V., Levine, P., Hughes, M., 2001. Modified constraint induced therapy: a randomized, feasibility and efficacy study. J. Rehabil. Res. Dev. 38, 583–590.

Page, S.J., Sisto, S., Levine, P., McGrath, R.E., 2004. Efficacy of modified constraint induced movement therapy in chronic stroke. Arch. Phys. Med. Rehabil. 85, 14–18.

Pang, M.Y., Eng, J.J., Dawson, A.S., Gylfadottir, S., 2006. The use of exercise training in improving aerobic capacity in individuals with stroke: a meta analysis. Clin. Rehabil. 20, 97.

Pariser, G., Madras, D., Weiss, E., 2006. Outcomes of an aquatic exercise program including aerobic capacity, lactate threshold and fatigue in two individuals with multiple sclerosis. J. Neurol. Phys. Ther. 30 (2), 82–90.

Ploughman, M., McCarthy, J., Bossé, M., et al., 2008. Does treadmill exercise improve performance of cognitive or upper-extremity tasks in people with chronic stroke? A randomized crossover trial. Arch. Phys. Med. Rehabil. 89, 2041–2047.

Pomeroy, V., King, L., Pollock, A., Baily-Hallam, A., Langhorne, P., 2006. Electrostimulation for promoting recovery of movement or functional ability after stroke (review). Cochrane Database Syst. Rev. (2) CD003241. DOI: 10.1002/14651858.CD003241. pub2.

Prange, G.B., Jannink, M.J., Groothuis-Oudshoorn, C.G., Hermens, H.J., Ijzerman, M.J., 2006. Systematic review of the effect of robot aided therapy on recovery of the hemiparetic arm after stroke. J. Rehabil. Res. Dev. 43 (2), 171–184.

Regnaux, J.P., Saremi, K., Marehbian, J., et al., 2008. An accelerometry-based comparison of 2 robotic assistive devices for treadmill training of gait. Neurorehabil. Neural Repair 22, 348–354.

Rietberg, M.B., Brooks, D., Uitdehaag, B. M.J., et al., 2004. Exercise therapy for multiple sclerosis. Cochrane Database Syst. Rev. 3, CD003980.

Royal College of Physicians, 2004. National Clinical Guidelines for Stroke Intercollegiate Stroke Working Party. R. C. o. Physicians, London. http://www.rcplondon.ac.uk/pubs/ books/stroke/stroke_guidelines_2ed. pdf.

Rogers, A., Furler, B.A., Brinks, S., Darrah, J., 2008. A systematic review of the effectiveness of aerobic exercise interventions for children with cerebral palsy: an AACPDM evidence report. Dev. Med. Child Neurol. 50, 808–814.

Sawaki, L., Butler, A.J., Leng, X., Wassenaar, P.A., Mohammed, Y.M., Blanton, S., et al., 2008. Constraint-induced movement therapy results in increased motor map area in subjects 3 to 9 months after stroke. Neurorehabil. Neural Repair 22, 505–513.

Scandalis, T.A., Bosak, A., Berliner, J.C., et al., 2001. Resistance training and gait function in patients with Parkinson's disease. Am. J. Phys. Med. Rehabil. 80, 38–43.

Schindl, M.R., Forstner, C., Kern, H., et al., 2000. Treadmill training with partial body weight support in non-ambulatory patients with cerebral palsy. Arch. Phys. Med. Rehabil. 81, 301–306.

Scianni, A., Butler, J.M., Ada, L., Texeira-Salmel, L.F., 2009. Muscle strengthening is not effective in children and adolescents with cerebral palsy: a systematic review. Aust. J. Physiother. 55 (2), 81–87.

Shepherd, R.B., Carr, J.H., 1999. Treadmill walking in neuro-rehabilitation. Neurorehabil. Neural Repair 13, 171–173.

Singer, B., 1987. Functional electrical stimulation of the extremities in the neurological patient: a review. Am. J. Physiother. 33 (1), 33–42.

Skidmore, F.M., Mackman, C.A., Pav, B., et al., 2008. Daily ambulatory activity levels in idiopathic Parkinson disease. J. Rehabil. Res. Dev. 45, 1343–1348.

Smith, G.V., Macko, R.F., Silver, K.H.C., et al., 1998. Treadmill aerobic exercise improves quadriceps strength in patients with chronic hemiparesis following stroke: a preliminary report. J. Neurol. Rehabil. 12, 111–117.

Smith, A.D., Zigmond, M.J., 2003. Can the brain be protected through exercise? Lessons from an animal model of parkinsonism. Exp. Neurol. 184, 31–39.

Smith, P.S., Thompson, M., 2008. Treadmill training post stroke: are there any secondary benefits? A pilot study. Clin. Rehabil. 22, 997–1002.

Snook, E.M., Motl, R.W., 2009. Effect of exercise training on walking mobility in multiple sclerosis: a meta-analysis. Neurorehabil. Neural Repair 23, 108–116.

Sterr, A., Freivogel, S., 2003. Motor-Improvement following intensive training in low-functioning chronic hemiparesis. Neurology 61, 842–884.

Stokes, E.K., 2009. Outcome measurement. In: Lennon, S., Stokes, M. (Eds.), Pocketbook of Neurological Physiotherapy. Churchill Livingstone Elsevier, Edinburgh, pp. 191–201.

Sunderland, A., Tuke, A., 2005. Neuroplasticity, learning and recovery after stroke: a critical evaluation of constraint-induced therapy. Neuropsychol. Rehabil. 15 (2), 81–96.

Sunnerhagen, K.S., Svantesson, U., Lonn, L., et al., 1999. Upper motor neurone lesion: their effects on muscle performance and appearance in stroke patients with minor motor impairment. Arch. Phys. Med. Rehabil. 80, 155–161.

Sutoo, D., Akiyama, K., 2003. Regulation of brain function by exercise. Neurobiol. Dis. 13, 1–14.

Tanaka, S., Hachisuka, K., Ogata, H., 1997. Trunk rotatory muscle performance in post-stroke hemiplegic patients. Am. J. Phys. Med. Rehabil. 76, 366–369.

Tang, A., Sibley, K.M., Thomas, S.G., Bayley, M.T., Richardson, D., McIlroy, W.E., et al., 2009. Effects of an aerobic exercise program on aerobic capacity, spatiotemporal gait parameters and functional capacity in subacute stroke. Neurorehabil. Neural Repair 23, 398–406.

Tasiemski, T., Bergstrom, E., Savic, G., Gardner, B.P., 2000. Sports, recreation and employment following spinal cord injury: a pilot study. Spinal Cord 38 (3), 173–184.

Tasiemski, T., Kennedy, P., Gardner, B.P., Taylor, P., 2005. The association of sports and physical recreation with life satisfaction in a community sample of people with spinal cord injuries. NeuroRehabilitation 20, 253–265.

Taub, E.M., Novak, T., Cook, E., et al., 1993. Technique to improve chronic motor deficit after stroke. Arch. Phys. Med. Rehabil. 74, 347–354.

Taub, E., Crago, J., Uswatte, G., 1998. Constraint-induced movement therapy: a new approach to treatment in physical rehabilitation. Rehabil. Psychol. 43, 152–1570.

Taub, E., Uswatte, G., 2006. Constraint-induced movement therapy: answers and questions after two decades of research. NeuroRehabilitation 21 (2), 93–95.

Tuke, A., 2008. Constraint-induced movement therapy: a narrative review. Physiotherapy 94, 105–114.

Taylor, N., Dodd, K., Damiano, D., 2005. Progressive resistance exercise in physical therapy: a summary of systematic reviews. Phys. Ther. 85 (11), 1208–1223.

Van den Berg, M.H., Ronday, H.K., Peeters, A.J., et al., 2006. Using internet technology to deliver a home-based physical activity intervention for patients with rheumatoid arthritis: a randomized controlled trial. Arthritis Rheum. 55, 935–945.

Van der Lee, J.W., Lankhorst, G.F., Vogelaar, T.W., Deville, W.L., Bouter, L. M., 1999. Forced use of the upper extremity in chronic stroke patients. Results from a single-blind randomised clinical trial. Stroke 30, 2369–2375.

van der Ploeg, H.P., Streppel, K.R.M., van der Beek, A.J., et al., 2006. Counselling increases physical activity behaviour nine weeks after rehabilitation. Br. J. Sports Med. 40, 223–229.

van der Slot, W.M.A., Roebroeck, M.E., Landkroon, A.P., et al., 2007. Everyday physical activity and community participation of adults with hemiplegic cerebral palsy. Disabil. Rehabil. 29, 179–189.

Voorips, L.E., Ravelli, A.C.J., Dongelmans, P.C.A., et al., 1991. A physical activity questionnaire for the elderly. Med. Sci. Sports Exerc. 23, 974–979.

Wahbeh, H., Siegward, M.E., Oken, B.S., 2008. Mind body interventions: applications in neurology. Neurology 70, 2321–2328.

Wandel, A., Jorgensen, H., Nakayama, H., Raaschou, H., Olsen, T., 2000. Prediction of walking function in stroke patients with initial lower extremity paralysis: the copenhagen stroke study. Arch. Phys. Med. Rehabil. 81, 736–738.

Wang, C., Cole, J.P., Lau, J., 2004. The effect of tai chi on health outcomes in patients with chronic conditions. Arch. Intern. Med. 164, 493–501.

Ward, N.S., Cohen, L.G., 2004. Mechanisms underlying recovery of motor function after stroke. Arch. Neurol. 61 (12), 1844–1848.

Winstein, C.J., Rose, D.K., Tan, S.M., Lewthwaite, R., Chui, H.C., Azen, S. P., 2004. A randomized controlled comparison of upper-extremity rehabilitation strategies in acute stroke: a pilot study of immediate and long-term outcomes. Arch. Phys. Med. Rehabil. 85 (4), 620–628.

Wittenberg, G.F., Chen, R., Ishii, K., Bushara, K.O., Taub, E., Gerber, L.H., 2003. Constrain induced movement therapy in stroke: magnetic stimulation motor maps and cerebral activation. Neurorehabil. Neural Repair 17, 48–57.

Wolf, S.L., Winstein, C.J., Miller, J.P., et al., 2008. The EXCITE trial: retention of improved upper extremity function among stroke survivors receiving CI movement therapy. Lancet Neurol. 7, (1), 33–40.

Wolf, S.L., Winstein, C.J., Miller, J.P., et al., 2006. Effect of constraint-induced movement therapy on upper

extremity function 3 to 9 months after stroke. JAMA 296 (17), 2094–2104.

Woodford, H.J., Price, C., 2007. Electromyographic feedback for the recovery of motor function after stroke. Stroke 38, 1999–2000.

World Health Organization, 2001. International Classification of Functioning, Disability and Health: ICF. WHO, Geneva.

Wu, C.Y., Chen, C.L., Tang, S.F., Lin, K. C., Huang, Y.Y., 2007. Kinematic and clinical analyses of upper extremity movements after constraint-induced movement therapy in patients with stroke: a randomized controlled trial. Arch. Phys. Med. Rehabil. 88, 964–970.

Yardley, L., Donovan-Hall, M., 2007. Predicting adherence to exercise-based therapy in rehabilitation. Rehabil. Psychol. 52, 56–64.

Zijdewind, I., Thomas, C., 2003. Motor unit firing during and after voluntary contractions of human thenar muscles weakened by spinal cord Injury J. Neurophysiol. 89, 2065–2071.

Chapter | **19** |

Self-management

Fiona Jones

CONTENTS

INTRODUCTION

The concept of self-management, including active involvement in decisions about care and shared responsibility with professionals has a confirmed place for many individuals living with the consequences of a long-term neurological condition (Department of Health (DoH), 2005b). Self-management not only involves the skills to cope with medical needs, such as dealing with self-catheterization or walking to reduce spasticity and stiffness, but also includes the emotional and social adjustments required by individuals over time. Although there is research on stages of adjustment and the development of self-management skills, this always has to be taken in the context of the nature of the neurological condition, which may be sudden as in the case of a spinal cord injury (see Ch. 4) or unpredictable in the case of multiple sclerosis (MS) (see Ch. 5).

Individuals and their families are often resourceful in the face of the challenges presented to them by their disability and frequently find solutions without the help of clinicians. However, for many individuals, the experience of a new neurological event such as stroke (see Ch. 2) or a changing disability such as MS requires guidance and support from a health professional. Yet the way in which the support is given, could have a profound effect on how successful a person is at being able to self-manage. As rehabilitation professionals, we have the opportunity to enable individuals to take control of their symptoms and develop a range of skills and strategies to live in an optimum way with their condition. We also have the potential to disempower and inhibit individuals' abilities to develop self-management skills so that they become more reliant on our help and expertise. To facilitate a departure from help and reliance on an 'expert physiotherapy clinician' toward a more collaborative approach which will sustain successful self-management is not an easy or straightforward process.

The evidence relating to successful self-management programmes, demonstrates the value of an interactive process between the heath professional and individual with a focus on shared decision-making and problem-solving (Newman et al., 2004). This would suggest that success would not be achieved through such actions of the therapists as:

1. providing information to the individual about their condition in one format with no opportunity to ask questions
2. providing a home exercise programme just before discharge from physiotherapy, with the expectation the individual will transfer the learning into another environment and continue to exercise.

Consequently, planning and developing appropriate programmes requires an appreciation of the many factors that act as barriers to or enablers of behaviour change and self-management. We can learn not only from relevant research trials, but also from the experiences of individuals and patient groups to help inform and develop suitable programmes. So what is self-management and is it in fact new?

SELF-MANAGEMENT: WHAT IS IT AND WHY NOW?

In definitive texts on self-management there are often assertions concerning changing demographics associated with ageing in the developed world. As population death rates decline, more people are likely to be living with the consequences and challenges of a long-term condition (LTC); as such, demand on health care is likely to grow. Sceptics have suggested that the economic pressures associated with large numbers of people living longer and requiring health care drive the advancement and popularity of self-management programmes. In the UK, people with a chronic disease or disability account for one in three of the total population; people with neurological conditions account for 20% of all hospital admissions and such conditions are the third most common reason for seeing a general practitioner (DoH, 2005b). Individuals with neurological conditions will continue to be intensive users of health-care resources and this number is likely to grow, considering the number of neurological conditions that are more prevalent amongst people over 65 years, e.g. stroke.

In the UK, the NHS Improvement Plan (Department of Health, 2004) highlighted the growing concern about the increasing number of people living with a chronic condition and proposed three levels of management. The NHS Long Term Condition Model included at the 'top level' case management for people with more complex (including neurological) conditions. A new form of specialist clinician was introduced to deliver case management to those with complex needs. At the second level, the plan offered disease management for those with specific conditions, e.g. those individuals requiring effective medication alongside care. Finally, at the third level, and thought to constitute 60–70% of the overall patient population, are those individuals that could be helped by self-management programmes, such as those using trained lay leaders to deliver generic group-based programmes, e.g. the Expert Patient Programme (EPP) (DoH, 2001).

Defining self-management

Many definitions of self-management reflect both the medical and social aspects of living with and managing a long-term chronic condition. One commonly used definition is that given by Barlow et al. (2002) referring to self-management as:

> ... *an individual's ability to manage the symptoms, treatment, physical and psychosocial consequences and lifestyle changes inherent in living with a chronic condition. Efficacious self-management encompasses ability to monitor one's condition and to affect the cognitive, behavioural and emotional responses necessary to maintain a satisfactory quality of life, thus, a dynamic and continuous process of self-regulation is established.*

Somewhat confusingly, the term 'self-management' is often used interchangeably with 'self-care'. A comprehensive definition of self-care given by the Department of Health (2005a), shows similarities with Barlow's definition but with a stronger focus on the medical aspects:

> *The actions individuals and carers take for themselves, their children, their families and others to stay fit and maintain good physical and mental health; meet psychological and social needs; prevent illness or accidents; care for minor ailments and long term conditions; and maintain health and wellbeing after an acute illness or accident.*

What these definitions both suggest is that self-management means greater responsibility on the part of the person for their own ongoing and, possibly, changing health needs. Self-management is seen as one aspect of the move towards encouraging patients to play a more active role in their own health, and aligns with other health-care policy in the UK, which emphasizes patient-centred care and engagement (Coulter & Ellins, 2006). But for individuals to become engaged in self-management practices it could be argued that there needs to be a greater concordance with the type of treatment being provided by health-care professionals. The transition towards successful self-management may also happen at different time points for each person; physiotherapists will therefore need to be able to assess an individual's readiness to take on more responsibility. This flexibility may be difficult when the amount of treatment and timing is pre-determined. More involvement, self responsibility and shared decision-making may be key components of self-management but, in some cases, organizations and services are unable to adapt and respond to what is needed.

A focused ethnographic study of individuals attending a stroke club revealed that individualized needs were not addressed during the rehabilitation process and that services were insufficient to ease the transition to community living (Sabari et al., 2000). This suggests that therapy services were not adequately preparing individuals for the transition from regular treatment to self-management, a concern echoed by other authors (Cott et al., 2007; Rittman et al., 2004).

Experts on self-management may not fully agree on all its components, but most agree on what it is not. Self-management is not simply providing the information and expecting the patient to get on with it, nor can we expect patients to adjust to a new or changing condition at the same rates or time points. An individual's involvement in self-management is (a) likely to fluctuate over time and (b) will depend on several factors (for example; the stage of life when a person receives their diagnosis, and knowledge that a neurological condition is only one part of a person's life). This will doubtless influence how much time, priority and importance a person gives to self-management – indeed, what they can or want to do. People's response to self-management is therefore unique (Corben & Rosen, 2005).

Self-management has also been defined according to a specified outcome, e.g. practicing specific health behaviours. It may be inhaler management in the case of people with asthma or controlling diet in people with diabetes (Newman et al., 2004). But the specific health behaviours needed to self-manage a neurological condition are more difficult to specify and generalize. This may be one reason why cohorts involved in research on generic self-management programmes rarely include participants with a neurological condition such as stroke.

Kate Lorig, the founder of a generic group-based programme known as the Chronic Disease Self-management Programme (CDSP), described self-management as distinct from medical care and involving the 'learning and practicing skills necessary to carry an active and emotionally satisfying life in the face of a chronic condition' (Lorig, 1993). What this definition adds is the aspect of learning, with the unique difference between self-management programmes and educational programmes being the need to facilitate behaviour change through different means. Clearly, much of health policy on self-management shows an emphasis on partnership and empowerment and this approach has been cited as one of the key components of a person-centred health service (DoH, 2000). But it has been argued that if self-management programmes are provided in clinical settings by health professionals, then the balance of power still lays with the professional not the individual (Wilson et al., 2007). It has also been suggested that implicit in many self-management programmes is an assumption that the best regimes are those suggested by a clinician and that the best outcome is achieved through optimum compliance (Kendall & Rogers, 2007).

Do therapists and patients see a good outcome in the same way, and does it always involve the individual adhering to advice and following treatment plans? Maclean et al. (2002) found that stroke patients perceived by health professionals to be highly motivated were more compliant with the aims and expectations of rehabilitation and more likely to understand and follow the advice of professionals. However, some patients perceived to have low motivation described the mixed messages given by therapists in discouraging their individual efforts. This raises some concerns about which patient is doing better and is more likely to learn the skills of self-management; the patient not complying with treatment and trying activities independently or the patient following advice and complying with rehabilitation (Maclean et al., 2002).

If an individual feels obliged to take part in and comply with a specified treatment strategy is this compliance a successful outcome? This could create a contradiction with the new group of self-managers, described as reflexive autonomous individuals and not passively accepting medical advice (Wilson et al., 2007). Against the rather negative predictions of the growing numbers of people living with a LTC likely to need medical care, there is also evidence from a recent survey that the majority of adults living with a LTC are comfortable taking responsibility for their condition (IPsos MORI for Department of Health, 2009). Again, it is worth remembering that many individuals self-manage without the support of a clinician or self-management training:

Lee, a 77-year-old stroke survivor, lives at home with his wife and no longer receives regular physiotherapy. He described his paretic leg as being unpredictable and no longer under his control, but he dealt with this by 'learning not to panic, and rely so much on my powerful stronger leg'. He achieved this by setting small tasks where the likelihood of success was high 'giving my leg a chance to succeed' (Jones, 2004). Self-management strategies in Lee's case, involve decision-making, setting targets, and reflecting on progress. He explained, 'Doing more walking at home is my goal, you must have a goal, and have measures which you can check against which are fairly objective, and I do roughly do that, how many yards I have walked each day, and I use note books and diaries to record how I am doing'.

The key to incorporating shared decision-making into rehabilitation involves inviting the individual to participate in the decision-making and the problem-solving, and not asking the individual to comply with an exercise or treatment. One model used an approach in which the care was a question of gaining insight into the patient decisions rather than the opposite (Zoffman et al., 2008). Ellis-Hill has also highlighted the importance of the shared discourse between the therapist and patient, to facilitate self-discovery and problem-solving on behalf of the patient. In this way, the therapist is acting more as a guide or coach, rather than an expert. Using this model, the balance of power between professionals and patients is recognized. Ellis-Hill and colleagues developed their Life Thread Model (2008), based on narrative theory and focusing on interpersonal relationships. The model includes:

a. endorsing a positive view of self
b. 'being' with somebody as well as 'doing' things for them
c. seeing acquired disability as a time of transition rather than simply of loss.

Table 19.1 The Virtual Ataxia Group	
WHO FOR?	WHAT IS IT?
People with hereditary or acquired ataxia	A group for people who have ataxia but may live in rural areas and cannot access local groups. There are chat sessions online, and all members are encouraged to take an active role in the group. Provides peer support and a forum for people with ataxia to exchange ideas, experiences and solutions about living with Ataxia http://www.ataxia.org.uk/page.builder/virtual_branch.html

Self-management is not new

The paradox of this growing interest in self-management is the knowledge that it is not a new phenomenon. Individuals have always found ways of coping with their chronic condition, showing resourcefulness both at an individual and community level. Sociologists such as Mike Bury and others have highlighted that models of coping with a chronic long-term condition, based on resilience and self-responsibility, have existed for many decades. They also argue that health-care professionals would make a case that they have long promoted self-management (Bury et al., 2005). There are a great many examples of how people with a neurological condition self-manage, not only at a personal level but also at a more collective/societal level. Peer support is one way that people with the same neurological condition can exchange ideas, experiences and gain advice. Peer support can consist of groups held in local communities, such as a stroke club, and there is a growth of online support groups, particularly when the neurological condition is less common and individuals are not readily able to meet. A good example of this is the Virtual Ataxia Group (Table 19.1).

The starting point for many individuals living with a neurological condition may not always be a medical issue, such as impairment. Social isolation, family life, work and adjustment to the changes over time may be a far more important influence on self-management (Kendall & Rogers, 2007). If we are to integrate self-management principles into therapy programmes for people with neurological conditions, then an agreed definition of what self-management is and what it is not is needed first before exploring the key components and specific interventions. Furthermore, as a therapy profession providing a service for patients with many different neurological conditions, should we also question whether our start point always needs to be about health? After stroke, self-management behaviours are often promoted to prevent a second event

and reduce risk factors through strategies such as increasing activity. But exercise and access to community groups can be challenging for stroke survivors who wish to adopt a healthier lifestyle (Rimmer et al., 2008). In this way, social isolation from an inaccessible environment may be more of a barrier to successful self-management. The role in the community played by both formal and informal self-help activities, such as stroke clubs, is also a vital aspect of a more collective approach to self-management (Ch'ng et al., 2008). But these groups are often not accessed by individuals with restricted mobility or communication impairments, or minority or ethnic groups, such as populations from Southern Asia (Davidson et al., 2008).

To understand all aspects of self-management, one needs to look beyond the challenges of specific impairments associated with neurological conditions, to consider the interactions between:

- individual health conditions, e.g. stroke
- personal characteristics (such as motivation)
- restrictions posed by the environment and societal barriers, such as inaccessible work conditions, transport and access to leisure facilities.

INDIVIDUAL RESPONSES TO SELF-MANAGEMENT PROGRAMMES: THEORY AND RESEARCH

Understanding responses to neurological disability

Traditionally, therapists have guided and supported patients to learn and to gain confidence in dealing with their neurological condition. However, the expectation that patients will follow the advice offered, and that increased information and support will lead naturally to self-management, does not fully take into account motivation, beliefs and other difficulties that might influence how this advice will be incorporated into individuals' daily lives.

Why is it important to gain more understanding of motivation, fears and beliefs? Before examining some of the theories underpinning self-management programmes, it is worth reviewing some of the findings from qualitative studies that have explored these concepts. Taking the experience of stroke as the main example, it could be argued that confidence and beliefs about self-management will be based on a diverse range of events occurring in the post stroke period. These may be personal experiences as a result of a change in independence and life circumstances, but equally could be shaped by external factors such as the environment and structure of rehabilitation and the nature of interactions with professionals and family (von Koch et al., 1998).

Fear and uncertainty perceived by individuals is also well documented in studies exploring the early poststroke period (Hafsteindóttir & Grypdonk, 1997; Robinson-Smith, 2002). Anxiety about bringing on a second stroke, or feeling out of control, may act as a barrier to setting goals and taking action. The sudden loss of independence and changes in identity associated with acute stroke also heighten individual concerns about potential losses and the restriction of future roles (Bendz, 2003; Faircloth et al., 2004). This early period of instability and uncertainty post stroke may have a profound influence on forming judgements and beliefs about the future. In addition, the high levels of depression and anxiety experienced by stroke survivors may be compounded by these feelings of dependency and loss of control (Hackett et al., 2005). Some of the practices in early stroke care can reinforce feelings of helplessness and dependency which would not be conducive to developing self-management skills (Andrews & Stewart, 1979; von Koch et al., 2000).

Another common theme in the literature is that individuals may not always follow well-defined stages of adjustment after stroke, and personal 'readiness' to take on concepts of self-management and self-responsibility may not coincide with the timing of rehabilitation. The perception of 'recovery' has been found to be personal to each individual taking into account a range of other factors such as age and previous health status (Faircloth et al., 2004). Some authors prefer to use the term 'biographical flow' to describe how individuals experience the stroke event in the context of their everyday lives. Stroke is not necessarily seen as a catastrophe, but part of a person's ongoing life narrative with many individuals describing an implicit expectation about continuing to do the things that were done before the stroke (Faircloth et al., 2004).

Benchmarking used by individuals to measure their own progress and adjustment to stroke is also a common finding in qualitative research, and the recovery experience is often constructed by individuals in relation to the practical reality of living with a stroke on a daily basis (Dowswell et al., 2000; Gubrium et al., 2003; Jones et al., 2007). The knowledge and understanding of rehabilitation professionals about individual's incentives and motivations relating to personal goals could also increase the likelihood of developing strategies and confidence to succeed. Higher levels of tenacious goal pursuit and flexible goal adjustment at 5 months has also been found to be a strong predictor of higher levels of quality of life at 12 months post stroke (Darlington et al., 2007).

Stroke is usually a sudden onset event, but with neurological conditions such as MS, the onset is more gradual but potentially less predictable (see Ch. 5). For many, diagnosis is a protracted experience with the challenge of making sense of the long-term implications of living with a changeable chronic condition. Focus groups carried out with people diagnosed with MS for 5 years or more to explore personal narratives and self-management strategies highlighted the key differences between the early and later stage experiences. The need to get a named diagnosis, lack of psychosocial support and concerns about the consequences in lifestyle dominated the early stages, along with stress and fear about the unpredictability and coping with major challenges. Nevertheless, after a period of time, individuals developed more proactive attitudes and strategies, gaining more knowledge about their own disease progression and accessing formal and informal support networks (Malcomson et al., 2008).

What these qualitative studies tell us is that whilst living with a neurological condition, individuals will experience a number of beliefs, emotional responses and barriers that could influence the successful rehabilitation and self-management (see Table 19.2).

Table 19.2 Factors influencing rehabilitation and self-management
Belief/behaviour
Fear and uncertainty about a second event or dependency on others
Worry about unpredictability of disease
Recovery is personal and perceived within a personal narrative
Concerns for the future challenges
Feelings of discontinuity with previous life
Personal benchmarks which may not match therapy goals
Importance of hope and the possibility of further improvement
(Sabari et al., 2000; Rittman et al., 2004; Jones et al., 2007; Bendz, 2003.)

Social Cognitive Theory and self-efficacy

What then is the best way of helping an individual to learn more about their own beliefs and responses to rehabilitation? Psychological theories provide a framework for understanding human behaviour, and many self-management interventions are now developed on the basis of different theories. The most commonly cited in the development of self-management programmes is Social Cognitive Theory (SCT), in which an individual's belief in their own capability to produce a change in a specific behaviour (self-efficacy) is said to be critical to the success (Bandura, 1989; Bandura, 1997). *Self-efficacy* is a construct introduced by Bandura (1997), and has been defined as 'people's beliefs about their capabilities to produce designated levels of performance that exercise influence over events that affect their lives' (Bandura, 1994, pp. 71). Self-efficacy beliefs can determine how people feel, think, motivate themselves and behave with regards to their health. For example, self-efficacy influences motivation and health behaviours, by determining the goals people set, how much effort they invest in achieving those goals, and their resilience when faced with difficulties or failure (Dixon et al., 2007). Individuals with strong self-efficacy tend to select challenging goals, and approach difficult tasks as challenges to overcome, rather than as threats to avoid. In the face of failure, such individuals may heighten and sustain their efforts, quickly recover their sense of efficacy, and even attribute failure to insufficient effort or deficient knowledge and skills that can be acquired (Bandura, 1994).

The difference between SCT and other theories is that Bandura provides a clear direction regarding how to influence self-efficacy, which can inform therapeutic interaction and self-management programmes. The construct of self-efficacy also appears to provide resonance with many aspects of sustaining progress and coping with setbacks whilst living with a neurological condition. The information and feedback that an individual obtains from the performance of a task are the sources of self-efficacy.

There are four main sources of self-efficacy (Bandura, 1997):

1. Mastery experiences
2. Vicarious experiences
3. Verbal persuasion
4. Physiological feedback.

Mastery experiences include positive experiences in a task or skill. As people's experiences of success may improve their self-efficacy, breaking the task into smaller achievable components may be useful, in order to build up and accumulate confidence (van de Laar & van der Bijl, 2001). For people with stroke, this could be gained following accomplishment of a small personal goal through independent effort (Jones et al., 2007). Mastery experiences are said to be the most reliable source of efficacy

information (Schwartzer, 1992) and have been targeted in neurological rehabilitation through a variety of methods (Johnston et al., 2007; Kendall et al., 2007, Watkins et al., 2007).

Vicarious experience is gained through the comparison and modelling of others, as it can be beneficial to observe someone perceived to be similar successfully performing the task, e.g. learning from another individual's experience of the recovery period post stroke. Seeing others' achievements, especially for individuals who are uncertain of their capabilities to perform certain tasks, may help the observers believe that they also possess capabilities to perform the same tasks (Bandura, 1997; Shapero Sabari et al., 2000).

Verbal persuasion serves to increase an individual's belief about their personal level of skill using persuasion and verification from a significant other (stroke professional or key family member). However, verbal persuasion needs to be directed in such a way that it enables the individual to interpret the experience of performing the skills as a success (Bandura, 1997).

Physiological feedback is where the efficacy beliefs are formed from feedback produced by an individual's own physiological state. Self-efficacy may be increased by the interpretation of the individual's physical and emotional feelings as positive, rather than negative, e.g. walking unaided post stroke without feeling unsteady (Bandura, 1997; Ewart, 1992).

Neurological rehabilitation could provide the opportunity to address a combination of these four sources of self-efficacy and enhance an individual's potential to self-manage. If there are multiple components of a personal goal, such as walking, individuals are likely to have a number of distinct, interrelated self-efficacy beliefs (Cervone, 2000). Practice to ensure transference of beliefs regarding capability to different situations and settings therefore requires a dynamic cognitive process (Cervone, 2000). However, there may be limited scope for individuals to practice their own personal tasks in some acute-care setting and receive sustained support to build self-efficacy and functional performance beyond a defined few weeks of rehabilitation. The development of effective self-management skills by enhancing self-efficacy is an approach which would need to be started early in the rehabilitation process.

The Stress Coping Model

Another theory used to inform self-management programmes is the *Stress Coping Model* (Lazurus, 1990), which focuses on the strategies people use to overcome the challenges and stresses of living with a chronic disease. Programmes based on this model usually incorporate the use of cognitive behavioural techniques to encourage individuals to develop more positive and active coping strategies. Passive and avoidant behaviours (such as evading activity or not taking medication) will usually have detrimental effects on health outcomes, and, as such, it will be important for therapists to recognize and explore unhelpful beliefs and anxieties that might be impeding progress. An example can be taken from cardiac rehabilitation, where self-management programmes involve individuals learning to perceive feelings of breathlessness and raised heart rate as a positive and necessary step towards fitness, as opposed to a negative experience indicative of a possible medical complication (Ewart, 1992).

The Transtheoretical Model of Behaviour Change and motivational interviewing

The Transtheoretical Model of Behaviour Change (Prochaska & Velicer, 1997) has been used in a large number of self-management programmes, and makes an assumption that behaviour changes involve movement through a specified number of stages (Serlachius & Sutton, 2009). The likelihood of change is also influenced by factors related to motivation and readiness to change. These include:

1. precontemplation: no intention to take any action
2. contemplation: intends to take action within the next few months
3. preparation: intends to take action within the next few days
4. action: change in behaviour which has been sustained for less than 6 months
5. maintenance: change in behaviour which has been sustained for more than 6 months.

Interventions should match the participant's stage of change. However, the model has been criticized in recent years because of problems defining the stages, and following suggestions that the stages are not real time periods and are difficult to operationalize. Nonetheless, a technique known as *motivational interviewing* (MI) based on the Transtheoretical Model of Change has been used successfully in the acute stroke care setting (Watkins et al., 2007). MI uses a counselling technique based on four principles:

1. To express empathy
2. To develop a discrepancy between unhealthy behaviour and patients' goals
3. To work with resistance by inviting new perspectives
4. To support self-efficacy.

MI requires therapeutic skills of reflective listening, asking open questions, affirming and summarizing (Levensky et al., 2007). By adopting these principles and skills, practitioners focus on encouraging patients to explore their reasons for behaviour change and help them to develop their own strategies to enable this change. The patient is empowered to make their own decisions, thereby maintaining self-efficacy and increasing their confidence in their abilities to make a change (Levensky et al., 2007).

The move away from didactic expert-led treatments for people with neurological conditions to a more collaborative problem-solving approach is as a positive step towards supporting self-management. But the theoretical basis of each approach requires careful consideration. SCT theory is the most commonly used theory, but in practice, it is likely that there is overlap between the different theories and self-management programmes. There are distinct differences though with SCT, for instance, focusing on behaviour change whilst others focus on the more cognitive aspects of living with the chronic condition, such as coping with stress.

Components of self-management programmes

It is important to appreciate the theoretical influences that guide the delivery and content of self-management programmes. This enables the variables and outcomes to be defined and tested using the relevant measures.

Key components of self-management programmes often include:

- Problem-solving
  This involves the individual deciding on the problem, breaking it down into smaller parts, thinking of various solutions, selecting a course of action, trying out the action or a strategy and evaluating success, or choosing an alternative action if necessary.
- Target- or goal-setting
  Involves translating thoughts into actions, or the difference between what people say and what they do and requires a selection of strategies which if successful can provide mastery experiences.
- Resource utilization
  This involves making use of what other resources may be available to sustain participation or enable further progress. It could include accessing local self-help groups, seeking expert advice if a problem emerges, using friends or family to support access to services or activities.
- Collaboration
  This involves working together with a health-care professional, to decide together on a course of action, or preferred direction to rehabilitation. The therapist and the individual share expertise; a shift from traditional thinking whereby the therapist is always seen as the expert.
- Knowledge
  Living with a neurological condition involves a continuous process of learning from new experiences, particularly when the condition can fluctuate and change over time, such as MS. Increased knowledge about the condition, symptoms and treatment is an important aspect of self-management, but should represent a more active process than just gaining knowledge. A key skill is being able to gather, to process and to evaluate the information.

It is worth restating that successful self-management should always involve 'doing', and 'taking action': whether mobilizing support or finding a new way of doing something, the action is on the part of the individual. Put more simply, if we are to promote self-management as part of rehabilitation, we need to consider ways of individuals discovering their own strengths and a difficulties, experimenting and trying out different strategies and activities; inevitably this requires an element of risk taking. If the activities are not achieved, then we need to support the individual to learn to set their target slightly differently or devise an alternative target (Creer & Holroyd, 1997).

The list of components provides some idea of the complexity and range of skills promoted and facilitated through self-management programmes. But if we remember a self-management intervention does not mean simply imparting and providing information, but an active collaborative process, then we can start to understand how a behaviour change may be possible. However, there can be many different interpretations of each process and skill. Consider the following two alternative approaches to goal setting:

Process A

1. Goals are discussed between physiotherapist and patient
2. A suitable goal is decided upon and written in the physiotherapy notes
3. Patient works with physiotherapist to achieve goal within a predetermined therapy time (no time is spent independently practicing activities outside of physiotherapy)
4. Patient achieves goal with the help of the physiotherapist
5. 'Goal achieved' recorded in the physiotherapy notes.

Process B

1. The patient's story (narrative) is discussed, what do they enjoy doing and what is important to them?
2. A list of long-term goals and hopes is written down (by the patient, if possible)
3. Patient is encouraged to think of what they would like to work on first, what could be something a little smaller, but still meaningful that they would like to do in the next few days
4. A smaller target or goal is written down with a time frame
5. Patient is asked how confident they feel about achieving the goal within the next few days, and if possible confidence is scored using a self-efficacy scale
6. The action needed by the physiotherapist and the patient is agreed upon together after each physiotherapy session, the patient is asked how they feel they are progressing towards their own goal, and asked to rate their confidence

7. Patient records when they have achieved the target and a record of successes is kept with the patient at all times
8. Families are invited to read the targets and progress made.

It is clear that the second process may take more time and skill, but if the key outcome is to enable confidence to self-manage in individuals with a neurological condition such as stroke, then the interaction is not straightforward, and requires time and patience on the part of the physiotherapist.

SELF-MANAGEMENT PROGRAMMES: THE EVIDENCE BASE FOR STROKE AND PROGRESSIVE NEUROLOGICAL CONDITIONS

The precise methods of delivery and features of self-management programmes are still subject to debate. The evidence for and against different types of intervention will be reviewed in this section in relation to conditions of sudden onset, such as stroke, and more progressive and unpredictable conditions, such as MS. The development of programmes for the latter has been slower to progress but this may reflect the complexity and range of challenges facing those living with and managing a changing neurological condition. The number of specifically designed self-management programmes for people with chronic diseases has grown over the past two decades. Programmes can be:

- for a generic group or disease-specific
- delivered by health-care professionals or by trained lay leaders
- group-based or individualized.

There have been few self-management programmes designed specifically for individuals with neurological conditions, the exception being stroke-specific programmes (discussed later in the chapter). Reviews comparing different types of interventions mostly focus on diabetes, asthma and arthritis (Newman et al., 2004; Newbold et al., 2006): Table 19.3 provides a brief critique of some of the different approaches.

Currently, health-care professionals lead most disease-specific programmes; lay leaders have tended to be more involved in the delivery of generic chronic disease programmes. Lay- and professional-led programmes show no differences in outcomes, which raises the possibility that favourable outcomes after self-management programmes are more to do with the effects of group participation than leadership. The mechanisms involved or active ingredients of self-management programmes remain uncertain (Newbold et al., 2006).

Table 19.3 Strengths and limitations of selected self-management interventions

INTERVENTION	STRENGTHS	LIMITATIONS
Group based interventions	• More cost-effective • Value of group learning, social and peer support	• Usually, educated women attend; under-privileged groups less likely • No scope for individuals learning and changing behaviour at different rates
One-to-one interventions	• Tailoring to individual needs • Some barriers to self-management can't be shared in a group setting • Can be delivered in non-clinical setting, and incorporated into rehabilitation	• More time needed, reduced opportunity for modelling/vicarious learning • Less cost-effective
Lay-leaders	• Can act as role models • Less costly • May not have to re-learn an approach to chronic disease self-management • Could be in a good position to encourage others to join groups	• Information about training and skills required by lay leader not reported • Some, difficulties recruiting suitable leaders, and providing the infrastructure for support
Professional leaders	• More able to address factual issues relating to condition and treatment • Easier to integrate into rehabilitation	• Health-care professionals traditionally deliver more didactic approaches, e.g. medical advice • Training needs often not recognized
Disease-specific	• Allows more focus on specific skills required for different conditions	• Emphasis on disease specific skills first rather than general skills, could reduce learning and management of subsequent heath challenges
Generic	• More cost-effective, and encourages practice of more generic problem-solving skills • Effective for individuals with multiple co-morbidities	• Difficulties of facilitating a group with wide ranging conditions, symptoms and disease trajectories • No disease specific advice

Self-management and chronic disease

There is an increasing emphasis on self-management as a component of clinical practice and rehabilitation. Arguably, many of the common components of a self-management intervention are included within most comprehensive rehabilitation programmes. However, a list of components advocated for a self-management programme for people with Parkinson's disease suggested by Doyle Lyons (2003), fails to emphasize the collaborative, shared approach to self-management advocated by most experts in the area and includes the following:

1. Teach participants to observe their behaviour
2. Teach participants to set measureable goals
3. Allow practice of skills and tasks
4. Target self-efficacy
5. Use a group format
6. Include family members and caregivers
7. Integrate with primary health care
8. Teach general problem-solving skills
9. Include disease education
(Doyle Lyons, 2003).

Self-management programmes are clearly distinct from simple patient education or skills training, in that they are designed to encourage people with chronic diseases to take an active part in the management of their own condition. Kate Lorig and researchers at Stanford University are the main pioneers of self-management research and developed what is perhaps the most well-known programme, the CDSP. The programme is a 6-week, lay-led, self-management skills training course for people with generic long-term physical conditions. Overall evaluations suggest improved outcomes and some cost reductions for chronic care following the programmes (Lorig et al., 1999, Lorig et al., 2001). Main outcomes include increase in exercise, improved coping strategies and symptom management, less fatigue, fewer hospital visits and fewer medical consultations at 6 months follow-up, as well as at 1 and 1 years' follow-up (Lorig et al., 2001).

The CDSP has been adopted in a number of countries, and in England and Wales has been adapted as the EPP (DoH, 2001). Lorig and others argue that the most empowering aspect of CDSP-based courses is that it is not facilitated by a health professional but by a lay volunteer who has a long-term condition themselves (Kennedy et al., 2005). However, the evidence for this claim is limited. In the UK attempts to integrate EPP into the National Health Service (NHS) has also had limited success (Bury & Pink, 2005), possibly due to the lack of engagement by health-care professionals, particularly general practitioners (Kennedy et al., 2005). Furthermore, trials have not provided convincing evidence of the generalizability of the programme, given that men and ethnic groups are greatly under-represented in most studies (Jordan & Osborne, 2007). One reason for this could be that active self-management is such a complex set of skills (Thorne et al., 2003), that generic approaches are unlikely to reach the depth required to develop these skills, particularly in individuals with more complex conditions such as stroke (Davidson, 2005).

Arguably, many key components of programmes such as the CDSP could be adapted for people with neurological conditions and there has been some success with disease-specific self-management initiatives. A self-management programme developed to encourage exercise behaviours for people with mild to moderate MS showed significant improvements in walking speed and quality of life in the study group. Despite the lack of a control group, the authors suggest this model provides evidence of the potential benefits of introducing an earlier self-management intervention for encouraging exercise in people with MS (Hartley, 2009).

Issues in self-management research

The main methodological issues associated with self-management research are:

- no explicit theory, and would be hard to replicate
- intervention is not self-management training, but has a more educational focus
- high levels of attrition, particularly from group-based programmes
- some seminal research is questionable; it lacked a control group and samples were self-selecting
- some groups such as those with lower educational level and men tend not to access self-management programmes
- many of the results report short-term benefits, but few studies report long-term outcomes.

Despite these issues, there are a number of positive outcomes from well-designed programmes, particularly those with a clear theoretical framework and well-described components (Marks, 2001).

Self-management and stroke

Stroke is, without doubt, under-represented in self-management research compared to chronic diseases such as asthma, arthritis and diabetes (Newman et al., 2004). Interventions such as the EPP do incorporate components common to many stroke rehabilitation programmes, such as goal setting, self-exercising and skills training to cope with set-backs (Newman et al., 2004). However, during stroke rehabilitation, there is evidence that these components are not consistently patient-centred or collaborative (Wressle et al., 1999). Self-management training could provide the forum to develop these skills, but the CDSP group setting may not be suitable for all individuals, particularly those with aphasia or mobility limitations (Wressle et al., 1999).

Moreover, conditions such as stroke have been traditionally viewed as acute events, and much of the focus has been on the front end of care. Although there is evidence of the potential for further functional improvement in the longer term this is coupled with a concern expressed by individuals about the lack of support once the early period of rehabilitation is completed (Kwakkel et al., 2004; Sabari et al., 2000). There is also a noticeable difference in the management post stroke compared to after cardiac events, with a much more coordinated programme of self-management education, and staged rehabilitation available for cardiac patients. This is even more puzzling considering that the causes of stroke mirror those of chronic heart disease and that the controllable risk factors, such as diet, activity and smoking, are identical. If we view stroke more as a chronic disease, it is reasonable to assume that self-management interventions may also be beneficial for individuals post stroke.

Research to evaluate programmes incorporating certain key principles of self-management training for stroke is emerging. A few studies have attempted to adapt the CDSP for stroke, with mixed results. A randomized controlled trial by Kendall et al. (2007) involving 100 people with stroke applied the CDSP (group/lay led) in Australia in an acute stroke setting. The intervention group avoided a decline in function in the first year post stroke, although the intervention failed to impact on self-efficacy and other outcomes such as mood and social participation. A Shanghai version of the CDSP was trialled for participants with various chronic diseases including stroke (Dongbo et al., 2003). The intervention group had significant improvements in weekly exercise, practice of cognitive management, self-efficacy and health status compared to the control group. However, treatment allocation was not concealed at baseline and large numbers were lost to follow-up in both groups. Neither study had long-term follow-up, a common criticism of self-management research (Taylor & Bury, 2007).

MI, based on the transtheoretical model of change (Prochaska & Velicer, 1997), was tested in a single centre open randomized controlled trial (Watkins et al., 2007). The aim of MI was to develop confidence in ability to adjust and identify realistic personal goals in the acute setting post stroke. The intervention group received up to four sessions of MI, from a randomly allocated therapist, trained by a clinical psychologist who also provided supervision. Subjects received between one and four sessions of MI; the majority of subjects (72%) received four. There were significant changes in mood at 3 months in the intervention group compared with the control group, and protective effect of MI on depression. This was a robust study, but the results were mixed, with no effect on function, and no long-term follow-up, so results may not be sustained.

A self-management workbook designed to modify control cognitions and based on a prototype for post myocardial infarction has more recently been tested with individuals post stroke (Johnston et al., 2007). The intervention group showed a significant difference in recovery from disability at 6 months after discharge from hospital. However, there was a large attrition rate from the intervention group, which could have biased findings. This study showed no change in the cognitive construct known as 'perceived control', which is similar to self-efficacy, despite previous findings by the authors. Although another measure of 'confidence in recovery' was affected by the intervention, again there was no immediate mediation effect. The authors suggest a change in confidence may produce more long-term value, and could help sustain belief and encourage the initiation of more self-management strategies (Johnston et al., 2007). Considering the criticisms levelled at generic, group-based programmes, there is some scope for developing and testing more individualized self-management interventions for stroke survivors (DoH, 2007). An intervention ('Bridges' – a stroke self-management programme) used a workbook based on self-efficacy principles. It incorporates the main sources of self-efficacy (mastery, vicarious experience and feedback), with content informed by qualitative research and contributions from a group of ten stroke survivors (Jones et al., 2007). Pilot work using a multiple-participant, single-subject design demonstrated significant improvement in self–efficacy (measured by the Stroke Self-efficacy Questionnaire) (Jones et al., 2008) and personal control (measured by the Recovery Locus of Control Scale) (Partridge & Johnston, 1989), but no significant changes in activity, participation or mood.

The measurement of self-management

Measuring self-management is not straightforward, as the behaviours that contribute are multifaceted and depend largely on each individual and the challenges of the particular condition. The most important consideration is to define the outcome of interest, for example activity or levels of fatigue, and then find a valid and reliable measure of the target outcome (DeVellis & Blalock, 2009). There are potentially many outcome measurements that can be used to measure self-management and it may not always be possible to gain direct observed evidence of change in target behaviour. Some measures are reported and cannot be directly observed and can include self-report scales that are about testing more factual information, e.g. knowledge of condition, or measurement of a more subjective state such as perceived competency or mood. Further many measures require a degree of cognitive competency, for example recalling past events, or rating one's own ability in a certain task, for example 'walk across the room without falling'.

There are specific scales to measure self-management behaviours, and these can be both generic and disease-specific. The Self-Management Behaviours Scale is a generic measure of self-management and was developed by Lorig and colleagues to evaluate the effectiveness of their chronic-disease self-management programme (Lorig et al., 1996). However, it has also been adopted for disease-specific programmes, such as the Arthritis Self-Management Programme (Barlow & Barefoot, 1996). Responses to different items relating to self-management behaviours, such as managing medication and self-exercise, are measured on either a 6-point Likert scale where 0=None or Never and 5=More than 3 hours/week or Always depending on the context of the question asked, or a dichotomous scale. Finally, two items require responses in frequency of self-management behaviour, e.g. Number of times or Total hours in the past 6 weeks, depending on the question asked (Lorig et al., 1996).

The effectiveness of programmes underpinned by Social Cognition Theory, are often measured using change in self-efficacy. However, Bandura supports a model of measurement in which it is suggested that efficacy beliefs should be measured in terms of specific judgements within the chosen area of activity (Bandura, 1997). Therefore, it is important to use a self-efficacy scale that is relevant to the target behaviours and specific to the context of living with the particular chronic condition. Examples of such scales within neurological rehabilitation are the Stroke Self-efficacy Questionnaire (Jones et al., 2008) and the MS Self-efficacy Scale (Airlie et al., 2001).

Overall, there have been some promising results from early studies of self-management programmes in stroke. But the methodological problems are similar to those for other self-management interventions. Further consideration is needed to identify ways of enhancing self-management within normal clinical practice while the evidence base for specific self-management interventions continues to develop. In addition, there needs to be careful consideration of the behaviours targeted by self-management programmes. Outcome measures may need to include both observed and self-report scales in order to capture fully all potential aspects of change.

ENHANCING SELF-MANAGEMENT: WHAT ARE THE SKILLS REQUIRED BY THERAPISTS?

One of the key determinants of success with the delivery of self-management programmes is the skill of the facilitator or trainer (Newman et al., 2004). To understand the factors that contribute to behaviour change, a therapist needs to have an appreciation over and above the biomedical aspects of the neurological condition, and have an in-depth understanding of social and psychological processes. The way in which rehabilitation is structured may also have to change to emphasize a more collaborative approach to include more focus on discursive/problem-solving strategies rather than physical training, and recognize that increasing knowledge and skills acquisition may not be enough to sustain confidence and progress in the longer term (Ellis-Hill et al., 2007).

A key component of self-management programmes is shared decision-making and this clearly involves a two-way process. Information given by the health-care professional should be relevant to the decision-making process. Achieving shared decision-making requires time, skill and effort by both the professional and patient. The provision of self-management information can be seen to be a quicker and easier method, and evidence suggests there is a tendency for health-care professionals to fall back on more didactic paternalistic methods if time is limited or constrained by other demands, such as the acute care setting (Bury, 2005).

Hardeman and Mitchie (2009) suggest that 'in the absence of training, health-care professionals do not usually posses the knowledge and skills to deliver self-management interventions' (p. 102). Therapists working in neurological rehabilitation will undoubtedly attend a great many post registration courses to enhance their skills and practice. However, there is very little emphasis given to the key communication skills required to effectively support self-management either within usual rehabilitation or delivering specific programmes (Hardeman & Mitchie, 2009). Efforts are being made to define the knowledge, characteristics and skills required for effective self-management training. Hardeman and Mitchie (2009) suggest the following:

- **Knowledge**: not just of the neurological condition; trainers should understand theories and techniques of behaviour change, and how to impart knowledge to enable optimal learning
- **Communication and relationship-building skills**: using simple non-technical language, active listening skills and encouraging interaction. Taking a person-centred collaborative approach rather than a 'mastery/expert' role in training. Promoting a trusting relationship through getting to know an individual's characteristics and life story, tailoring information and feedback to each individual

- **Managing groups**: using different methods to facilitate learning, e.g. working in pairs, and feeding back to larger group, role-play and observing each other. Providing positive leadership, deflecting a negative atmosphere and demonstrating enthusiasm. In addition understanding the needs of the group as a whole and its individuals, dealing with differences and bringing out the best of each individual
- **Specific behaviour change skills**: using key processes, such as goal setting, and exploring beliefs and confidence, such as those described within Bandura's Social Cognition Theory (Bandura, 1989). Using modelling skills to encourage vicarious learning and support. Introducing a key structure to encourage involvement in goal setting, such as breaking down tasks, developing an action plan, and recording and reflecting on progress.

The growing body of work that has helped to highlight patient needs also highlights the skills needed by professionals to support self-management. A paper published by the Kings Fund in 2005 reviewed patients' perceptions about managing their own LTC and relevant literature (Corben & Rosen, 2005). Three key themes emerged from interviews with patients about how providers of health care can support self-management in a more effective way:

1. Good relationships between professionals and patients
   - Understanding how individuals perceive their condition
   - Listening and identifying main concerns
   - Allowing time for discussion and ensuring care is planned with them, not for them
2. Clear accessible information and signposting
   - Providing enough information after initial diagnosis, and support to understand the condition, treatment and services available
   - The use of key workers and peer support to provide support about services, voluntary organizations and benefits
3. Flexibility in serviced provision
   - Individuals need different support at different times
   - Having enough time to talk with individuals is important
   - Being able to fit support from professionals with the rest of daily life, e.g. evening groups, etc.
   - Having access to assistive technology to facilitate self-management across different age groups, e.g. online support systems.

In summary, supporting individuals to self-manage may require a change in how therapists currently work in neurorehabilitation. In addition to the key skills required to deliver self-management programmes, it is also necessary for therapists to reflect on some of the values that underpin their practice. Common core principles produced by the

Department of Health (2008) may be a good place for therapists and neurorehabilitation teams to examine how they are currently enabling and supporting self-management. These include principles outlined in the document *Common Principles to Support Self-care* (Skills for Health and Skills for Care, 2008) for supporting and enabling individuals to:

- make informed choices
- assess their own needs and develop confidence to self-care
- access appropriate information to manage needs
- develop skills to self-care
- use technology to support self-care
- access support networks, and participate in the planning and development of services
- undertake risk management and risk taking to maximize independence and choice.

Overall, policy and research strongly support the need for health-care professionals working with individuals with long-term conditions to adopt a more collaborative approach. Therapists working in neurorehabilitation should be no different and need to be ready to learn new skills, work in different ways, and challenge practice that is not consistent with these principles:

As Terry, a stroke survivor explained, 'I mean sometimes physiotherapy it can be a very passive thing, but I enjoyed it the most when I was putting equal into it as well, and I felt we, things were being achieved'.

KEY POINTS

- The key outcome of many self-management programmes is a positive change in behaviour and better health.
- Self-management centres on the problems identified by the person; the clinician's role is to support problem-solving and decision-making, to set goals and, most importantly, to take action.
- Self-management is not new, and individuals have always found creative ways of managing problems and living with a chronic condition.
- Self-management includes gaining knowledge, but it also concerns behaviour change and developing strategies to manage life with a chronic disease (Newman, 2004).
- Self-management interventions are fundamentally different from education programmes.
- Self-management will depend on not only personal factors such as beliefs and motivation, but also environmental factors such as access to equipment, groups, etc.
- The skills required by therapists to not only deliver specific self-management interventions, but also embed some of the principles into their current management, should not be underestimated.

REFERENCES

Airlie, J., Baker, G., Smith, S., Young, C., 2001. Measuring the impact of multiple sclerosis on psychosocial functioning: the development of a new self-efficacy scale. Clin. Rehabil. 15, 259–265.

Andrews, K., Stewart, J., 1979. Stroke recovery: he can but does he? Rheumatol. Rehabil. 18, 43–48.

Bandura, A., 1989. Human agency in social cognition theory. Am. Psychol. 44, 1175–1184.

Bandura, A., 1994. Self-efficacy. In: Ramachaudran, V. (Ed.), Encyclopedia of Human Behavior. Academic Press, New York.

Bandura, A., 1997. The nature and structure of self-efficacy. In: Bandura, A. (Ed.), Self-efficacy: The Exercise of Control. W.H Freeman and Company, New York.

Barlow, J., Barefoot, J., 1996. Group education for people with arthritis. Patient Educ. Couns. 27, 257–267.

Barlow, J., Sturt, J., et al., 2002. Self-management interventions for people with chronic conditions in primary care: examples from arthritis, asthma and diabetes. Health Edu. J. 61 (4), 365–378.

Bendz, M., 2003. The first year of rehabilitation after stroke - from two perspectives. Scand. J. Caring Sci. 17, 215–222.

Bury, M., 2005. Health and Healthcare. Health and Illness. Polity Press, MA, USA.

Bury, M., Newbould, J., Taylor, D., 2005. A rapid review of the current state of knowledge regarding layled self-management of chronic illness. The National Institute for Health and Clinical Excellence, London.

Bury, M., Pink, D., 2005. The HSJ debate: self-management of chronic disease doesn't work. Health Serv. J. 18–19.

Cervone, D., 2000. Thinking about self-efficacy. Behav. Modif. 24, 30–56.

Ch'ng, A., French, D., Maclean, N., 2008. Coping with the challenges of recovery from stroke. J. Health Psychol. 13, 1136–1146.

Corben, S., Rosen, R., 2005. Self-management for long-term conditions: patients' Perspectives on the Way Ahead. Kings Fund, London.

Cott, C.A., Wiles, R., Devitt, R., 2007. Continuity, participation and transition:preparing clients for life n the community post stroke. Disabil. Rehabil. 29, 1566–1574.

Coulter, A., Ellins, J., 2006. QEI Review: patient-focused interventions, Chapter 3, 8–142. The Health Foundation, London.

Creer, T., Holroyd, K., 1997. Self Management. In: Baum, A., Newman, S., Weinman, J., Mcmanus, C. (Eds.), Cambridge Handbook of Psychology, Health and Medicine. Cambridge University Press, Cambridge.

Darlington, A.S., Dippel, D.W., Ribbers, G.M., van Balen, R., Passchier, J., Busschbach, J.J., 2007. Coping strategies as determinants of quality of life in stroke patients: a longitudinal study. Cerebrovascular. Disease. 23, 401–407.

Davidson, B., How, T., Worral, L., Hickson, L., Togher, L., 2008. Social participation for older people with aphasia – the impact of communication disability on friendships. Top. Stroke Rehabil. 15, 325–340.

Davidson, L., 2005. Recovery, self management and the expert patient - Changing the culture of mental health from a UK perspective. J. Ment. Health 14, 25–35.

Department of Health, 2000. The NHS Plan: A plan for investment, a plan for reform. The Stationary Office, London.

Department of Health, 2001. The expert patient: a new approach to chronic disease for the 21st century. The Stationary Office, London.

Department of Health, 2004. The NHS Improvement Plan: Putting people at the heart of public services. The Stationary Office, London.

Department of Health, 2005a. Self-Care: A real choice. The Stationary Office, London.

Department of Health, 2005b. The National Service Framework for Long Term Conditions. The Stationary Office, London.

Department of Health: Skills for Care, Skills for Health, 2008. Common Core Principles to Support Self-care: a guide to support implementation. DH Publications, London.

Department of Health: Vascular Programme-Stroke, 2007. National Stroke Strategy. DH Publications, London.

DeVellis, R., Blalock, S., 2009. Outcomes of self-management interventions. In: Newman, S., Steed, L., Mulligan, K. (Eds.), Chronic physical illness: self-management and behavioural interventions. Open University Press, Berkshire.

Dixon, G., Thornton, E., Yound, C., 2007. Perceptions of self-efficacy and rehabilitation among neurologically disabled adults. Clin. Rehabil. 21, 230–240.

Dongbo, F., Hua, F., Mcgowan, P., et al., 2003. Implementation and quantitative evaluation of chronic disease self-management programme in Shanghai, China: Randomized controlled trial. Bull. World Health Organ. 81, 174–182.

Dowswell, G., Lawler, J., Dowswell, T., Young, J., Forster, A., Hearn, J., 2000. Investigating recovery from stroke: a qualitative study. J. Clin. Nurs. 9, 507–515.

Doyle Lyons, K., 2003. Self-management of Parkinson's Disease: guidelines for program development and evaluation. Phys. Occup. Ther. Geriat. 21, 17–31.

Ellis-Hill, C.S.L., Payne, S., Ward, C., 2008. Using stroke to explore the Life Thread Model: an alternative approach to understanding rehabilitation following an acquired disability. Disabil. Rehabil. 1–10.

Ewart, C., 1992. The role of physical self efficacy in the recovery from a heart attack. In: Schwarzer, R. (Ed.), Self-efficacy: Thought control of action. Taylor and Francis, Philadelphia, USA.

Faircloth, C., Boylstein, C., Rittman, M., Young, M., Gubrium, J., 2004. Sudden illness and biographical flow in narratives of stroke recovery. Sociol. Health Illn. 26, 242–261.

Gubrium, J., Rittman, M., Williams, C., Young, M., Boylstein, C., 2003. Benchmarking as everyday functional assessment in stroke recovery. J. Gerontol. B Psychol. Sci. Soc. Sci. 58B.

Hackett, M., Chaturangi, Y., Varsha, P., Anderson, C., 2005. Frequency of depression after stroke: a systematic review of observational studies. Stroke 36, 1330–1340.

Hafsteindóttir, T., Grypdonk, M., 1997. Being a stroke patient: A review of the literature. J. Adv. Nurs. 26, 580–588.

Hardeman, W., Mitchie, S., 2009. Training and quality assurance of self-management interventions. Open University Press, Berkshire.

Hartley, S., 2009. Developing a self-management and exercise model for people with multiple sclerosis. Int. J. Ther. Rehabil. 16, 34–42.

IPsos MORI for Department of Health, 2009. Long Term Conditions 2009: Research conducted for the Department of Health. Available online at: http://www.dh.gov.uk/en/PublicationsandstatisticsPublications/Publications/PolicyAndGuidance/DH_101090 (accessed 30.07.09.).

Johnston, M., Bonetti, D., Joice, S., et al., 2007. Recovery from disability after stroke as a target for a behavioural intervention: results of a randomized

controlled trial. Disabil. Rehabil. 29, 1117–1127.

Jones, F., 2004. A memorable patient: an individual approach to stroke recovery. Physiother. Res. Int. 9, 147–148.

Jones, F., Mandy, A., Partridge, C., 2008. Reasons for recovery after stroke: a perspective based on personal experiences. Disabil. Rehabil 30, 507–516.

Jones, F., Reid, F., Partridge, C., 2008. The Stroke Self-Efficacy Questionnaire (SSEQ): measuring individual confidence in functional performance after stroke. J. Nur. Healthcare Chronic Illn. 17, 244–252.

Jordan, J., Osborne, R., 2007. Chronic disease self-management education programs: challenges ahead. Med. J. Aust. 186, 84–87.

Kendall, E., Catalano, T., Kuipers, P., Posner, N., Buys, N., Charker, J., 2007. Recovery following stroke: the role of self-management education. Soc. Sci. Med. 64, 735–746.

Kendall, E., Rogers, A., 2007. Extinguishing the social?: state sponsored self-care policy and the Chronic Disease Self-Management Programme. Disabil. Soc. 22, 129–143.

Kennedy, A., Rogers, A., Gately, C., 2005. From patients to providers: prospects for self-care skills trainers in the National Health Service. Health Soc. Care. Community 13, 431–440.

Kwakkel, G., Kollen, B., Lindeman, E., 2004. Understanding the pattern of functional recovery after stroke: facts and theories. Restor. Neurol. Neurosci. 22, 281–299.

Lazurus, R., 1990. Stress, coping and illness. In: Friedman, H. (Ed.), Personality and Disease. John Wiley and Sons, Oxford.

Levensky, E., Forcehimes, M., O'donoghue, W., Beitz, K., 2007. Motivational interviewing: An evidence based approach to counselling helps patients follow treatment recommendations. Am. J. Nurs. 107, 50–58.

Lorig, K., 1993. Self-management of chronic illness: A model for the future. Generations 17 (3), 11–14.

Lorig, K., Sobel, D., Ritter, P., Laurent, D., Hobbs, M., 2001. Effect of a self-managment program on patients with chronic disease. Eff. Clin. Pract. 4, 256–262.

Lorig, K., Sobel, D., Stewart, A., Byron, W., Bandura, A., Ritter, P., et al., 1999. Evidence suggesting that a chronic disease self-management program can improve health status while reducing hospitalisation: A randomized trial. Med. Care 37, 5–14.

Lorig, K., Stewart, A., Ritter, P., González, V., Laurent, D., Lynch, J., 1996. Outcome measures for health education and other health care interventions. SAGE Publications.

Maclean, N., Pound, P., Wolfe, C., Rudd, A., 2002. The concept of patient motivation. A qualitative analysis of stroke professionals' attitudes. Stroke 33, 444–448.

Malcomson, K., Lowe-Strong, A., Dunwoody, L., 2008. What can we learn from the personal insights of individuals living and coping with multiple sclerosis? Disabil. Rehabil. 30, 662–674.

Marks, R., 2001. Efficacy theory and its utility in arthritis rehabilitation: review and recommendations. Disabil. Rehabil. 23, 271–280.

Newbold, J., Taylor, D., Bury, M., 2006. Lay-led self-management in chronic illness: a review of the evidence. Chronic Illn. 2, 249–261.

Newman, S., Steed, L., Mulligan, K., 2004. Self-management interventions for chronic illness. Lancet 364, 1523–1537.

Partridge, C., Johnston, M., 1989. Perceived control of recovery from physical disability: measurement and prediction. Br. J. Clin. Psychol. 28, 53–59.

Prochaska, J., Velicer, W., 1997. The transtheoretical model of health behaviour change. Am. J. Health Promot. 12, 38–48.

Rimmer, J., Wang, E., Smith, D., 2008. Barriers associated with exercise and community access for individuals after stroke. J. Rehabil. Res. Dev. 45, 315–322.

Rittman, M., Faircloth, C., Boylstein, C., et al., 2004. The experience of time in the transition from hospital to home following stroke. J. Rehabil. Res. Dev. 41, 259–268.

Robinson-Smith, G., 2002. Self-efficacy and quality of life after stroke. J. Neurosci. Nurs. 34, 91–98.

Sabari, J.S., Meisler, J., Silver, E., 2000. Reflections upon rehabilitation by members of a community based stroke club. Disabil. Rehabil. 22, 330–336.

Schwartzer, R., 1992. Self-efficacy in the adoption and maintenance of health behaviours: theoretical approaches and a new model. In: Schwartzer, R. (Ed.), Sel-Efficacy: Thought control of action. first ed. Taylor and Francis, Philadelphia.

Serlachius, A., Sutton, S., 2009. Self-management and behavioural change: theoretical models. In: Newman, S., Steed, L., Mulligan, K. (Eds.), Chronic Physical Illness: self-management and behavioural interventions. Open University Press, Berkshire.

Shapero Sabari, J., Meisler, J., Silver, E., 2000. Reflections upon rehabilitation by members of a community based stroke club. Disabil. Rehabil. 22, 330–336.

Skills for Health & Skills for Care, 2008. Common core principles to support self-care. In: Department of Health, London.

Taylor, D., Bury, M., 2007. Chronic illness, expert patients and care transition. Sociol. Health Illn. 29, 27–45.

Thorne, S., Paterson, B., Russell, C., 2003. The structure of everyday self-care decision making in chronic illness. Qual. Health Res. 13, 1337–1352.

van de Laar, K., van der Bijl, J., 2001. Strategies enhancing self-efficacy in diabetes education: a review. Sch. Inq. Nurs. Pract. 15, 235–248.

von Koch, L., Holmqvist, L., Wottrich, A., Tham, K., De Pedro-Cuesta, J., 2000. Rehabilitation at home after stroke: A descriptive study of an individual intervention. Clin. Rehabil. 14, 574–583.

von Koch, L., Wottrich, A., Holmqvist, L., 1998. Rehabilitation in the home versus the hospital: The importance of context. Disabil. Rehabil. 20, 367–372.

Watkins, C., Auton, M., Deans, C., et al., 2007. Motivational interviewing early after acute stroke: a randomized, controlled trial. Stroke 38, 1004–1009.

Wilson, P., Kendall, S., Brooks, F., 2007. The Expert Patients Programme: a paradox of patient empowerment and medical dominance. Health Soc. Care Community 15, 426–438.

Wressle, E., Oberg, B., Henriksson, C., 1999. The rehabilitation process for the geriatric stroke patient an exploratory study of goal setting and interventions. Disabil. Rehabil. 21, 80–87.

Zoffman, V., Harder, I., Kirkevold, M., 2008. A person-centred communication and reflection model: shared decision making in chronic care. Qual. Health Res. 18, 670–685.

Chapter | **20** |

Falls and their management

Dorit Kunkel, Emma Stack

CONTENTS

INTRODUCTION

Falls are 'events which cause you to come to rest on the ground or other lower level unintentionally, not due to seizure, stroke/myocardial infarction or an overwhelming displacing force' (Tinetti et al., 1988). Similar definitions abound but the common phrase 'come to rest' is misleadingly genteel. Anyone who has heard or seen an adult crash to the floor will be under no illusion: falls can be calamitous and terrifying.

FALLS AND FALLING

KEY POINTS

- When stability is challenged we may fear falling, almost fall or actually fall.
- Do not underestimate their seriousness: falls can be calamitous, terrifying events.
- Falls are high on the agenda of those who fund and provide rehabilitation.
- The literature, common sense and thorough assessment will identify individuals at risk.
- Elderly people and neurological patients are at high risk of falling.
- There are over 400 interacting risk factors for falling.
- The consequences of falling are various and costly, from activity restriction to death.

Any situation that challenges our postural stability has the potential to:

a. instil within us (and those who care for us) a swiftly passing or enduring fear of falling

b. give rise to a 'near miss' (if a fall feels imminent but does not actually occur)

c. result in a fall (which may have devastating consequences, including death).

Falls are high on the agenda of those who fund and provide health care. They are a major cause of disability and the leading cause of mortality due to injury in people aged over 75 years (Department of Health (DoH), Website). The economic impact of falls among elderly people in the UK is considerable and increasing. In 1999, there were more than 600 000 A&E attendances, 200 000 hospital admissions and nearly 5000 fatalities in people aged 60 years and over following falls. The total cost to the UK government was almost £1 billion. The National Health Service incurred 59% of the cost (equivalent to the total budget for one Strategic Health Authority, or 3.3 times the total funding earmarked for mental health, coronary heart disease, cancer, and primary care in England) and the Personal Social Services for long-term care incurred the remainder (Scuffham et al., 2003).

Falls should also be high on the agenda of everyone involved in the rehabilitation of an elderly person or someone with a neurological disorder: it takes less of a challenge to threaten the postural stability of someone with a neurological disorder, for example, than it does someone with an intact system. In the model below (Figure 20.1) someone with good postural stability is likely to fall only after a major challenge; a moderate threat may challenge their stability and register a near-miss; any lesser threat may not even cause a near-miss. Conversely, someone with poor postural stability may fall when faced by even a minor threat. If they have negligible saving reactions, such as someone with acute stroke or advanced PD, almost any threat to their postural stability may result in a fall. As patients progress through rehabilitation, they may acquire the skills to survive the type of moderate threat that previously generated near-misses before they acquire the skills to survive greater perturbation. This may explain the reduction in near-misses, but not in falls observed in a recent fall-prevention trial in Parkinson's disease (PD) (Ashburn et al., 2007).

To identify *patient groups* at high risk of falling, consult the extensive literature on the risk factors for falling (see below). People with neurological disorders and elderly people are clearly more vulnerable to falls than are healthy young people and they form the focus of this chapter. Other populations vulnerable to falls and likely to form part of the rehabilitation caseload include:

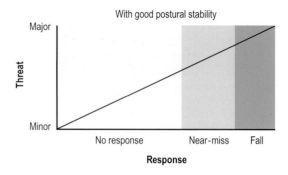

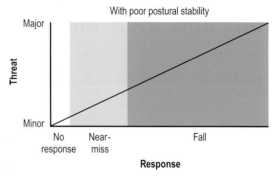

Figure 20.1 A theoretical model of the relationship between challenges to stability and response.

- People with dementia
  In a recent Swedish study (Pellfolk et al., 2009), 40% of the people with dementia living in residential homes fell during a 6-month period. Fall frequency peaked in the evening (which suggests that careful supervision at this time may reduce falls) and following episodes of anxiety and confusion, the causes of which may be treated to further reduce falls. Residents who were mobile were among the most likely to fall. Anyone involved in physical rehabilitation aimed at increasing mobility must be aware that, across all patient groups, increased mobility equates with increased opportunities to fall. This is worth discussing with the patient and their carers. Although cognitively impaired elderly patients may make considerable functional gains during rehabilitation, they remain at greater risk of falling than their cognitively intact peers and have a greater need for supervision, both in hospital and at discharge (Vogt et al., 2008).
- Inpatients and people recently discharged from hospital
  Tzeng and Yin (2008) argued that 'safety-driven design with a goal to prevent inpatient fall-related

injuries should be a hospital design principle'. They identified a number of clinical (nurse-led) interventions that may reduce in-patient falls relating to the environment, caregiver communication, assessment and reassessment, and care planning and provision. Stapleton et al. (2001) and Mackintosh et al. (2005) found that a high proportion of falls among people with stroke happened during weekend home visits from hospital and following discharge; again this suggests that falls happen when the opportunity to be mobile arises. Some ward policies may minimize patient falls by limiting patient mobility, so do not assume that someone who has not fallen during their hospital stay will not fall at home.

To identify *a patient* at high risk of falling, be aware of the risk factors, use common sense (Haines et al., 2009, showed that physiotherapists were highly accurate in predicting patient falls during rehabilitation) and complete a comprehensive patient assessment (see below). There is no such thing as 'a faller'; every patient who has fallen is an individual: while an individual carries their risk factors for falling with them 24 hours a day, they only fall at particular moments. The path to preventing someone falling (or, at least, falling again) stems from understanding their fall history in detail (see below), i.e. the circumstances (Stack & Ashburn, 1999) in which they fear falling, have nearly fallen or have actually fallen. It is important not to overlook near-misses, which Skelton (2005) defined as 'a potential fall corrected'.

Extent of the problem

It is widely believed that approximately one-third of elderly people fall annually. People with neurological conditions also fall frequently and stroke is one of the greatest risk factors (see Ch. 2). Between one-quarter and three-quarters of community-dwelling elderly people with chronic stroke fall over 6 months, with approximately half falling repeatedly, and this population is at high risk of experiencing a fracture. Impairments such as muscle weakness, impaired cognition, sensorimotor dysfunction, and balance and mobility problems presumably contribute to the large number of falls among people with stroke (Marigold and Misiaszek, 2009). Hyndman et al. (2002) identified an association between repeated falls after stroke and impaired mobility, reduced arm function and impaired ability to carry out activities of daily living (ADL). People with PD are twice as likely as are other elderly people to be recurrent fallers (see Ch. 6). As these falls have devastating consequences, there is an urgent need to identify and test innovative interventions with the potential to reduce falls in people with PD. Falls are common in Huntingdon's disease (see Ch. 7) and targets for physical intervention include gait bradykinesia, stride variability and chorea leading to increased sway, cognitive decline and behavioural change (Grimbergen et al., 2009). Gait disorders, among the most common symptoms in neurology, may play a part in half the falls among these patients (Stolze et al., 2005). Among inpatients, Stolze et al. identified gait symptoms in 93% of patients with PD and 83% with MND. One survey of neurological inpatients suggests that falling leads to 7% of neurological inpatient admissions and that one-third of inpatients fall annually (Stolze et al., 2004).

Causes of falling

Grouped simply, some of the most frequently cited risk factors for falls are:

- **Nutritional status**, e.g. vitamin D or calcium deficiency
- **Environmental hazards**, e.g. loose carpets, poor lighting, poor footwear
- **Lack of exercise**, e.g. muscle weakness, poor balance, gait disturbance, bone loss
- **Medication**, e.g. antidepressants, hypnotics, diuretics
- **Age & medical condition**, e.g. visual impairment, cognitive impairment, osteoarthritis.

For a fuller description of the risk factors for falls among elderly people, see the 1996 Effective Health Care Bulletin. The literature mentions more than 400 risk factors for falling. The more risk factors an individual has, the more likely they are to fall (Nitz & Choy, 2008), but, encouragingly, many risk factors are amenable to intervention. In many cases, a multidisciplinary assessment will be necessary, drawing on the skills and expertise of those trained to assess factors ranging from balance and mobility to underlying medical conditions, and multidisciplinary intervention may follow. People who are in pain or who are acutely unwell are at higher than usual risk of falling. Among elderly people with mobility disorders, pain predicts decreased balance and mobility, as demonstrated by Bishop et al. (2007) using the Berg Balance Scale (Berg et al., 1989) and Dynamic Gait Index (Whitney et al., 2003). Falls can be a symptom of urinary tract infection (Rhoads et al., 2007).

Of more importance than the risk factors in themselves is the *interaction* between them. As Berry and Miller (2008) stated, 'falls result from an interaction between characteristics that increase an individual's propensity to fall and acute mediating risk factors that provide the opportunity to fall'. To reduce falls, therapists target the hazardous interactions by identifying the circumstances in which the patient falls and relating them to the pathology, to determine the factors causing falls: these factors are likely to be disease-specific.

Box 20.1 **Consequences of falling**

Fear of falling

This may be associated with a fear of dependency.

Half of the 200 elderly residents interviewed by Sharaf and Ibrahim (2008) had moderate to severe concern about falling, particularly those:
- who used a walking device
- with depression or anxiety
- with balance impairment or a history of falls.

Intervention can decrease these sources of fear. A fear of falls can lead to activity restriction and increase the risk of falls or prompt potential fallers to take extra care. Fear, alongside other factors that restrict activity, should feature in fall-prevention programmes (Lee et al., 2008).

An enduring fear can also affect carers (Liddle & Gilleard, 1995).

Dependence

Anything from requiring support at home to requiring long-term care.

Injury

Fall descent, impact and bone strength are important determinants of whether a fall will result in a fracture (Berry & Miller, 2008). Fractured femur is one of the most costly and debilitating consequences of falling. Cummings and Nevitt (1989) hypothesized that four factors increased the likelihood of a fall resulting in a hip fracture:
- Faller orientation – moving slowly, with little forward momentum, a fall would result in direct application of impact energy to the femur
- Protective response – grabbing something or stumbling might prevent a fall, change the faller's orientation or dissipate impact
- Local shock absorption – muscle or fat would be protective, whereas a hard landing surface would increase fracture risk

- Bone strength – a number of disorders would weaken the bone around the hip and increase the risk of fracture.

There is supportive evidence that the 'nature of the fall' may determine the type of fracture (Nevitt and Cummings, 1993): elderly women with hip fractures are likely to have fallen 'sideways or straight down' and those with wrist fractures are likely to have fallen backward. The pattern of excessive proximal humerus, pelvis and hip fractures in PD suggests that the increased risk is due to specific types of backward or sideways falls (Johnell et al., 1992).

Costly intervention

Injurious falls may require medical attention. Costs include:
- ambulance journey
- A&E attendance
- hospital stay
- outpatient attendance
- GP consultations
- long-term care.

Carer strain/injury

Davey et al. (2004) interviewed 14 spouses of repeat fallers with PD. Most were frightened about their spouse falling; they had received little information about falls, felt unprepared for their role and expressed a need for more support and advice about managing falls. Carers can be injured attempting to prevent falls and helping someone up after a fall: rehabilitation must not overlook them.

Death

Falls are the direct cause of most limb and femoral neck fractures and the fifth most frequent cause of death among elderly people (Czerwinski et al., 2008).

A minority of fallers lie for long periods after falling before anyone finds them (4% in the Stolze et al. (2004) series).

Consequences of falling

The consequences of falling are wide-ranging, interconnected, costly and they may be devastating (Box 20.1).

ASSESSING PEOPLE WHO HAVE FALLEN

KEY POINTS

- Take a thorough fall history before observing the patient move.
- Identify the circumstances surrounding previous falls and near-misses.

- Interview the person who fell (or witnesses) and consider using a falls diary.
- Observe the person who fell performing their fall-related activities in a functional way.
- Consider the careful use of a video camera.
- Complete a battery of appropriate tests and outcome measures.

It would be dangerous not to take a good fall history (with the patient in a safe, stable position) before asking the patient to perform any mobility tests. When, for example, a person who has fallen reports 'turning is fatal' or 'all falls are to do with turning' (Stack & Ashburn, 1999), the therapist will be suitably alert to the risks inherent in asking that patient to perform a turn test. In the same way that a thorough history from a patient with low back pain should leave the therapist almost able to *feel* the pain, a thorough history after a fall should leave the therapist almost able to recreate the event in their mind. Some researchers have asked people who have fallen to re-enact the events leading to a fall (for example, Connell & Wolf, 1997), but this is potentially risky and there is no guarantee of a more accurate recall than there is with a verbal account.

Falls are distinct events that happen in a specific time and place and for a specific reason. Although people with neurological conditions fall more frequently than people without, they do not fall continuously. An individual's risk factors for falling act on them *all-day-every-day*, but people only fall occasionally, when they cannot preserve their postural stability as they move about their environment. In 1997, Berg et al. wrote that 'relatively little research has addressed what fallers are actually doing at the time of a fall'. That is changing and we are increasingly illuminating the circumstances in which people (with PD and stroke, at least) fall (Ashburn et al., 2008; Hyndman et al., 2002; Mackintosh et al., 2005; Stack & Ashburn, 1999).

Time spent interviewing the person who has fallen (or a carer or witness) is time well spent, as it will guide intervention. Unfortunately, in the case of inpatient falls, the person documenting the fall may not have witnessed it: Morse et al. (1985) found that staff witnessed only 23% of inpatient falls. While a witness can easily record the location in which they found the faller, the time and evident injuries, they can only surmise what had happened (i.e. the fall-precipitating circumstances).

Interviewing patients and carers

Previous falls are not always well documented in patients' medical records; patients may not share the same ideas as health-care professionals about what constitutes a fall (e.g. 'I didn't fall, I slipped'); nor may they wish to disclose a fall. It is imperative that therapists use all their interviewing skills to talk to patients about previous falls and to probe carefully if a patient denies falling. We strongly disagree with Wild et al. (1981) who claimed that 'fallers are rarely sufficiently aware of what happened or sufficiently articulate in their description to provide doctors with the necessary information'. The key to understanding what has happened (and thus being able to prevent a repetition) is being able to identify the circumstances in which the individual has fallen.

In other words, the therapist must attempt to discover, through questioning and observation:

1. where the patient fell
2. what they were trying to do at the time: the 'fall-related activity'
3. what might have caused them to fall at that instant

4. whether they were able to break their fall in any way
5. what happened when and after they hit the floor.

Even the act of taking a detailed falls history may be a fall-preventive intervention, boosting insight and confidence. Elderly people who reflect on their falls and seek understanding are better able (than are their non-reflecting peers) to develop strategies to prevent future falls, face their fear of falling and remain active (Roe et al., 2008). Self-reported impaired balance is a readily assessed risk factor for future fractures in elderly people (Wagner et al., 2009). On completion of the interview, refer patients to other specialists if their input is necessary.

Falls diaries

The same questions that one might ask a patient directly can form the basis of a falls diary. Research participants often complete diaries, sometimes for several months. In a recent study (Ashburn et al., 2008), repeated fallers with PD recorded the circumstances in which they fell over a 6-month period. On a calendar sheet, they marked any day on which they had a fall or a near-miss. On separate dated sheets, they noted where they fell, the suspected cause, what they were doing at the time, how they landed and what happened next. The example diary entries in Table 20.1 outline some injurious falls in which turning was the fall-related activity.

Clinically, someone who falls frequently or experiences frequent near-misses can keep a record of the events while they are on a physiotherapy waiting list, for example, or in active rehabilitation. The document can assist professionals with their assessments (and guide intervention) by:

a. detailing the circumstances in which a patient is unstable
b. illuminating the patient's level of insight: multiple 'Don't Know' or 'No Idea' type responses may suggest that the patient lacks insight or interest or was not conscious.

Having someone who has fallen recently jot down the circumstances shortly after the incident may seem a promising way of recording the details before they fade from memory, but there is no guarantee. Diaries will not suit everyone. Interviews, re-enactments and diaries all have strengths and weakness, but ultimately they all rely on the patient's perception.

Observing fall-related activities

Now that the reader is clear about what type of activities cause the patient to fear falling or have previously caused near-misses or actual falls, it is time to observe the patient attempting such activities:

- Embed the activities within representative 'real-life' activities, rather than ask the patient to perform isolated movements outside a functional context. For

Table 20.1 Examples of injurious falls during turning requiring health service input: an example of falls diary use

LOCATION	ACTIVITY/ CAUSE	LANDING	INJURY	GETTING UP	INTERVENTION
Hotel	Turned too quickly	Right side	Fractured hand, bruises	Wife and son helped me	X-ray; surgery
Descending stairs	Twisted	On back	Fractured ribs, concussion		Husband called ambulance 10 hours in hospital
Putting food in fridge	Turned	Very hard on back	Fractured ribs, bruises		Friends called ambulance; GP called 2 days later
Sitting room	Turned too sharply	Left side	Hurt left shoulder	With help of chair	Called GP; sent to A&E
Shop	Turned quickly	Face first	Cut face, nose bleed	Two ambulance men helped me	Ambulance
Kitchen	Turned quickly opening door	Heavily on side	Banged head, arm and shoulder	Crawled to lounge; used chair	Paramedics called

(From Ashburn et al., 2008, reprinted by permission of Taylor & Francis Group, http://www.informaworld.com.)

example, if a patient reports having fallen reaching, watch them reach for something off a high shelf and/ or from a low cupboard rather than ask them to perform the Functional Reach Test (Duncan et al., 1990).

- Functional tasks replicate more closely the type of challenge that meaningful action poses, whereas outcome measures are likely to impose certain limitations on the way patients move. Certain turn tests, for example, dictate where the subject should turn and in what direction; such a test will not reveal how subjects spontaneously turn when it is necessary so to do.
- Another advantage of observing functional tasks rather than relying on standard tests is that the patient has something on which to focus other than the movement of interest. You could ask a patient who has fallen turning and reaching to perform the Timed Up and Go Test and the Functional Reach Test or you could ask them to make a cup of tea (ideally in their own environment) while you observe them. The former will give you the time taken and distance reached. The latter will illuminate how the person moves during challenging tasks, whether they compensate and to what hazards they may be exposing themselves.

Video

We recommend using a video camera as a record of a patient assessment and for feedback to the patient. A video record allows repeated playback, which facilitates the rating, timing or step counting required by certain outcome measures. It also facilitates discussion with colleagues who may not have been able to attend a patient assessment in person. Always secure the permission of a patient to make, store and use a video record, and take all reasonable precautions not to record other patients' images or conversations inadvertently. Remember that a camera with a trailing power lead is in itself a trip hazard and that a hand-held camera prevents the therapist's hands being free to catch a falling patient. Be careful (Stack et al., 2005); we recommend batteries and tripods.

Standard tests and outcome measures

In assessing patients who have fallen, there is certainly a place for standardized measures. Armed with a detailed fall history and having observed the patient perform the culprit activities naturally, the therapist can progress to evaluating aspects of the patient's mobility and balance that:

1. may be contributing to their risk of falling
2. will form the focus of intervention.

While there has been considerable interest in developing screening tools to identify people at risk of falling, the results are contentious. Remembering the variety of risk factors for falling, it is apparent that predicting who will and who will not fall within a given time is no simple task; see Oliver et al. (2008). Most readers will know that their patients are at risk of falling (if those patients are elderly and/or have neurological conditions) and, indeed,

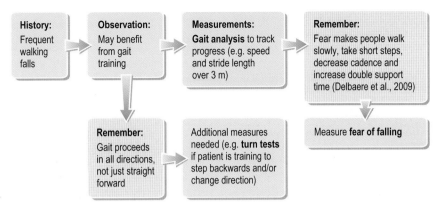

Figure 20.2 Example of connection between history, observation and choice of measure.

many of their patients will already have fallen. Therefore, we will not discuss the issue of population screening tools here but focus instead on the type of tools that will help a therapist track their patient's progress as their condition changes and/or they progress through rehabilitation. In summary, no single tool will suffice; therapists should consider a battery of measures that record the scope of their patient's abilities.

The choice of outcome measures will reflect what is key to the patient's physical rehabilitation. Bear in mind the *connections* between the problems identified from the fall history and through observation, the treatment plan and the reason for measurement (Figure 20.2).

See Ryerson (2009) and Stokes (2009) for further guidance and recommendations for outcome measures.

PREVENTING FALLS AND MANAGING PEOPLE WHO HAVE FALLEN

KEY POINTS

- Target the hazardous interactions between the individual and their environment.
- Exercise can reduce risk of falling and stimulate continued physical activity.
- Developing new movement strategies can make everyday activities safer.
- Appropriate foot wear reduces the risk of falling.
- Modifying the environment reduces falls where hazards play a part.
- Not everyone is interested in falls prevention and some falls are unavoidable.

Following a comprehensive assessment, the therapist will be able to target the interactions between the individual and their environment that place them at risk of falling. For a patient with a condition (or other risk factor for falling) that will be ongoing, the therapist must consider the challenges that person will face over 24 hours and address each one: the history of falls, near-misses and fears will highlight the priorities. Targets for intervention include people and the environment.

The person at risk of falling

Exercise and other training programmes

In the prevention of falls among elderly people (Rose, 2008), physical activity (or exercise) can:

- prevent the pathology and impairments that lead to disability and increased fall risk
- slow the progression of disease and system impairments
- restore function to a level that allows for more autonomy in the activities of daily living.

Options for exercise content and delivery change as the risk of falling increases (see Box 20.2).

A meta-analysis of 44 trials (with more than 9000 participants) by Sherrington et al. (2008) revealed that exercise reduced the rate of falling by 17%. Programmes that included a high dose of exercise (over 50 hours) with challenging balance exercises (e.g. conducted while standing with feet together or on one leg, with minimal hand support

---

Box 20.2 **Risk of falling and appropriate options for exercise**

Risk of falling

Low - Many exercise choices are available

Increasing - Tailored, progressive programmes target the risk factors for falls

High - Multifactorial intervention with an integral exercise component

---

Box 20.3 Example programme 1

- Part of a multifaceted intervention in German nursing homes
- Balance exercises and progressive resistance training with ankle weights and dumbbells
- Groups (of six to eight) exercised twice weekly for 75 minutes per session (including breaks)
- Entry criteria: able to stand while holding a chair and to lift one's foot
- To begin: 20 minutes of balance exercise in standing (and walking if possible)
- Nine exercises (all major limb muscle groups), two sets at 10 repetition maximum (10RM)
- Progressed as tolerated to a maximum of 10 kg ankle weights and 5 kg for the upper extremity

(Adapted from Becker et al., 2003.)

Box 20.4 Example programme 2

- A balance and strength retraining group and home exercise programme
- 36 weeks of 'falls management exercise' classes once a week for 1 hour: balance specific, individually-tailored and targeted dynamic balance, strength, bone, endurance, flexibility, gait and functional skills, 'righting' or 'correcting' skills, backward-chaining and functional floor exercises (Skelton & Dinan, 1999).
- Home exercise programme (20–40 minutes duration, twice a week) aimed at reducing asymmetry in strength of the lower limbs.
- Progressive OTAGO exercises (Robertson et al., 2001) were core.
- Hip protectors were supplied for wear during the exercise sessions.

(Adapted from Skelton et al., 2005.)

Box 20.5 Example programme for people with stroke

- A challenging, but safe, 'agility' programme:
  - appropriately graded (and supervised) fast, dynamic movement
  - multisensory integration.
- A 'stretching and weight-shifting' programme:
  - increasing use of the paretic limb
  - incorporates the useful challenge of getting down to and up from the floor.
- Training thrice weekly for 10 weeks.

(Adapted from Marigold et al., 2005.)

Box 20.6 Example programme for people with Parkinson's disease

- Home-based exercise programme
- Exercises taught and progressed by a physiotherapist (at weekly, hour long visits)
  - ○ Muscle strengthening
    - ▪ Knee and hip extensors, hip abductors
  - ○ Range of movement
    - ▪ Ankle, pelvic tilt, trunk and head
  - ○ Balance training
    - ▪ Static, dynamic and functional
  - ○ Walking
    - ▪ Inside and outside
  - ○ Strategies for fall prevention, movement initiation and compensation.

(Adapted from Ashburn et al., 2007.)

---

and controlled movements of the centre of mass) were most effective. Muscle strength contributes to postural control and training (as part of a multifactorial intervention) often shows a reduction in fall rates (Horlings et al., 2008). While not all the example programmes outlined (in Boxes 20.3–20.7) have been adequately tested in fully powered fall-prevention trials, each one contains ideas for intervention that may suit specific patients.

Exercise may improve balance and mobility and reduce falls after stroke (also see Ch. 2).

Some small, recent studies have shown improvements in strength and balance after people with PD participated in exercise two or three times per week for between 6 weeks and 3 months (Hirsch et al, 2003; Kluding & Quinn McGinnis, 2006; Toole et al., 2005). The exercise trial for repeated-fallers with PD summarized below reduced near-misses. A fully-powered trial is underway (Canning et al., 2009) to determine whether exercise targeting reduced balance, reduced leg strength and freezing (plus standardized falls prevention advice) can reduce fall rates in people with PD at risk of falling (and the cost effectiveness of the programme). See also Chapter 6.

With a change of emphasis, working with the individual who has fallen (or a group) moves from exercise to balance retraining. When balance is disturbed in standing or walking, whole-body responses emerge. These responses may be exploited for rehabilitation purposes; preliminary results indicate that training programmes designed to elicit whole-body responses effectively reduce falls and improve functional mobility in older adults with and without neurological impairment (Marigold & Misiaszek, 2009). Nitz and Choy (2004) piloted the following programme with elderly people who had fallen and achieved a significant reduction in falls.

- Participants attended 10 sessions of 1-hour duration at weekly intervals
- Some activities were individual
  - Sit–stand–sit; stepping all directions; reaching to limits
  - Step up and down; balance strategy practice; sideways reach task
- Some activities involved working (for fun and competition) as a group
  - Ball games; treasure hunt
- All challenges were progressed (see their paper for a comprehensive description)
- Participants also received a booklet on reducing the risk of falls.

(Adapted from Nitz & Choy, 2004.)

Continued physical activity

Falls prevention programmes have the potential to stimulate continued involvement in physical activity (Laforest et al., 2009), particularly when the programme includes a focus on enhancing both physical activity and confidence in performing daily activities (Ziden et al., 2008). Keep balance, strength and flexibility in the forefront of your mind when you encourage patients to adopt the types of exercise and activity that may reduce their risk of further falls. But remember, too, that different people are motivated in different ways towards exercise; patients will probably abandon boring home exercises very quickly. Think about the various reasons you enjoy exercise (spending time alone or with other people; relaxing or competing; being outdoors or achieving obvious results) and think about finding ways for your patients to experience the same satisfaction; see also 'Being active with a neurological condition' in Chapter 18.

Movement strategies

During rehabilitation, a patient may acquire the physical fitness needed to function well (by pursuing the types of exercise described in Boxes 20.3–20.7, above) and they may manipulate their own environment to reduce the hazards therein (see 'Physical Environment', below), but in itself fitness and a safe home is no guarantee of not falling at home or beyond. The third strand to fall prevention in people at ongoing risk of falling is for them to learn to move through their world safely in light of the risk. For example, someone with PD who has tripped and fallen may have good dorsiflexion and a home clear of clutter, but remain at risk of falling if they:

- forget to heel-strike
- cross an uneven pavement without keeping a hand free to grasp something solid if they stumble.

For a person with PD prone to tripping falls, 'conscious heel-striking' and 'keeping a hand free' are movement strategies: ways of minimizing the risk of falling while performing challenging activities in a way that takes into account the abilities of the individual. Movement strategies can make both sudden destabilizations (such as tripping) and self-induced perturbations (such as reaching) safer. The patient and therapist work together to instigate new movement strategies, with the therapist drawing on their assessment and teaching skills (see 'skill acquisition' in Ch. 11).

Step 1: Extract the fall-related activities from an individual's fall history

Step 2: Devise suitable movement strategies

Step 3: Help the person at risk of falling to learn these strategies.

Do not seek to 'normalize' a patient's posture or movement if an apparent abnormality (e.g. flexed posture; short stride) may be an appropriate compensation for impaired postural stability (imagine yourself walking across an icy pavement). On the contrary, it may be necessary to promote compensation in a way that improves patient safety (e.g. slow down; take several small steps).

A picture of the activities commonly surrounding falls in PD is emerging from the interview-based study of Stack and Ashburn (1999) and the diary-based study of Ashburn et al. (2008). In Table 20.2 we list examples of these activities and suggest suitable movement strategies.

In all cases people at risk of falling should attempt to avoid distractions while tackling challenging activities. Therapists and carers should avoid dividing the patient's attention by talking to them during tasks. It is impossible to avoid multi-tasking in every situation, so the complexity of tasks negotiated should increase progressively throughout rehabilitation.

Physical environment

Footwear

Footwear is a bridge between the person and their environment. It can influence balance by:

a. altering feedback to the foot and ankle

b. modifying friction at the shoe/floor interface (Menant et al., 2008).

In a recent study (Horgan et al., 2009), wearing their own footwear improved participants' Berg Balance Scale score compared to being barefoot. Footwear brought the greatest benefit to those with the poorest balance. Many elderly people wear suboptimal shoes. Walking indoors barefoot or in socks, and walking anywhere in high-heels, increase the risk of falls; wearing shoes with low heels and firm slip-resistant soles may reduce falls (Menant et al., 2008).

Table 20.2 Strategies that may enhance stability during common fall-related activities

FALL-RELATED ACTIVITY	STRATEGIES THAT MAY PREVENT FALLS
Tripping	• Install AND USE stable support around known trip hazards • Optimize dorsiflexion and remember to heel strike • Don't occupy both hands: keep one free for saving reaction
Turning	• Visualize and follow wide arcs, not tight turns • One direction may be easier; turn that way when possible • Slow down; pause between walking and turning
Reaching	• Reach forward, using visual guidance • Reach with one hand, while using the other for support • Keep both feet planted firmly on the floor
Transferring	• Remember that both sit-to-stand and stand-to-sit are challenging • Pause between movements • Use support
Walking	• Use well-maintained aids IF THEY HELP or keep a hand free • Plan the route from A-to-B and focus
Washing and dressing	• Sit down for stability, particularly when vision is obscured

The external environment

Key hazards for people at risk of falling (Becker et al., 2003) include:

- poor lighting
- chair and bed heights
- floor surfaces and clutter
- insufficient grab rails (toilets and bathrooms)
- improperly used and maintained walking aids.

The importance of environmental hazards in falls is debatable: Norton et al. (1997) implicated them in only one-quarter of falls at home, Sattin et al. (1998) in only one-fifth and Mackintosh et al. (2005) found that two-thirds of falls by people with stroke happened without any involvement from external hazards. The pooled analysis of six fall-prevention studies based on environmental interventions (Clemson et al., 2008) demonstrated a significant reduction of falls among those at highest risk. Lord et al. (2006) demonstrated similar findings: home hazards pose the greatest risk for people with fair balance (those with poor balance are less exposed; those with good mobility are more able to cope), so hazard reduction is effective if targeted at those with a history of falls and mobility limitations (alongside other interventions).

With a patient at high risk of falling it may be helpful to sketch the layout of their home and mark on the sketch the environmental hazards and hazardous activities that are unavoidable (Figure 20.3). This exercise will identify the challenges to patient and therapist and may guide rehabilitation.

Engagement with falls prevention

Culture, lifestyle and the extent to which people are willing to engage in falls prevention activities varies, so there is no 'one-size-fits-all' approach to fall prevention.

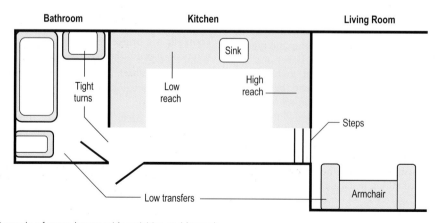

Figure 20.3 Example of room layout with activities and hazards.

In practice, you will encounter people who fall very frequently and are happy to continue doing so. As Becker et al. (2003) emphasized, safety alone (and injury prevention) should never be the only quality indicator for mobility-associated quality of life. In Yardley et al.'s (2008) survey of people aged over 54 years, home-based strength and balance training appeared more acceptable than classes but neither option appeared in great demand: 36% said they would definitely train at home; only 23% would definitely attend group sessions. A recent fall was associated with a greater willingness to train at home and accept help with home hazards. Horne et al. (2009) further argued the futility of urging a sedentary UK population to adopt exercise to prevent falls. They found that young older adults (unlike those who had fallen) did not feel they were at risk of falling, so lacked motivation to exercise to prevent falls. Whitehead et al. (2006) found that elderly people at risk of falling were most likely to take up the intervention with least impact on their lifestyle (i.e. daily osteoporosis medication rather than a home safety assessment or course of exercise classes). Hip protectors may prevent fractures, but not everyone wants to wear them (Becker et al., 2003). As with all aspects of rehabilitation, progress depends on participation and commitment: be prepared for people to opt out.

Not every fall is preventable

When a patient is clearly at risk of further injurious falls (for example a repeat faller with PD who has minimal saving reactions, but remains mobile; see Ch. 6) therapists must raise the priorities of injury prevention and death prevention over fall prevention. Expecting the patient to fall again, attention needs to turn to the landing and to what happens next. Could the environment be safer? Could the patient learn to get up from the floor alone? Expecting the patient to be unable to get up again alone, attention needs to turn to preventing a long lay or at least minimizing the consequences of one. How will the person who has fallen attract help? How will they stay warm, nourished and alive?

EFFECTIVE FALLS SERVICES AND TEAMS

Service models

In 2001, the NHS began to focus on developing service provision to prevent falls in older people. The introduction of integrated falls services designed to reduce falls (and their consequences for health-care providers and users) has been patchy. A recent Help the Aged survey of 94 primary care trusts found that few were on their way to an integrated service but most were developing falls prevention programmes (DoH, Website). In 2008, Lamb et al. surveyed three-quarters of the 303 falls clinics in existence (most in acute or community hospitals, with a few in primary care or emergency departments). Most services undertook a multi-factorial assessment, the content and quality of which varied substantially, as did intervention delivery: interventions for vision, home-hazard modification, medication review and bone health caused greatest concern in terms of meeting the NICE recommendations. Existing fall prevention programmes vary from single intervention strategies to comprehensive multifactorial approaches and while some target groups at high risk of falling, others target non-select groups of community-dwelling elderly people.

A multifactorial approach

There is a consensus that taking a multifactorial approach is the most effective way to prevent falls. In Example 1 (Box 20.8), set in a nursing home, residents could participate in any combination of intervention options for any time they wanted. In Example 2 (Box 20.9), the authors highlighted the variation in uptake of recommendations across the participating care homes and general practitioners.

A variety of community-based fall prevention programmes for elderly people exists; Costello and Edelstein (2008) make the following recommendations:

1. Multifactorial fall prevention programmes appear more effective for older individuals with a previous fall history than a non-select group

---

Box 20.8 Example 1: a multifaceted non-pharmaceutical intervention

- Staff training and feedback
  A 60-minute course plus written information on falls (including modifiable risk factors) and monthly feedback on fallers, fall rates and severe injuries.
- Information and education of residents
  All residents received written information on fall prevention and all mobile residents received a personal consultation from a nurse or exercise instructor. Residents were informed it would take months to see the effects of exercise and that hip protectors should be worn daily from arising until bedtime.
- Environmental adaptations
  See above.
- Exercise
  See above.
- Hip protectors
  All residents who could stand were offered two different types of hip protectors and their use was checked monthly.

(Adapted from Becker et al., 2003.)

Box 20.9 Example 2: a multifactorial risk factor modification programme

- Exercise programme

  Experienced exercise assistants supported by a physiotherapist visited each home thrice weekly.

  Exercise sessions aimed to improve balance and gait, flexibility, strength and endurance.

  If possible, exercises were linked to tasks such as transfers, dressing and using walking aids.

  Group sessions (40 minutes) consisted of a warm-up, a targeted circuit and a warm-down. Sessions included dancing and games.

  Exercises were progressed as appropriate, using weights and thera-bands.

  Individual sessions were provided for residents with physical frailty and cognitive impairment.

  Participants were encouraged to carry out individual exercise outside of the visits.

- Staff education

  All staff were encouraged to be involved in the interventions, and each care home manager received written information.

- Medical reviews

  Residents with suspected medical risk factors were examined, and recommendations were reported by letter to general practitioners (notably sedative and diuretic medication, poly-pharmacy, orthostatic hypotension and osteoporosis).

- Environmental modification

  An occupational therapy assistant visited each home to assess risk factors on an individual basis, and provided each home with a written report. Environmental health teams also visited the homes to carry out their routine assessments and to alert homes to any major risks.

- Optician and podiatry

  A review from an optician was arranged for residents with a visual acuity of 6/12 or less, or if they had not seen an optician in the previous year. Podiatry was arranged for residents whose foot condition was of concern.

(Adapted from Dyer et al., 2004.)

---

2. Medication and vision assessment with appropriate health practitioner referral should be included in a falls screening examination
3. Exercise alone is effective in reducing falls and should include a comprehensive programme combining strength, balance, and/or endurance training for a minimum of 12 weeks
4. Home hazard assessment with modifications may be beneficial in reducing falls, especially in a targeted group of individuals.

Falls prevention is an expanding area of health care. The already extensive literature is growing to incorporate falls prevention in a wide range of settings. Taken as a whole, the literature shows that the coordination of multidisciplinary assessment and intervention is possible (but challenging) everywhere from the hospital emergency department to community care, both with cognitively intact and cognitively impaired patient groups. A few recent publications illustrate the scope of falls prevention services (see Table 20.3).

The concluding message of this chapter is that falls necessitate thorough investigation and a coordinated approach to intervention. When skilled practitioners and committed teams tackle falls, many are preventable and the reduction in fear, injury, dependence and intervention is significant.

Table 20.3 Falls prevention services in different settings

IN HOSPITAL	DAY HOSPITAL	IN THE COMMUNITY	IN THE NURSING HOME
Emergency departments focus on injuries rather than consequences. But with prevention an emerging role, a multidisciplinary team should evaluate fallers and intervene as required for those discharged after their visit (Bloch et al., 2009).	Fewer recurrent fallers fall again if they receive multidisciplinary assessment followed by appropriate interventions in comparison with community assessment and targeted referral (Spice et al., 2009).	An inter-professional falls prevention programme for elderly people with a history of falls achieved persistent improvements in physical function and balance and reduced the fear of falling (Banez et al., 2008).	Among psycho-geriatric patients, a structured multifactorial fall prevention intervention (medical assessment, multidisciplinary fall risk evaluation and general and individual fall prevention activities) significantly reduced falls (Neyens et al., 2009).

REFERENCES

Ashburn, A., Stack, E., Ballinger, C., Fazakarley, L., Fitton, C., 2008. The circumstances of falls among people with PD and the use of Falls Diaries to facilitate reporting. Disabil. Rehabil. 30, 1205–1212.

Ashburn, A., Fazakarley, L., Ballinger, C., Pickering, R., McLellan, L.D., Fitton, C., 2007. A randomised controlled trial of a home based exercise programme to reduce the risk of falling among people with Parkinson's disease. J. Neurol. Neurosurg. Psychiatry 78, 678–684.

Banez, C., Tully, S., Amaral, L., Kwan, D., Kung, A., Mak, K., et al., 2008. Development, implementation, and evaluation of an Interprofessional Falls Prevention Program for older adults. J. Am. Geriatr. Soc. 56 (8), 1549–1555.

Becker, C., Kron, M., Lindemann, U., Sturm, E., Eichner, B., Walter-Jung, B., et al., 2003. Effectiveness of a Multifaceted Intervention on Falls in Nursing Home Residents. J. Am. Geriatr. Soc. 51, 306–313.

Berg, W., Alessio, H., Mills, E., Tong, C., 1997. Circumstances and consequences of falls in independent community-dwelling older adults. Age Ageing 26, 261–268.

Berg, K., Wood-Dauphinee, S., Williams, J.I., Gayton, D., 1989. Measuring balance in the elderly: preliminary development of an instrument. Physiother. Can. 41 (6), 304–311.

Berry, S.D., Miller, R.R., 2008. Falls: epidemiology, pathophysiology, and relationship to fracture. Curr. Osteoporos. Rep. 6 (4), 149–154.

Bishop, M.D., Meuleman, J., Robinson, M., Light, K.E., 2007. Influence of pain and depression on fear of falling, mobility, and balance in older male veterans. J. Rehabil. Res. Dev. 44 (5), 675–683.

Bloch, F., Jegou, D., Dhainaut, J.F., Rigaud, A.S., Coste, J., Lundy, J.E., et al., 2009. Do ED staff have a role to play in the prevention of repeat falls in elderly patients? Am. J. Emerg. Med. 27 (3), 303–307.

Canning, C.G., Sherrington, C., Lord, S.R., Fung, V.S., Close, J.C., Latt, M.D., et al., 2009. Exercise therapy for prevention of falls in people with Parkinson's disease: a protocol for a randomised controlled trial and economic evaluation. BMC Neurol. 9, 4.

Clemson, L., Mackenzie, L., Ballinger, C., Close, J.C., Cumming, R.G., 2008. Environmental interventions to prevent falls in community-dwelling older people: a meta-analysis of andomized trials. J. Aging Health 20 (8), 954–971.

Connell, B., Wolf, S., 1997. Environmental and behavioural circumstances associated with falls at home among healthy elderly individuals. Arch. Phys. Med. Rehabil. 78, 179–186.

Costello, E., Edelstein, J.E., 2008. Update on falls prevention for community-dwelling older adults: review of single and multifactorial intervention programs. J. Rehabil. Res. Dev. 45 (8), 1135–1152.

Cummings, SR, Nevitt, MC., 1989. A hypothesis: the causes of hip fractures. J. Gerontol. 44, M107–M111.

Czerwinski, E., Bialoszewski, D., Borowy, P., Kumorek, A., Bialoszewski, A., 2008. Epidemiology, clinical significance, costs and fall prevention in elderly people. Ortopedia Traumatologia Rehabilitacja 10 (5), 419–428.

Davey, C., Wiles, R., Ashburn, A., Murphy, C., 2004. Falling in Parkinson's disease: the impact on informal caregivers. Disabil. Rehabil. 26 (23), 1360–1366.

Delbaere, K., Sturnieks, D.L, Crombez, G., Lord, S.R, 2009. Concern about falls elicits changes in gait parameters in conditions of postural threat in older people. J. Gerontol. A Biol. Sci. Med. Sci. 64 (2), 237–242.

Department of Health, Website: http://www.dh.gov.uk/en/SocialCare/Deliveringadultsocialcare/Olderpeople.

Duncan, P.W., Weiner, D.K., Chandler, J., Studenski, S., 1990. Functional Reach: a new clinical measure of balance. J. Gerontol. 45 (6), M192–M197.

Dyer, C., Taylor, G., Reed, M., Dyer, C. A., Robertson, D., Harrington, R., 2004. Falls prevention in residential care homes: a randomised controlled trial. Age Ageing 33, 596–602.

Grimbergen, Y., Knol, M., Bloem, B., Kremer, B., Roos, R., Munneke, M., 2009. Falls and gait disturbances in Huntington's disease. Mov. Disord. 23 (7), 970–976.

Haines, T., Kuys, S.S., Morrison, G., Clarke, J., Bew, P., 2009. Cost-effectiveness analysis of screening for risk of in-hospital falls using physiotherapist clinical judgement. Med. Care. 47 (4), 448–456.

Hirsch, M., Toole, T., Maitland, C.G., Rider, R.A., 2003. The effects of balance training and high-intensity resistance training on persons with IPD. Arch. Phys. Med. Rehabil. 84, 1109–1117.

Horgan, N.F., Crehan, F., Bartlett, E., Keogan, F., O'Grady, A.M., Moore, A.R., et al., 2009. The effects of usual footwear on balance amongst elderly women attending a day hospital. Age Ageing 38 (1), 62–67.

Horlings, C.G., van Engelen, B.G., Allum, J.H., Bloem, B.R., 2008. A weak balance: the contribution of muscle weakness to postural instability and falls. Nat. Clin. Pract. Neurol. 4 (9), 504–515.

Horne, M., Speed, S., Skelton, D., Todd, C., 2009. What do community-dwelling Caucasian and South Asian 60–70 year olds think about exercise for fall prevention? Age Ageing 38 (1), 68–73.

Hyndman, D., Ashburn, A., Stack, E., 2002. Fall events among people with stroke living in the community: circumstances of falls and characteristics of fallers. Arch. Phys. Med. Rehabil. 83, 165–170.

Johnell, O., Melton, L., Atkinson, E., O'Fallon, W., Kurland, L., 1992. Fracture risk in patients with parkinsonism: a population-based study in Olmstead County, Minnesota. Age Ageing 21, 32–38.

Kluding, P., Quinn McGinnis, P., 2006. Multidimensional exercise for people with PD: a case report. Physiother. Theory Pract. 22, 153–162.

Laforest, S., Pelletier, A., Gauvin, L., Robitaille, Y., Fournier, M.,

Corriveau, H., et al., 2009. Impact of a community-based falls prevention program on maintenance of physical activity among older adults. J. Aging Health 21 (3), 480–500.

Lamb, S.E., Fisher, J.D., Gates, S., Potter, R., Cooke, M.W., Carter, Y.H., 2008. A national survey of services for the prevention and management of falls in the UK. BMC Health Serv. Res. 8, 233.

Lee, F., Mackenzie, L., James, C., 2008. Perceptions of older people living in the community about their fear of falling. Disabil. Rehabil. 30 (23), 1803–1811.

Liddle, J., Gilleard, C., 1995. The emotional consequences of falls for older people and their families. Clin. Rehabil. 9, 110–114.

Lord, S.R., Menz, H.B., Sherrington, S., 2006. Home environment risk factors for falls in older people and the efficacy of home modifications. Age Ageing 35 (S2), ii55–ii59.

Mackintosh, S.F.H., Hill, K., Dodd, K.J., Goldie, P., Culham, E., 2005. Falls and injury prevention should be part of every stroke rehabilitation plan. Clin. Rehabil. 19, 441–451.

Marigold, D.S., Misiaszek, J.E., 2009. Whole-body responses: neural control and implications for rehabilitation and fall prevention. Neuroscientist 15 (1), 36–46.

Marigold, D.S., Eng, J.J., Dawson, A.S., Inglis, J.T., Harris, J.E., Gylfado, S., 2005. Exercise leads to faster postural reflexes, improved balance and mobility, and fewer falls in older persons with chronic stroke. J. Am. Geriatr. Soc. 53, 416–423.

Menant, J.C., Steele, J.R., Menz, H.B., Munro, B.J., Lord, S.R., 2008. Optimizing footwear for older people at risk of falls. J. Rehabil. Res. Dev 45 (8), 1167–1181.

Morse, J., Prowse, M., Morrow, N., Federspiel, G., 1985. A retrospective analysis of patient falls. Can. J. Public Health 76, 116–118.

Neyens, J.C., Dijcks, B.P., Twisk, J., Schols, J.M., van Haastregt, J.C., van den Heuvel, W.J., et al., 2009. A multifactorial intervention for the prevention of falls in psychogeriatric nursing home patients, a randomised controlled trial (RCT). Age Ageing 38 (2), 194–199.

Nevitt, M.C., Cummings, S.R., 1993. Type of fall and risk of hip and wrist fractures: the study of osteoporotic fractures. J. Am. Geriatr. Soc. 41, 1226–1234.

Nitz, J.C., Choy, N.L., 2008. Falling is not just for older women: support for pre-emptive prevention intervention before 60. Climacteric 11 (6), 461–466.

Nitz, J.C., Choy, N.L., 2004. The efficacy of a specific balance-strategy training programme for preventing falls among older people: a pilot randomised controlled trial. Age Ageing 33, 52–58.

Norton, R., Campbell, A.J., Lee-Joe, T., Robinson, E., Butler, M., 1997. Circumstances of falls resulting in hip fractures among older people. JAGS 45 (9), 1108–1112.

Oliver, D., Papaioannou, A., Giangregorio, L., Thabane, L., Reizgys, K., Foster, G., 2008. A systematic review and meta-analysis of studies using the STRATIFY tool for prediction of falls in hospital patients: how well does it work? Age Ageing 37 (6), 621–627.

Pellfolk, T., Gustafsson, T., Gustafson, Y., Karlsson, S., 2009. Risk factors for falls among residents with dementia living in group dwellings. Int. Psychogeriatr. 21 (1), 187–194.

Rhoads, J., Clayman, A., Nelson, S., 2007. The relationship of urinary tract infections and falls in a nursing home. Director 15 (1), 22–26.

Robertson, M.C., Devlin, N., Gardner, M.M., Campbell, A.J., 2001. Effectiveness and economic evaluation of a nurse delivered home exercise programme to prevent falls. 1: Randomised controlled trial. BMJ 322, 697–701.

Roe, B., Howell, F., Riniotis, K., Beech, R., Crome, P., Ong, B.N., 2008. Older people's experience of falls: understanding, interpretation and autonomy. J. Adv. Nurs. 63 (6), 586–596.

Rose, D.J., 2008. Preventing falls among older adults: no "one size suits all" intervention strategy. J. Rehabil. Res. Dev. 45 (8), 1153–1166.

Ryerson, S., 2009. Neurological assessment: the basis of clinical decision making. In: Lennon, S., Stokes, M. (Eds.), Pocketbook of Neurological

Physiotherapy. Churchill Livingstone, Edinburgh, pp. 113–126.

Sattin, R.W., Rodriguez, J.G., DeVito, C.A., Wingo, P.A., 1998. Home environmental hazards and the risk of fall injury events among community-dwelling older persons. Study to assess falls among the elderly (SAFE) group. J. Am. Geriatr. Soc. 46 (6), 669–676.

Scuffham, P., Chaplin, S., Legood, R., 2003. Incidence and costs of unintentional falls in older people in the United Kingdom. J. Epidemiol. Community Health 57, 740–744.

Sharaf, A.Y., Ibrahim, H.S., 2008. Physical and psychosocial correlates of fear of falling: among older adults in assisted living facilities. J. Gerontol. Nurs. 34 (12), 27–35.

Sherrington, C., Whitney, J.C., Lord, S.R., Herbert, R.D., Cumming, R.G., Close, J.C., 2008. Effective exercise for the prevention of falls: a systematic review and meta-analysis. J. Am. Geriatr. Soc. 56 (12), 2234–2243.

Skelton, D., Dinan, S., Campbell, M., Rutherford, O., 2005. Tailored group exercise (Falls Management Exercise — FaME) reduces falls in community-dwelling older frequent fallers (an RCT). Age Ageing 636–639.

Skelton, D.A., Dinan, S.M., 1999. Exercise for falls management: rationale for an exercise programme to reduce postural instability. Physiother. Theory Pract. 15, 105–120.

Spice, C.L., Morotti, W., George, S., Dent, T.H., Rose, J., Harris, S., et al., 2009. The Winchester falls project: a randomised controlled trial of secondary prevention of falls in older people. Age Ageing 38 (1), 33–40.

Stack, E., Ashburn, A., Jupp, K., 2005. Postural instability during reaching tasks in Parkinson's disease. Physiother. Res. Int 10 (3), 146–153.

Stack, E., Ashburn, A., 1999. Fall-events described by people with PD: implications for clinical interviewing and the research agenda. Physiother. Res. Int. 4, 190–200.

Stapleton, T., Ashburn, A., Stack, E., 2001. A pilot study of attention deficits, balance control and falls in the subacute stage following stroke. Clin. Rehabil. 15, 437–444.

Stokes, E.K., 2009. Outcome measurement. In: Lennon, S., Stokes, M. (Eds.), Pocketbook of Neurological Physiotherapy. Churchill Livingstone, Edinburgh, pp. 191–201.

Stolze, H., Klebe, S., Baecker, C., Zechlin, C., Friege, L., Pohle, S., et al., 2005. Prevalence of gait disorders in hospitalised neurological patients. Mov. Disord. 20 (1), 89–94.

Stolze, H., Klebe, S., Zechlin, C., Baecker, C., Friege, L., Deuschl, G., 2004. Falls in frequent neurological diseases. J. Neurol. 251, 79–84.

Tinetti, M.E., Speechley, M., Ginter, S.F., 1988. Risk factors for falls among elderly persons living in the community. N. Engl. J. Med. 319, 1701–1707.

Toole, T., Maitland, C.G., Warren, E., Hubmann, M.F., Panton, L., 2005. The effects of loading and unloading treadmill walking on balance, gait, fall risk and daily function in Parkinsonism. Neurorehabilitation 20, 307–322.

Tzeng, H.M., Yin, C.Y., 2008. Nurses' solutions to prevent inpatient falls in hospital patient rooms. Nur. Econ. 26 (3), 179–187.

Vogt, L., Wieland, K., Bach, M., Himmelreich, H., Banzer, W., 2008. Cognitive status and ambulatory rehabilitation outcome in geriatric patients. J. Rehabil. Med. 40 (10), 876–878.

Wagner, H., Melhus, H., Gedeborg, R., Pedersen, N.L., Michaelsson, K., 2009. Simply ask them about their balance–future fracture risk in a nationwide cohort study of twins. Am. J. Epidemiol. 169 (2), 143–149.

Whitehead, C., Wundke, R., Crotty, M., 2006. Attitudes to falls and injury prevention: what are the barriers to implementing falls prevention strategies? Clin. Rehabil. 20, 536–542.

Whitney, S., Wrisley, D., Furman, J., 2003. Concurrent validity of the Berg Balance Scale and the Dynamic Gait Index in people with vestibular dysfunction. Physiother. Res. Int. 8 (4), 178–186.

Wild, D., Nayak, U., Isaacs, B., 1981. How dangerous are falls in old people at home. Br. Med. J. 282, 266–268.

Yardley, L., Kirby, S., Ben-Shlomo, Y., Gilbert, R., Whitehead, S., Todd, C., 2008. How likely are older people to take up different falls prevention activities? Prev. Med. 47 (5), 554–558.

Ziden, L., Frandin, K., Kreuter, M., 2008. Home rehabilitation after hip fracture. A randomized controlled study on balance confidence, physical function and everyday activities. Clin. Rehabil. 22 (12), 1019–1033.

Appendix | 1 |

GLOSSARY OF TERMS

Acidosis increased acidity

Afferent nerve transmits impulses centrally from tissues towards the brain and spinal cord (sensory nerve).

Agnosia inability to recognize objects.

Akinesia inability to initiate movement due to difficulty selecting and/or activating motor pathways in the central nervous system. Common in severe Parkinson's disease.

Allodynia meaning 'other pain'. Exaggerated response to non-noxious stimuli. Can be either static or mechanical.

Anaesthesia dolorosa pain in an area which is anaesthetic

Aneurysm a localized, blood-filled dilatation (bulge or ballooning) of a blood vessel (usually of an artery) caused by disease or weakening of the vessel wall.

Anoxia complete deprivation of oxygen supply.

Aphasia inability to communicate. Either a receptive or expressive problem affecting the understanding and use of correct words (content) in speech or writing.

Apnoea cessation of breathing (see OSA).

Apraxia loss of ability to carry out learned purposeful movements, despite having the desire and physical ability to perform movements. A disorder of motor planning.

Aspiration inhalation of food particles or fluids into the lungs.

Assessment process of understanding a measurement in a specific context.

Associated reactions involuntary activation of muscles remote from those normally engaged in a task, e.g. upper limb flexion during sit to stand (see Ch. 14, Table 14.3).

Ataxia disturbance of movement coordination. Occurs with disorders of the cerebellum or its brainstem connections, e.g. multiple sclerosis, Friedreich's ataxia, posterior fossa tumours.

Atelectasis collapse of part or all of a lung.

Autonomic nervous system (ANS) or visceral nervous system the part of the peripheral nervous system that acts as a control system, maintaining homeostasis in the body. Primarily operates without conscious control or sensation. The ANS regulates body functions including: blood pressure, heart rate, respiration rate, bowel and bladder emptying, perspiration, pupil diameter in the eyes, salivation and digestion. The ANS has three components: the sympathetic nervous system, parasympathetic nervous system and enteric (gut) nervous system.

Autonomic dysteflexia/hyperreflexia or sympathetic hyperreflexia or paroxysmal hypertension an over-activity of the ANS in response to an irritating stimulus below the level of spinal cord injury, such as an over-full bladder. The stimulus sends nerve impulses to the spinal cord which are blocked by the lesion at the level of injury, activating a reflex that increases activity of the sympathetic portion of the ANS. This results in spasms and increased blood pressure. Nerve receptors in the heart and blood vessels detect this rise in blood pressure, which cannot be regulated due to the spinal lesion. Occurs predominantly in patients after spinal cord injury at T5 level and above. Can develop suddenly and become a possible emergency situation. If not treated promptly and correctly, it may lead to seizures, stroke, and even death.

Ballismus violent, large amplitude involuntary movements of limbs. Sometimes affecting one side of the body – *hemiballismus*. Occurs in Huntington's disease.

Barotrauma damage to body tissues caused by a difference in pressure between an air space inside or beside the body and the surrounding gas or liquid. Occurs when the body moves to or from a higher pressure environment, such as in sea diving or during uncontrolled decompression of an aircraft.

Bradycardia heart rate below 60 beats per minute (bpm).

Bradykinesia slowness in execution of movement.

Bullae bubble-like cystic lesions. Ruptured pleural bullae (singular bulla) can lead to a pneumothorax.

Bullous emphysema abnormal increase in size of air spaces arising from destruction of airway walls.

Capnometry measures carbon dioxide at the end of expiration, known as end-tidal carbon dioxide ($ETCO_2$).

Cardiovascular accident (CVA) see 'Stroke'.

Central nervous system (CNS) brain and spinal cord.

Cerebral palsy (CP) an umbrella term for a range of causative factors producing a disorder of posture and movement, as a result of damage to the developing nervous system before or during birth, or in early infancy.

Chorea brief, irregular contractions that are not repetitive or rhythmic, but appear to flow randomly from one muscle to the next. Occur in basal ganglia disorders, e.g. Huntington's disease.

Clasp-knife phenomenon response of a muscle with spasticity to passive stretch (see Ch. 14, Table 14.3).

Client-centred practice an approach to rehabilitation that seeks to respect clients' right to autonomy – ability to act on choices and be in control of one's own life.

Clinical hypertonicity increase in tone that occurs during voluntary movement resulting from, e.g., insufficient trunk control during a task or compensatory training patterns. May be fluctuating or persistent.

Clinical practice guidelines represent the consensus opinion of experts based on explicit and objective reviews of the scientific literature.

Clonus rhythmical contraction of a muscle in response to a brisk stretch (see Ch. 14, Table 14.3).

Continuity of care refers to patients experiencing some form of transition or transfer of care.

Contracture shortening of a muscle or tendon.

Critical appraisal the process of methodically examining research evidence to assess its validity, importance and applicability to clinical practice.

Constraint-induced (forced-use) movement therapy (CIMT) the contralateral limb is constrained with a glove or sling so that the patient is forced to use their affected limb.

Decerebrate posture/rigidity abnormal body posture with arms extended by the sides, legs extended and toes pointing downward and backward arching of the head – usually indicates brainstem damage.

Decorticate posture/rigidity abnormal body posture with arms flexed and turned inward towards the body, hands clenched into fists held on the chest and legs extended. Indicates damage to the corticospinal tract (pathway between brain and spinal cord).

Demyelination immune-mediated destruction of the myelin sheath insulating nerve fibres. Characteristic of some neurodegenerative disorders, such as multiple sclerosis and Guillaine-Barré syndrome.

Diplopia double vision. Simultaneous perception of two images of a single object.

Dynamometer apparatus for measuring force, torque or power of skeletal muscles.

Dysaesthesia uncomfortable sensation, often described as burning, tingling or numbness.

Dysarthria motor disorder of speech, characterized by poor articulation. Difficulty in producing or sustaining the range, force, speed and coordination of movements needed to achieve appropriate breathing, phonation, resonance and articulation for speech.

Dysphagia difficulty with swallowing due to disruption in the swallowing process.

Dyskinesia an involuntary movement distinguished by the underlying cause, e.g. myoclonus, chorea, ballismus, dystonia, tic, tremor. The term hyperkinesia also used, but is misleading as it implies movements are faster and this is not the case.

Dysmetria lack of coordination of movement typified by the undershoot and/or overshoot of intended position (see Ch. 14, Table 14.7).

Dysphasia impaired ability to communicate, usually used synonymously with aphasia but the latter is a total inability to communicate.

Dystonia movement disorder characterised by involuntary and repetitive contraction of muscle groups, resulting in twisting movements, unusual postures and possible tremor. (Previously known as athetosis.)

Efferent nerve transmits impulses away from the central nervous system to a muscle (motor neuron) or organ.

Enteric nervous system (ENS) directly controls the gastrointestinal system. It is capable of autonomous functions such as the coordination of reflexes, but receives considerable innervation from the autonomic nervous system and thus is considered a part of it.

Evidence-based practice a systematic process for finding, appraising and applying current best evidence to inform clinical practice.

Fasciculation or 'muscle twitch' is a small, local, involuntary muscle contraction (twitching) visible under the skin arising from the spontaneous discharge of a bundle of skeletal muscle fibres. Fasciculations have a variety of causes, the majority of which are benign, but can also be due to disease of the motor neurons.

Fatigue describes a range of abnormal functions or states, varying from a general state of lethargy to a specific work-induced sensation in muscles. Fatigue can be both physical and mental. *Physical fatigue* is the inability to continue functioning at the level of one's normal abilities. *Mental fatigue* manifests as somnolence (drowsiness). Physiological classification of *neuromuscular fatigue*: central and peripheral. *Central fatigue* occurs in the brain or spinal cord; *peripheral fatigue* occurs at or distal to the anterior horn cell, at the neuromuscular junction or muscle cell membrane.

Goniometry measurement of joint angles to assess range of movement.

Guillain-Barré syndrome (GBS) an acute inflammatory demyelinating neuropathy. Time from onset to peak disability is less than 4 weeks (see polyneuropathies in Ch. 9).

Hemianopia visual field defect – blindness or reduction in vision in one half of the visual field due to damage of the optic pathways in the brain.

Hemiplegia the paralysis of muscles on one side of the body affecting the arm, trunk, face and leg (contralateral to the side of the lesion in the brain i.e. stroke).

Heterotopic ossification (HO) development of bone in abnormal areas, usually in soft tissues, particularly muscles, around joints or long bones. Results from traumatic injuries, commonly spinal cord injury.

Huntington's disease an inherited (autosomal dominant) progressive degenerative disease featuring a triad of a movement disorder, an affective disturbance and cognitive impairment.

Hydrocephalus abnormal accumulation of cerebrospinal fluid (CSF) in the ventricles of the brain. May cause increased intracranial pressure (ICP).

Hyperalgesia an exaggerated painful response to a normally painful sensation.

Hypercapnia/hypercarbia increased levels of carbon dioxide in the blood ($PaCO_2$ >6kPa/ >45 mmHg).

Hyperesthesia increased sensitivity to stimulation.

Hyperpathia an abnormally painful reaction to a stimulus, especially a repetitive stimulus.

Hyperplasia increase in number of normal cells. In the context of strength training, there is an increase in muscle cells.

Hyperreflexia greater than normal reflex response.

Hypersomnolence excessive daytime sleepiness. Patients are compelled to nap repeatedly during the day, often at inappropriate times, e.g. at work or during a meal, usually without relief from symptoms.

Hypertonia increased muscle tone – spasticity and rigidity.

Hypocapnia state of reduced carbondioxide in the blood ($PaCO_2$ <4.7 kPa/ <35 mmHg). Usually results from deep or rapid breathing, known as hyperventilation.

Hypokinesia slowness in initiation of movement or diminished (small amplitude) movement, as occurs with Parkinson's disease.

Hypotonia reduced muscle tone, occurs in central or peripheral nervous system disorders.

Hypoxaemia reduced oxygen level in the blood (PaO_2 <8 kPa / <60 mmHg).

Hypoxia deprived of adequate oxygen (whole or part body).

Impairment a problem in body function or structure such as a significant deviation or loss.

Incidence probability that a patient without disease develops the disease during an interval, referring only to new cases, e.g. incidence of stroke for people aged 55 years or more ranges from 4.2 to 6.5 per 1000 population per annum.

INVOLVE a government supported organization that aims to improve patient, carer and public involvement in research (www.invo.org.uk).

Ischaemia restriction in blood supply resulting in damage or dysfunction of tissue.

Kyphoscoliosis curvature of the spine in both a coronal and sagittal plane; a combination of both a kyphosis and scoliosis.

Kyphosis spinal curve that results in an abnormally rounded upper back, either due to bad posture or a structural abnormality of the spine.

Labyrinth vestibular sense organ in the inner ear. See proprioception.

Measurement application of standard scales or instruments to variables, giving a numerical score, which may be combined for each variable to give an overall score.

Micutrition bladder emptying

Motor learning the process of improving motor skills, the smoothness and accuracy of movements.

Motor re-learning (adaptation) regaining motor performance.

Motor neurone disease (MND) progressive degeneration of upper and lower motor neurones (UMN & LMN). Most patients aged 50 to 70 years. Three main forms: Amyotrophic lateral sclerosis (ALS) 65% of MND cases; progressive bulbar palsy 25% of cases; progressive muscular atrophy 10% of cases.

Motor skill ability to use skeletal muscles effectively in a goal directed manner, as a result of practice of specific tasks. Indicator of quality of performance.

Multiple sclerosis a chronic progressive demyelinating disease, characterized by focal disturbance of function, with a relapsing and remitting course (periods of attacks and remission), usually presenting between the ages of 20 and 40 years and occurring more commonly in females than males.

Muscle disorders inherited or acquired, classified according to site of defect in the motor unit. Often progressive conditions leading to physical disability and in cases, reduced life expectancy.

Myoclonus brief shock-like jerks of a limb or body part.

Myometer instrument for measuring skeletal muscle contraction force (also see dynamometer).

Neurological weakness loss of central ability to produce and sustain force.

Neuromuscular junction (NMJ) the synapse (junction) between a nerve fibre and muscle tissue. The axon terminal of the motorneuron joins with the motor end plate (highly excitable region of the muscle fibre membrane) responsible for initiation of action potentials, causing the muscle to contract. The signal passes through the NMJ via the neurotransmitter acetylcholine.

Neuron(e) (nerve cell) electrically excitable cells in the nervous system that process or transmit information. Neurons are the core components of the brain, spinal cord and peripheral nerves.

Nystagmus rapid, repetitive movement of the eye in one direction, alternating with a slower movement in the opposite direction.

Obstructive sleep apnoea (OSA) cessation of airflow during sleep preventing air from entering the lungs caused by an obstruction.

Oedema swelling. Increase of insterstitial (intercellular) fluid in any tissue or organ.

Orofacial paresis partial paralysis of the muscles of facial expression. Leads to problems with drooling, swallowing and feeding.

Orthopnoea inability to breathe easily unless one is sitting up straight or standing erect.

Orthosis an external device used to correct deformity or assist/improve function by modifying the structural or functional characteristics of the neuromusculoskeletal system.

Paralysis complete loss of muscle function for one or more muscle groups. Often includes loss of feeling in the affected area. Caused by damage to the central (brain or spinal cord) or peripheral nervous (nerve cells or fibres) systems.

Paraplegia impairment or loss of motor, sensory and/or autonomic function in thoracic, lumbar or sacral segments of the spinal cord. Upper limb function is spared.

Parasympathetic nervous system (PNS) regulates actions that do not require immediate reaction, complimenting the actions of the sympathetic nervous system. The PNS is concerned with conservation and restoration of energy, as it causes a reduction in heart rate and blood pressure, and facilitates digestion and absorption of nutrients, and, consequently, excretion of waste products. The preganglionic outflow of the PNS arises from cranial nerves III, VII, IX and X in the brain stem and the 2nd–4th sacral segments of the spinal cord, known as the cranio-sacral outflow. The PNS uses only acetylcholine (ACh) as its neurotransmitter.

Paresis partial loss of movement or impaired movement.

Paresthesias abnormal sensations, spontaneous or evoked, including numbness, tingling ('pins and needles'), burning, prickling, and increased sensitivity, or hyperesthesia.

Parkinson's disease (PD) a chronic progressive neurodegenerative disorder. Involves degeneration of the basal ganglia and reduced production of the neurotransmitter dopamine by the substantia nigra, resulting in rigidity and releasing the inhibition of tremor, as well as increasing inhibition to the thalamus leading to bradykinesia.

Pes cavus high arch or high instep; sole of the foot is hollow on weight bearing; foot is in fixed plantar flexion.

Percutaneous endoscopic gastrostomy (PEG) a tube placed through the abdominal wall into the stomach of a patient unable to eat.

Peripheral nervous system (PNS) extends outside the central nervous system to serve the limbs and organs. The PNS is divided into the somatic nervous system and the autonomic nervous system.

pH measure of acidity or alkalinity.

Plasticity ability to permanently change or deform. *Neuroplasticity or neural plasticity* – any enduring changes in neuron structure or function to better cope with the environment. When an area of brain is damaged, another area may take over the same function. *Synaptic plasticity* – a property of a neuron or synapse to change its internal parameters in response to its history. *Muscle plasticity* – adaptability. Ability to change to accommodate specific stressors.

Pneumothorax air or gas is present in the pleural cavity (the space around the lung) causing collapse of lung tissue. A pneumothorax can occur spontaneously or due to chest trauma with a puncture to the lung or disease. A pneumothorax can be created therapeutically to collapse a lung.

Poikilothermic reaction inability to maintain body temperature due to autonomic disruption in patients with tetraplegic spinal cord injury, resulting in the person taking up the surrounding temperature.

Polyneuropathies a group of disorders affecting peripheral nerves in one or more pathological processes, resulting in motor, sensory and/or autonomic symptoms.

Positive reinforcement method for improving behaviour employing praise, rest breaks, positive social attention and meaningful (tangible) rewards.

Prevalence probability of disease in the entire population at any point in time, e.g. prevalence of stroke is 500–800 cases per 100 000.

Proprioception sensory modality that provides feedback on the status of the body internally for self-regulation of posture and movement. Feedback originates in receptors imbedded in the joints, tendons, muscles and labyrinth.

Prosopagnosia inability to recognize faces.

Ptosis drooping eyelids.

Pulmonary barotrauma damage to the lung from rapid or excessive pressure changes.

Quadraparesis/tetraparesis weakness of all four limbs.

Rehabilitation a process of learning to live well with an impairment in the context of one's own environment.

Reliability extent measurement is consistent and free from error.

Reciprocal inhibition inhibition of antagonists that would otherwise inhibit voluntary movement.

Rigidity increase in muscle tone, leading to resistance to passive movement throughout the range of motion. Common in Parkinson's disease.

Romberg's test or Romberg maneuver is a postural balance test of proprioception, which requires healthy functioning of the dorsal columns and spinal cord. The patient stands with feet together, and maintains balance with eyes open. The eyes are then closed and a loss of balance is a positive, abnormal response.

SMART framework goals are Specific, Measurable, Achievable, Realistic and Timed.

Somatic nervous system the part of the peripheral nervous system associated with voluntary control of body movements and with reception of external stimuli, which helps keep the body in touch with its surroundings (e.g. touch, hearing and sight).

Spasticity velocity dependant increase in resistance to passive (stretch reflex hyperactivity) of a muscle, with exaggerated tendon reflexes.

Spina bifida a neural tube defect (NTD) in which the neural tube fails to fuse somewhere along its length in the spine.

Spondylosis spinal degeneration and deformity of the joint(s) of two or more vertebrae that commonly occurs with aging. Can involve compression of nerve roots and, less commonly, direct pressure on spinal cord.

Stroke a rapidly developed loss of cerebral function of presumed vascular origin and of more than 24 hours' duration. Also termed cardiovascular accident (CVA).

Subrachnoid haemorrhage (SAH) bleeding into the subarachnoid space, usually from ruptured aneurysm at or near the Circle of Willis.

Sympathetic nervous system (SNS) responsible for automatic regulation of many homeostatic mechanisms in the body. The SNS enables the body to be prepared for fear, flight or fight. Sympathetic responses include: increased heart rate, blood pressure and pupil size, contraction of sphincters. The cell bodies of the preganglionic fibres are in the lateral horns of the spinal cord at T1–L2, the so-called thoraco-lumbar outflow. The preganglionic fibres enter the sympathetic ganglia, arranged in two paravertebral chains lying anterolateral to the vertebral bodies, called the sympathetic ganglionic chains. Several transmitter substances are involved in the SNS, including adrenaline, noradrenaline and acetylcholine.

Talipes equinovarus or club foot. Heel is elevated, the foot inverted and the person appears to be walking on their ankle.

Tenodesis grip wrist actively extended, fingers and thumb pulled into flexion to produce a functional 'key-type' grip.

Tetraparesis/quadraparesis weakness of all four limbs.

Tetraplegia impairment or loss of motor, sensory and/or autonomic function in cervical segments of the spinal cord, primarily from traumatic causes, affecting all four limbs.

Titubation (1) head tremor or nodding or (2) staggering, bobbing, stumbling or ataxic gait: cerebellar in origin.

Tracheostomy or trachiotomy surgical procedure on the neck to created a direct airway through an incision in the trachea.

Transcranial magnetic stimulation non-invasive method to excite neurons in the brain used to study the circuitry and connectivity of the brain.

Transient ischaemic attack (TIA) a stroke like syndrome in which recovery is complete within 24 hours.

Traumatic brain injury (TBI) insult to the brain caused by an external force which may alter level of consciousness. Injury may be closed (intact skull) or penetrating (risk of infection).

Tremor an unwanted, rhythmic, sinusoidal movement of a limb or body part, classified according to the situation in which it occurs. Types include: *resting tremor* (when limb relaxed and fully supported, occurs in Parkinson's disease); *action tremor* (during movement) associated with cerebellar dysfunction and includes *postural tremor* (when limb is held against gravity), *kinetic tremor* (during any type of movement) and *intention tremor* (worsens at the end of a goal-directed movement).

Urinary incontinence inability to hold urine in the bladder due to loss of voluntary control over the urinary sphincters resulting in the involuntary, unintentional passage of urine.

Validity ensures a test measures what it is intended to measure.

Valsalva's manoeuvre forced exhalation (strain) against a closed airway (closed lips and pinched nose) forcing air into the middle ear.

Vasovagal response/syncope (fainting) characterized by the common faint, resulting from 'vagally' mediated cardioinhibition and vasodepression. Caused by excessive venous pooling (commonly from prolonged standing or upright sitting) that paradoxically results in vasodilatation and bradycardia rather than the appropriate physiologic responses of vasoconstriction and tachycardia. The resulting bradycardia reduces cerebral blood flow to a level inadequate to maintain consciousness.

Appendix | 2 |

Associations and support groups

This appendix lists some national charities and professional groups which provide support to those with neurological disabilities and their carers. The list is not exhaustive, as other groups exist locally and there may also be national groups for rarer disorders. National offices will have contact details for different parts of the UK and internationally, where they exist. Some of these charities also fund medical research.

ATAXIA

Ataxia
(formally known as Friedreich's Ataxia Group)
Rooms 10–10A Winchester House
Kennington Park
Cranmer Road
London SW9 6EJ
Tel: 020 7582 1444
e-mail: office@ataxia.org.uk
www.ataxia.org.uk

BALANCE DISORDERS

Brain and Spine Foundation
See 'Brain injury', below.

Ménière's Society
The Rookery
Surrey Hills Business Park
Wotton
Dorking

Surrey RH5 6QT
Admin & minicom tel: 01306 876883
Fax: +44 (0)1306 876057
Helpline: 0845 120 2975
e-mail: info@menieres.org.uk <info@menieres.org.uk>
www.menieres.org.uk
Royal National Institute for Deaf People
See 'Communication', below.

BRAIN INJURY

Basic
The Neurocentre
554 Eccles New Road
Salford M5 5AP
Tel: 0161 707 6441
Fax: 0161 206 4558
Helpline: 0870 750 0000
www.basiccharity.org.uk

Brain & Spine Foundation
General Administration
Brain & Spine Foundation
3.36 Canterbury Court
Kennington Park
1–3 Brixton Road
London SW9 6DE
Tel: 020 7793 5900
Fax: 020 7793 5939
e-mail:info@brainandspine.org.uk
www.brainandspine.org.uk
Helpline tel: 0808 808 1000
helpline@brainandspine.org.uk

British Epilepsy Association
New Anstey House
Gate Way Drive
Yeadon
Leeds LS19 7XY
Tel: 0113 210 8800
Helpline: 0808 800 5050
www.epilepsy.org.uk

Headway
The Brain Injury Association
Bradbury House
190 Bagnall Road
Old Basford
Nottingham NG6 8SF
Tel: 0115 924 0800
Helpline: 0808 800 2244
e-mail: enquiries@headway.org.uk
www.headway.org.uk

National Meningitis Trust
Fern House
Bath Road
Stroud
Gloucester GL5 3TJ
Tel: 01453 768000
24-hour helpline UK. 0800 028 18 28
e-mail: info@meningitis-trust.org
www.meningitis-trust.org.uk

UKABIF (United Kingdom Acquired Brain Injury Forum)
PO Box 355
Plymouth
PL3 4WD
Tel: 01752 601318
e-mail: ukabif@btconnect.com
www.ukabif.org.uk

CARE AND RESPITE

Crossroads – Caring for Carers
Association Office
10 Regent Place
Rugby
Warks CV21 2PN
Tel: 0845 450 0350
e-mail:through website
www.crossroads.org.uk
(see local support contacts via website)

Leonard Cheshire Disability
66 South Lambeth Road
London SW8 1RL
Tel: 020 3242 0200

Fax: 020 3242 0250
Email: info@LCDisability.org
www.lcdisability.org

CEREBRAL PALSY

Scope
6 Market Road
London N7 9PW
Tel: CPHelpline: 08088 003333
e-mail: response@scope.org.uk
www.scope.org.uk

COMMUNICATION (ASSISTIVE DEVICES AND COMMUNICATIONS AIDS)

Ability Net
PO Box 94
Warwick CV34 5WS
Tel: 01926 312847
Helpline: 0800 269545
E-mail: enquiries@abilitynet.org.uk
www.abilitynet.org.uk

Royal National Institute for Deaf People
19–23 Featherstone Street
London EC1 Y8SL
Tel: 0808 808 0123
Textphone: 0808 808 9000 (freephone)
Fax: 020 7296 8199
e-mail: infomationline@rnid.org.uk
www.rnid.org.uk

Typetalk
RNID Typetalk
PO Box 284
Liverpool L69 3UZ
Text helpline: 0800 500 888
Voice helpline 0800 7311 888
e-mail: helpline@rnid-typetalk.org.uk
www. rnidtypetalk.org.uk

GENERAL SUPPORT SERVICES

Association of Medical Research Charities (AMRC)
61 Gray's Inn Road
London WC1X 8TL
Tel: 020 7269 8820
Fax: 020 7242 2484
e-mail: info@amrc.org.uk
www.amrc.org.uk

Capability Scotland ASCS (Advice Service Capability Scotland)
11 Ellersly Road
Edinburgh EH12 6HY
Tel: 337 9876
Textphone: 0131 346 2529
Fax: 0131 346 7864
e-mail: ascs@capability-scotland.org.uk
www.capability-scotland.org.uk

Disability Action – Northern Ireland
Portside Business Park
189 Airport Road West
Belfast BT3 9ED
Tel: 028 9029 7880
Textphone: 028 9029 7882
Fax: 028 9029 7881
e-mail: hq@disabilityaction.org
www.disabilityaction.org

Disabled Living Foundation (DLF)
380–384 Harrow Road
London W9 2HU
Tel: 020 7289 6111
Fax: 020 7266 2922
e-mail: dlf@dlf.org.uk
www.dlf.org.uk

Physically Handicapped and Able Bodied (PHAB)
Summit House
50 Wandle Road
Croydon
London CR0 1DF
Tel: 020 8667 9443
Fax: 020 8681 1399
e-mail: info@phab.org.uk
www.phab.org.uk

Royal Association for Disability and Rehabilitation (RADAR)
12 City Forum
250 City Road
London EC1V 8AF
Tel: 020 7250 3222
Fax: 020 7250 0212
e-mail: radar@radar.org.uk
www.radar.org.uk

HUNTINGTON'S DISEASE

Huntington's Disease Association
Neurosupport Centre
Norton Street
Liverpool L3 8LR

Tel: 0151 298 3298
Fax: 0151 298 9440
e-mail: info@hda.org.uk
www.hda.org.uk

MOTOR NEURONE DISEASE (MND)

Motor Neurone Disease Association
PO Box 246
David Niven House
10-15 Notre Dame Mews
Northampton NN1 2BG
Tel: 01604 250505
Fax: 01604 24726
Helpline MND Connect: 08457 62 62 62
e-mail: enquiries@mndassociation.org
www.mndassociation.org.uk

MOTOR NEURONE DISEASE CARE AND RESEARCH CENTRES

Contact the MND helpline or website (see above) for up to date contacts and their telephone numbers (see Ch. 4 for addresses):
Belfast – Royal Hospital
Cambridge – Addenbrooke's Hospital
Birmingham – Queen Elizabeth Hospital
Cardiff – University Hospital of Wales (Rookwood Hospital)
Leeds – The Leeds Teaching Hospitals (Leeds General Infirmary)
London – Barts & London
London – King's College Hospital
London – National Hospital
Liverpool – The Walton Centre
Manchester – Hope Hospital
Newcastle – Newcastle General Hospital
Nottingham – Queens Medical Centre University Hospital
Oxford – Radcliffe Infirmary
Plymouth – Peninsula MND Network
Preston – Royal Preston Hospital
Sheffield – Royal Hallamshire Hospital
Southampton – Wessex Neurological Centre

REGIONAL CARE ADVISERS (RCAs) FOR MND

Listed on the MND website: e-mail: care@mndassociation.org

MULTIPLE SCLEROSIS

Multiple Sclerosis Society of Great Britain
MS National Centre
372 Edgware Road
London NW2 6ND
Tel: 020 8438 0700
Fax: 020 8438 0701
e-mail: on-line through website
www.mssociety.org.uk

Multiple Sclerosis Society in Scotland
National Office
Ratho Park
88 Glasgow Road
Ratho Station
Edinburgh EH28 8PP
Tel: 0131 335 4050
Fax: 0131 335 4051
e-mail: through the website

Multiple Sclerosis Society Wales/Cymru
Temple Court
Cathedral Road
Cardiff CF11 9HA
Tel: 029 2078 6676
Fax: 029 2078 6677

Multiple Sclerosis Society In Northern Ireland
The Resource Centre
34 Annadale Avenue
Belfast BT7 3JJ
Tel: 02890 802 802

NEUROCUTANEOUS DISORDERS

Dystrophic Epidermolysis Bullosa Research Association (DEBRA)
DEBRA House
13 Wellington Business Park
Dukes Ride
Crowthorne
Berks RG45 6LS
Tel: 01344 771961
Fax: 01344 762661
e-mail: debra@debra.org.uk
www.debra.org.uk

The Neurofibromatosis Association
Quayside House
38 High Street

Kingston on Thames
Surrey KT1 1HL
Tel: 020 8439 1234
Fax: 020 83439 1200
Minicom: n020 8481 0492
e-mail: info@nfauk.org
www.nfauk.org

NEUROMUSCULAR DISORDERS

Muscular Dystrophy Campaign
61 Southwark Street
London SE1 0HL
Tel: 020 7803 4800
e-mail: info@muscular-dystrophy.org
www.muscular-dystrophy.org

Myasthenia Gravis Association
The College Business Centre
Uttoxeter New Road
Derby DE22 3WZ
Tel: 01332 290219
Helpline UK: 0800 919922
Helpline Republic of Ireland: 1800 409672
Fax: 01332 293641
e-mail: mg@mga-charity.org
www.mgauk.org

PARKINSON'S DISEASE

Parkinson's Disease Society of the UK
215 Vauxhall Bridge Road
London SW1V 1EJ
Tel: 020 7931 8080
Helpline: 0808 800 0303
Fax: 020 7233 9908
e-mail: enquiries@parkinsons.org.uk
www.parkinsons.org.uk

POLYNEUROPATHIES

Charot–Marie–Tooth (CMT)
CMT United Kingdom
98 Broadway
Southbourne
Bournemouth
NH6 4EH
Tel: 0800 852 6316
e-mail: info@cmt.org.uk
www.cmt.org.uk

Guillain–Barré Syndrome (GBS) Support Group
GBS Support Group of the UK
Lincolnshire County Council Offices
Eastgate
Sleaford
Lincolnshire NG34 7EB
Tel/fax: 01529 304615
Helpline UK: 0800 374803
Helpline Republic of Ireland: 00 44 1529 415278
e-mail: admin@gbs.org.uk
www.gbs.org.uk

SEXUAL COUNSELLING

Outsiders/Sex and Disability Helpline
(Formerly SPOD – Association to Aid Sexual and Personal
Relationships of People with a Disability.)

BCM Box Lovely
London
WC1N 3XX
Tel: 0707 499 3527
Helpline: 020 7354 8291 – Self Help Groups
e-mail: sexdis@outsiders.org.uk
www.outsiders.org.uk

SPINA BIFIDA

**Association for Spina Bifida and Hydrocephalus
(ASBAH)**
ASBAH House
42 Park Road
Peterborough
Cambridgeshire PE1 2UQ
Helpline: 0845 4507755
Fax: 01733 555 985
e-mail: helpline@asbah.org
www.asbah.org

SPINAL CORD INJURY

**Association of Spinal Injury Research, Rehabilitation
and Reintegration (ASPIRE)**
Wood Lane
Stanmore, Middlesex
London HA7 4AP
Tel: 020 8954 5759
e-mail: info@aspire.org.uk
www.aspire.org.uk

Back Up Trust
Jessica House

Red Lion Square
191 Wandsworth High Street
London SW18 4LS
Tel: 020 8875 1805
Fax: 020 8870 3619
www.backuptrust.org.uk

Spinal Injuries Association
SIA House
2 Trueman Place
Oldbrook
Milton Keynes MK6 2HH
Tel: 0845 678 6633
Fax: 0845 070 6911
e-mail: sia@spinal.co.uk
www.spinal.co.uk

SPORT

WheelPower (British Wheelchair Sports Foundation)
WheelPower
Stoke Mandeville Stadium
Guttman Road
Stoke Mandeville
Aylesbury
Bucks HP21 9PP
Tel: 01296 395995
Fax: 01296 424171
e-mail: info@wheelpower.org.uk
www.wheelpower.org.uk

Pashby Sports Fund Concussion Site
www.concussionsafety.com

**Riding for the Disabled Association (RDA)
Incorporating Carriage Driving**
Norfolk House
1a Tournament Court
Edgehill Drive
Warwick CV34 6LG
Tel: 0845 658 1082
Fax: 0845 658 1083
e-mail: through website
www.riding-for-disabled.org.uk

STROKE

Chest, Heart and Stroke Association (Scotland)
65 North Castle Street
Edinburgh EH2 3LT
Tel: 0131 225 6963
Fax: 0131 220 6313
e-mail: admin@chss.org.uk
www.chss.org.uk

Northern Ireland Chest, Heart and Stroke Association
21 Dublin Road
Belfast BT2 7HB
Tel: 028 9032 0184
Advice Line: 08457 697 299
Fax: 028 9033 3487
e-mail: mail@nichsa.com
www.nichsa.com

The Stroke Association
Stroke House
240 City Road
London EC1V 2PR
Tel: 020 7566 0300
Helpline: 0303 303 3100
Fax: 020 7490 2686
Textphone: 200 7251 9096
e-mail: info@stroke.org.uk
www.stroke.org.uk

OTHER LOCAL SERVICES

Crossroads (Care Attendants Scheme Ltd)
Dial-a-ride
Meals on wheels
Stroke clubs

PROFESSIONAL GROUPS FOR PHYSIOTHERAPISTS

These groups are relevant to neurological rehabilitation and are contactable via:

The Chartered Society of Physiotherapy
14 Bedford Row
London WC1R 4ED
Tel: 020 7306 6666
Fax: 020 7306 6611
e-mail: through the website
www.csp.org.uk

AGILE – Chartered Physiotherapists Working with Older People
Association of Chartered Physiotherapists Interested in Neurology (ACPIN)
Association of Chartered Physiotherapists in Oncology and Palliative Care (ACPOPC)
Association of Community Physiotherapists
Association of Paediatric Chartered Physiotherapists for People with Learning Disabilities
Association of Chartered Physiotherapists in Mental Health Care
Association of Chartered Physiotherapists in Riding for the Disabled
Association of Chartered Physiotherapists in Women's Health
Association of Chartered Therapists Interested in Electrotherapy
Association of Chartered Physiotherapists Interested in Vestibular Rehabilitation (ACPIVR)
British Association of Bobath Trained Therapists
British Association of Hand Therapists
Hydrotherapy Association of Chartered Physiotherapists
Physiotherapists interested/specializing in balance and vestibular disorders – list of names available.

CONFERENCES FOR PROFESSIONALS

Organizations holding conferences/seminars relevant to neurological rehabilitation include:

Association of Chartered Physiotherapists Interested in Neurology (ACPIN)
c/o Chartered Society of Physiotherapy
www.csp.org.uk

British Society of Rehabilitation Medicine (BSRM)
www.bsrm.co.uk

Society for Research in Rehabilitation (SRR)
www.srr.org.uk
Other organizations can be found in various physiotherapy and rehabilitation journals, in sections listing conferences.

Index